"Insightful and eye-opening . . . a must-read for anyone who thinks they know what they're eating!"
—Michael Eades, MD and Mary Dan Eades, MD, authors of *The Protein Power Lifeplan: A New Comprehensive Blueprint for Optimal Health* and hosts of PBS "CookwoRX"

"A well-researched and reader-friendly book on the increasing dangers of modern factory food. A wake-up call to boycott supermarket food in favor of certified organic."
—Samuel S. Epstein, MD, Professor emeritus, Environmental & Occupational Medicine, University of Illinois at Chicago School of Public Health; Chairman, Cancer Prevention Coalition

"One of the most important books written on nutrition and health. Deville presents a powerful analysis of what is wrong with one of the major suppliers of our foods, the supermarket, and how you can protect yourself and your loved ones from this eminent danger. Everyone concerned with the health of their loved ones should study this most important book."
—Russell L. Blaylock, MD, Advanced Nutritional Concepts, Inc., Visiting Professor of Biology, Belhaven College, Jackson, Mississippi

"Nancy Deville's Death by Supermarket *is a must-read for anyone interested in health and wellness. She has painstakingly researched the ugly realities of our food industry and exposes the real causes of the American health crisis."*
—Maoshing Ni, PhD, DOM, Dipl. ABAAP, co-founder of the Tao of Wellness and the author of *The Secrets to Longevity.*

DEATH BY
SUPERMARKET

The Fattening, Dumbing Down, and
Poisoning of America

NANCY DEVILLE

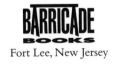

BARRICADE
BOOKS
Fort Lee, New Jersey

Published by Barricade Books Inc.
185 Bridge Plaza North
Suite 308-A
Fort Lee, NJ 07024

www.barricadebooks.com

Library of Congress Cataloging-in-Publication Data
A copy of this title's Library of Congress Cataloging-in-Publication Data is available on request from the Library of Congress.

ISBN 13: 978-1-56980-332-5
ISBN 1-56980-332-3

First Printing
Manufactured in the United States of America

Contents

Acknowledgments

I AM GRATEFUL to my agent Gary Heidt and my publisher Carole Stuart for believing in this book. I would also like to thank my editor, Ivy McFadden, for her support and insights. I'm deeply thankful to Nadine Saubers, RN, who helped me with the research and endnotes with tenacity and perfectionism. I have numerous experts to thank who graciously granted interviews and contributed quotes and otherwise helped me through the process of putting this book together: Carol Simontacchi, MS, CNN; Daniel E. Lieberman, PhD; the late David Kritchevsky, PhD; David R. Allen, MD; David Zava, PhD; Edward Giovannucci, PhD; Henry Han, OMD; John Komlos, PhD; John W. Olney, MD; Joseph and Brenda Cochran; Kaayla T. Daniel, PhD, CCN; Maoshing Ni, PhD, LAC, DOM; Mark McAfee; Mary Dan Eades, MD; Mary Enig, PhD; Michael Eades, MD; Michele L. Trankina, PhD; Mike Katke; Robin Marzi, RD, MA; Ron Schmid, ND; Russell Blaylock, MD; Sally Fallon; Samuel Epstein, MD; Stephanie Gunning; and Uffe Ravnskov, MD, PhD.

The lion's share of my gratitude goes to my husband, John Davis, who is my partner in all things, and whose love and support make all things possible.

Dedication

For you, Grandma.

Introduction

IN RECENT FILM, after most of Los Angeles is destroyed by aberrant tornados, a climatologist warns the president of the United States that he must immediately enforce mass evacuations to save millions of Americans from an impending storm brought on by global warming. The president dismisses the urgency and refuses to take action. True to the climatologist's predictions, a devastating storm and accompanying ice age obliterate the Northern Hemisphere.

The epidemic of obesity in the United States is as ominous as tornados ripping across Los Angeles. Americans are the fattest people walking the earth today. In a population of 300 million, nearly 68 percent of our citizens are overweight. Some are so large they can't fly on airplanes, go to a movie theater, or otherwise function in society. New industries have sprung up to accommodate "people of size" by manufacturing larger seats for restaurants, wheelchairs, and toilets; mega hospital beds; and XL coffins. It's gotten so surreal that we hardly blink an eye at people being hoisted around with *cranes*.

I believe that the American diet of processed, convenience, junk, fast, and otherwise industrialized "factory" food is the major contributing factor in our obesity epidemic. And this diet is also responsible for our skyrocketing rates of degenerative disease and ugly death. Yet because our medical community and government are not protecting us, the epidemic escalates, with millions of people on a trajectory that is certain to culminate in apocalyptic human tragedy.

The message we should be hearing is that if Americans stopped eating all factory food and ate only real food we would calm the irrational craving that compels us to eat these injurious substances. Real food is organically produced meat, fish, poultry, dairy, vegetables, fruits, grains, legumes, seeds, and nuts that could (in theory) be picked, gathered, milked, hunted, or fished. By giving our bodies and brains the necessary nutritional building blocks found in real food, Americans would be healthy, fit, and sexy, with each individual fully realizing his or her unique physical and mental potential—we'd be as intelligent, tall, and physically and emotionally gifted as our genetics predispose us to be. This would dramatically reduce the number of patients flocking to obesity clinics, ERs, and shrinks' offices. As it stands, though Americans worship youth and beauty, we are aging more rapidly than we have to because we eat factory food instead of real food.

I initially held my beliefs about real food because of the influence of my grandmother, Stella, who taught me about nutrition. In the last ten years I have coauthored books on weight loss, adrenal burnout, and Chinese medicine. The common thread was that the first step in resolving weight and health problems was to stop eating factory food and to eat real food. But I also believe that our health and weight problems are not just because of factory food.

Before World War II much of our population suffered from malnutrition due to lack of food, which manifested in emaciation, depression, lowered IQ, disease, and ugly death. Since WWII, our food chain has become permeated with factory foods, diets, and drugs; we are now suffering from a new type of malnutrition that manifests in *obesity,* depression, lowered IQ, disease, and ugly death. An unhealthy symbiotic relationship ultimately developed among our medical establishment; government; the food, diet, and pharmaceutical corporations; and us—American consumers. The food industry addicts us to their products, fattens us up, makes us depressed and sick, and then, backed by our medical community and government, the diet and drug industries profit by selling us diet products that perpetuate malnutrition and drugs that exacerbate our health problems.

The agencies that should be protecting us are complying with the moneymakers. While the Food and Drug Administration (FDA) is supposed to be responsible for protecting the public health by ensuring the safety and efficacy of the substances we ingest, the fact is, Americans are killing themselves and their loved ones by supermarket—with FDA approval. In addition, our medical community has evolved a health care system that acquiesces to government policies that in turn support the food industry, and has summarily rejected nutrition as "standard of care" (accepted modes of medical practice). This health care system actually encourages people to eat products that have contributed to the epidemic of disease.

All of this may seem very hard to believe. Americans have been subjected to intense conditioning from infancy through adulthood, and like other types of abusive relationships, the food, diet, and drug industries, as well as the medical community and our government, use wooing, denial, ridicule, and threats to keep us from breaking away. And so we remain addicted to factory food, desperately dieting and taking drugs to try to fix the health problems caused by this unnatural diet.

Do Americans even care? Reportedly, the factory foods that have the worst nutritional value sell the most briskly in the United States. When it comes to suggesting health changes, health educators continue to set the bar lower and lower, ostensibly because Americans are too lazy to make any substantive changes. After three years of research, I'm convinced that our fat and disease epidemic is no more our fault than it would be if we were caged lab rats being subjected to mind control, force-feeding, and bizarre experiments. That said, we have given in to the industries that have made us fat and sick, without much of a fight. As a path of least resistance, we attempt to make ourselves feel better about our fatness, our dumb-and-dumberness, our unhealthiness, and our addiction to factory food by adopting a "we are all in this together" mentality about our diet. We laugh to cope, but unfortunately, this dismissive attitude perpetuates our role as victims.

I want to make it perfectly clear that this book is not a condemnation for being fat, sick, or weak-willed. My purpose is to share with you what I have learned about nutrition and the influences of the food, diet, and drug industries so that you can make the healthiest choices.

There is a division of the classes occurring in America that has less to do with money and more to do with personal choice. Increasingly, two distinct groups are emerging: the overweight, depressed, sick eaters of factory food, who constantly diet and rely on a cocktail of over-the-counter and prescription drugs; and the eaters of organic, real food, who don't diet, avoid taking drugs, and are healthy, fit, and happy.

What's about to happen in America is analogous to an apocalyptic movie. Picture a few survivors blinking at the devastation they have escaped and brimming with hope for a future utopia. You and your family could be numbered among the survivors.

All it takes is turning the page.

I

How Factory Food Changed the Way We Live. . . and Die

CHAPTER 1

America's Missed Opportunity for Utopia

FORTY YEARS AGO, on the TV sitcom *Green Acres*, socialite Lisa just added boiling water to prepare "Dee Dee's 'dehydroficated' Mason Dixon Southern Fried Chicken Dinner" for her husband, Oliver. This 1960s parody of the modern American diet is a reality today. Instead of breastfeeding, we feed our newborns industrialized infant formula and wean them on scary "kid foods" like Nabisco Teddy Grahams, Clifford the Big Red Dog Cinnamon Graham Sticks, Danimals SwingN' Strawberry Banana Flavored Yogurt, Keebler Scooby-Doo! IronKids No-Crust White Bread, X-Treme Jell-O Pudding Sticks, and Kool-Aid.

American children go off to school on breakfasts of Hostess Ding Dongs, Pillsbury Cinnamon Rolls, Cap'n Crunch, and Reese's Puffs. They eat Fritos and McDonald's for lunch, and snack on movie popcorn, Hot Pockets, Fat-Free Pringles, Crystal Light Sugar-Free Lemonade, Nickelodeon Fruit Snacks, and Coke.

Americans have evolved an "every man for himself" system for dinner, swinging through fast food drive-thrus, 7–Elevens and AM/PMs, calling Domino's, or foraging in the kitchen for Kellogg's Eggo Buttermilk Waffles, Campbell's Soup, Chef Boyardee Ravioli, and Lean Cuisine and Hungry Man frozen dinners.

Back when our country was founded, Thomas Jefferson idealized the family farm as the backbone of American democracy.

But over the last one hundred years, family farms and ranches have been taken over by behemoth corporations, and the production of poultry and meat has been industrialized. Livestock were moved from their natural habitats and were incarcerated in cramped, dark factories, pens, and cages to live short, miserable lives eating species-inappropriate food, being pumped with genetically modified growth hormones, and kept alive on drugs before being slaughtered in the cruelest (i.e., cheapest) ways. Since it's more profitable and less of a headache to ride herd on hair-netted factory workers than it is to manage the farms and ranches that historically fed us, the food industry developed products that have long shelf lives and can be easily shipped thousands of miles—unlike "real" food, which spoils and is difficult to transport.

Factory food products are made, for the most part, from real food that is broken down in laboratories and factories, using heat and chemical solvents, into its basic components. The components are then mixed with colored dyes, preservatives, synthetic vitamins, and hundreds of other substances. Teams of chemists and "food flavorists" manipulate the chemical composition of recipes so the resulting products titillate taste buds, have appealing "bite characteristics" and "mouth feel," along with a maximum shelf life. Although factory foods promise good health, beauty, and satisfaction, they lack the life-sustaining nutrients necessary to maintain healthy metabolic processes and are mostly foreign and toxic to human physiology. The sad reality is that rather than feeling sated by eating these products, the resultant "hysterical" hunger provokes us to binge insatiably—and we get fat.

Industrialized animal products (meat, dairy, fish, chicken, and eggs) that are produced in Concentrated Animal Feeding Operations (CAFOs) also contribute to obesity and ugly death. In CAFOs animals are deprived of sunlight, clean water, and space to move, swim, or lie down. They are fed species-inappropriate food (for example, herbivores are fed soybeans and chicken poop), are injected with hormones, and, because of the depraved conditions in

CAFOs, they must be given drugs to keep them alive long enough to fatten for slaughter. They are lonely, frightened, and crazed from birth to death. Since the way animals are treated and their nutrition determines the nutritional value of their meat, milk, and eggs, CAFO foods contain fewer life-sustaining nutrients. Because of the poisons in animal feed and the drugs they are given, CAFO products contain toxins that can harm human beings.

On the other hand, real food (including humanely raised animal products) contains life-sustaining nutrients necessary to maintain healthy metabolic processes. Real food is recognized and utilized by human physiology. As I said in the Introduction, I learned this initially from my grandmother. Stella was a dark-haired beauty, a Polish immigrant who came through Ellis Island in 1911 and suffered her fair share of health problems as a result of inadequate early nutrition. In 1942, at age thirty-nine, Stella happened upon a "health" lecture, became a health food devotee, and was henceforth labeled the family kook. When I was a child, I often found her in the basement, lying in the dark on her "slant board," blood rushing to her head as she meditated. She was famous for her delicious cooking, juicing, and canning homegrown vegetables, dispensing vitamin C capsules, and dog-earing pages in nutritional pioneer Adele Davis's books for us to read.

Stella was an example of someone who did not start out with an adequate diet because her family was poor, but rebounded later in life by providing her body and brain with the necessary building blocks of nutrition. In so doing, she was able to salvage some of her genetic gifts. Among Stella's unique gifts were her physical beauty, strength, energy, and—her most remarkable quality—a positive attitude about life, despite hardship and tragedy. By giving our bodies and brains the necessary building blocks of nutrition, Americans living today could also take advantage of their genetic gifts. Future generations would benefit to a much greater extent in that adequate nutrition from conception on would allow them to *fully realize* their genetic potential.

As research for this book I read numerous diet and health books and I have to admit I felt somewhat indignant when I read in Mireille Guiliano's *French Women Don't Get Fat: The Secret of Eating for Pleasure* that "being a French woman is mostly a state of mind." I thought she sounded really superior—after all, Americans are supposed to be the top dogs. In fact, our nation has its own well-established superiority complex being that we are the richest, macho-est, most technologically advanced nation in the world. At the same time, we are falling behind in world health. Of thirteen countries in a 2002 World Health Organization (WHO) comparison, the United States ranked twelfth for sixteen important indicators, such as low birth weight, infant mortality, life expectancy, and mortality. In a 2005 WHO study, the United States had fallen to thirty-seventh in the world in terms of overall health performance.[1] (WHO is a United Nations agency dedicated to global health.)

In addition, although studies have demonstrated that tall people enjoy a positive bias in society, get promoted faster in their careers, earn more money, and have better luck than short people in relationships and politics, American men are not growing taller, as are other men all over the world. As for American women, they are actually shrinking. According to John Komlos, PhD, the leading expert in the field of anthropometric history (which tracks how populations around the world have changed in stature), the average adult height attained by a population is a historical record of the overall nutrition of that population. Dr. Komlos's twenty years of research has documented the height of almost a quarter of a million people from the 1700s to the present.

"Americans were the tallest people in the world until right after World War II, which was a reflection our healthy eating habits," Dr. Komlos told me. "Because of our poor diet, Americans have gone from being tallest in the world—one to three inches taller than Western and Northern Europeans—to being towered over by the Dutch, Swedes, Norwegians, Danes, British, and Germans by one to three inches. Today, Americans are, on average, the same height of the men and women of the Czech Republic."[2] In other words, Americans are now the same height as the citizens of an eastern European country that has been economically repressed and nutritionally deprived for hundreds of years.

But what about the French? "The French have not yet overtaken us, but they are getting there," Dr. Komlos replied. "They are about an inch shorter. And that is saying a lot for a population whose men were between five-foot-three to five-foot-five in 1690!"

So we are still taller than the non-fat French (the average American man is five-foot-nine and the average woman, five-foot-four). That is nothing to brag about when you consider that our industrialized diet has resulted in more American kids being at higher risk for a host of health problems, including precocious puberty and neurological disorders, such as attention deficit hyperactivity disorder (ADHD) and attention deficit disorder (ADD)—diseases characterized by inattention, impulsivity, and hyperactivity—and autism, a disorder of mental introversion, aloneness, inability to relate, repetitive play, and rage reactions. Type 1 diabetes, an autoimmune disorder of absolute insulin deficiency, is on the rise in children.[3] Also occurring more frequently in children are the degenerative diseases usually associated with aging: cancer, heart disease, and Type 2 diabetes—a chronic disorder of carbohydrate metabolism formerly known as "adult onset" diabetes.

In all age groups, there is an alarming increase in incurable autoimmune conditions such as Hashimoto's thyroiditis (chronic inflammation of the thyroid gland), lupus (progressive ulcerative skin disease), Crohn's disease (chronic inflammation of the intestines), rheumatoid arthritis (chronic inflammation of the joints), Grave's disease (overactive thyroid), myasthenia gravis (progressive muscular weakness), interstitial cystitis (chronic inflammation of the bladder), and Sjogren's disease (white blood cells attack moisture-producing glands, causing numerous health problems). Autoimmune conditions occur when the immune system loses the ability to distinguish between normal healthy cells and destructive foreign invaders and attacks healthy cells. People who develop autoimmune conditions are often condemned to a lifetime of chronic pain, the despair of being characterized as hypochondriacs, and the plight of being guinea pigs at the hands of doctors who don't know how to help them.

Millions of factory food-eating Americans today suffer from lack of "feel good" neurotransmitters, which are chemicals that carry messages between cells. Imbalances of these neurotransmitters cause the hysterical hunger that drives us to eat injurious substances. Neurotransmitter imbalances can also result in problems such as ADD, ADHD, insomnia, exhaustion, depression, obsessive or even suicidal thoughts, panic disorders, anxiety, rage, agitation, anorexia nervosa, bulimia, and lack of sex drive.

To add insult to injury, Americans are also dying ugly deaths.

On her deathbed at age ninety-seven, Stella's skin glowed and was virtually wrinkle free, and her hair was radiant. When a nurse came in to check her vitals, Stella demonstrated her famous bicycle kick exercise. The next day, she died peacefully. At her eulogy, my husband John compared her with an 1858 Oliver Wendell Holmes poem on old age called "The Deacon's Masterpiece" about a one-horse carriage that survived one hundred years in perfect shape and then on its last day disintegrated into a heap of sawdust. Holmes writes about an ideal life of good health and peaceful death that few Americans experience today. But Stella did, largely because she ate real food.

Eating only real food exponentially increases your chances of dying a peaceful death, like Stella. This is something to think about, as death from degenerative diseases has risen spectacularly in the last one hundred years. And dying from a degenerative disease is not like the pretty, soft-focus pharmaceutical commercials you see with Grandpa fishing with his grandchildren and Mom gardening with her daughter in idyllic settings with poignant music, and perfect hair and makeup. Dying of a degenerative disease is torture that ravages the family as it brings its victim down.

Historically, Americans did not suffer or die on a massive scale from degenerative diseases. Prior to the year 1900, hygiene—the basic practice of cleanliness—was an advancement yet to be "discovered." Raw sewage ran in city streets, contaminating drinking water. Doctors with filthy fingernails blew their noses during surgery. People and their habits were essentially dirty. Prior to the year 1900, the primary cause of death was infectious disease.

In the late 1850s, French chemist and bacteriologist Louis Pasteur promoted the "germ theory of disease": all infectious diseases have a causative agent—a bacteria, virus, fungus, or parasite. The discovery of microorganisms precipitated scientific advancements such as the use of personal hygiene, antibiotics, sanitation, and refrigeration, which systematically eradicated many infectious disease plagues. In addition, for the first time in the history of humankind, a population as vast as ours was gaining the capacity to produce enough life-sustaining meat, fish, poultry, dairy, vegetables, fruits, grains, legumes, seeds, and nuts to feed our nation. At the turn of the twentieth century, the United States was poised to evolve into a utopia filled with healthy, strapping people. But this did not occur. Instead, obesity and degenerative disease rose throughout the twentieth century and are now epidemic.

There are current statistics that demonstrate our epidemic of degenerative diseases, but I believe Americans have become numb to numbers on pages. We have not become inured to the fear of disease, however. Over fifty years ago, Adele Davis wrote in *Let's Eat Right to Keep Fit: The Practical Guide to Nutrition Designed to Help You Achieve Good Health Through Proper Diet,* "Statistics can tell so little. The number of new cancer cases discovered each year tells nothing of the fear and dread in the hearts of millions of Americans who already know that some day they themselves will suffer from the disease."[4]

The more immediate focus should be, why are we experiencing this radical rise in degenerative diseases?

Beginning one hundred years ago, as medical advancements

in fighting infectious diseases developed, two factors thwarted our potential for utopia. First, we didn't take advantage of the perfect opportunity to thrive with less infectious diseases by eating real food. As factory food usurped real food in our food chain, more people started dying of degenerative diseases.

Factory food is not the only contributing factor to the epidemic of obesity and disease. There are industrial chemicals and solvents, volatile organic compounds, exhaust, radiation, heavy metals, cigarette smoke, and harmful pharmaceuticals among other toxic insults, as well as genetic predispositions, bacteria, viruses, and other biological causes. But these other factors would not have the same devastating impact on our health if we were eating an exclusive diet of real food. Eating real food—containing protein, fats, vitamins, minerals, and enzymes (catalysts necessary for internal chemical reactions)—fuels cellular processes; imparts energy for the muscles and the brain; supplies the building materials for the ongoing replenishing of cells, tissues, muscle, and bone; and keeps endocrine systems, including our immune system, functioning optimally, to at least give our bodies a fighting chance.

The second factor that thwarted America's potential for utopia was that Pasteur's germ theory of disease unfortunately influenced our medical community to drop the pursuit of *disease prevention*. Beginning in the nineteenth century, chemicals with drug actions were isolated from plants, and increasingly drugs were made by chemical synthesis. Our medical community became convinced that the newly discovered drugs were the most advantageous modality with which to practice medicine (i.e., combat germs and other disease causing agents). Nutrition as "standard of care," which had been accepted doctrine from the time of Greek physician Hippocrates (the "father of modern medicine," B.C. 460 to 377), was unilaterally rejected by "modern" medicine. Since then, medicine has virtually ignored the impact of nutrition on the building up or breaking down of the body and shifted its focus to treating disease after it occurs—primarily with drugs.

The medical community's dismissal of nutrition as standard of care in favor of a drug approach was the first step in our becoming a nation of factory food eaters. It was the first time in history that people abdicated responsibility for their own health and placed their utter trust into the hands of the medical community. As we became a nation of drug takers following the advice of the medical community—which had shunned nutrition—the old wisdoms of food and nutrition were lost. Today few people remember their grandmothers advising them what to eat or drink to prevent or correct illness. That's because most grandmothers did not learn the simple truths about nutrition from *their* grandmothers.

Our reliance on doctors to tell us what to do and the accompanying acceptance of drugs provided a natural segue for our acceptance of chemical additives to our food supply. Fifty years ago, DuPont sold us on "better living through chemistry," and many people today do not see a problem with ingesting foods made from ingredients that we cannot pronounce, much less define. In the past one hundred years, as Americans increasingly adopted a chemicalized diet, we also took over-the-counter medications and prescription drugs to treat the resulting chronic conditions and diseases. It's proven to be a bad mix. Yet, because of the marvels of modern medicine, people are living longer—with tubes hanging out of them and beepers going off.

The fact that medicine abandoned the research, teaching, and employment of nutrition as a medical modality was an important factor in the rise to power of the factory food industry. As our food culture shifted from the real foods produced by Thomas Jefferson's ideal small family farm to "Dee Dee's 'dehydroficated' Mason Dixon Southern Fried Chicken Dinner," American brains became neurotransmitter-imbalanced, and we found ourselves hysterically hungry. The World Health Organization politely referred to our bingeing as "excess intake," and linked mass gorging to our epidemic of obesity and degenerative diseases of aging.[5] This excess thereby created a market for the diet and drug industries to flourish.

PART one

As you'll learn in the next chapter, keeping us dependent on factory food is paramount to keeping the cash flowing into the coffers of the food, diet, and drug industries. Has it ever occurred to you that heroin, cocaine, white sugar, and refined white flour have three things in common? They are all white, powdery—and highly addictive.

II

Hysterical
Hunger

CHAPTER 2

Socially Acceptable Sugar Addiction

IN 1984, RIGHT AFTER the release of Arnold Schwarzenegger's *Terminator*, my childhood friend, Mary Jane, took her two-year-old daughter, Rosemary, to the dentist. To M. J.'s horror, Rosie was diagnosed with "bottle mouth," which in simple terms meant that her baby teeth were rotting out as a result of too much sucking on bottles of juice. In order to save her permanent teeth from the damage that would ensue if her teeth were left to decay any further, under anesthesia, Rosie had her front teeth ground down to nubs and capped in silver. After the trauma of the ordeal began to wear off, I taught Rosie how to say "Terminator baby."

Like my friend M. J., millions of Americans think they are doing the healthy thing by handing their babies bottles of juice. Families say grace over breakfasts of Count Chocula, Ho-Hos, and Kellogg's Chocolate Chip Cookie Dough Pop Tarts because it's socially acceptable to be addicted to sugar. Americans became addicted to sugar through a slow, insidious campaign by the food industry, much like a pusher addicts a junkie to drugs. First they supplied us with small doses of sugar, then larger and larger doses, and pretty soon we were clamoring for more.

Sugar is a white, crystalline stimulant that offers zero nutritional value. Since refined white sugar is devoid of the vitamins and minerals necessary to digest and metabolize itself, your body ends up depleting vitamins and minerals from your diet or from internal stores in order to digest it. A short explanation of macronutrients and micronutrients might help explain why depleting vitamins and minerals is a bad thing.

Macronutrients (proteins, fats, and carbohydrates) provide energy and are the materials used in the breaking down and building up of the body's metabolic processes.

Micronutrients (vitamins A, B, C, D, E, and K; minerals, such as calcium and phosphorous; and trace elements, such as iron, zinc, and manganese) are the essential cofactors for metabolism to function. In other words, your body cannot properly utilize macronutrients without micronutrients.

The vitamins A, D, E, and K are classified as fat-soluble because they dissolve in fat before being absorbed in the bloodstream. Fat-soluble vitamins that are not immediately used are stored in the liver, and, because they can be stored, they do not need to be consumed every day. B complex and vitamin C are water-soluble vitamins and are easily washed out of the body through urination, and so they must be consumed every day. The vitamins A, C, D, E, and K are antioxidants that neutralize free radicals in your body (more is said about free radicals on page 46).

If you eat a lot of sugar and don't eat a lot of foods containing B vitamins every day (meats, whole grains, legumes, green leafy veggies, dairy, citrus, and so on), you will become depleted of B vitamins and may ultimately suffer from a burning sensation on your tongue, wrinkles surrounding your lips, exhaustion, gastrointestinal problems, thinning, graying hair, and chronic blues. These are only some of the problems that occur as a result of the vitamin and mineral depletion that occurs from overconsumption of sugar.

Eating sugar also depletes antibodies, which roam your body eliminating foreign viruses, bacteria, and yeasts. In your depleted state, you get every cold and flu that goes around.

Few Americans are in need of yet another laundry list of the health problems associated with eating sugar. However, many aren't versed in exactly how sugar contributes to hysterical hunger. Irrational hunger is the reason why sugar is holy to factory food manufacturers.

Hysterical hunger is the result of neurotransmitter imbalances, and these imbalances can begin at conception.

Our brains are more than 60 percent fat. From conception to birth human beings need essential fatty acids for proper brain formation.[1] (Essential fatty acids are discussed on page 122.) Also imperative for proper brain formation is cholesterol.[2] (Cholesterol is covered on pages 252–255.) Equally crucial for brain formation and development are amino acids.[3] Nine amino acids are essential for life. Another eight amino acids are considered conditionally essential. Amino acids are obtained by eating protein such as eggs, dairy, fish, poultry, and meat. They are the chemical building blocks used to make cell membranes, tissues, enzymes, antibodies, hormones, and neurotransmitters. Healthy neurotransmitters are crucial for happiness.

Here's how they work: Your endocrine system generates hormones, which comprise the chemical communication system that controls every function in your body. Your nervous system is actually an endocrine gland that generates impulses (chemical messages) and conveys these messages by jumping from neuron to neuron. Synapses are gaps between neurons, which are jumped by the chemical messengers called neurotransmitters. This jumping of the gaps is known as the "firing" of a synapse, a process through which your brain choreographs the complex orchestra of speech, hearing, sight, emotions, and trillions of metabolic functions that comprise human physiology. A healthy brain will have a healthy supply of the neurotransmitters such as dopamine, which acts as a stimulant (you feel energized); endorphins, which are your brain's painkiller and pleasure chemical (pains of life are diminished and you instead feel a sense of joy); serotonin, which is responsible for a sense of well-being (you feel high on life); and gamma amino butyric acid (GABA), which promotes a sense of calm (you feel calmly in control).

If a pregnant woman eats a high-sugar, chemicalized diet of factory food instead of eating a diet of real food that includes essential fatty acids, cholesterol, and amino acids, her baby's brain won't get the building materials it needs, and that baby risks being born without the fully developed brain he or she could have had.[4] Nor will the baby have balanced brain feel-good neurotransmitters.

Breastfeeding is the next step in the process of brain development and neurotransmitter production. Breast milk is *real food* for babies. But most Americans aren't breastfed, or are, but only briefly. They are fed factory formula. Instead of being raised on a diet of real, whole food, most American kids are fed substances that are permeated with sugar. From conception on, the majority of Americans' brains do not get the essential fatty acids, cholesterol, and amino acids we need to fully develop and to make neurotransmitters. So we are set up for lifelong brain neurotransmitter imbalances.

When brain neurotransmitters are in short supply, you are more prone to suffer from all the neurological problems we reviewed on page 8. Accompanying these symptoms are addictions to sugar, drugs, and stimulants such as caffeine, alcohol, and nicotine. The reason we have these addictions is because we learn very quickly that consuming those substances makes us feel better *temporarily*.

Every visit to a restaurant or market is an anthropological research expedition for me. At Spangler, the cafeteria at Harvard Business School (where my husband John teaches), I sat down to a lunch of steak, chicken, and vegetables. An obese woman next to me was eating her lunch that consisted of a small bowl of fruit salad and a Rice Krispie square. Fruit, while healthy, is all sugar, and so, obviously, is a Rice Krispie square. I could not help imagining the binge that woman was destined to go on later in the afternoon.

This is what happened inside that woman's body after she consumed that all-sugar lunch: Eating sugar triggers the pancreas to secrete the "nutrient-storing" hormone insulin. The secretion of insulin stimulates an excessive "rush" of stored neurotransmitters in the brain.[5] Thus the woman experienced the infamous sugar high. Since excess sugar damages cells, insulin's primary directive was to stow all that sugar away into cells. Now there was not enough sugar in her bloodstream to satisfy her brain's need for an ongoing drip of sugar, so her brain demanded more sugar. At the same time, her neurotransmitter rush ended, and unless she had superhuman self-control, she was guaranteed to binge, as the craving for more sugar was intense. Meanwhile, all this stress alerted her adrenals to release the stress hormones adrenaline and cortisol. These chemical messengers mobilized sugar into her bloodstream to be utilized by her body and brain during this time of stress: Adrenaline released glycogen—sugar that is stored in the liver and muscles for immediate fuel needs—and cortisol began breaking down her lean muscle mass (muscle and bones) to convert it into sugar. All this internally generated sugar, along with the sugar she most likely binged on after lunch, propelled her back into her sugar high. But this dangerous influx of sugar into her bloodstream again triggered the secretion of insulin, which immediately stored this new sugar away into cells. The woman's blood sugar crashed again.

For some people, this roller coaster ride goes on all day long.

You might think that since eating sugar facilitates an excessive rush of stored neurotransmitters in your brain, that continually eating sugar is a permanent solution to keeping your brain supplied with feel-good neurotransmitters. But the fact is, brain neurotransmitters are finite and will eventually become depleted if you do not eat the foods necessary to make more. You will feel terrible sooner or later no matter how much sugar you eat. Unfortunately, the brain does not say to you, "Please feed me food so that I can make more neurotransmitters." No, the brain is only focused on its immediate needs and so it screams feverishly, "GIVE ME SUGAR." Thus you are led around by your dumb brain. In a futile attempt to balance your brain neurotransmitters, your body desperately extracts whatever minute amount of nutrients it can from your factory diet.

And your doctor will likely be happy to write you a prescription for antidepressant selective serotonin reuptake inhibitors (SSRIs) that will allow your brain to eke a little more good feeling out of its pathetic levels of neurotransmitters. (SSRIs inhibit the disposal of serotonin from the brain, thus leading to longer-lasting normal levels of serotonin.)

Eating refined grains is the same thing as eating refined white sugar, and the food industry has slam-dunked our sugar addiction by permeating our food supply with refined grain products. In the fall of 2004, the *New York Times* ran a front-page article, "These Days, the College Bowl Is Filled with Milk and Cereal." College students, the *Times* said, are eating cereal and milk for breakfast, lunch, dinner, and snacks. A new restaurant chain called Cereality Cereal Bar and Café is rolling out on college campuses, featuring thirty cereals, seven milk options and toppings like marshmallows and M&Ms, which will be served by pajama-uniformed "cereologists" while the Cartoon Network plays on TV monitors. David Roth, a cofounder and the president of Cereality, said, "The ubiquity of Starbucks is what we aim for."[6]

The fact that cereal shops are springing up around universities is alarming since young Americans already have so many strikes against them when it comes to developing their brains. The brain is not fully formed at puberty, but continues to develop and mature until the age of twenty-four.[7] This means that students who graduate after four years of eating cereal, sodas, chips, and other sugary garbage for breakfast, lunch, and dinner are going to have lesser brains than those who suck it up and figure out how to forage for real foods that contain brain-healthy nutrients.

Americans overeat refined grains, not because we have a stupid gene that other cultures do not. Rather, our culture is oversaturated with these products. Consider that every single culture on the face of the earth has a version of the donut (fried dough). In Japan, where American *donhnatsu* franchises have proliferated, they also eat traditional *age pan*—a deep-fat fried blob with sweet fillings. In

Mexico it's *churro,* fried dough in a long, serrated breadstick-shape rolled in sugar. In India, it's *papad,* a deep-fried, crispy, spicy, thin dough round. The difference is that in other countries real food is a prevalent part of the diet (although the world is rapidly catching up to the United States in factory food consumption). In the United States, refined grains are readily accessible; they are easy to eat, good tasting, and addictive.

Grains were not part of the Paleolithic (hunter/gatherer) diet, and were not eaten by humans until ten thousand years ago when agriculture was first developed. Prior to that time, humans consumed carbohydrates in the relatively indigestible forms of nuts, berries, and roots. In other words, grains are a recent addition to our food chain and physiology, and refined grains are brand new.[8] But ten thousand years seems like long enough for human physiology to adjust to whole grains as part of the diet. Given that we understand that whole grains are part of a healthy diet, food companies like to capitalize on this belief. For example, Post, which produces Honey Bunches of Oats, Oreo Os, Pebbles, Post Toasties, Honeycomb—and, in all fairness, also makes "healthy" cereals like Shredded Wheat and Raisin Bran—actually bills their company as "whole grain experts for over 100 years." And so we accept refined grain products as "whole grain." Taking it a step further, Americans have been told by food manufacturers that such products as Eggo Homestyle Waffles, Pillsbury Enriched Wheat Bread, Sunshine Krispy Saltines, and cereals like Kellogg's Frosted Flakes, Post Banana Nut Crunch, and Rice Krispies are good for us because they are made from "enriched" grains (i.e., refined flour). In the immortal words of Adele Davis, "Such flour is 'enriched' just as you would be enriched by someone stealing 25 dollars from you and returning 99 cents."[9]

So-called enriched flour is typically made from genetically modified grain with its coarse outer husks removed, which are rich in vitamins, minerals, and fiber. The resultant stripped flour is combined with synthetic vitamins and minerals that were created in a laboratory.

Real foods contain the perfect ratios of naturally occurring vitamins, minerals, trace minerals, enzymes, amino acids, and fatty acids that are necessary to maintain healthy metabolic processes. This perfect ratio is never duplicated by food manufacturers. Instead, synthetic vitamins are added to factory foods in arbitrary amounts.

If that is not bad enough, most cereals are manufactured in a process called "extrusion" that subjects grains to extreme pressure at high temperatures, rendering the proteins in the grains into neurotoxins. These neurotoxins are even more prolific in "whole-grain" (read: "health food") cereal.[10]

In the 1960s, the hippie-baby boomer generation was into natural foods and nourishing grains such as barley, brown rice, whole grain buckwheat, corn grits, couscous, millet, oats, polenta, quinoa, rye, whole grain semolina, whole grain wheat, wheat germ, and wild rice. These youthful idealists reintroduced Americans to cool recipes like granola. But of course, factory food manufacturers immediately sensed a market like a shark senses a severed limb in bloodied waters. They hooked onto the concept of "natural" and hit the ground running with it. Since the first hippie girl made a batch of granola, factory food purveyors have been offering their factory food junk to a public eager for "natural" foods.

For example, today we have refined grain products that are packaged to appear healthy and have natural-sounding names like Kellogg's Nutri-Grain Yogurt Bars, a name that implies this product is nutritious. The company's Web site proclaims, "Calcium-rich cereal bars with yogurt filling provides smart nutrition for those on the go. In three creamy flavors, Vanilla, Strawberry, and Peaches and Crème. So when you are on-the-go and need a nutritious breakfast solution, go ahead and grab Kellogg's Nutri-Grain Bars and Respect Yourself in the Morning."[11]

In addition to genetically modified enriched wheat flour, Nutri-Grain Yogurt Bars contain high fructose corn syrup (highly addicting, manmade sugar), partially hydrogenated soybean and cottonseed oil (trans fats), natural and artificial flavor (possible MSG), mono- and diglycerides (on the FDA list to be studied for links to severely deformed fetuses and other reproductive effects), diacetyl tartaric acid esters of mono- and diglycerides (ditto), soy lecithin (a soy oil waste product, see page 93), yellow #6, yellow #5 (can cause allergic reactions), natural and artificial vanilla flavor (may contain MSG), corn starch (may cause allergic reactions including skin rashes and asthma), carrageenan (may contain MSG, and was found to cause ulcerations and malignancies in the gastrointestinal tract of animals), guar gum (may cause nausea, flatulence, and abdominal cramps).[12]

Rather than respecting yourself in the morning by eating this highly refined, chemicalized grain product, you may ultimately have people paying their respects to your surviving loved ones.

In addition to their claims of "enrichment," refined, sugary cereals are notorious for claiming to have fiber. In 1984, the Kellogg Company, with the endorsement of the National Cancer Institute, launched a campaign for All-Bran cereal, which supposedly reduced the risk for certain types of cancer. This campaign was the first time a factory food company used a "health" claim to market a product. Since that time, food makers have had the assistance of the FDA and the American Heart Association (AHA), as well as other "health" agencies, to sell us on the merits of their refined grain cereals. (The AHA is a national voluntary health organization whose mission is to reduce disability and death from cardiovascular diseases and stroke.) Claims like the one for Kellogg's All-Bran sound convincing because we know that we need fiber.

Normal elimination is once or twice a day. Primitive humans likely didn't have problems with constipation because their rough, fibrous foods stimulated peristalsis, the organized rhythmlike movement that moves foodstuffs from the mouth through the digestive system to elimination. But since refined food products immediately turn into soft, smooth, slippery, sugary sludge upon entering your system, there's no stimulation to get peristalsis moving. Refined grain products contain toxins such as the aforementioned nerve damaging protein fragments created by the extrusion process and chemical additives such as those listed in Nutri-Grain Bars. Compounding this problem is that fact that many of us have undiagnosed sensitivities to the actual grains in these products because we have simply eaten too much refined grain—and it has become toxic to our bodies. Toxins in the factory food you eat sit in your colon where they can be reabsorbed through your intestinal walls. Those toxins must go somewhere. Since most toxins are fat-soluble, they permeate and are stored indefinitely in your fat cells, where they kill and damage cells.

If you pay attention to your body, it will tell you that eating sugar doesn't feel good. In his book, *It's Not About the Bike: My Journey Back to Life*, Lance Armstrong said, "In one of the first pro triathlons I entered, I made the mistake of eating badly beforehand— I downed a couple of cinnamon rolls and two Cokes—and I paid for it by bonking, meaning I ran completely out of energy. I had an empty tank. I was first out of the water, and first off the bike. But in the middle of the run, I nearly collapsed. My mother was waiting at the finish, accustomed to seeing me come in among the leaders, and she couldn't understand what was taking me so long. Finally, she walked out on the course and found me, struggling along."[13]

Lance Armstrong, who is arguably one of the most impressive athletes to have ever lived, was brought down by cinnamon rolls and Cokes.

Sugar is sugar whether you eat a candy bar or a bowl of cereal. But there is a worse addiction than sugar and refined grains. In January of 2004, American Sugar Refining, an operation that had been in business since the 1880s in Brooklyn, New York, closed due to lack of demand for sugar! The closing of that sugar plant was like closing down a marijuana farm (American Sugar Refining) because of an increased demand for heroin (high fructose corn syrup). In other words, we went from a bad habit to an out-and-out lethal addiction, as you'll read next.

CHAPTER 3

Addicted to High Fructose Corn Syrup

"IN MY OPINION, Shape Up! products can play an important role in the support of an individual's physiology, which is often disrupted during the nutritional changes associated with weight loss," TV psychologist Phil McGraw was quoted as saying on www.shapeup.com. "Thirty years of work with obesity have taught me that psychological, lifestyle, and physiological balance are all essential to lasting success. Shape Up! can contribute to that balance."[1]

Dr. Phil entered into a licensing deal for Shape Up! products in 2003 with CSA Nutraceuticals[2] and made so much money on his weight loss business that in the fall of 2004 he was able to purchase a Beverly Hills home for $7.5 million in cash.[3] He writes in his book *The Ultimate Weight Solution: The 7 Keys to Weight Loss Freedom*, "So if you truly want to manage your weight, you must program your environment in every possible way to avoid difficult foods, binge foods, and reminders to eat . . . . Toss this stuff out, feed it to the garbage disposal, take it to the Dumpster, or at least get it out of your sight. Do this now, do this right away, so that it is impossible to fail. Begin today to reprogram your environment and set yourself up for success."[4] I guess he meant binge foods other than the Shape Up! "nutritional" Chocolate Peanut Butter, Oatmeal Raisin,

Fudge Brownie, and Chocolate Toffee Crunch bars he endorsed that contained high fructose corn syrup (HFCS), a factory-made substance that is not found in nature and can provoke a hysterically hungry individual to go into a frenzied binge.

In the two years or so that these products were on the market, many of his faithful followers unwittingly consumed a substance that was counterproductive to weight loss.

HFCS registers to the taste buds exactly like cane or beet sugar in sweetness and taste. Eighty percent of HFCS is extracted from genetically modified corn and is made using enzymatic fermentation, fungus, and chemicals. It's then pumped into tanker trucks and dispersed all over America to be manufactured into thousands of factory food products. Since its introduction in the 1970s, the consumption of HFCS has risen over 1,000 percent.

Like sugar, fructose has no nutritional value, and so it must rob your body of nutrients in order to be metabolized. HFCS causes all kinds of bad things to occur within the human body. It has been said that feeding kids HFCS produces exactly the same results as the force-feeding of geese: Both end up with fatty livers. Only most parents would not like to think of their children having *pâté de foie gras.* The introduction of HFCS parallels the 47 percent spike in Type 2 diabetes and the 80 percent increase in obesity in that same time period. Because HFCS has permeated our food chain, making it likely that we will consume it throughout each and every day, it contributes to hysterical hunger like no other food additive on the market.

Overweight bingers are not the only HFCS consumer targets. Optimal sports and integrative medicine factory foods—the latest spin-off in the "natural" factory foods market—are blatant exploitations of people's interest in the emerging field of integrative medicine and in optimal performance athletics. Athletes are eating and drinking HFCS sports products in an ironic quest for good health and optimal athletic performance.

Labeling and advertising imply that we are getting the benefits of herbs when we consume alternative medicine products that contain herbs along with HFCS. But drinking, say, Snapple Ginseng Tea, which contains HFCS along with small amounts of hibiscus and ginseng, is not the same thing as taking the Chinese medicinal herbs hibiscus and ginseng in appropriate doses to treat a particular illness or to promote optimal wellness.

The fact that Chinese medicinal herbs are mixed with HFCS is an insult to this incredible four thousand–year old medicine. Chinese medicine is energy-based and centered on the concept of wholeness and balance. When you go to a doctor of Chinese medicine, he or she is truly interested in all the reasons why your energy is imbalanced. In fact, one of the reasons Chinese medicine is so popular with Americans is because, while studies show that MDs interrupt within *eighteen seconds* of asking the patient to explain his or her problem,[5] doctors of Chinese medicine will listen raptly to a nonstop, graphic monologue about a person's poo, pee, snot, farts, and so on. All symptoms are important. After diagnosing a problem, the doctor designs an individualized herbal formula especially to rebalance a person's energy system.

This simple explanation of a complex and dynamic medicine should be enough to demonstrate why factory products containing herbs are not the same as using herbal medicine to treat a particular illness or to promote optimal wellness, and furthermore only serve to imbalance your energy system. Incidentally, doctors of Chinese medicine don't just hand out herbs. A treatment plan always includes prescriptives to one's diet. For Americans this *always* includes counseling to stop eating factory food, especially food containing HFCS.

"Emotional eating" and "emotional triggers" are terms bandied about by weight loss psychobabbleists who are furthering our obesity problems by ignoring our factory food pathology. Emotional eating refers to bingeing in an attempt to assuage one's emotions. Emotional triggers are upsetting events or experiences that "trigger" emotional eating.

But saying we are overeating because of our emotions is totally missing the larger picture. We're overeating because we have been addicted to unnatural food and our brains have gone understandably haywire, causing us to gobble everything in sight in an insane attempt to satisfy our bodies' and brains' needs for sustenance.

To break it down further, emotional eating is the result of severe, prolonged neurotransmitter imbalances caused by a chronic diet of sugary factory food (and exacerbated by diets and drugs). Years of consuming sugar and not eating enough real food has created chemically imbalanced brains that are addicted. However, as much we hate ourselves for our addiction to sugar, it is not the result of a weak-willed nation. It is a normal physiological response to a purposely systematic overfeeding of sugar to us by the food industry. In the nineteenth century, dairy cows were fed the "distillery slop" left over after the refining of whiskey. Prohibitionist Robert Milham Hartley likened distillery cows to alcoholics. At first, he writes, the cows resisted eating the slop, but ultimately, "generally learn to love the nauseous slush as men acquire a relish for intoxicating drinks. Eventually, indeed, they become voraciously fond of this kind of food; and if they fail of their usual supply, they will paw and rave and indicate all the unhappiness of the drunkard who is deprived of his accustomed drams."[6]

Like the addicted dairy cows of old, our neurotransmitter depleted brains are permanently on code red, so that we paw and rave and act out our extreme anxiety if we don't have our sugar fix.

Emotional triggers are the result of "conditioned response." The classic study of conditioning was conducted by Russian physiologist and experimental psychologist Ivan Petrovich Pavlov, who discovered the conditioned response. Pavlov began by ringing a bell (conditioned stimulus) and presenting his dogs with food. At first the dogs salivated at the sight and scent of the food (unconditioned response). But after a number of trials the dogs salivated as soon as the bell had been rung (conditioned response) even without the presentation of food. It took a very short time for Pavlov to detect the conditioning of his dogs to the bell. Reinforced conditioning for sugary factory foods begins in infancy with Americans and continues through childhood and adulthood. To many Americans, eating sugar is associated with alleviating (however fleetingly) any type of pain. Because our brains lack feel-good neurotransmitters, we feel pain a lot. We crave, we feel insecure, unconfident, tired, cranky, depressed, obsessive, and so on. And because we've conditioned our brains over and over again to associate ingesting sugar with a temporary high that makes us feel so much better, that bell of Pavlov's is always ringing. We are a hysterically hungry society that is "conditioned" to knee-jerk react to any type of pain by ingesting horrendously unhealthy junk.

Hysterical hunger was rare rather than the norm before our country became a nation of factory food eaters. Binge eating should be addressed by keeping Americans' brain neurotransmitters replenished so that people do not feel as much emotional pain. Purging our culture of sugary factory food and making real food abundant, affordable, and convenient so that people can eat a regular diet of real food, including organically produced protein, fats, and cholesterol, would stop the cycle of so-called emotional eating for most people.

In the Introduction I said that by avoiding factory food and eating only real food we would stem the number of patients who are now flocking to obesity clinics, ERs, and shrinks' offices. Taking these steps would also dramatically reduce our prison population. This is a bold statement for some to swallow, as many people do not believe that food can affect us that much or do not believe that food can do what antidepressants can do.

By the end of 2003, 6.9 million Americans were either on probation, in jail, prison, or on parole.[7] Between 1985 and 1993, the number of homicides committed by fifteen- to nineteen-year-old boys increased in the United States by 150 percent.[8] It stands to reason that we can't possibly be all of a sudden mutating into a society of hostile people for no reason at all. People like to point fingers at violence on TV and movies, but if you think about it, those brutal ideas didn't just spring out of the air. There's a reason Americans don't feel well and that many feel the rage that permeates our society.

Consider that the majority of Americans are not gestated or brought up on real food, which would provide them with the crucial nutrients their brains and bodies need to develop. Instead, many women consume soft drinks and eat chemicalized, HFCS-laden factory foods during pregnancy, do not breastfeed at all or long enough, and then feed their children sugary, synthetic foods. So we are a nation that does not have the fully developed brains we were genetically predisposed to having. On top of that, we do not give our underdeveloped brains the nutrients necessary to produce feel-good neurotransmitters.

Some neurotransmitter imbalanced people self-medicate on sugary chemicalized factory foods. Others act out, cutting themselves, smoking cigarettes, abusing drugs, being sexually promiscuous, and otherwise directing their pain inward. Some neurotransmitter imbalanced people project their pain outward and their rage lands them in prison, where their chemical imbalances are further cultivated on a diet of the cheapest, most noxious substances in the American food supply.

What if the entire population of the United States—including drug addicts and prisoners with the potential for rehabilitation—stopped eating all factory food and ate only real food that provided amino acids, essential fatty acids, cholesterol, and other nutrients needed to fully develop their brains and make neurotransmitters?

Keeping the neurotransmitters of the entire American population balanced should be a top priority of the U.S. government. Unfortunately, our country's most trusted health agencies and our government are the factory food manufacturers' best allies in keeping us hooked on sugary factory food.

CHAPTER 4

The Government Protects the Sugar Industry

CARDIOVASCULAR DISEASE is the leading cause of death for men and women in the United States. According to the Centers for Disease Control (CDC), nearly one-quarter of all Americans have some form of cardiovascular disease, and each year about seven hundred thousand Americans die of heart disease. (The CDC is a government agency whose mission is to prevent and control disease, injury, and disability.)

Since over half of those who die of heart disease-related deaths each year are women, on January 4, 2004, the American Heart Association published new guidelines, written by a panel of experts, for preventing heart disease and stroke in women. The story was all over the news so I decided to investigate further and logged onto the AHA Web site, which states: "The guidelines are based on the highest-quality evidence from all the available research related to [cardiovascular disease] prevention."[1]

Recommendations for women included eating a "heart-healthy" low-fat, low-cholesterol diet to reduce current risk and to prevent major risk factors from developing. To assist us in eating such a diet, the AHA offered an invitation to make a heart-healthy Valentine's Day cake and provided three options: Espresso Ice Cream Cookie Wrap-Ups, Crispy Strawberry Napoleons, or Fudgy Chocolate Walnut Pie.[2]

Fudgy Chocolate Walnut Pie's "heart-healthy" ingredients included vegetable oil spray (riddled with free radicals, see page 46); reduced-fat, thin chocolate wafer cookie crumbs or chocolate graham crackers (sugar, MSG, and trans fats); white sugar; fat free evaporated milk (sugar); light corn syrup (sugar); unsweetened cocoa powder (heart-healthy if organic, see page 36); semisweet chocolate chips (sugar, trans fats); egg substitutes (stripped of most nutritional value); and a few chopped walnuts (the only other "heart-healthy" ingredient).

These recipes from the supposed paragon of preventing heart disease would be more appropriately referred to as "Recipes Especially Designed to Give You Heart Disease." If the AHA were some dinky, grassroots organization existing on the proceeds from the friendly neighborhood bake sale, I would say, okay, we'll give you a pass on this, but this is the *American Heart Association.*

To make matters worse, the AHA allows their "American Heart Association Tested and Approved" heart-check mark on factory foods that meet the FDA criteria for a "healthy" food. FDA labeling rules allow food companies to use the words "healthy" if their substances meet the following criteria: low-fat (less than or equal to 3 grams); low saturated fat (less than or equal to 1 gram); low cholesterol (less than or equal to 20 milligrams); sodium value of less than or equal to 480 milligrams for individual foods; contains at least 10 percent of the Daily Value of one or more of these naturally occurring nutrients: protein, vitamin A, vitamin C, calcium, iron or dietary fiber, .5 grams or less of trans fat and 51 percent by weight of the "Reference Amount Customarily Consumed (RACC)" of whole grain.[3]

When I contacted the AHA, I was informed that the heart-check mark was created "as a first-step in building a heart-healthy lifestyle. The mark continues to be an easy and reliable tool in selecting heart-healthy foods. Most importantly, it comes from the most respected source for health and nutrition." According to the AHA, 84 percent of consumers say the heart-check mark is important in making food choices or buying decisions. Of third-party programs, the AHA heart-check mark is the most respected by consumers. The AHA heart-check mark is a powerful marketing tool that fulfills shoppers' needs—"with it on your packaging and in your promotions, the heart-check mark can help move your product."[4] Fees to obtain the heart-check mark are $7,500 per product and $4,500 annually. Factory food makers get a discount if they enroll more than twenty-five products.

Out of one side of its mouth, the AHA assures food manufacturers that by employing the trusted AHA heart-check mark, "We can help move your product," and from the other side of its mouth, the AHA reassures consumers that, "You can rely on our mark because the American Heart Association is your most trusted source of heart-health information."[5]

The AHA Web site offered a list of over eight hundred factory food products bearing the trusted AHA heart-check mark, such as Healthy Choice Brownie Bliss Premium Low Fat Ice Cream; Chocolate Cherry Mambo Premium Low Fat Ice Cream; General Mills Berry Burst Cheerios-Strawberry Banana, Cocoa Puffs, Cookie Crisp, French Toast Crunch, Frosted Cheerios, Golden Grahams, Lucky Charms, Trix; Kellogg's Frosted Mini-Wheats Big Bite; Smart Start-Soy Protein; and Brain Twist Slap Chocolate Drink.[6] So if you are among the "84 percent of consumers [who] say the heart-check mark is important in making food choices or buying decision," you trustingly eat up all that refined white flour, chemical flavoring, factory milk, aspartame, MSG, industrially processed soy, hydrogenated fat, colored dye, and, most of all, *refined white sugar* and *high fructose corn syrup*.

On January 12, 2005, the Health and Human Services Department (HHS) issued their "nutritional guidelines," which are revamped every five years. (The HHS is a government agency founded to protect the health of Americans.) The guidelines affect what goes into school lunch programs and government dietary education such as the U.S. Department of Agriculture (USDA) food-guide pyramid and factory food labeling. (The USDA is a government agency founded to help farmers and ranchers and to keep our animal food products safe.)

The panel that composed the guidelines reviewed scientific evidence submitted by an advisory committee linking sugar to obesity and demonstrated that eating sugar reduces the consumption of nutritious food. The panel chose not to include the specific guideline, "Reduce added sugars," but watered it down to, "Choose carbohydrates wisely for good health."[7] As you now know, you are free to make "wise choices" from the eight hundred unhealthy carbohydrates that have been assigned the "American Heart Association Tested and Approved" heart-check mark by the AHA.

A few years ago, the International Obesity Task Force estimated that one billion people worldwide were overweight or obese, including 22 million overweight or obese children *under the age of five*. The World Health Organization recognized this alarming worldwide epidemic of obesity and the accompanying degenerative diseases of aging as "malnutrition" attributable to "excess." In the spring of 2003, a group of internationally respected scientists attempted to address this problem by drafting a global strategy on diet, physical activity, and health entitled "The Expert Consultation on Diet, Nutrition, and the Prevention of Chronic Diseases."[8]

The simple strategy focused on cutting down on sugar consumption and factory food, and replacing those items with real food. They also mentioned limiting advertising directed toward children. When the Sugar Association read these suggestions, they threatened to use "every avenue available to expose the dubious nature" of the WHO report and pressured members of Congress to get the United States to threaten to withdraw $406 million in contributions to WHO.

Responding were two of the world's leading experts in nutrition policy, Kelly D. Brownell, PhD, director of the Yale Center for Eating and Weight Disorders and author of *Food Fight: The Inside Story of the Food Industry, America's Obesity Crisis and What We Can Do About*

It, and the world's leading nutrition policy advisor, Marion Nestle, PhD, MPH, author of *Food Politics: How the Food Industry Influences Nutrition and Health*. "Senators Larry Craig [R–ID] and John Breaux [D–LA], co-chairmen of the Senate Sweetener Caucus, asked [Bush appointee] Health and Human Services Tommy Thompson to call on the WHO to 'cease further promotion' of the report, while trade associations for the sugar, corn refining and snack food industries questioned the report's legitimacy and asked for Mr. Thompson's personal intervention. They got it."[9]

Rather than support WHO's simple strategy, Thompson had his department issue a line-by-line, twenty-eight page critique, accusing the organization of shoddy sugar research, and he demanded that WHO "cease further promotion" of their report. In short, Thompson did not allow WHO to release the report to the mainstream so that people could read that eating too much sugar is making us fat and sick.

Not long after the WHO report, the CDC issued a report in the *Journal of the American Medical Association* (JAMA) that obesity may soon overtake tobacco as the leading cause of preventable death in the United States. In response, at a March 12, 2004, news conference, Thompson had the gall to say, "Americans are literally eating themselves to death."[10] He proceeded to write to Dear Abby: "I know you care passionately about individuals taking steps each day to improve the quality of their lives. Please help me spread the word about improving the health of millions of Americans . . . . Please encourage your readers to see for themselves how small steps can lead to big health benefits . . . . Eating only half portions of dessert can add up to giant steps on the path to a healthier life."[11]

This from a man who sided against the American people so that the sugar industry would not lose profits.

That said, my grandma, Stella, was a health advocate, but she wasn't a zealot. Her motto was, "Do your best and don't worry about the rest." She was never intent on robbing her family of life's pleasures. Eating healthfully means eating real food, not living like a monk. On many research expeditions in restaurants, I've noted a phenomenon with which I'm sure you're familiar. The waiter brings out everyone's entrées. Note the anticipatory moans that greet hot plates of steak, chicken, or fish. But it's very different when the waiter clears the plates and brings around the tray loaded with crème brûlée, chocolate cheesecake, apple raisin pie *à la mode,* coconut cream tart. Everyone giggles. Eyes dart around. Hands wring napkins. We know sugar is not exactly healthy, but it's all in fun.

A delicious dessert, a glass of wine, or a beer lend pleasure to life, and it's only making matters worse that we are feel guilty about indulging. It is better to eat a balanced diet of real food, and then indulge in moderation on occasion. If you're going to have dessert, for goodness sake, have a real dessert. White sugar from time to time is not going to kill you, but factory dessert products will. Brown sugar and turbinado are to white sugar what wheat bread is to white bread. But if you decide you want to bake your own desserts, there are a few healthier alternatives to refined white and brown sugar.

I doubt if any of us will be trading Martha Washington's recipes via e-mail any time soon, but "old-fashioned" sugars such as maple sugar and molasses contain minerals and are delicious in traditional recipes such as gingerbread and cookies. Unrefined honey contains healthy enzymes (see page 155 for more on enzymes) and antioxidants (which neutralize free radicals) and is a healthy addition to a balanced diet. Sucanant or Rapadura are dehydrated cane sugar juice, which also contain minerals and are thus superior to refined white sugar. *Stevia rebaudiana,* a South American herb, is a new popular sugar substitute that has the same science fictiony aftertaste as aspartame, but does not kill brain cells. Stevia is 200 times sweeter than sugar but does not trigger an insulin response or have any calories or carbohydrates. (There are no long-term studies on stevia, so moderation is suggested.)

Dark chocolate is loaded with flavonoids, which are plant compounds that keep your blood vessels clear of plaque and inhibit other responses that lead to heart attack. Dark chocolate contains more flavonoids than any other flavanoid-containing food (green tea, black tea, red wine, or blueberries).

Wineries are getting hip to the fact that more people want organic everything these days, so sooner or later we'll have more organic wine choices than we currently do. In the meantime, red wine contains the highest amount available today of the polyphenol (a plant compound) resveratrol, which is concentrated in the grape skins and made available by the alcohol in wine. Resveratrol has been found to be both a potent cancer preventative agent while improving cardiovascular health. (Resveratrol is perishable when exposed to light and air and so the dark, corked bottles help preserve it.)[12]

Commercial beers are generally made with genetically modified ingredients and are pasteurized—heated to kill microorganisms—which kills life-giving enzymes. Unpasteurized "live" beer is actually a better choice than non-organic wine, as it provides healthy enzymes. In fact, it is surprisingly nutritious food, as long as you don't drink a keg of it. You can find breweries of live beer on www.beertravelers.com.

Enjoying small amounts of sugar in the form of desserts, wine, and live beer in an otherwise balanced diet of real food is not going to kill anyone, but eating HFCS on a regular basis will. Unfortunately, high fructose corn syrup is not the only scary additive to inundate our food supply. Monosodium glutamate (MSG) has virtually permeated our food chain, and millions of Americans are unaware that they are eating this brain-damaging flavor enhancer every day.

III

Science Fiction Food Additives

CHAPTER 5

MSG Keeps Us Coming Back for More

WHO HASN'T BITTERLY complained about the obnoxiousness of TV ads? Commercials run so repetitively that you feel like Alexander De Large in the 1968 movie *A Clockwork Orange*—eyes propped open, forced to watch the same images over and over until you're ready to lose your mind. Even though we hate commercials—and it's safe to say that no one really believes advertisers have our best interests in mind—we continue to consume their products. That's because factory food is addicting.

Factory foods whose virtues are extolled as tasting good and being satisfying, affordable, and convenient are in nearly every kitchen pantry, refrigerator, freezer, desk drawer, locker, purse, briefcase, backpack, and glove compartment in America. But what does it mean to be satiated? To many it means tasting a yummy flavor and experiencing instant gratification. But factory food is designed to make you want to eat more. And wanting to eat more is the polar opposite of being satisfied. How does the factory food industry get you to want to eat more? The primary addicting ingredient is sugar, but the deal clincher is the flavor enhancer monosodium glutamate (MSG).

MSG, made from the seaweed kombu (sea tangle), has been used for thousands of years by Japanese cooks to enhance the taste of foods. After WWII, military powers heard through the grapevine that American GIs were raving that Japanese military rations were truly edible, even delicious. The military, interested in learning how to improve the palatability of military K-rations, met with factory food executives to discuss the flavor enhancer MSG. At this meeting, they learned that this additive enhances any flavor it is added to. If you want a cheeseburger to be more beefy and cheesier, add MSG. If you want ice cream to be creamier, add MSG. If you want chicken broth to be deeper, richer, add MSG. And so the light bulbs went on. Food execs understood that they could boil spaghetti noodles to mush, add some crummy sauce made from nutrient deficient, tasteless tomatoes and let their concoctions languish for months in a tin can if only they added some handy-dandy MSG to spark up the flavor. Since that watershed meeting, the food industry has continually increased the quantity of MSG added to factory fare so that today it permeates our food chain.

But right after military and food bigwigs met in 1948, scientists began to note freaky experiments that should have halted MSG additives to our food supply. In one of the original experiments conducted by a Japanese scientist in 1950, MSG was repeatedly injected into a dog's brain. Each time, the dog fell down convulsing uncontrollably. The conclusion: The amino acid glutamate caused the dog's neural cells to become overexcited, firing out of control.

John W. Olney, MD, is a neuroscientist and researcher at the Washington University School of Medicine. Thirty-five years ago, Olney also conducted experiments on glutamate and aspartate (aspartame) and dubbed these amino acids "excitatory amino acids" or "excitotoxins" because these amino acids excited neural (brain) cells to death.

After the food industry glommed onto MSG as the panacea for their bland fare back in 1948, they started adding it to baby food. More and more studies appeared showing alarming health hazards of MSG and aspartame. Olney took notice. His own studies on MSG repeatedly confirmed that MSG caused severe damage to the neurons of the retina of the eye, as well as massive destruction of neurons in the brain, including the hypothalamus, which regulates most endocrine glands and numerous systems that determine growth, the onset of puberty, and circadian rhythm.

"I testified [before Congress] on many occasions," Dr. Olney said. "Thirty-five years ago when [food companies] were dumping large amounts of MSG into baby foods that were ingested by babies throughout the world. Babies are vastly more sensitive to the neurotoxic effects of MSG than are adults, so it was a matter of urgency to get them to stop adding MSG to baby foods."[1] Dr. Olney's testimony before Congress resulted in MSG being removed from baby foods in 1969. Still nothing was done to remove MSG from the rest of our food supply, so pregnant women have continued ingesting it—despite Dr. Olney's repeated experiments that demonstrated brain damage in the offspring of pregnant monkeys who were fed MSG.

Russell Blaylock, MD, a board-certified neurosurgeon, made use of over five hundred scientific references to illustrate how MSG and aspartame cause serious neurological damage in his book *Excitoxins: The Taste That Kills*. I asked Dr. Blaylock, "What made you pursue the subject of excitotoxins, which is outside the realm of conventional medicine?" Dr. Blaylock replied, "Actually excitotoxins are within the realm of conventional medicine. Excitotoxins are considered the central mechanism for most neurological diseases, and are covered in all texts of neuroscience. It has just taken the rest of physicians so long to catch up and most still have never heard of excitotoxins. Physicians are not known to keep up with new discoveries outside their field of expertise."[2]

I stand corrected. But if neuroscientists understand the damaging effects of MSG why did MSG receive FDA approval in 1959?

Dr. Blaylock explained, "One of the reasons it is so difficult to convince skeptics and the FDA about the toxic effects of MSG and other food-borne excitotoxins is that the effects can be subtle and major damage may take years or even decades to manifest. Long periods of accumulative damage by excitotoxins are generally necessary to produce observable clinical effects on behavior, memory and learning. We now know that in the case of the infant brain some of the injuries can be immediate and some may not appear until later developmental milestones are scheduled to appear."[3]

As far as the general public is concerned, there are two major misconceptions about MSG. First, when most people think of MSG, they think of fragile individuals who suffer from MSG sensitivity, known as the "Chinese restaurant syndrome." But MSG affects everyone to lesser or greater degrees, and, as Dr. Blaylock said, the effects of MSG may not be apparent for decades.

Equally important is that people believe they have a choice whether or not to ingest MSG. But this is a delusion brought to us by the FDA which bent to the Glutamate Association, making it possible for factory food manufacturers to add monosodium glutamate to products in concentrations less than 100 percent without having to notify the consumer on the label. (The Glutamate Association was formed to provide communication among its members, industry, and the government about the "use and safety" of glutamates.) This means that you could be regularly ingesting a product that contains 99 percent MSG. To give you an example of how you unwittingly and regularly ingest MSG, just think back to your last Chinese restaurant experience. Many people understand that MSG isn't healthy—though they could not tell you why exactly—and they know enough to ask the waiter in Chinese restaurants if there is MSG in the food. Although the waiter will tell you no, they do not add MSG to the food, that isn't necessarily true. If the restaurant used, say, ready-made chicken broth, you are likely going to get MSG in your food as MSG is added to most chicken broths today. At home if you make tuna salad with Bumble Bee Tuna, you may be ingesting MSG as this product contains vegetable broth, which often contains MSG. If you ate Dr. Phil's so-called nutritional bars when they were on the market, you ingested glutamate, as Shape Up! bars contained soy protein isolate, which is an ingredient that contains naturally-occurring glutamate.

According to Blaylock, additives are often euphemisms for MSG. Additives that *always* contain MSG are hydrolyzed vegetable protein, hydrolyzed protein, hydrolyzed plant protein, plant protein extract, sodium caseinate, calcium caseinate, yeast extract, textured protein, autolyzed yeast, and hydrolyzed oat flour. Additives that *frequently contain* MSG are malt extract, malt flavoring, bouillon, broth, stock, flavoring, natural flavoring, natural beef or chicken flavoring, seasoning, and spices. Additives that *may contain* MSG or that can be high in naturally-occurring glutamate are carrageenan, enzymes, soy protein concentrate, soy protein isolate, and whey protein concentrate.[4]

To understand how MSG and aspartame affect your brain, you must first understand the basics of brain chemistry. As we looked at in our discussion of brain chemistry balance in chapter 2, your body's chemical communication system controls bodily functions. It has been said that a butterfly flapping its wings in Shanghai affects weather patterns in Los Angeles. That's what neurological activity is like, as one neuron firing impacts countless other neurons in the exquisitely complex interconnected circuitry of your nervous system.

However, once a synapse has fired and accomplished its task, your brain has mechanisms to deactivate neurotransmitters to prevent the synapse from firing over and over uncontrollably and burning itself out.

Amino acids are the chemical building blocks the human body uses to make protein. When they are slightly altered by metabolic processes, they are classified into different categories or groups. One such group is the acidic neurotransmitters, to which glutamate and aspartate belong. Your brain naturally contains low concentrations of both. In fact, glutamate is the most common neurotransmitter in your brain. Glutamate and aspartate are excitatory neurotransmitters that stimulate your brain. Other neurotransmitters act as inhibitors. A combination of excitatory and inhibitory neurotransmitters results in balanced brain chemistry.

All cells and neurons in the human body are guarded in a lock and key fashion. This lock and key system enables the trillions of actions within the human metabolism to operate in an orderly fashion. In other words, everything goes where it is supposed to go. Hormones go where they are supposed to go, sugar goes where it is supposed to go, neurotransmitters go where they are supposed to go, and so on. In your brain, neurotransmitters are the keys that activate receptors (the locks), which allows entry into the neurons so that the neurotransmitters can fire synapses.

Excess glutamate and aspartame in your brain will facilitate a cascade of chemical reactions resulting in the rapid and uncontrollable firing of synapses—culminating in brain cell death. Your brain has regulation systems to rid itself of the excess, but this system requires high levels of energy. Lack of energy is the outcome of dieting, extreme exercise, and hypoglycemia (which occurs when blood sugar levels dip too fast and too low because of eating too much sugar, or as a result of going hungry).

Let's say you eat a diet heavily weighted in factory food containing MSG. You drink diet drinks as well as coffee and iced tea laced with NutraSweet. You eat very little fruit or vegetables (antioxidants). You either don't take supplements or you take an inferior drugstore, supermarket, or Big Box brand. Since blood levels of glutamate remain high for three hours after ingestion, if you eat three meals, plus snacks containing aspartame and MSG, you will have high glutamate blood levels all day long, resulting in the above-mentioned cascade of chemical reactions that end in neural death.

It gets worse. "Once this cascade of destruction is triggered...the whole process proceeds with the explosiveness of a nuclear chain reaction," Dr. Blaylock writes.[5] Specifically, in addition to neurons firing to death, free radicals also reproduce like crazy, bouncing around and further damaging brain cells and destroying neural connections.

Free radicals have been written about extensively in recent

years, but let's review here just so we are all clear about why they are to be avoided. Molecules consist of a positively charged nucleus and negatively charged electrons that orbit the nucleus in pairs. Free radicals are molecules with a missing electron. When an electron is lost, the molecule becomes extremely reactive and is referred to as a "free radical" because it frantically seeks electrons to pair up with its unpaired electrons. Free radicals ravage the molecules in your body, stealing electrons from complete molecules. This process, called oxidation, is essentially a domino effect of molecules becoming free radicals and further rampaging to obtain paired electrons, causing more free radicals. Free radicals kill cells, damage DNA, cause chromosomal damage, create arterial plaque, accelerate aging, and are the key factor in almost every degenerative disease, including brain diseases such as Parkinson's and Alzheimer's.

Free radicals are produced in your body through normal, healthy metabolic processes and are regularly eliminated by antioxidants (also known as free radical scavengers). Antioxidant vitamins A, C, D, E, and K are allowed through your blood brain barrier and can be obtained by eating food or by taking quality supplements.

Your brain is a chemical laboratory where all actions are tightly scripted. Because your brain's life or death depends on tight controls, your body has a blood brain barrier that allows desirable substances in, and bars toxic substances from entering. But, said Dr. Blaylock, "The blood brain barrier is not fail-safe. It can be weakened by numerous factors including excessive physical stress, elevated core body temperatures, infection, trauma, head injuries and certain drugs and metals, as well as the conditions of aging, such as hardening of the arteries, diabetes, hypertension, poor blood oxygenation and tumors. When the blood brain barrier is weakened it can be breached."[6]

According to Blaylock, because of the many factors that weaken the blood brain barrier, people have, at one time or another, a porous blood brain barrier. When your blood brain barrier is porous and you ingest MSG or aspartame, they pass readily through to brain. Also, said Blaylock, even if your blood brain barrier is not weakened, if there is chronic prolonged exposure to a flooding of MSG or aspartame, excitotoxins will ultimately seep past the blood brain barrier to the brain.[7] If excitotoxins are in even a minute overconcentration in the brain, they cause brain cells to become excited to death.

Consider the fact that if a pregnant woman ingests MSG or aspartate her blood levels can reach high enough concentrations to cross the placenta barrier—or the placenta barrier can be breached if there is a defect. Dr. Blaylock said, "MSG does most of its damage during the last trimester of pregnancy and the first two years after birth in humans. This is when the infant brain is undergoing its normal fluctuations in concentration. An excess of glutamate during critical neuronal migrations can cause significant developmental dysfunction—many of which are delayed until later in life." Exposure in the womb and in the first few years of life may affect brain development, resulting in autism, learning disorders, hyperactive behavior, or even schizophrenia. Moreover, as Dr. Blaylock said, these effects may not be evident until puberty or early adulthood.

I asked Dr. Blaylock if MSG has been used for thousands of years in Japan, why are they not having the same neurological problems as Americans? Dr. Blaylock explained: "[For] several reasons. One, the Japanese consume a diluted form of MSG and less volume. Unlike Americans, they also eat a diet that is known to reduce excitotoxic injury—such as a diet high in flavonoids [compounds with therapeutic effects found in fruits and vegetables], foods that are high in omega-3 fats, which directly block excitotoxicity, as well as magnesium, which blocks the glutamate receptor, among other factors. Yet they are suffering from excitotoxic disorders, including Alzheimer's dementia, in increasing numbers."[8]

It's important to note that excitotoxins have a compounding effect on your brain. A fast food meal adulterated with MSG from McDonald's, Wendy's, Taco Bell, or the like that is washed down with a Diet Coke containing aspartame will do compounded damage to your brain. For many it's hard to imagine eating a burger without drinking a diet soda.

CHAPTER 6

Aspartame Poisoning: Urban Legend or Fact?

FUZZY THINKING, memory loss, ringing in the ears, numbness and tingling of the extremities, blindness, multiple sclerosis, brain tumors, and (perhaps the most alarming) grand mal seizures suffered by commercial airline pilots—these and other serious neurological disorders are part of the aspartame urban legend. I had not researched aspartame in depth until I started working on this book. When I did probe into the aspartame world, it was a short-click journey to innumerable, highly energetic Internet pages on aspartame that took me back to the good old days of reading and deciphering the fine print on a bottle of Dr. Bronner's soap.

Despite vociferous warnings, books that have been published on so-called aspartame poisoning do not reach the bestseller list, and the alleged dangers of aspartame do not appear newsworthy to the mainstream media. In fact, doctors advocate the use of aspartame, and many use it themselves (think of that box of free samples of sugar-free Metamucil in your doctor's office). Another example is Arthur Agatston, MD's bestselling diet book, *The South Beach Diet: The Delicious, Doctor-Designed, Foolproof Plan for Fast and Healthy Weight Loss*, in which he recommends the use of Equal, "sugar free" yogurt, and such. What's more, aspartame has the endorsement of the FDA, CDC, the American Diabetic Association (ADA), the American Dietetic Association (ADA) and the majority of the medical establishment. (These associations are, respectively, the nation's leading nonprofit health organization that provides diabetes research, information, and advocacy, and the nation's largest organization of food and nutritional professionals.)

Yet despite these endorsements and the thinly veiled, exasperated assertions by the aspartame industry and the FDA that we have nothing to worry about, there are reputable medical doctors and research scientists, hundreds of peer-reviewed research papers, mountains of empirical (anecdotal) evidence, and clinical experience that tell a different story.

When aspartame first came on the scene, I asked a doctor friend of mine what he thought of it. He replied, "It's just a couple of amino acids, so it's probably okay." This was partly true, but as it turns out, not that simple.

Dr. Blaylock told me, "Aspartame is a compound made from three components: phenylalanine (an amino acid), aspartic acid (an excitotoxic amino acid), and joined chemically by methanol, a toxic alcohol. When consumed, aspartame is metabolically broken down into its three component parts—all three of which are toxic to the nervous system as well as to all cells. In addition, further metabolism occurs producing dozens of other potentially toxic compounds and even carcinogenic compounds.

"Three new studies have shown that the methanol component is metabolically converted into formaldehyde and formic acid, both powerful toxins, even in very small doses. Formic acid is the toxin that causes the intensely painful bite of the fire ant and blindness when methanol is ingested in sufficient quantities. [As evidenced in alcoholics who ingest methanol to get drunk.] Formaldehyde is known to be a powerful cancer-causing agent, even in very small doses. In one of these studies it was shown that aspartame's formaldehyde accumulates near the DNA of cells, severely damaging this critical cell component. This can lead to neurodegenerative diseases and cancer.

"Because formaldehyde is tightly bound to the DNA and

accumulates, drinking even one aspartame-sweetened drink a day can eventually lead to one of these diseases—especially in a cancer prone person. Another new study found that aspartame dramatically increased leukemias and lymphomas in experimental animals in doses equal to that seen with human consumption of aspartame products. The highest intake of aspartame is in children and pregnant women, which would greatly increase the risk of these two highly malignant diseases in the children.

"There is also evidence that one of the other breakdown products, called diketopiperizine, is also carcinogenic and may account for the 4,700 percent increase in brain tumors seen in the original safety studies of aspartame. Combined with the formaldehyde, this would also explain the dramatic increase in breast, pancreatic, prostate, thyroid, liver, lung, uterine, and ovarian tumors seen in aspartame exposed test animals."[1]

Considering that these factors are in addition to the excitotoxin effects outlined in the previous chapter, one would think that it would be enough to stop a reasoned individual from ingesting aspartame—or feeding it to children. But again, we have FDA approval, which still packs tremendous clout for many Americans.

The saga of aspartame began in December 1965, when a chemist at G. D. Searle discovered a substance that is two hundred times sweeter than sugar with no calories. Naturally, Searle was eager to get aspartame FDA approved. The goal was to get aspartame classified as an inert substance. The reason is that any compound that affects physiological systems is classified as a drug by the FDA, which means that it's subject to more demanding regulatory procedures than a food additive. But if a compound is shown to be inert, it's exempted from the ongoing safety monitoring imposed on drugs (such as it is). Factory food manufacturers are not obligated to monitor adverse reactions associated with the additive, submit reports of adverse reactions to the FDA, or required to carry out additional research to confirm the additive's safety.

In November 1970 the popular artificial sweetener cyclamate

was linked to cancer and yanked from the market. Saccharin was subsequently put under scrutiny, throwing the market wide open for the introduction of aspartame.

From that time on, numerous experts, including neuroscientist John Olney, informed the FDA of studies demonstrating the deleterious effects of ingesting aspartame. The drama that ensued over the next two decades involved independent researchers such as Olney, a dogged consumer interest attorney, Searle's own researchers as well as their legal and PR firms, an FDA task force, various FDA commissioners, Democrat and Republican senators, U.S. attorneys, grand juries, the then-president of Searle, Donald Rumsfeld, and the newly inaugurated POTUS Ronald Reagan in an incredibly convoluted story of sloppy science of epic proportions, intrigue, self-interest, ambition, greed, and shenanigans.[2]

Despite the valiant efforts of those who wanted to halt FDA approval of aspartame, greed did manage to get its foot in the door, resulting in FDA approval of aspartame for limited use on July 26, 1974. It was approved specifically as a free-flowing sugar substitute, as tablets for sweetening hot beverages, and in cereal, gum, and dry bases (coating on products such as pills). And in 1983, the incredibly lucrative aspartame was FDA-approved for use in carbonated beverages and carbonated beverage syrup bases. In 1985, Searle sold out to the chemical company Monsanto, which has a long and checkered history in the field of deadly chemicals. (Among its many sordid affiliations was Monsanto's 1967 joint venture with I. G. Farbenfabriken, the manufacturer of a lethal nerve gas used in Hitler's Final Solution.[3]) After acquiring aspartame, Monsanto created the nutritious-sounding subsidiary the NutraSweet Company.

On June 27, 1996, the FDA removed all restrictions and authorized aspartame use in all products—even heated and baked goods, although studies had demonstrated that that aspartame breaks down into free methanol in temperatures above 86 degrees Fahrenheit (like say when you cook no-cal Jell-O Pudding or leave a case of Diet Dr Pepper in your car).

Since the aspartame patent expired in the early 1990s, this fake sugar is now sold under the brand names Equal, Spoonful, Equal-Measure, as well as generically, but the brand is essentially owned by NutraSweet. Like MSG, even those who want to avoid aspartame may be ingesting in products like toothpaste, laxatives, wine coolers, vitamins, and *prescription drugs.*

By 1994, the Department of Health and Human Services had documented ninety-two adverse medical symptoms attributed to aspartame use, including anxiety attacks, arthritis, asthma, brain cancer, chronic fatigue, depression, insomnia, memory loss, migraines, numbness of extremities, seizures, tachycardia, tinnitus, vertigo, vision loss, and weight gain.[4]

In addition, aspartame use is thought to worsen or mimic the symptoms of Alzheimer's disease, arthritis, attention deficit disorder, chronic fatigue syndrome, depression, diabetes, epilepsy, fibromyalgia, lupus, Lyme's disease, lymphoma, multiple chemical sensitivities, multiple sclerosis, panic disorders, and Parkinson's disease.[5]

Since the introduction of aspartame in the mid 1970s, the incidence of brain tumors has risen exponentially.[6] Evidence indicates that one particular type of brain tumor, primary lymphoma of the brain, may be associated with aspartame use. According to Dr. Blaylock, "It is a particularly nasty tumor with a high mortality rate."[7]

The medical establishment and the aspartame industry argues that the precipitous rise in the incidence of brain tumors does not correspond to the introduction and rise in use of aspartame, but rather it is due to better diagnostic techniques. Not true, Dr. Blaylock told me. "The original studies by the G. D. Searle Company found a 47 percent increase in brain tumors in rats exposed to the highest dose of aspartame. My personal investigation, using the SEER brain tumor registry, found an increase in primary brain tumors, unexplained by better diagnosis or an aging population. Dr. John Olney, using the SEER tumor registry, also found an increase in malignant brain tumors in those consuming aspartame-containing diet products."[8] (The National Cancer Institute's Surveillances, Epidemiology and End Results [SEER] is considered the state-of-the-art brain tumor database.)

In December 1996, *60 Minutes* aired an exposé on aspartame titled "How Sweet Is It?" Mike Wallace opened with, "Last month, the *Journal of Neuropathology and Experimental Neurology* published a scientific paper that says, in effect, that the ingestion of the widely used artificial sweetener called aspartame, better known as NutraSweet or Equal, may just be responsible for what the authors say is a dramatic increase in the number of people who develop brain tumors. In recent weeks, there's been a spate of media activity about this, because a small but outspoken group of consumer advocates and researchers have become more vocal about what they say may be aspartame's adverse effects. These consumer groups and scientists are not calling for a ban, but they are asking the Food and Drug Administration, the FDA, to take another look at aspartame."[9]

Wallace was referring to Dr. John Olney's study "Increasing Brain Tumor Rates: Is There a Link to Aspartame?" Olney went on record on *60 Minutes*, that although "three to five years after aspartame was approved, there's been a striking increase in the incidence of malignant brain tumors," he was not calling for a ban on aspartame, but that "the FDA needs to reassess [aspartame], and this time around, FDA should do it right."[10]

Olney's study provoked the proverbial less than zero interest within the FDA to reassess the safety of aspartame.

Regarding the rise in brain tumors, Dr. Blaylock said, "As a neurosurgeon I see the devastating effects a brain tumor has, not only on its victim, but on the victim's family as well. To think that there is even a reasonable doubt that aspartame can induce brain tumors in the American population is frightening. And to think that the FDA has lulled them into a false sense of security is a monumental crime."[11]

Since the mid-1980s I have personally known several people

who have been diagnosed with brain tumors. I wonder how many people you have known who have met the same fate?

So why do we use aspartame? Simply put, we want to be thin. Turn the TV on anytime, night or day, and you'll see beautiful, thin women with glossy lips drinking diet sodas. But how many beautiful girls do you really see drinking diet sodas? None of the beautiful, thin women I know would so much as use diet sodas to remove the lime deposits on their shower doors. That's because diet sodas do not make you thin or beautiful.

Way back in 1983, Richard Wurtman, an MIT neuroscientist, researched the weight loss effects of aspartame and concluded that using aspartame may actually result in cravings for foods high in calories and carbohydrates.[12] The reason is that although aspartame is calorie free, it's sweet, and so it triggers the release of insulin, which stows away sugar. If food is not forthcoming, hypoglycemia (low blood sugar) attacks and severe hunger follows.[13]

In 1986, after tracking eighty thousand women for six years, the American Cancer Society documented that the women who used artificial sweeteners gained more weight than those who avoided them.[14]

One of the biggest quandaries in the obesity issue today is that some people are obese on *normal amounts of food*. Aspartate has been established as an excitotoxin that causes neurons to fire out of control until death. Numerous studies on excitotoxins in mice (closest to humans in glutamate and aspartate sensitivity) have concluded that the hypothalamic damage caused by MSG and aspartate resulted in the test subjects and their offspring being shorter than normal in stature *and obese on normal amounts of food*.[15]

Now that's depressing. But if packing on more pounds doesn't get you down, the use of aspartame just might. Excessive levels of the amino acid phenylalanine in your brain cause serotonin to dip. And if you recall from our discussion of neurotransmitters, serotonin is the one that gets you high on life. Without enough serotonin in your brain, it's doom and gloom *plus* carb craving.[16]

Brain tumors, Lou Gherig's disease, severe mental retardation, seizures, multiple sclerosis, obese on normal amounts of food. To date, studies continue to confirm that aspartame is a dangerous, neurotoxic substance that should never have been released into our food chain and at the very least should be illegal to give to pregnant women and children.[17] How in the world did aspartame ever get FDA approval?

CHAPTER 7

FDA-Approved Murder by Supermarket

MY GRANDMA STELLA set an admirable example and was a major influence on my lifelong attitudes about nutrition, but growing up I didn't always take her seriously. One of the reasons she didn't get the credit she deserved for being so ahead of her time in her views about nutrition might have had something to do with her somewhat apocryphal presentation. Like the story she liked to repeat about a friend of hers who murdered her husband by feeding him nothing but hot dogs. We used to roll our eyes back then.

About the time Grandma was telling us about the hot dog murder, forensic science was just beginning to develop. Today we have DNA testing, advanced computerization, and laser light scattering technology to help solve murders. You would have to be an idiot to try to murder someone using arsenic or cyanide. But police agencies and the FBI don't care if you feed your family carcinogenic, neurologically damaging, toxic food products, as long as the ingredients are approved by the FDA; the agency that brags that it is "the Nation's Foremost Consumer Protection Agency." Today, millions of Americans are unwittingly killing their families by supermarket—with FDA approval.

Factory foods are manufactured or raised with toxic substances that have either received the FDA approval or have slipped through the cracks in their loose screening process. There are many reasons for this lack of monitoring. First, policing the food industry takes money. In 1996, Michael Friedman, MD, deputy commissioner of the FDA testified, "Given the current constraints on government resources, it is unlikely the FDA will ever have sufficient resources to inspect, sample and analyze more than a small percentage of all food products, domestic, as well as imported." Friedman went on to say, "The current system generally relies on detecting and correcting problems after they occur rather than preventing them in the first place."[1]

Then there's the meaningless FDA status of "Generally Recognized as Safe" (GRAS), which is the status that was granted to MSG way back in 1959. The status, established by Congress in 1958, was granted to additives that had previously existed in the food supply based on unmonitored, inadequate, hit-or-miss surveys and nonexistent follow-up. After the initial structuring of the GRAS list, for a manufacturer to obtain a new GRAS status for a substance, a formal petition was required by the FDA that provided evidence that supported the safety of the substance.

In 1997, the FDA decided that GRAS food ingredients would no longer be required by law to go through the same "review" process just described. Now factory food manufacturers must only notify the FDA that such and such additive is GRAS and provide some evidence that the FDA can then file into a drawer. This eliminated pesky paper shuffling for the FDA and allowed the agency to "gain increased awareness of ingredients in the nation's food supply and the cumulative dietary exposure to GRAS substances."[2] Given that industry now has carte blanche to put anything they want into their products, the FDA "Generally Recognized as Safe" status for food additives would be more appropriately labeled, "Wha? Huh? Um, I Guess It's Okay If Food Companies Say So."

Although drug companies are required to report adverse reactions to the FDA, food companies are not required to report adverse reactions to GRAS additives to the FDA. So we don't really know what GRAS additives are problematic. For all the "safe"

GRAS ingredients included in factory food products, some noxious substances have slipped into our food supply. But let's say that some GRAS substances are safe, some are moderately safe, some are safe in small amounts, and some are toxic, especially when accumulated in your body with prolonged use. But we are not just eating one little thing that is GRAS every day. We are bombarding our bodies with GRAS substances over the prolonged period of a lifetime.

In addition to this flimflam "review" process to obtain GRAS status for food additives, the FDA has fallen into a truly sorry state of disorganization, ineptness, and corruption that ultimately affects many other decisions rendered by the FDA regarding food products, diet products, and drugs. In recent years, our nation has been rocked by the scandalous realization that the FDA might be too lackadaisical about drug approvals, which has led to the unleashing of dangerous drugs onto the market that generate billions of dollars of profits for drug companies. For example, the FDA allowed the painkillers Vioxx, Celebrex, Bextra, and Aleve on the market although these drugs increase the risk for heart attack and stroke. In 1999, *The New England Journal of Medicine* reported that arthritis sufferers dying each year from the side effects of nonsteroidal anti-inflammatory drugs numbered up to 16,500— the same number as were dying from AIDS. In addition, more than 100,000 people were hospitalized every year due to gastrointestinal problems associated with these drugs.[3] Of the 25 million Americans who took Vioxx between 1999 and 2004 (as of this writing), up to 4,600 of these—or their family members—are suing the maker, Merck, claiming Vioxx caused strokes and heart attacks.

Samuel Epstein, MD, is a professor emeritus of environmental and occupational medicine at the University of Illinois Medical Center in Chicago, an internationally recognized authority on cancer causes and prevention, and the author of 260 peer-reviewed scientific articles and fifteen books on this subject. Dr. Epstein told me, "Six or seven years ago I urged the use of aspirin, which is a Cox-2 inhibitor, and is as effective as Celebrex and all the other

Cox-2 inhibitor drugs, but without all the dangerous side effects." But the FDA did not heed this warning.

Subsequent to the initial yanking of Cox-2 inhibitors from the shelves, we learned that FDA "drug advisors" were lobbying for some of these drugs to be returned to the market—despite their known problems. The press reported that ten of the thirty-two drug advisors to the FDA just so happened to have consulted in recent years for the drugs' manufacturers. Nine of these ten had voted to return the potential deadly Cox-2 inhibitors to market. CBS reported, "If these ten 'experts' had not been drafted for the panel, neither Bextra nor Vioxx would have received enough votes to get the panel's thumbs up."[4]

The *New York Times* reported, "Researchers with ties to industry commonly serve on Food and Drug Administration advisory panels, but their presence has long been contentious issue; several of panel members flagged with conflicts say most or all of money from drug makers went not to themselves but to their universities or institutions." (An indirect route to their salaries, bonuses, and perks.) The *Times* also mentioned that shares of Merck and Pfizer soared after the panel's vote was announced.[5] You have to wonder if the nine FDA drug advisors also held stocks in Merck and Pfizer.

How did these drug advisors ultimately arrive at their conclusions that unsafe drugs should be re-released in the market? In 2000 Merck found itself in an untenable situation when they were faced with the death of a seventy-three-year-old participant in a clinical trial, who had likely died of a heart attack. The woman's death, writes Merck's top scientist Edward M. Scolnick, MD, in an e-mail, "put us in a terrible situation." (As it turns out, in this twelve-week drug trial, called "Advantage," eight out of 5,500 participants suffered a heart attack or sudden cardiac death.) The major issue appeared to be that Scolnick did not want the FDA to demand Vioxx carry a warning for cardiac risks as it would not sell as well as its competitor Celebrex, which did not warn of cardiac risk on its label. In fact, in other e-mails Scolnick "fiercely criticized the FDA and said he would personally pressure senior officials at the agency if it took action unfavorable to Vioxx."[6] And so Scolnick got his way and thousands of people were harmed.

In 2006 juries sided with the Vioxx takers with multimillion dollar judgments handed down against Merck.[7]

David Graham, MD, MPH, who has been with the FDA for twenty years, is currently the associate director for science and medicine in the Office of Drug Safety. In November 2004, Dr. Graham appeared before the Senate Finance Committee and subsequently appeared on *PBS Online News Hour Program* to tell the country that the FDA was "incapable of protecting America from another Vioxx. Simply put, the FDA and the Center for Drug Evaluation and Research (CDER) are broken."[8] (The CDER, a branch of the FDA, responds to written inquires regarding prescription and over-the-counter drugs.)

In the movie *Beyond Borders* renegade relief doctor Nick Callahan attempts to illustrate the difference between people in the developed world who indulge in every means at their disposal to relieve misery and African refugees who embrace suffering because it is inescapable for them. He asks bleeding heart American socialite Sarah Jordan, "What is the first thing you do when you get a cold?" She replies, "Chicken soup, aspirin, scotch." "You never just have the cold?" he asks. Well, actually, no Dr. Callahan, most of us in the West do not just have the cold, nor do we endure any other malady without at least seeking comfort in OTC [over-the-counters]. And this is where the trouble lies. Because OTCs are FDA approved, we blithely self-prescribe without pondering the prospect of acute liver failure. Partly as a result of the Cox-2 inhibitor debacle, Americans have been lulled into a false sense of security over the use of OTC pain relievers containing acetaminophen (the active ingredient in Tylenol). A study in the December 2005 issue of *Hepatology* reveals that, because the FDA has not made even the most laid-back effort to educate Americans about acetaminophen poisoning, most of us have no clue how easy it is to overdose on it. People with cluster symptoms can end up taking a variety of OTCs all containing acetaminophen without realizing they've reached or exceeded the maximum adult daily dose of 4,000 milligrams. Tim Davern, MD, who is a gastroenterologist with the liver transplant program of the University of California at San Francisco and a coauthor of the above-mentioned study, concluded this scenario: "It's extremely frustrating to see people come into the hospital who felt fine several days ago, but now need a new liver."[9]

Today more than a half a million children suffer from autism, and every year more than forty thousand are diagnosed. In *The Rolling Stone*, attorney and environmentalist Robert F. Kennedy writes, "Since 1991, when the CDC and the FDA had recommended that three additional vaccines laced with the [mercury based] preservative [thimerosal] be given to extremely young infants—in one case, within hours of birth—the estimated number of cases of autism had increased fifteenfold, from one in every 2,500 children to one in 166 children .... Rep. Dan Burton, a Republican from Indiana, oversaw a three-year investigation of thimerosal after his grandson was diagnosed with autism. 'Thimerosal used as a preservative in vaccines is directly related to the autism epidemic,' his House Government Reform Committee concluded in its final report. 'This epidemic in all probability may have been prevented or curtailed had the FDA not been asleep at the switch regarding a lack of safety data regarding injected thimerosal, a known neurotoxin.'"[10]

In addition to Cox-2 inhibitors, acetaminophen, and thimerosal, the FDA failed to protect Americans from the serious risk of heart valve damage from the weight loss miracle-in-a bottle Fenfluramine and Phentermine (Fen-Phen). The FDA failed to restrict the acne drug Accutane, even though it is known to cause Thalidomide-like birth defects when taken by pregnant women. The FDA allowed the sale of the cholesterol-lowering medication, Crestor, even though it can lead to kidney failure, and did not warn doctors and parents about the risk of suicide among children taking antidepressants.

The FDA's problems are not exclusive to the pharmaceutical industry, said Dr. Epstein, "Whether you want to look at it from the standpoint of indifference, conspiracy, or conflict of interest, the FDA poses a great danger to consumers. What's happening now with these drugs is symptomatic of the FDA."[11]

While the recent drug scandal may make it appear as if the FDA has all of a sudden sunk to an all-time low, it appears that this government agency has had problems for a very long time. Herbert L. Ley, MD, FDA commissioner from 1968 to 1969, said, "The thing that bugs me is that the people think that the FDA is protecting them—it isn't. What the FDA is doing and what the public thinks it's doing are as different as night and day."[12]

Richard Crout, former director of the FDA's Bureau of Drugs, testified way back in 1976 that the FDA was in bad shape. "I want to describe the agency as I saw it. Now one knew where anything was . . . . There was absenteeism; there was open drunkenness by several employees . . . . There was intimidation internally . . . . People—I'm talking about division directors and their staffs—would engage in a kind of behavior that invited insubordination; people tittered in the corners, throwing spitballs—now I'm describing physicians; people would slouch down in their chairs and not respond to questions; and moan and groan, [making] sleeping gestures. This was a kind of behavior I have not seen in any other institution from a grown man . . . . the FDA has a long-term problem with the recruitment of personnel, good, scientific personnel."[13]

In June 2006, after reviewing the results of a fifteen-month inquiry he had initiated, Representative Henry A. Waxman (D-CA) said, "Americans have relied on the FDA to ensure the safety of their food and drugs for 100 years. But under the Bush administration, enforcement efforts have plummeted and serious violations are ignored."

When it comes to our food supply, the FDA is greatly responsible for our evolution from a real food diet to a supermarket food diet, but not solely responsible. Food additives would not be getting FDA approval in the first place if companies weren't applying for approval. And within those businesses are people who possess a single-minded purpose: making as much money as they can. It's widely known that Washington players hop from government positions to law firms to corporate positions to elected office and back again. Career advancement in Washington and the biotech industry (an industry with far-reaching implications in food production) is predicated on favors and back scratching. In researching this book, I found dozens of references of people who went from White House careers to positions at Monsanto, from Congress to Monsanto, from federal agencies to Monsanto and the biotech industry, and from Monsanto and the biotech industry to government employment. When decisions are made about public health and safety, career and financial interests often influence these decision makers.

The sad state of affairs concerning our food supply has been developing since the late 1800s as the food, diet, and pharmaceutical industries systematically cultivated a complex and inextricable web of relationships with (some, not all) FDA scientists and other researchers, administrators and attorneys, biotech attorneys, elected officials, government agencies, lobbyists, medical associations, medical and scientific journals, and doctors. This tangled, powerful network of relationships has influenced what you have been putting in your mouth and what you will put in your mouth in the future. The billions of dollars in profits wracked up by these industries through the sales and consumption of their products wouldn't be possible if it weren't for tickets and invitations to sports events, operas, symphonies, theater performances, and invitations to prestigious movie premiers, lunches, dinner parties, birthday parties, weddings, golf games, and exotic vacations, as well as the honorariums, grants, donations, kickbacks, payoffs, and miscellaneous and sundry "favors" accepted by the support players listed above.[14]

Clearly, there are innumerable independently operating moving parts that buoy the activities of these industries. Not everyone involved is corrupt. Some people in government and industry are simply trying to make a living at their careers. And many Americans—including elected and appointed officials—still have a "better living through chemistry" mentality. We can only assume that at least some of our elected and appointed officials and their families are as much in the dark as we are. If they knew the facts about our food supply, one can only hope that our elected and appointed officials would revise their current diversionary strategy of health care reform to shift the primary focus instead on reforming the food supply that is causing so many people to need health care in the first place.

Industries have gained a powerful foothold in America because of the efforts of a relative handful of very wealthy, extraordinarily powerful, self-interested inside players, their paid-off hench-people, agencies such as the FDA, as well as the unwitting participation of millions of bit players and trusting consumers. So we can't really say that this is a conspiracy—except insomuch as it is a conspiracy to protect shareholder profits. Nevertheless, the end results (our epidemic of obesity and disease) are just as horrendous as if these contributing players had gathered in a back room and agreed, "Let's get rich at the expense of Americans' health."

Corporations are able to hawk injurious substances like MSG and aspartame to Americans because of FDA approval. For example, the public is continually assured by the FDA that aspartame is an inert compound that does not affect physiological systems. In 1984, FDA spokesperson Robert Shapiro said, "The FDA concluded that [aspartame] is one of the most thoroughly tested food additives they'd ever seen. And it's safe."[15] Indeed, as recent as the summer of 2006, Laura Tarantino, PhD, director of the Office of Food Additive Safety in the FDA's Center of Food Safety and Applied Nutrition, maintained, "At this time, our position that aspartame is safe is based on the large body of information previously reviewed. Our conclusions are based on a detailed review of more than 100 toxicological and clinical studies on safety."[16]

It might be useful to take the FDA's stance on aspartame in the context of its overall mentality about dangerous substances. Every year more than one hundred thousand Americans are killed from adverse reactions to prescription and over-the-counter medicines and an additional 2.1 million are seriously injured (and this does not include prescribing errors).[17] Is it any wonder that the FDA is not bothered that aspartame is one of two additives that have consistently generated the most consumer complaints of adverse reactions?[18]

However, given the mountains of empirical evidence and hundreds of peer-reviewed research studies that demonstrate the dangers of aspartame use, it appears that the FDA approval of aspartame may have been a tad premature. Dr. Blaylock told me that the FDA handling of aspartame "is what one would expect of a federal regulatory agency. They have ignored all studies and complaints."[19] I would go a step further and say that if any substance is "FDA approved" the best course of action is to run screaming from the room.

Because it's common sense that factory food is a primary cause of many of our obesity and health problems, many stalwart Americans are turning to "health food." Instead of supplying us with real, organic food, factory food makers have flooded the market with pretend "health food," like meat "analogs"—fake meat products made from soy (tagged with FDA "health" claims). It may come as a shock, but everyone is not as "go soy go" as you may have been led to believe.

IV

Science Fiction Food

CHaPTeR 8

Soy: Internet Paranoia—Or Fact?

WHEN I WAS FIFTEEN in 1966, my family packed up and moved to a Navy base in Japan. Only twenty years after WWII, Japan was still a developing country. Kimono-swathed Japanese shuffled along on geta. Homes were made of rice paper and tatami mats. There was no such thing as fast food. A ravenous teenager, I learned to navigate the train system to better eat my way across Japan in soba shops and sushi bars. Never once did I see a single Japanese sit down to a meal of soy. It's true that, along with their traditional diet, the Japanese ate a number of soy foods. But mostly I remember Japanese chop-sticking teeny pieces of soy out of their soup, like condiments.

Flash forward to the 1990s. All of a sudden soy hits the scene. Medical experts said that eating soy protein reduces your risk for heart disease by lowering cholesterol levels, the isoflavones in soy reduce or alleviate hot flashes in menopausal women, the isoflavones in soy prevent osteoporosis, and that numerous components in soy have anticancer properties. A clever public relations campaign by the soy industry massaged this message into the brains of busy Americans as, "Asians are healthier because they eat soy, soy, soy and more soy." And I'm thinking, *Hmmm. Call me crazy, but that is not my recollection of the Japanese diet.*

I get suspicious when big businesses, the media, and doctors start aggressively telling us that any product or substance is "healthy." I start to wonder when I'm being told I should eat soy hot dogs, soy cheese, soy yogurt, soy ice cream, soy pasta, soy chips, soy low-carb pancakes, and soy burgers, and to drink soy milk and feed soy to my pets. That I should take soy supplements instead of using real, bioidentical estrogen replacement, shampoo my hair with soy, and rub soy cream into my hands. I started getting curious. Very curious.

Did those involved in soy have our best interest in mind when they introduced new industrially processed soy foods into our food chain? Or could it be that those friendly, neighborhood, behemoth purveyors of scary substances, like Monsanto—which produced Agent Orange for the Vietnam War and is now sunnily saturating Earth with the herbicide Roundup—those types of companies might have accidentally on purpose planted nearly the entire planet with soybeans and now they've got to convince you to brush your teeth with it?

Since we're inundated with gung-ho soy propaganda, it may come as a surprise to you that not everyone is upbeat about soy. I can't say that I was entirely objective about soy as I launched my investigation. Nevertheless, my motivation was to get to the truth. My biases included these five facts: One, I lived in Japan and didn't witness evidence to back up the claims that the historical Asian diet was heavily weighted in soy. Two, Americans do not eat whole soy foods as Asians do; rather, they eat factory foods containing industrially processed soy substances. Three, 80 percent of these soy substances are made from "Roundup Ready" soybeans created by Monsanto (soybeans genetically engineered to withstand the spraying of the weed and grass killer Roundup). Four, the FDA, which has given its blessing to soy, appears to be inept and corrupt. And five, big businesses are notoriously more interested in shareholder profits than Americans' health.

The pro-soy camp comprises the soy industry, the food processing industry, some vegetarians and vegans, the powerful contingency of administrators at the FDA, soy researchers whose research is funded by the soy industry, and celebrity nutritionists and doctors with best-selling books.

To get a well-respected opinion from the soy camp, I began by e-mailing Christiane Northrup, MD, celebrity women's doctor and author of *The Wisdom of Menopause: Creating Physical and Emotional Health and Healing During the Change*, who is also a spokesperson for Revival, a company that manufactures high-isoflavone soy protein powders, energy bars, and other soy products. Dr. Northrup replied, "The health benefits are very well documented . . . [soy] helps support nearly the entire body and its systems, including hormone regulation, breast health, the heart, the bones, the brain, and the colon and bowels.

"Many women know first hand that this phytoestrogen complex, or plant-based estrogen, is a safe alternative to synthetic hormone replacement therapy. They've seen first hand what the studies have shown: Soy helps reduce many of the common symptoms reported during perimenopause and menopause, including the frequency and intensity of hot flashes, mood swings, and vaginal dryness. These same women have also noticed changes on the surface, enjoying more youthful looking skin, healthier hair, and even weight loss. Soy has other benefits: As you may know, free radicals from oxygen, pollution, and various toxins are what actually cause the tissue damage we call 'aging.' So eating foods with antioxidant properties is one way to prevent this damage and maintain health. And as it turns out, in addition to all its other benefits, soy has some well-documented antioxidant properties."[1]

For a second opinion, I turned to Bradley J. Willcox, MD, M Sc, co-investigator of the Okinawa Centenarian Study and coauthor of *The Okinawa Program: How the World's Longest-Lived People Achieve Everlasting Health—and How You Can Too*. Dr. Willcox e-mailed me his opinion. "The best evidence suggests that adding more soy foods to the Western diet may reduce the risk of heart disease through beneficial effects of soy on cholesterol levels and artery health. More research is needed before definitive recommendations can be made about increasing the consumption of soy for other health claims .... Our studies suggest that soy may have contributed to [the Okinawan populations'] overall health and that it may be implicated in their low risk for heart disease and hormone-associated cancers such as breast, prostate and colon cancers."[2]

These testimonies sounded convincing. But I decided to look into the anti-soy camp, which happens to be viewed as fringy fanatical by the group listed above. Indeed, integrative medicine advocate and celebrity author Andrew Weil, MD, whose word is gospel to many Americans, referred to the questioning of the safety of soy as "Internet paranoia."[3]

As it turned out, clinical nutritionist and soy expert, Kaayla T. Daniel, PhD, CCN, had very different experiences with her soy-consuming patients than did Dr. Northrup. She told me, "About ten years ago I started reading newspaper and magazine articles with titles like 'The Joy of Soy,' and 'Soy of Cooking,' but the hype didn't correspond with reality. I knew many vegetarians and vegans, most of whom were eating soy as their primary protein source, but very few of them looked healthy and many complained about fatigue, brain fog, poor skin, hair loss, and other problems. Also, as a health educator I worked with people privately and in classes. I couldn't help but notice that many of the most health conscious people ate and drank a lot of soy and were developing many health problems, particularly thyroid problems. This piqued my interest. If soy was so healthy, why were these people doing so poorly?"

Daniel's curiosity instigated four years of research, which culminated in the book *The Whole Soy Story: The Dark Side of America's Favorite Health Food*. Dr. Daniel told me, "Contrary to Dr. Northrup's claim, the health benefits of soy are not well documented. The studies are inconsistent and contradictory at best. Possible benefits are outweighed by proven risks. Hundreds of epidemiological, clinical, and laboratory studies link soy to malnutrition, digestive distress, thyroid dysfunction, cognitive decline, reproductive disorders, immune system breakdown, and even heart disease and cancer."[4]

Dr. Daniel wasted no time dousing the flames of Dr. Willcox's enthusiasm, "The authors of the *Okinawa Program* claim that soy was the key to lowered cancer risk in Okinawans, but a careful reading of the text indicates that they came to that conclusion based on three possibly unrelated factors: the presence of some soy in the Okinawan diet, the lower incidence of cancer there, and the pro-soy findings from several unrelated but well-publicized studies, most of which were funded by the soy industry."[5]

Dr. Daniel is not alone in her stance against soy. Those in the anti-soy camp include a number of scientists from the FDA laboratories of toxicological research whose research findings on soy have been ignored by the consumer protection division of the FDA; scientists whose research is not funded by the soy industry; scientists who *are* funded by the soy industry, but whose findings get buried; clinical nutritionists and other nutritional experts; doctors of Chinese medicine; authors of alternative health and wellness books; not to mention unhappy ex-soy consumers who attribute health problems to eating soy.

Those in the anti-soy camp refute the health claims made by the pro-soy camp and assert a litany of serious health problems associated with soy—everything from weight gain to birth defects.[6]

Soy entered our radar screen in the early nineties, but wasn't officially launched into our collective consciousness until—in response to a petition submitted to the FDA by Protein Technologies International—on October 26, 1999, the FDA issued a press release: "FDA's conclusion that foods containing soy protein included in a diet low in saturated fat and cholesterol may reduce the risk of CHD [coronary heart disease] by lowering blood cholesterol levels." This claim was supposedly based on "evidence that including soy protein in a diet low in saturated fat and cholesterol may also help to reduce the risk of CHD" and, "Scientific studies show that 25 grams of soy protein daily in the diet is needed to show a significant cholesterol lowering effect. In order to qualify for this health claim, a food must contain at least 6.25 grams of soy protein per serving."

This authorization had been fought by two FDA toxicologists, Daniel Sheehan, PhD, and Daniel Doerge, PhD, who were concerned about the inconclusiveness of the alleged cholesterol-lowering effect and also about known health hazards. On February 18, 1999, Drs. Sheehan and Doerge wrote a protest letter to the FDA saying, "There exists a significant body of animal data that demonstrates goitrogenic [thyroid inhibiting] and even carcinogenic effects of soy products. Moreover, there are significant reports of goitrogenic effects from soy consumption in human infants and adults."[7]

Nevertheless, the FDA ruling urged consumers, "Because soy protein can be added to a variety of foods, it is possible for consumers to eat foods containing soy protein at all three meals and for snacks."[8] As if Americans need to hear shouted, "MORE IS MORE," the factory food industry aggressively proceeded to scream, "MORE IS MORE," as they blasted soy into the marketplace. The pharmaceutical and supplement industries quickly followed with aggressive marketing campaigns for soy isoflavone supplements. A boisterously enthusiastic press initially spurned both efforts on.

In this whole-hearted, blanket acceptance of the health benefits of soy, vegetarians, vegans, menopausal women, eaters of low-carb factory food products, mothers of infants, and those at risk for heart disease fell into step with the multibillion dollar-a-year soy industry.

But why was soy touted as having health benefits?

CHAPTER 9

Isoflavone Supplementation

THE WORDS PHYTOESTROGEN and isoflavone have entered our lexicon. Phytoestrogens are plant compounds that have estrogen-like effects, and isoflavones are a type of phytoestrogen, which are believed to have both estrogenic and antiestrogenic capabilities. In other words, they are thought to both fit into to the estrogen receptor sites *and* block estrogen receptors. Phytoestrogens can either inhibit or stimulate the growth of certain cells.

Before the early ninth century the doctor and pharmacist were one and the same. The herbalist both prescribed and prepared medical compounds. But in the late eighteenth century, pharmacology developed with advances that enabled pharmacologists to isolate active ingredients thought to have the primary healing property for a given condition. Isolating the specific active ingredient responsible for a therapeutic effect has since been the focus of Western medicine. This mentality of isolating active ingredients from their whole plant form drives the soy isoflavone supplement industry, which isolates isoflavones from the whole soybean and then markets them in supplement form as a panacea for preventing heart disease, cancer, bone loss, and the symptoms of menopause.

It's worth noting that isoflavones are a factor in the bitter taste of soybeans and products such as soy milk taste much better with isoflavones removed. With this financial incentive to go to the trouble of removing the isoflavones, more companies have tried to sell the isolated isoflavones as supplements.

According to Dr. Daniel, isoflavones are "hormonally active substances," or "estrogen mimickers," that are endocrine disrupters that can cause thyroid damage, reproductive system disorders, and other problems. In men these endocrine disrupters lower testosterone levels, sperm count, and sex drive, "estrogenize" baby boys (resulting in tiny penises and breast development); cause premature puberty in boys and girls; and, in women, disrupt menstrual cycles and cause infertility and vulvodynia (swelling and pain in the external genitalia). Boys born to soy-eating mothers can have a birth defect called hypospadias (the opening of their urethra is in the wrong place).[1]

I would think that hearing this would be enough to stop anyone in their tracks. However, we're not hearing these messages about soy isoflavones.

In the past, women going through menopause bit the bullet and hoped for the best outcome in their postmenopausal years. This ultimately depended on their genetic predispositions, lifelong diet, and lifestyle habits. Today, women have four choices: One, bite the bullet and let menopause take its course. Two, use drugs like Prempro that pretend to be hormone replacement therapy (HRT). Three, use bioidentical HRT to actually replace the sex hormones that are no longer being supplied by the ovaries. Or four, bite the bullet and use various alternative medicine modalities, including soy isoflavone supplementation, in an attempt to alleviate the symptoms of sex hormone decline and cessation.

Millions of boomer women decided not to follow in their mothers' footsteps of zero sex, "pattern" balding, hot flashes, facial hair, weight gain, emotional roller coasters, and insomnia, and have opted not to bite the menopause bullet. First they tried the very lucrative estrogen drug concoction that was illegitimately billed as HRT. (These drugs are made from the urine of pregnant mares mixed with drugs and therefore cannot be "replaced" in a woman's body that never made horse pee and drugs in the first place. In fact, the horse-urine drug was never FDA approved as "HRT," but rather was approved to alleviate hot flashes and to reduce bone loss.) But in July 2002, the results from the Women's Health Institutive—an eight-year study—was halted early when results concluded that Prempro, made by Wyeth, didn't prevent heart disease or breast cancer; rather, it increased the risk for breast cancer, heart attack, stroke and blood clots—and also it did not prevent Alzheimer's or memory loss. So millions of women decided against the pretend-HRT drug.

Since the definition of hormone replacement is to replace the hormones lost when a woman's own sex hormone production declines and ultimately ceases, some of these women switched to bioidentical HRT. Bioidentical hormones have the same molecular structure as the hormones made by the human body and can therefore legitimately be referred to as bioidentical hormone replacement. (Pharmaceutical companies do not study bioidentical HRT, as natural substances can't be patented and therefore do not produce the same extravagant returns on their research investment that drug companies have enjoyed with the sales of drugs.)

Many women feel that using bioidentical HRT is still "unnatural" and choose to go through menopause with the help of various alternative medicine approaches, including soy isoflavone supplements. Soy is the most concentrated dietary source of the phytoestrogen isoflavones genistein and daidzein. These phytoestrogens were touted as the natural way to replenish declining estrogen levels and said to relieve menopausal symptoms such as hot flashes, as well as to decrease the risk of heart disease and osteoporosis. Although isoflavone supplementation is a booming business, studies have shown that soy isoflavone supplementation does not consistently alleviate hot flashes or other menopausal symptoms. And as Dr. Daniel said, when women use soy isoflavone supplementation during menopause they risk damaging their thyroid glands, which are already vulnerable in midlife women.[2]

I e-mailed Dr. Northrup again, "There appears to be many studies that dispute the claims that soy relieves menopausal symptoms and that, in fact, this claim is not authorized by the FDA." She replied, "My position that [soy] relieves menopausal symptoms is based on my clinical experience with hundreds of women. The studies vary widely on what type of soy was used, how much was used, over what period of time, etc. I generally recommend soy powders made from whole soybeans that contain over 100 milligrams of soy isoflavones per day. Any dose that's lower than that doesn't give much benefit. But at doses of 100 to 180 milligrams per day, you see a decrease in hot flashes, an increase in vaginal moisture, and also a nice effect on skin."

Again, Dr. Daniel disagreed, "As a clinical nutritionist, I have seen many premenopausal and menopausal women who trace hypothyroidism, weight gain, depression, fatigue, poor skin, and hair loss to 'health food' regimens including 'natural hormone replacement' programs based on soy. Dr. Northrup's newsletter promotes the consumption of immoderate amounts of soy every day and throughout the day—Revival soy shakes, Revival soy snacks, tofu for dinner, soymilk for drinks. I hear more health complaints associated with Revival than any other soy product."[3]

But what about taking soy isoflavone supplements to ward off cancer and heart disease? Some studies on the cancer preventative properties of soy suggest that soy isoflavones might ward off some cancers, but other studies indicate that soy isoflavones may actually increase the risk of cancer, especially breast cancer.

In fact, there is a growing uneasiness within the scientific community that soy isoflavone supplements and products have been unleashed on Americans (in a one-year period ending in October 1999, sales of isoflavone pills jumped by 246 percent) without iron-clad proof of the health benefits and, more important, the potential health risks of consuming *arbitrary amounts of isoflavones.* Dr. Margo Woods, an associate professor of medicine at Tufts University School of Medicine, who specializes in nutrition and breast cancer, said,

"As a food, soy does a lot of great things, but once you start looking at different components like phytoestrogens, you are talking about pharmacological things. It's wiser to talk about soy and soy foods. A whole food behaves very differently in the body than when you take one compound. We are looking into the components, but we haven't been studying in the area long enough. I would not recommend to anyone that they take isoflavones."[4]

Nevertheless, Earl Mindell, RPh, PhD, the author of numerous books on vitamins, minerals, and other aspects of nutrition, including *Earl Mindell's Soy Miracle* (1998), told me, "I take [isoflavone supplements] every day, because I can't eat soy every day, so I think that anywhere from about 60 to 100 milligrams of isoflavones would be great for the average person to take in on a daily basis."[5] Soy advocate Clare M. Hasler, PhD, MBA, said, "I don't think isoflavone supplements are dangerous at a reasonable level but if you consume 1,000 milligrams a day it might be a problem .... I think there's the potential [for risk] if you took [soy isoflavone supplements] at very, very high levels in certain scenarios, but in other cases they could be fine if taken at a modest level."[6]

Mike Fitzpatrick, PhD, is an environmental scientist whose research on phytoestrogens led him to the conclusion that soy isoflavones disrupt the endocrine system. Fitzpatrick found that high daily doses increase the risk for hypothyroidism. "There is potential for certain individuals to consume levels of isoflavones in the range that could have goitrogenic [thyroid inhibiting] effects," Fitzpatrick writes. "Most at risk appear to be infants fed soy formulas, followed by high soy users and those using isoflavone supplements."[7]

Hypothyroidism currently affects up to 40 percent of our population—though many go undiagnosed—and the incidence of hypothyroidism is increasing. The thyroid is a small, butterfly-shaped endocrine gland located just below your Adam's apple. Every cell, tissue, and organ of your body is affected by the actions of your thyroid gland. Symptoms of low-functioning thyroid are anemia and bruising easily; weight gain and inability to lose weight;

constipation; depression or extreme agitation/anxiety, feeling cool to the touch, having dry skin and no sex drive, dull facial expression and droopy eyelids; emotional instability; fatigue; feeling cold; low body temperature (under 98.6 degrees Fahrenheit), having a hoarse, husky voice; slow reflexes; impaired memory; brain fog; infertility; migraines; tinnitus; vertigo; muscle cramps; muscle weakness; puffiness in the face and hands; thinning, coarse, dry hair; and a yellow cast to skin.

Hypothyroidism is a life-altering condition that is very difficult to reverse. If you develop hypothyroidism, you will likely spend your life in an uphill battle with your weight, and you will suffer the symptoms listed above which can contribute to Type 2 diabetes and heart disease.

Eating soy is not the only cause of our rise in hypothyroidism. Fluoride, mercury, and other xenohormones (environmental estrogen mimickers) have also been implicated. Still, as Fitzpatrick said, we are "most at risk" when consuming soy formula and a lot of soy products or soy isoflavone supplements.

Isolated active ingredients have their place in health care, and we have all benefited from the wonders of drug and supplement therapy. But oftentimes it's better to obtain the synergistic properties contained in the whole plant, as the whole food can contain dozens of active ingredients that all have chemical or physiological effects on the human body. Take the simple saying, "An apple a day keeps the doctor away." The truth in this saying lies in the fact that the many active ingredients within the apple interact within the body. We don't completely understand the synergy that occurs with these active ingredients. We do know that if we isolate all of the active ingredients from an apple and ingest them individually, we will never get the same health benefits as eating the real apple. It's one of the marvels of nature.

We eat soy, in part, because we are told that Asians have less disease because they eat a lot of soy. But how much soy do Asians really eat?

CHAPTER 10

So Asians Do Eat Soy

IN ANCIENT TIMES, farmers cultivated soybeans to instill nitrogen into the soil so that other crops would thrive. When they did begin to eat small amounts of soy, they subjected it to a long fermentation process to make foods such as miso and shoyu (soy sauce). Historically, Asians understood that it was imperative to soak and naturally ferment soy to rid it, at least in part, of naturally occurring anti-nutrients (compounds that decrease the nutritional value of the plant) and toxins (which serve to protect plants from annihilation by insect and animal predators). The fermenting process, aided by healthy microorganisms, deactivated or eliminated most anti-nutrients and toxins, improved the soybean's nutritional profile, made the resulting food item more digestible, and imparted disease-fighting microorganisms to the intestinal track.

Naturally occurring anti-nutrients and toxins include allergens, which can cause a range of reactions from sneezing to death; lectins, which can affect the functioning of your immune system; oligosaccharides, which cause painful gas; oxalates, which block calcium absorption and contribute to kidney stones, and, in women, the aforementioned condition called vulvodynia; phytates, which impair absorption of minerals; isoflavones (see previous chapter); protease inhibitors which interfere with digestion and stress the pancreas; saponins, which may lower cholesterol, but also may damage your intestinal lining; and goitrogens, which damage the thyroid gland and can lead to hypothyroidism and cancer.

Since my experience in Japan was contrary to the claims of the soy industry, I felt it was important to understand where the claims that Asians ate a lot of soy were coming from. According to Dr. Willcox, "Our studies of the Okinawan population, who are among the world's healthiest and longest-lived people, show that adults consume between 60 to 120 grams per day of soy (ten to one hundred times what Americans consume)."[1]

Dr. Daniel, however, said that there is inconsistent and contradictory data in *The Okinawa Diet Plan* regarding the consumption of soy products by Okinawans. In addition, she told me, "Although reported levels of soy consumption in China, Indonesia, Korea, Japan, and Taiwan vary from study to study, Asians eat small amounts of soy, as condiments in the diet, not as staple foods."[2]

Suffice it to say, there is much debate about how much soy Asians eat or don't eat, but everyone agrees that Asians are eating whole, mostly naturally fermented soy food condiments as part of a whole foods diet. In agreement was David Zava, PhD, a biochemist with twenty-five years of experience in breast cancer research and the coauthor of *What Your Doctor May Not Tell You About Breast Cancer*, who told me, "I believe [soy] should be consumed in the manner that Asians have consumed it for thousands of years— well complemented with animal protein and a broad variety of vegetables."[3] But what exactly comprised this whole foods diet historically eaten by Asians?

The daughter of missionaries, Pearl Buck (1892–1973) was born in West Virginia but raised in China. With her agricultural economist husband, Buck lived her adult life in Nanhsuchou in the rural Anhwei province. In 1931, Buck won the Pulitzer Prize for her bestselling novel *The Good Earth,* the story of the principled subsistence farmer, Wang Lung, and his selfless former slave bride, O-lan, who through hard labor and determination rose to prominence in prerevolutionary China.

Throughout the story, Wang Lung and O-lan were driven by survival—growing, buying, or scrounging enough food to keep themselves and their family alive. Food was the focal point of the book, yet soybeans are mentioned only once in the context of describing Wang Lung's astonishment over the marketplace when, to escape starvation in a time of famine, his family left their mud hovel and traveled south. "Here in the city there was food everywhere," Buck writes. "The cobbled streets of the fish market were lined with great baskets of big silver fish, caught in the night out of the teeming river; with tubs of small shining fish, dipped out of a net cast over a pool; with heaps of yellow crabs, squirming and nipping in peevish astonishment; with writhing eels for gourmands at the feasts. At the grain markets there were baskets of grain that a man might step into them and sink and smother and none know it who did not see it; white rice and brown and dark yellow wheat and pale gold wheat, and yellow soybeans and red beans and green broad beans, and canary-colored millet and grey sesame. And at the meat markets whole hogs hung by their necks, split open the length of their great bodies to show the red meat and the layers of goodly fat, the skin soft and thick and white. And duck shops hung row upon row, over their ceilings and in their doors, the brown baked ducks that had been turned slowly on a spit before coals and the white salted ducks and the strings of duck giblets, and so with the shops that sold geese and pheasant and every kind of fowl."[4]

In the forty-plus years the story spanned, as Wang Lung rose from dirt-poor farmer to wealthy landowner, he and his family ate all types of foods—moreover, they *coveted* all types of foods. Not once did Wang Lung sip soy milk, munch soy nuts, or break off bits of tofu for his children. Nor did O-lan stir cauldrons of soybeans.

Pearl Buck was able to demonstratively infuse her modern classic with authenticity because she lived most of her eighty-one years in China, conducted extensive research, literally in the trenches, and undoubtedly bounced ideas off her agricultural economist husband who must have known a thing or two about the Chinese diet. It stands to reason that if soybeans were commonplace in the Chinese diet—as modern soybean industrialists would have us believe—Buck's characters would have eaten soy, or desired to eat soy, at least once.

Since space doesn't allow the analysis of every single Asian diet, let's take a quick look at the Japanese diet as another example of the whole foods diet Asians historically consumed. While the Japanese traditionally ate more soy than Westerners, the traditional Japanese diet did not comprise soy, soy, soy, and more soy. The average Japanese consumes a diet of over one hundred biologically different foods per week. (In Western countries the recommended minimum is only thirty.)

The traditional Japanese diet includes meguro (raw tuna), shiokara (pickled squid guts), kusaya (dried fish), eggs, pork, beef and chicken; white rice, linseeds and wholegrain bread, sesame seeds, soba (buckwheat noodles), seitan (seasoned wheat gluten) and udon (wheat noodles); bamboo shoots, eggplant, sweet potato, Chinese cabbage, seaweed, sea vegetables, shitake and matsutake mushrooms, ginger, broccoli, garlic, onions, lotus root, yam, taro, ginger, chicory, truffles, welsh onion, shallots, corn, sansai (garlic, bamboo grass shoots and fiddlehead fern), green leafy vegetables, carrots, burdock root, diakon radish, cucumber; nankusu (rice porridge); tofu, bean paste, bean curd, nato (fermented soy cheese), okara (pulp from soy milk), tempeh, edamame (steamed soy pods); azuki beans; toasted sesame oil, coconut oil, rice-bran oil, butter, talo, lard; wasabi, miso, curry, lemon, kuzu root, pickled ginger, sesame seed, mustard, rice based sake wine, dashi-stock and seasoning made from kelp and mackerel, shoyu, pickled plums, tea twig, brown rice vinegar and tamari; sake, soy coffee, and ocha (green tea); and all types of fruits.[5]

This whole foods diet, which as you can see includes some soy, provides combined chemical or physiological effects on the human body. But Americans are most certainly not eating the whole foods that Asians traditionally ate. We are eating highly industrialized soy substances. Dr. Daniel writes, "The old-fashioned traditional products bear little or no resemblance to the modern soy protein products promoted by the soy industry and sold in grocery stores."[6]

CHAPTER 11

The Weird Science of Modern Soy

IN THE YEAR 2022, 40 million people inhabit New York City. Unemployment is at 50 percent, and homelessness is the norm. The temperature is stifling, and the air almost too filthy to breathe. Government rationing of a food substance made by the Soylent Corporation invariably instigates rioting by the starving masses, requiring the dispatch of riot police. When Detective Thorn is called in at the death of a Soylent Corporation executive, his investigation leads him to the realization that Soylent green is not plankton and soy, but rather, "Soylent Green is people . . . . We're eating people!"

While soy products do not contain human flesh, my investigation has revealed that, aside from the naturally occurring anti-nutrients and toxins outlined in the previous chapter, like all foods subjected to industrialization, soy is adulterated with substances that are bad for humans.

And most soy is genetically modified.

Remember the print ad for the adorable, little Chinese girl with the perfectly white teeth and shining eyes—the ad that would have us believe that genetically modified rice was going to turn all Chinese children into glowingly healthy angels who incidentally weren't blind? If you recall, they didn't use some rotten-toothed, emaciated, wall-eyed kid who is really a Chinese peasant. You can just imagine the casting call it took to find that girl. Advertising such as this serves only one purpose, and that is to soften the hearts and minds of Americans so big corporations can foist genetically modified foods on us.

In *Seeds of Deception: Exposing Industry and Government Lies About the Safety of the Genetically Engineered Foods You're Eating*, Jeffrey M. Smith writes, "On May 23, 2003, President Bush proposed an Initiative to End Hunger in Africa using genetically modified (GM) foods. He also blamed Europe's 'unfounded, unscientific fears' of these foods for hindering efforts to end hunger. Bush was convinced that GM foods held the key to greater yields, expanded U.S. exports, and a better world ....The message was part of a master plan that had been crafted by corporations determined to control the world's food supply. This was made clear at a biotech industry conference in January 1999, where a representative from Arthur Anderson Consulting Group explained how his company had helped Monsanto create that plan. First, they asked Monsanto what their ideal future looked like in fifteen to twenty years. Monsanto executives described a world with 100 percent of all commercial seeds genetically modified and patented. Anderson Consulting then worked backward from that goal, and developed the strategy and tactics to achieve it. They presented Monsanto with the steps and procedures needed to obtain a place of industry dominance in a world in which natural seeds were virtually extinct."[1]

They didn't count on Europeans who viewed GM foods as anathema. And besides, the United States was not going to control the world's food supply if the Europeans had anything to do with it. Meanwhile, as Europeans continue to fight genetic engineering of their food supply, U.S. companies have succeeded in getting government approval for forty varieties of genetically engineered crops and putting these genetically modified mutations into 60 percent of the factory foods Americans eat.

DNA is the unique blueprint of an organism. An organism relies on the information within its DNA to conduct every biochemical process necessary for its survival. Genes are the elements of the DNA that contain specific features or functions of the organism. For example, the genes within your DNA will dictate if you have blue eyes or brown, or if you will be stocky or lanky. In crops, DNA dictates whether a fruit or vegetable is wind resistant or loves hot sun, among other qualities.

Genetic engineering, which is also known as recombinant DNA technology, is a two-step process. Molecular biologists use enzymes to dissect specific genes from the structure of DNA in living organisms. They then insert vectors (such as viruses and bacteria) into these genes to create desired characteristics, and insert these altered genes into the DNA of the organism they wish to alter. They are essentially creating new genetic DNA, which will dictate if a crop will be frost-, bug-, or drought-resistant and so on. This new crop is now "genetically modified."

Genetic engineering has created corn that resists insect infestation, Monsanto Roundup Ready wheat and soybeans, and fruits and vegetables that are devoid of nutritional value but don't rot. It has instilled "anti-freeze" genes into vegetables to extend the growing season, and created genetic pesticides within the DNA of crops, which essentially kill or ward off predators.

Humans, animals, birds, fish, insects, organisms, microorganisms, and so on have always lived and died in a seemingly random, but actually highly organized, pattern of coexistence. No one knows what altering the natural DNA of organisms will do to the natural food chain, our future health, or the environment. Genetic engineering occurs purely for the profit of big business. Small farmers do not need genetic engineering, and, in fact, small farming thrives by using time-tested, old-fashioned methods of agriculture and animal husbandry.

Genetic engineering may be creating new and more dangerous toxins in our food supply, including allergens, and it may be contributing to human resistance to antibiotics. GM foods are foreign to human physiology and have never previously existed on the face of this earth. No long-term tests have been conducted on GM foods, and the tests they have undergone are reminiscent of the flimflam review process the FDA uses to grant "Generally Recognized as Safe" (GRAS) status to food additives. Moreover, GM foods are not labeled, so you have no idea if you are eating genetically engineered organisms.[2]

Although we don't yet understand the repercussions of eating GM food, we do have some understanding of the dangers of unleashing these organisms into our environment. Genetically altered organisms and seeds are not stagnantly and obediently sitting where scientists assign them. They are carried by insects, birds, and wind into neighboring fields and beyond, and the pollen from genetically modified crops cross-pollinates with natural crops. In the Introduction to the bestselling novel *Prey*, which tells the story of escaped, mass-replicating clouds of nanoparticles hell-bent on destroying humans, Michael Crichton writes, "Sometime in the twenty-first century, our self-deluded recklessness will collide with our growing technological power. One area where this will occur is in the meeting point of nanotechnology, biotechnology, and computer technology. What all three have in common is the ability to release self-replicating entities into the environment.

"We have lived for some years with the first of these self-replicating entities, computer viruses. And we are beginning to have some practical experience with the problems of biotechnology. The recent report that modified maize genes now appear in native maize in Mexico—despite laws against it, and efforts to prevent it—is just the start of what we may expect to be a long and difficult journey to control our technology. At the same time, long-standing beliefs about the fundamental safety of biotechnology—views promoted by the great majority of biologists since the 1970s—now appear less secure. The unintended creation of a devastatingly lethal virus by Australian researchers in 2001 has caused many to rethink old assumptions. Clearly we will not be as casual about this technology in the future as we have been in the past."[3]

One can only hope that's true. In the meantime, we continue to eat GM foods. Eighty percent of all soy substances originate as GM soybeans that are resistant to Monsanto's weed killer Roundup. When you eat a "Roundup Ready" soy product, you are eating both the genetic organism that made it resistant to Roundup and you are eating the Roundup. So when you put a soy substance into your mouth or into the mouths of your children, the most important question to ponder is, do you really want to eat something that is made by Monsanto?

Much of the U.S. soybean crop today is processed into oil which accounts for 80 percent or more of the edible fats and oils consumed in this country in the form of shortening, margarine, cooking oil, and salad dressings. When you see the term "vegetable oil," assume it is close to, or all, soy oil. Oil manufacturers use the chemical and heat processes described on page 119, which create oxidizing free radicals that are then deposited into your coronary arteries as plaque. When you see the word "partially hydrogenated," bet on the fact that you are eating soy oil, which has been rendered into dangerous trans fats (described on page 120). Prior to recent mandatory trans fat labeling, all fried foods in this country were fried in partially hydrogenated soybean oil.

Lecithin, extracted from soybean oil, is a natural emulsifier and lubricant used in many foods. As an emulsifier, it can make fats and water compatible with each other as in say, keeping chocolate and cocoa butter in a candy bar from separating. Because we have been told for decades that lecithin prevents a number of diseases, including brain aging, consumers are gobbling up soy lecithin, thinking its a miracle food. But again, we have the problem of the damaging processing of lecithin out of soybeans. Dr. Daniel writes, "Soybean lecithin comes from sludge left over after crude soy oil goes through a 'degumming' process. It is a waste product containing solvents and pesticide residue and has a consistency ranging from gummy fluid to plastic solid."[4] In other words, the oil industry did not know what to do with the massive amounts of sludge left over after refining soybean oil, so they came up with an industrialized process that could turn it into so-called "healthy" soy lecithin and put it into every conceivable factory food product.

The chemical processing used to refine soy protein isolate—a very popular additive used to bulk up protein in products—infuses the soy protein with known carcinogens, such as nitrites and nitrosamines among other toxins. High temperature processing denatures some of the protein, rendering it largely ineffective as a metabolic building material. Although soy naturally contains aluminum (toxic to the nervous system and kidneys) processing imparts even more. Soy also naturally contains fluoride and processing impregnates soy with extra doses of it, which may be playing a role in the epidemic of childhood neurological disorders and adult osteoporosis.[5] Soy protein isolate also contains minute residues of up to thirty-eight petroleum compounds,[6] and is also often "enhanced" with MSG.

Clinical nutritionists are beginning to side against soy. Carol Simontacchi, MS, CNN, author of ten books including *Weight Success for a Lifetime,* told me that although she has recommended eating soy in previous books she is now backing away from recommending soy. "My first indication that something was wrong came several years ago when I was putting lots of people on soy and they called to complain they were gaining weight. I too gained about five pounds doing nothing other than drinking a soy-based breakfast drink each morning."[7]

Robin Marzi, RD, MA, a clinical nutritionist in private practice in Santa Barbara, who has taught me a lot about nutrition over the years, said, "The main problem with soy is what we are doing to it. We're not eating edamame, we're eating something so processed it's so far away from what it ever was. Who knows what this new type of soy does in the body? Processed soy isoflavone could be blocking estrogen receptors or over-saturating them. We don't know. I'm telling patients to stop eating refined soy altogether because of problems with allergies, weight gain, thyroid, cancer and because ultimately we don't know what soy does to hormone balance and my practice centers on balancing people's hormones."

In agreement was my good friend, Maoshing Ni, PhD, LAc, DOM, called Dr. Mao, who traces his lineage in the Chinese medical healing arts back to the thirteenth century. He is among the top doctors of Chinese medicine in the country and is the author of numerous books on the subject, including *Secrets of Longevity*. "As most things go in America, something wholesome and good comes along with promising benefits, a whole industry jumps on and industrializes it," he said. "Soy protein is not soy. The soy that Asians have eaten for 3,000 years is whole soy that is eaten in balance with other foods. Processed and concentrated soy protein products are not healthy."

Unlike the Japanese who consume one hundred biologically different foods per week, the average American does not even consume the recommended thirty biologically different foods per week. Many health-minded Americans today have virtually switched from real food to fake soy foods. As Robin Marzi said, "I have patients who eat soy egg substitute and soy sausage with a soy latte for breakfast, a tofu burger for lunch and soy tacos with soy cheese for dinner." But let's say a person ate the typical American diet of cereal, hamburgers and fries, and diet drinks, along with a soy hot dog or a daily soy isoflavone supplement. This meal plan would also not contain the dozens of active ingredients that instigate the chemical or physiological effects on the human body contained in the traditional Chinese and Japanese diets outlined in the previous chapter.

On his Web site, Dr. Weil recommends one cup of soy foods, such as soy milk, per day. However, unlike all the wholesome ads we see for soy milk, as it turned out in my investigation, soy milk is really a ghastly brew that few people would willingly drink without the added sugar that covers up the natural greasy, beany taste of soybeans. Also added is vitamin D_2, although, as internationally recognized biochemist and nutritionist, Mary Enig, PhD and Sally

Fallon, president of the Weston A. Price Foundation (a nonprofit organization devoted to educating the public about nutrition), point out in their book *Eat Fat, Lose Fat: Three Delicious, Science-Based Coconut Diets*, "Research indicates that synthetic vitamin D_2 has the opposite effect of natural vitamin D, causing softening of the bones and hardening of soft tissues such as the arteries. The dairy industry used to add D_2 to milk but quietly dropped it in favor of the less toxic (but not completely natural) D_3 when they realized how dangerous it was."[8] (Calling all menopausal women who drink soy milk to prevent osteoporosis.)

Some brands of soymilk also contain canola oil, which is a chemical and heat processed monounsaturated fat that contains oxidizing free radicals, which cause coronary artery plaquing. Another additive often used to thicken soy milk is carrageenan, which is suspected to cause ulcerations and malignancies.[9] Soy milk naturally contains high levels of glutamate (an excitotoxin),[10] and can contain hydrolyzed vegetable protein, an additive that always contains MSG. Soy milk must never be given to infants in place of formula as it is so deficient in vital nutrients that near fatal incidences have occurred. "The myth that soy is a health food has led many parents to believe that soy milk is a complete and nourishing food not only for adults but for babies and children," writes Daniel in her October 25, 2005 newsletter that discusses the possible link between soy milk and the death of three-month old Brooklyn twins.[11]

Regarding the assertion that only fermented soy is healthy to eat, Dr. Weil writes, "That is simply not true. Some of the best forms of soy—edamame, tofu, and soy nuts—are unfermented and are much more likely to help you than hurt you."[12] (A very strange choice of words.)

According to Dr. Daniel, edamame, which are boiled green vegetable soybeans, are safe to eat—in moderation—since the soybeans are harvested young before developing mature levels of anti-nutrients and toxins. Tofu is made by soaking and slow boiling soybeans then curdling the resulting mash. Outside of monasteries where impotence caused by eating large amounts of soy was desirable, tofu has always been eaten in very small amounts in Japan. It is a distant choice after favored animal proteins like pork and seafood. Tofu has actually been studied here in the United States, and Dr. Daniel writes of a study detailing, "Men and women who eat two or more servings of tofu per week in midlife are more likely to experience cognitive decline, senile dementia, and brain atrophy later in life than those who eat little or none."[13] She also said, "Tofu is a whole food product but contains antinutrients, toxins, and soy phytoestrogens and should be eaten only occasionally."

Weil recommends eating soy nuts, and Mireille Guiliano, author of *French Women Don't Get Fat,* suggests soy nuts as a snack when your flight is delayed or some such event occurs that allows traditionally nonsnacking Frenchwomen to eat between meals. According to Dr. Daniel, soy nuts are notoriously hard to digest and may cause cramps and flatulence, and are among the soy foods that contain the highest level of isoflavones (phytoestrogens).

Because fermenting does not remove the isoflavones, Dr. Daniel recommends that fermented soy foods such as miso, natto, tempeh, and shoyu be eaten only occasionally and in small amounts. Soy sauce is a classic example of the difference between traditional Asian soy and Americanized soy. Supermarket soy sauce is not the shoyu created by the traditional long, healthy fermenting process; rather, it's made by a fast, cheap industrial process, which imparts chemicals, artificial dyes, and MSG. Dr. Daniel told me, "I recommend raw, (unpastuerized) old-fashioned naturally fermented tamari or shoyu such as Ohsawa Namo Shoyu." You can find naturally fermented tamari and shoyu in health food stores or online at www.qualitynaturalfoods.com and www.naturalizing.com.

If you really want to get an idea of the true nature of soy, buy a bag of soy flour, as I did, and try to bake something out of it. Doing so was by far the foulest experience I've had in the kitchen. Soy is not very appetizing, to say the least. And the soy industry has had to work hard to convince us to eat it.

The soy industry told us soy was a prestigious health food, and we bought that message. So instead of eating small handfuls of edamame, tiny pieces of tofu in our miso soup, a few sprinkles of naturally fermented shoyu on our meals of real food, Americans are consuming inordinate amounts of chemical-processed soy—and babies are now being fed soy formula instead of breast milk.

CHAPTER 12

Feeding Babies Soybean Formula

ELEVEN-YEAR-OLD KEVIN was a tall, slim and attractive all-American boy. His mother delighted in his articulate, quick wit. The joy his mother felt was dampened only by self-doubt and remorse over feeding his twin brother, Dennis, soy formula. Dennis had developed into a sluggish, underachieving, overweight, gawky adolescent with large breasts. Brittany had also fed her baby soy formula, and agonized over her seven-year-old son's small stature. The kids at school were merciless about his small penis. Marc and Jennifer finally decided to take matters into their own hands when eleven-month-old Chrisy's pediatrician refused to see anything out of the ordinary about her developing breasts, pubic fuzz, and premenstrual spotting. The young parents were incredulous when they read that soy formula had estrogenizing capabilities.[1]

Although breast milk is real food for babies, today only about 60 percent of American mothers breastfeed their babies, and most stop breastfeeding by the time their babies are two months old. Breastfeeding, however, is a crucial step in your baby's ability to achieve his or her genetic gifts, and it is also the most important preventative measure for breast cancer for both mother and baby. Studies show that a woman's risk of breast cancer decreases by 7 percent for every birth she experiences, another 3 percent for each year under twenty-eight years old she is when that child is born, another 4.3 percent for every twelve months of her life that she breast feeds, and yet another 23 percent for whether or not she was personally breast fed by her mother.[2] (Note that breast cancer is rising today in men.)

Other benefits of breastfeeding range from boosting your infant's immune system to boosting his or her IQ. No matter how much the baby formula companies try to paint a benevolent picture of vibrant health, they just do not have the goods. According to Carol Simontacchi, "When the untrained eye reads the ingredient listing on the back of the baby bottle or the advertisements from the baby food companies, it is difficult to see that there is a problem at all. Formulas seem similar to mother's milk; nutrients are measured in a few milligrams or grams. When we look closely at the fine print and compare the composition of artificial formulas with mother's milk, however, we see that the differences are great and can, in some cases, translate into tangible, permanent physical deficits."[3]

Mother's first milk contains protein and mineral-rich colostrum vital for your baby's immune system. From then on, breast milk delivers good bacteria, immunoglobulins (a type of antibody), digestive enzymes, growth factors, hormones, and nonessential fatty acids—about one hundred elements that are not contained in baby bottle formula—nutrients that are vital for the full development of your baby's fully formed brain.[4] The composition of breast milk changes over time. The ratio of nutrients on day one is very different than eight to twelve months later. Baby bottle formula ratios are stagnant.

Although the pros and cons of breastfeeding versus baby bottle formula extend into every area of brain and body health for your baby, our focus here is soy formula.

Breast milk contains brain-healthy essential fatty acids (EFAs), which are crucial for neurotransmitter production, and brain and nervous system development. Soy formulas either do not contain any EFAs or only trace amounts.[5] Breast milk also contains cholesterol, imperative for a baby's growing brain and nervous system. Soy formula contains no cholesterol. According to Dr. Enig, "Infants who don't get enough cholesterol in their diets during the first years when their brains are developing risk a loss of cognitive function."[6] Breast milk also contains lactose, which is used for, among other things, brain development. "In reality, very few infants are lactose intolerant," Dr. Daniel writes, "although many are allergic to the processed proteins and other ingredients in milk-based formula."[7] In breast milk the balance of lactose and fats creates a healthy, happy baby with balanced brain neurotransmitters.

Soy formula, which incidentally is not "milk" but rather heat and chemical processed juice from a legume, possesses a number of problems: Soy formula is not as digestible as breast milk and may cause loose stools and gas. Soy estrogens from soy formula have been linked to rising rates of ADD/ADHD and learning disabilities. Soy formula contains high amounts of manganese, which can cause brain damage resulting in learning disorders, ADD/ADHD, and even violent behavior.[8] It may also contribute to the development of cancer[9] and thyroid damage.[10] As soy formula delivers to your baby the equivalent amount of estrogen of three to five birth control pills each day, soy formula may contribute to precocious puberty in girls and delayed puberty or feminization in boys; and soy formula may contribute to the development of Type 1 diabetes.[11]

A January 2006 study demonstrated that the isoflavone genistein can disrupt the development of the ovaries of newborn female mice, causing reproductive problems and infertility. "This is a wakeup call for parents and pediatricians," said Dr. Daniel."[12]

Soy formula contains a natural protein called phytic acid that blocks the absorption of calcium, magnesium, iron, copper, and zinc. These minerals are important for brain health. Depletion of magnesium and calcium is associated with neurological malfunctions such as depression, anger, and learning disabilities to name a few problems.

Soy advocate Dr. Hasler disagrees that soy formula is dangerous for babies. "There's no problem with soy formula," she told me. "Soy infant formula has been approved. It's recommended. It's been fed to millions of infants."[13]

While American parents may find it confidence inspiring to hear assurances from the soy industry that Asian babies have been raised on soy milk for centuries, as it turned out, this claim turned out to be false. Soy milk is a very recent aberration in Asia that was first promoted by well-meaning Seventh Day Adventists missionaries and subsequently by American soy industries attempting to infiltrate new markets. If you think questioning the potential health hazards of soy formula as is nothing more than Internet paranoia, you have to ask yourself, are any scientists ringing alarm bells about the health risks of breast milk? If not, then you have to ask yourself, is breast milk the very best food for my baby?

Mothers who can't breastfeed can find recipes for healthy infant formula in Sally Fallon's cookbook, *Nourishing Traditions.*

Vegetarian or vegan women often rely on soy foods as an alternative to animal proteins during pregnancy and breastfeeding, and so finding out that soy is not a good alternative might be deflating. The logical next option would be rice and beans, which is a complete protein. A complete protein is one that contains adequate amounts of all of nine amino acids—that are essential for life—as well as the additional eight amino acids that are considered conditionally essential. Although rice and beans together do make a complete protein, one cup of brown rice contains 5 grams of protein but also contains 46 grams of carbohydrate, and one cup of kidney beans contains 15 grams of protein but also contains 40 grams of carbohydrate. So eating two cups of the rice and bean combo provides a mere 20 grams of protein but packs 86 grams of carbohydrate. Unless you are an extreme athlete like some of the vegan Ashtanga yogis I know, or engage in comparable vigorous activity every day, 86 grams of carbohydrate is too much sugar entering the system at one meal. Equally important, rice and beans do not contain cholesterol or essential fatty acids.

Women who eat a vegetarian or vegan diet may want to consider making concessions during pregnancy and breastfeeding for the sake of their baby's optimal health. Drinking vitamin-, mineral-, enzyme-, and protein-rich natural milk and eating organically produced eggs for cholesterol, cod liver oil for essential fatty acids, and small fish such as herring, sardines, and anchovies for amino acids will guarantee that your baby's brain is getting the nutrients it needs for proper formation and development. (Small fish feed on even smaller fish and so have not consumed as much mercury as, say, tuna or salmon.)

Despite all we have covered in these chapters on the topic of soy, there are those who do not want to discuss the possibility that soy might not be healthy for adults or babies. Why not a reasoned discussion?

CHAPTER 13

No Reasoned Discussion About Soy

WE ARE EATING SOY today because studies were submitted to the FDA and the conclusions of those studies were accepted at face value. Once FDA approval is granted, that approval then becomes the pivotal arguing point. In fact, many soy advocates I contacted and nearly every pro-soy source I investigated used FDA claims to back up their pro-soy stance. Dr. Hasler said, "Soy's safe— it's been approved by the FDA, it's got a health claim on it, as part of a total dietary approach to managing cholesterol. I think it's a good thing." When I asked, "Are you saying because the FDA says it's okay, that it's okay?" Dr. Hasler replied, "I can already tell by the way you're couching this that you have some issues with the Food and Drug Administration."

Many issues indeed. Just because the FDA—an agency that bends so easily to pressures from big business—says something is okay does it mean it really is. There are many FDA scientists who do not believe that soy is healthy and who were against the FDA allowing factory food producers to use soy-healthy claims on their packaging. In fact, in January 2006 the American Heart Association, after concluding a review of a decade studies, announced that there was no evidence that soy affords us any of the purported miraculous health benefits, essentially debunking the FDA-approved cholesterol lowering claim.

Besides the fact that we must worry about the dangerously inept and corrupt "protection" we are getting from "The Nation's Foremost Consumer Protection Agency," we also must contend with health experts' animosity regarding soy. Throughout the course of my investigation of soy, I wondered—if both pro- and anti-soy camps are truly interested in the health and welfare of Americans— why can't there be a civilized dialogue about soy?

If you had a prized rose garden and you heard about a new rose food that would ward off aphids and other rose blights but you attempted to talk to the rose food advocates about some negative reviews you heard and they were frosty, hostile, dismissive, even ridiculing, wouldn't you question why these rose food advocates could not have a civil, reasoned discussion about rose food? Would you rush home and lather your prize roses with this new plant food?

It's up to you to decide whether questioning of the embracement of highly refined soy into America's food supply is rash or prudent. You must decide whether you want to eat old-fashioned whole soy foods, modern industrially processed soy products, take soy isoflavone supplements, or feed soy formula to your baby. You must decide if experts for and against soy are motivated by your best interests or by personal gain. (Bear in mind, it was empirical evidence—the health problems of her soy-eating patients—that led Dr. Daniel, who has been falsely accused of being "paid off" by the beef and dairy industry, to spend four years researching the effects of soy on human physiology, to mortgage her home and incur $90,000 of personal debt to get the facts about soy out to the American public.)

The fact that soy, soy, soy has permeated our factory food chain should be enough to give anyone pause. We are no longer talking about thousands of factory food products that scream SOY! on their labels. We're talking about virtually every factory food on the market today. Today it's nearly impossible to find a loaf of supermarket bread, a can of tuna, or any other supermarket product that doesn't contain a refined soy ingredient. Even products I previously thought were sacrosanct, like See's Candy and Ben & Jerry's and Häagen-Dazs ice creams, contain soy. Is it just me, or is the wholesale takeover of livestock feed, the infant formula market, and the factory food supply not just a little body-snatcherish?

Over the past fifty years, Americans have been force-fed factory foods made out of bizarrely refined junk, and now the medical establishment mentality of isolating active ingredients from their whole plant form has resulted in our factory food supply becoming permeated with bizarrely refined additives. But just because we're able to isolate an allegedly healthy property from a food doesn't mean that we should eat it in every single food we consume.

In the first chapter on soy, I said that I get suspicious when big businesses, the media, and doctors start aggressively telling us that any product or substance is "healthy." I devoted a lot of space to soy because it's important for us to understand how virtually any substance can be slipped under our noses under the banner of "healthy" while we are busy living our lives. Industrially processed soy is not the first unhealthy substance to be foisted on Americans, and with billions invested in food technology, it definitely will not be the last. Consider that there are three types of phytoestrogens: isoflavones found in soy, coumestans found in clover and alfalfa sprouts, and lignans mainly found in flaxseeds. Flax is another substance we need to watch, as, like soy isoflavone phytoestrogens, flaxseed lignan phytoestrogens can dampen thyroid function, and, in addition, flax is highly prone to rancidity (caused by oxygen, light, and heat), which creates free radicals. Putting flax in products that are cooked or otherwise heated, and that sit on the shelf—like bread, let's say, would be a very bad thing. But if corporations get it into their heads that Americans want flax—or any thing else— they will begin to hammer us with every imaginable form of food product. If we do not protest with our wallets, we are likely to soon see flaxseed-enhanced infant formula, flax milk, flax cheese, flax margarine, flax shortening, flax salad dressing, flax power bars, flax cereal, flax baked goods, flax dog and cat kibble. Every single fast food restaurant in the nation may someday, God forbid, deep fat fry french fries in flaxseed oil.

Why are Americans so gullible about what we put in our mouths? This question takes us back to the inception of the food industry so that we can begin to understand the logical progression of the development of the factory food, diet and drug industries, and how Americans fell under their spell. It began early in the twentieth century when doctors, researchers, and our government recognized that we had an epidemic rise in heart disease. Unfortunately, the efforts to arrest this epidemic through dietary measures only made matters worse by foisting on us the biggest crock of the century: the belief that saturated fat causes heart disease. We'll consider the ramifications of this erroneous belief next.

V

The Fat Fiasco

chapter 14

Fat Kills!

THE LARD CRISIS HIT Britain hard in the Christmas season of 2004. The supply of pork fat, traditionally used to bake the flakiest of holiday piecrusts, had run low due to a snafu with European Union production regulations. Prices for lard climbed 20 percent and eBay bids were up to $18 per container. British Lard Marketing Board founder, Tim Allen, was quoted in *Newsweek,* "If you launched [lard] as a product now, no one would touch it because it's not healthy."[1] Such is the enduring sentiment of most of the developed world: fat kills.

This belief began fifty years ago with the wholesale embracement of the so-called "lipid hypothesis" by the medical community: the belief that elevated blood cholesterol levels were a risk factor for heart disease, and that blood cholesterol levels were elevated by eating cholesterol-laden foods and saturated fat. The lipid hypothesis vilified historically consumed saturated fats, promoted the consumption of processed polyunsaturated vegetable oils, and instigated the low-fat diet. These three factors worked in concert to prime the marketplace to be receptive to the introduction of thousands of factory products into our food supply, which dramatically increased the incidence of disease and obesity in our country.

Meanwhile, the French never stopped gorging on butter,

cheese, and cream, which led researchers to coin the term the "French paradox." To researchers, it's a mystery why the French can consume so much dietary fat and be so thin and have lower heart disease rates. The only solution they could come up with is that it must be all the red wine that the French drink.

But today not all Americans shudder at the thought of lard (pork fat, which is made up of 50 percent monounsaturated fat, 40 percent saturated fat and 10 percent polyunsaturated fat). A growing contingency of renegade researchers, clinical nutritionists, MDs, and naturopathic physicians, would return Americans to the same diet—rich in organic saturated fats and cholesterol laden foods—that we ate prior to the year 1900, when heart disease was virtually nonexistent in the United States. Many of these rebels are followers of the obscure research of a little known dentist named Weston A. Price.

Born in Ontario, Canada, in 1870, Price earned a degree in dentistry and immigrated to the United States in 1893, settling in Cleveland, Ohio. In his practice, he was continually taken aback at the crowded, crooked, rotten teeth of the children of the relatively well-to-do. Concluding that nutrition was most likely the problem, Price and his intrepidly sturdy wife, Florence, set out in 1931 on "difficult expedition" to study the effects of nutrition on human health and disease by examining the indigenous diets of fourteen "savage" groups of people: Swiss alpine villagers, Gaelics in Scotland, Eskimos of Alaska, North American Indians, Peruvian Indians, the Melanesians and Polynesians in the South Pacific, African tribes, Australian aborigines and Malay tribe and the Maori of New Zealand. Whenever possible, Price also studied "members of the primitive tribes who have been in contact with modernized white races."[2] The results of his ten-year study were published in his meticulously documented tome (with photographs, thank goodness) entitled *Nutrition and Physical Degeneration* (1939).

The long and the short of it was that the primitive people who ate historically indigenous diets almost always had all thirty-two perfectly aligned teeth and cavities were a rarity. The photographs of these native people show smiles out of *People* magazine. These people were attractive, cheerful, robust, fertile, and free from mental, dental, and degenerative diseases. The photographs of native people who ventured out to live on "white man's food"—sugar, flour, pasteurized milk, hydrogenated vegetable oils, and other factory foods—were more reminiscent of the backwoods folks in the 1972 movie *Deliverance*. Without exception, primitive people who became "civilized" in their eating habits developed infertility problems and suffered with gnarly, rotten teeth and rank gums, as well as infectious, mental, and degenerative diseases and obesity.

The diets that promoted robust health consisted of primarily foods that are forbidden by our modern medical establishment: fat, fat, and more fat from the organ meat of wild or grass-fed domesticated animals, insects (including such savory treats as fly and ant eggs), birds, sea mammals, guinea pigs, bears and hogs, and the egg yolks from various birds, whole raw milk, cheese, butter, and other dairy products, as well as the more conventionally acceptable fish, shellfish, fish organs, fish liver oils, and fish eggs.

Price shipped twenty thousand food samples back to America for analysis, including deep yellow butter—a product of grass-eating cows—which was a prized food of many of the cultures studied. When Price analyzed the butter, he found it to be exceptionally high in fat-soluble vitamins, particularly vitamins A and D. (Without these fat-soluble vitamins, humans cannot properly utilize minerals or absorb water-soluble vitamins.) From grass-fed dairy products, fatty organ meats, and some seafood, Price also isolated another biochemical catalyst for the absorption and utilization of minerals—which was also an immune system enhancer—a substance that he dubbed with the Flash Gordonish name Activator-X. In addition, his research determined that the "savages" consumed four times the minerals and water-soluble vitamins and about ten times the fat-soluble vitamins that Americans were eating at that time (roughly seventy years ago).

Francis Pottenger, MD, had just finished his residency at LA County Hospital in 1930, the year before Weston and Florence Price set out on their journey. During the years the Prices trekked the globe, Pottenger engaged in parallel research and became known for his 1932 to 1942 research on more than nine hundred cats.

Pottenger compared the effects of two diets on cats. Cats that were fed diets of raw milk and raw meat had shiny, pettable fur, sound bones, and good teeth, and were parasite free, healthy, fertile, and lovable. The cats that were fed cooked meat and pasteurized milk gave birth to weak, puny kittens. These cats were riddled with fleas, ticks, intestinal parasites, skin diseases, and allergies. The females were she-devils, the males meek and cringing. They had terrible bone structure, and, in fact, Pottenger observed the same types of facial and dental degeneration in his cats that Price found his "civilized" native people.[3]

Pottenger maintained, like Price, that where there is smoke there is fire. In other words, terrible bone structure and messed-up teeth indicate poor nutrition, just as sound bone structure and pearly whites indicate healthy nutrition. (This is not to say that, in this book, we are headed toward gnawing on raw meat. But only to point out that both Price's and Pottenger's research demonstrates that nutrient dead foods—i.e., "civilized" diets—produce poor health, while untampered with, real food produces robust health.) However, because of the prior rejection of nutrition as standard of care, neither Price's nor Pottenger's research made lasting impressions on the medical community. On the contrary, events unfolded within the American population that spurred the medical community in the opposite direction so that dairy and meat would be vilified, and factory fats that were made in laboratories would be glorified as health giving.

From 1900 to the end of WWII, the rise in myocardial infarction brought the medical community together in an attempt to figure out the cause. Atherosclerosis is the stiffening of the coronary arteries combined with plaque, which is a coating on the artery walls. In some people with advanced atherosclerosis, arterial plaque becomes so thick and protruding that it blocks off the blood and accompanying oxygen supply to the heart, thus causing radiating discomfort called angina. If blood and oxygen flow to part of the heart is completely blocked, the part of the heart that is affected will die. This condition is known as myocardial infarction or a heart attack.

Today, according to the CDC, 2,600 Americans die of cardiovascular disease every day, an average of one death every thirty-four seconds. Each year 10 million Americans are disabled by cardiovascular diseases, including heart disease, stroke, and disorders of the circulatory system. *Children* now suffer from heart disease, a degenerative condition related to aging.

Prior to 1900, when Americans ate butter, cheese, whole milk, red meat, beef and lamb tallow, chicken fat and lard, heart disease caused only 9 percent of all deaths. The first reported incidence of myocardial infarction did not occur until 1926. By then Americans' diets were changing rapidly with factory foods infiltrating our food chain. But our medical community did not use research like Price's and Pottenger's to determine ways to get Americans eating real foods again. Instead, they fixated on cholesterol as the culprit in the rise of heart disease and discouraged the consumption of historically eaten animal fats.

In 1953, when biochemist Ancel Keys, PhD, argued that heart attacks could be prevented by avoiding cholesterol-laden foods, the scientific community was primed to embrace this message.[4] Scientists had already observed that the incidence of heart disease was low in occupied Europe after WWII at a time when Europeans were eating less cholesterol (meat, dairy, eggs). Ignored was the fact that sugar, flour, alcohol, cigarettes, and gas were scarce after the war and so people were eating less sugar and refined white flour, drinking and smoking less and walking more. Then there was the obvious fact that butter and other animal fats are yellow and viscous, just like the fatty deposits found in the arteries of autopsied heart attack victims. It stood to reason, cut out the cholesterol from animal fat in your diet, and you would not have plaque in your arteries (even though it only contains an insignificant amount of cholesterol along with collagen, calcium, and other materials).

Keys arrived at his lipid hypothesis in his famous "Seven Countries Study," in which he maintained that countries with the highest fat intake had the highest rates of heart disease.[5] Keys was accused of handpicking data from the countries that supported his hypothesis and ignoring those that didn't (data were available from twenty-two countries). And just as he ignored data from the countries that didn't support his hypothesis, Keys ignored the fact that in 1936, pathologist Kurt Landé and biochemist Warren Sperry of the Department of Forensic Medicine at New York University conducted an extensive study that found no correlation between the degree of atherosclerosis and blood cholesterol levels.[6] These findings were repeated by Indian researchers in 1961, Polish researchers in 1962, Guatemalan researchers in 1967, and Americans in 1982.[7]

Lipid biochemist David Kritchevsky, PhD, was a young Russian immigrant in 1954 when he conducted studies that demonstrated that rabbits fed artificial cholesterol had elevated blood cholesterol levels while rabbits fed polyunsaturated vegetable oils had lowered cholesterol levels.[8] Similar studies, also done on animals, were said to prove the lipid hypothesis. But by the late fifties, scientists understood the flaws inherent in studies that force-fed plant-eating rabbits an artificial, species-inappropriate carnivorous diet. Dr. Kritchevsky agreed that artificial cholesterol is an unnatural food for a rabbit and remarked, "Alexander Pope said, 'The proper study of mankind is man.' But I don't think the average guy would submit to a diet and let me tear his aorta out after six months. Animal experiments are just animal experiments." Nevertheless, animal experiments using inappropriate vegetarian test subjects were used to promote the lipid hypothesis.

It didn't take much to frighten people into believing that

saturated fats caused heart disease. America originated with Puritanism after all. Like sex (that feels good), if food tastes good, it must be bad. So millions of Americans stopped eating eggs and butter and pushed away their steaks.

Next came the instruction to eat polyunsaturated vegetable oils to lower your risk for heart disease. This pronouncement was easy to swallow too because polyunsaturated fats *were* found to lower cholesterol levels in animal studies. What was not understood at the time was that polyunsaturated fatty acids lower blood cholesterol because when these fatty acids, which are soft, are deposited into cell membrane, the body must stabilize the membrane by pulling cholesterol, which is denser, out of the bloodstream and putting it into cell structure. But because polyunsaturated fats were found to lower cholesterol levels in animal studies, the edible oil industry began heavily promoting polyunsaturated fats to the American public as "heart healthy."

"The trouble is that science moves rather slowly, but promoters move quickly," Dr. Kritchevsky told me. "If you publish six papers that said horse manure is good for you, two days later it would be on the market." And so it was with polyunsaturated fat research. The edible oil industry hit the ground running with their polyunsaturated fats, and their wallets open to all government and health agencies that could help them promote these fats. Meanwhile science was left plodding slowly behind.

Today the health benefits of small amounts of polyunsaturated fats as found in whole foods or fresh, nonrancid oils are well known. But the edible oil industry did not market *naturally occurring polyunsaturated fats* to Americans in *small amounts.* The oil industry manufactured and marketed factory fats *made* from polyunsaturated vegetable oils and virtually inundated our food supply with these fats.

CHAPTER 15

So What Are Polyunsaturated Fats Anyway?

PRIOR TO 1900, vegetable oil was processed out of its natural state (such as corn oil made from corn) by small, slow, cold temperature batch presses. But in the 1920s, industrialists realized that human-dependent, small batch, cold-pressing was too slow and not profitable enough, so they switched automated heat and chemical processes that produced high volumes of oil at a greater profit.

Unfortunately, these new processes did very bad things to oils. In simple terms, fatty acids are chains of carbon atoms with hydrogen atoms filling the available bonds. A fatty acid is considered "saturated" when all available carbon bonds are occupied by a hydrogen atom. Monounsaturated fatty acids lack two hydrogen atoms and polyunsaturated fatty acids lack still more. The level of hydrogen atom "saturation" determines how "stable" a fatty acid is when exposed to heat, light, and oxygen. Saturated fatty acids are the least likely to oxidize (create free radicals), monounsaturated fatty acids are the second most stable, and polyunsaturated fatty acids are the most fragile under these conditions.

The heat and chemical processing of polyunsaturated oils goes like this: Seeds, kernels, fruits, and nuts are hulled and ground, which exposes their oils to air and light and begins the rancidity process, creating free radical oxidation, which you read about on page 46.

After hulling, the pulp is cooked for up to two hours at high temperatures—creating more free radical oxidation. Subsequent pressing also exposes the oil to heat, causing a chemical reaction that essentially creates the same chemical constituent as plastic, varnish, and shellac. Another method of removing the oil from raw sources uses chemical solvents, which also infuses the oil with free radicals.

After the initial heat and chemical processing of vegetable oils, the oils are then often "de-gummed" using phosphoric acid (used in bathroom cleaners) and high temperatures to remove impurities and nutrients, a process that increases rancidity. To remove free fatty acids and minerals from the oil, sodium hydroxide (i.e., lye, which is also used in Drano and Easy Off oven cleaner) and high temperatures are used. Subsequent bleaching removes undesirable pigments from oils. At this point, the oils may possess pungent odors and tastes that must be removed through a high temperature deodorizing process.

Some of these oils end up in rows upon rows of glistening, sanitary looking cooking oils on your supermarket shelves. But much of this heat and chemical processed oil is then hydrogenated or partially hydrogenated. This alters the molecular structure of the fatty acid by adding hydrogen atoms, changing the chemical structure from a "cis" shape that is recognized and utilized by human cells, to a "trans" shape that is foreign and lethal to human physiology. Hydrogenation turns polyunsaturated vegetable oil into a hardened butterlike product, which holds up better than liquid oils in food production processes and has a longer shelf life.

The industrialized fats that were introduced into our food chain were a far cry from the organic, saturated animal fats eaten by Price's native peoples. But these factory polyunsaturated vegetable fats were touted as healthier than butter and other historically consumed animal fats. And in the minds of Americans, the word "polyunsaturated" became synonymous with protection against heart disease. However, back when scientists first decided the lipid hypothesis was the black-and-white answer to heart disease and began their campaign to eradicate saturated fat and cholesterol-laden foods from the American diet and to replace these fats with polyunsaturated vegetable oils, in their haste, they overlooked one simple and very important fact: By the 1950s people had already, for personal economic reasons, significantly decreased consumption of butter and increased consumption of factory polyunsaturated vegetable fats.[1]

In 1900, the average American consumed eighteen pounds of butter per year, but only three pounds of polyunsaturated vegetable fat in shortening and margarine. By the 1950s, Americans were eating ten pounds of polyunsaturated vegetable fat and only ten pounds of butter per year.[2] With the decreased consumption of butter and the increased consumption of polyunsaturated vegetable fats, *heart disease had increased correspondingly.*

Some scientists questioned whether there might be a connection between the rise in polyunsaturated vegetable oil consumption and the rise in heart disease. But these rumblings were mere squeaks compared with the roar coming out of Madison Avenue—a din paid for by factory fat makers who coined the slogan, "Healthy for Your Heart," whose sole interest was influencing Americans to eat factory polyunsaturated vegetable oils.

Yet empirical evidence was mounting against the lipid hypothesis and the introduction of polyunsaturated vegetable fats. Empirical evidence is derived from observation. Let's say you notice that your begonias do better with one fertilizer over another. You don't need a study to tell you what you see with your own eyes. Empirical evidence demonstrated that we had been healthier and had less heart disease before we traded our traditionally consumed diet that included saturated fats for a factory diet including factory fats. Still, the AHA launched the Prudent Diet in 1956, which encouraged Americans to replace saturated fats with polyunsaturated vegetable oils.

The expression "you are what you eat" aptly describes what

happens when you eat any type of fat. "Dietary fat . . . is absorbed pretty much as it goes in and is then burned for energy, stored as adipose tissue, or incorporated into cell membranes and other tissues in just about the same form in which you ate it," write Michael Eades, MD, and Mary Dan Eades, MD, in their book *The Protein Power Lifeplan: A New Comprehensive Blueprint for Optimal Health.* "If you go out to a ball game and eat a hot dog, the next day . . . if you look in the mirror, the fat in the hot dog will be staring back at you, unchanged, in the lipid bilayers of your skin, in the whites of your eyes, and even in your brain. That's why it pays to be careful about the types of fat that you eat."[3]

Salad dressing, cheese "foods," deep-fried foods, vegetable cooking oils, imitation meat products, mayonnaise and mayo-like products, ersatz sour cream and dessert toppings, margarine, movie popcorn and microwave popcorn, non-dairy artificial cream products, soy spreads, and vegetable shortening are all examples of lethal factory fats. But just because food makers have processed polyunsaturated oils into poisons doesn't mean that you should avoid polyunsaturated fats altogether, because naturally occurring polyunsaturated fats are health giving.

Within the polyunsaturated fatty acid are omega-3 and omega-6 and gamma-linolenic acid (GLA) properties. Omega-3 and omega-6 are essential fatty acids, which means they are required by the body but can only be obtained through eating the right foods.[4]

Studies show that omega-3 promotes lean body mass, which means that including omega-3 fatty acids in your diet will help you burn fat and build muscle.[5] Omega-3 fats are essential to cellular health. Without omega-3 you will likely end up with dry skin; premature wrinkles; thin, brittle hair and nails; depression and other neurotransmitter imbalances, chronic constipation and a malfunctioning immune system, leading to muscle and joint pain and arthritis. Of course with omega-3, you will enjoy the opposite effects.

The ideal and traditional ratio of omega-3 to omega-6 polyunsaturated fatty acids is about 1:1. Today Americans consume a 1:20 to 1:50 ratio. And this is not good, as an imbalanced omega-3:6 ratio has been shown to be a major contributing factor in the development of cancer and other degenerative diseases.

The reason the ratio has gotten so skewed is that since the 1950s, the meat industry gradually moved cattle and chickens from the range to CAFOs. Instead of feeding cattle their natural diet of grass and weeds and chicken their natural diet of weeds, insects, and worms, these animals are fattened on corn and grain. Like humans, animals are what they eat. Cattle and chickens' natural diet contains a close to optimal ratio of omega 3:6 and so subsequently their meat and eggs contain a close to optimal ratio. But grains have a greater quantity of omega 6 polyunsaturated fatty acids. Consequently the meat from grain-fed cattle and chickens contains an omega-3:6 ratio of 1:14 and 1:19, respectively. The same holds true for eggs and dairy products. Consuming these animal products has contributed to our radically imbalanced ratio of omega-3:6. The consumption of corn, soy, canola, safflower, and sunflower oils also contribute excess omega-6.

Now that people are becoming aware of the health-giving properties of omega-3 fatty acids, factory fat makers are jumping on the bandwagon to produce their factory omega-3 "spreads." However, it's important to note the distinction between factory omega-3 spreads and naturally occurring polyunsaturated fats. We now understand the fragile nature of the polyunsaturated fatty acids. These oils should be protected from heat, light, oxygen, and chemical processes. But edible oil makers do not seem prepared to change their manufacturing mentality. Just like the polyunsaturated vegetable oils that were hydrogenated, oxidized, and turned into shellac, omega-3 polyunsaturated fats are now being subjected to unnatural industrialization. Omega-3 fortified butterlike spreads like SmartBalance OmegaPlus are not the same healthy polyunsaturated omega-3 fatty acids found in foods, no matter what the ads say, because manufacturing processes always alter, reduce, or deaden the healthy biological properties of oils.

Not to forget, gamma linolenic acid (GLA), is an omega-6 polyunsaturated fatty acid used in the production of prostaglandins. Prostaglandins are essential to the proper functioning of each cell and play a role in many biological processes, including regulating your immune system. Prostaglandins maintain homeostasis in your body—the body's adaptive responses that attempt to return the body from an abnormal state back to status quo. GLA is an anti-inflammatory agent, inhibits the growth of some cancer cells, aids fat metabolism, and helps prevent rheumatoid arthritis, cardiovascular disease, high blood pressure, premenstrual syndrome, and neurological problems related to diabetes. The GLA oils black current, borage, and evening primrose can be taken in supplemental capsule form.

The polyunsaturated oils, corn, cottonseed, safflower, soy, and canola are subjected to degumming, refining, bleaching, and deodorizing processes and should not be eaten until the public can be assured that these oils are being processed in high-quality, cold-pressed plants. (I personally will never knowingly eat soy oil.) However, since we have to live on what we have in our food chain, choosing less toxic oils is the best we can do for now. Look for cold-pressed oils bottled in dark glass or plastic. "Cold pressing" is still heat processing, but for now, it's the best we can expect from our food manufacturers.

Examples of healthy polyunsaturated fats are cold-water fish such as cod, herring, mackerel, salmon, and sardines and their oils; eggs; butter; cream; pumpkin seeds and oil; sesame seeds and oil; sunflower seeds and oil; walnuts and walnut oil; wheat germ and wheat germ oil; and flaxseed oil (experts recommend cod liver oil over flaxseed oil, as flax tends to go rancid more quickly). Sesame oil is the only polyunsaturated oil that can be used safely in cooking.

My grandma was a believer in the power of healthy oils and chugged olive oil directly from the bottle every day and more if she needed to "fix herself." Olive oil is a monounsaturated oil. Monounsaturated fats lower LDL-cholesterol in the blood, are necessary for healthy skin, maintain the structural integrity of neural membranes, are high in the antioxidant vitamin E, which boosts immunity and provides protection against certain cancers such as breast and colon cancer. Monounsaturated fats are more prone to the creation of oxidizing free radicals than are saturated oils when they are cooked, so it's best to eat monounsaturated foods and oils at room temperature, with the exception of olive and peanut oils, which can be used for cooking. Examples of healthy monounsaturated oils are almonds and oil, avocados and oil, hazelnuts and oil, peanuts, peanut butter and oil, olives and oil, rice bran oil, "high oleic" safflower and sunflower oils, and sunflower seeds.

(Saturated fat is the subject of chapter 18.)

It seems crazy in retrospect that anyone could be convinced that fats made in a laboratory were healthier than butter, a naturally occurring dietary fat that was historically eaten by humans. But as a friend of mine said, "Eighty percent of Americans believe that wrestling on TV is real." In other words, if there's enough pomp and press—or in this case *studies*—we'll go along.

CHAPTER 16

How Studies Influence What We Put in Our Mouths

IN THE EARLY SEVENTIES, I visited a friend who was going through medical school. He fixed himself instant Top Ramen for dinner and offered me some too, but I declined. "I can't believe you're going to eat those chemicals," I said. "The human body is made up of chemicals," he replied. That statement—from a medical student—blew my mind and has stayed with me all these years.

Modern medicine has advanced beyond our wildest dreams and expectations to where the impossible is now possible, and many brilliant, caring, hardworking MDs are able to perform seeming miracles on a daily basis. As extraordinary as medical feats are today, the advancements that are clearly obtainable in the near future boggle and excite the mind. To achieve this level of medical competence takes years of dedicated, tenacious hard work and sacrifice. However, there is one area that most doctors have no experience with and should not lecture us about. That is nutrition. Since Louis Pasteur's germ theory of disease influenced Western medical schools to reject nutrition as an important aspect of medicine, doctors have not seen fit to learn about nutrition. And I say this with all due respect as I have many doctor friends and am confident that none of them would profess to be qualified to give nutritional advice.

If a person wanted to go into the business of winemaking and become a vintner of fine wines, that person might end up at a school like UC Davis studying viticulture. The study of viticulture includes how and what to feed the grapevines in order to produce the best quality grape. But somehow, modern medicine has felt it unnecessary to understand—and teach—how and what to feed the human body to produce *the best quality human being.*

After medical training, MDs are required to obtain continuing education credits every year. Other than these required courses, doctors learn from drug reps, medical journals, conferences and lectures, books, and the media. Sixty to 70 percent of nonsurgical continuing education comes to doctors via drug reps, referred to as "detail people," as in that's where docs get the details on which new drugs have hit the market, not about how to prevent patients from having to take drugs in the first place. (Now that the feds have squeezed pharmaceutical companies to knock off the "gifts" to doctors, this industry has cleverly turned to recruiting beautiful, sexy, former cheerleaders as drug reps.)[1]

Very few doctors independently pursue an education in nutrition.

Shockingly, nutritional information in medical journals is highly tainted. According to Dr. Nestle, author of the aforementioned *Food Politics,* nutritional research is often funded by the food industry. A 1996 survey disclosed that nearly 30 percent of university researchers investigating food products accepted funding from the food industry. Another survey demonstrated that 34 percent of the lead authors of eight hundred papers in molecular biology and medicine were involved in patents, served on advisory committees, and/or held shares in the companies that would benefit from their research. The *Journal of Nutritional Education,* writes Nestle, accepts financial contributions from eight "corporate patron friends," and four "corporate sustaining friends," and the *American Journal of Clinical Nutrition* accepts financial assistance from twenty-eight companies that support "selected educational activities." Such sponsors are Coca-Cola, Gerber,

Nestlé/Carnation, Monsanto, Proctor & Gamble, Roche Vitamins, Slim-Fast Foods, and the Sugar Association. In addition, drug advertising contributed $20 million per year to prestigious journals such as the *New England Journal of Medicine* and the *Journal of the American Medical Association,* which, according to Nestle, "both of which publish the 'hottest' of nutrition research."[2]

Concurring with Nestle was a July 2005 National Institutes of Health (NIH) survey that demonstrated that 33 percent of U.S. scientists admitted that they engaged in "unethical practices" such as manipulating or hiding data, designing their studies to reach certain conclusions, or altering the conclusions of their studies to satisfy sponsors.[3] (The NIH is the primary federal agency for conducting and supporting medical research.)

With nutritional education coming from factory food manufacturers, our medical community's collective consciousness has deteriorated to the point where *diseased* and *injured* patients in hospitals are served Ensure, Jell-O, Diet 7-Up, Better'n Eggs, Kellogg's Corn Flakes, and coffee with Coffee-Mate Creamer and NutraSweet. Hospitals are also the new frontier for fast food franchises.

In defense of medical doctors, they are discouraged by medical school indoctrination, peer pressure, and threats of lawsuits not to stray from standard of care nutritional doctrine, such as the lipid hypothesis that generated the low-fat diet. If a doctor advised his or her patient to eat more saturated fat and that person had a heart attack, because the doctor had strayed from the standard of care, he or she would be liable for litigation. So it's easy to see why doctors toe the ideological line when it comes to nutrition.

At the same time, doctors are notoriously skeptical of empirical evidence, which they refer to as "anecdotal." If you went into your doctor's office claiming that ingesting a certain substance caused you a health problem, he or she would not likely agree with you unless you provided evidence that that substance caused said symptoms. The evidence they want is at least one double-blind, peer-reviewed study that is published in a peer-reviewed medical journal. A double-blind study means that neither the test subjects nor the researchers know what treatment the test subjects are receiving. At the conclusion of the study, the code is broken and the data analyzed. This method eliminates observer and test subject bias. Peer-reviewed means that researchers of equal standing to the investigators evaluate the quality of study. Once a double-blind study is published in a peer-reviewed medical journal, the conclusions of the study are considered medical truth.

Over the course of fifty years, medical doctors have given Americans devastating nutritional advice about fats. This advice has encouraged Americans to eschew the historical human diet of real fat in favor of highly industrialized fats. Much of this advice was based on the results of studies.

Unfortunately, there are many problems with studies. For one, it's only with absolutes that you can even begin to approach an absolute conclusion. The variables of human experience, genetics, and behavior automatically render results of human trials inconclusive, even if your test subjects were selected from a pool of virtually identical individuals, either male or female, sharing the same race, height, weight, dietary and exercise history, sleep patterns, cigarette and alcohol use, baseline cholesterol numbers, prescription and OTC use, sex lives, TV habits, golf scores, and number of children. You would still have to have a team of unbiased scientists from another planet examine the results because, when a researcher sets out to prove a hypothesis, he or she is looking for that proof of that hypothesis in the results of whatever study he or she conducts. Research protocols are not perfect, and data can be juggled or ignored, corners cut and so on, so that a researcher is likely to get the results he or she is looking for. Especially if they stand to make money from any ventures that rely on a hypothesis being correct. And scientists and doctors who have spent their entire careers hyping a hypothesis and perhaps have lucrative clinics, books, and other products based on this premise are not likely to back down from their original position.

I have cited studies throughout this book, but it's my opinion that nutritional studies should always be weighed against empirical evidence because there are just too many problems with studies. As Nestle reported, most studies are paid for by the industries that stand to profit by the results of the studies. For example, over the past twenty years, soy symposiums where researchers present their finding are funded by multibillion dollar soy producing corporations such as Archer Daniels Midland Company (the world's dominant soybean processor), Monsanto, Central Soya Company, United Soybean Board, Cargill Soy Protein Products/ Cargill Nutraceuticals, and the Illinois Soybean Association. Many of the studies presented are made possible by grants from these and other soy producing corporations.

And it's not just the soy industry. Most scientists rely on funding from industries to do research. If they do not provide research results that are consistent with the views of their benefactors, they have their funding (salaries) cut off.

There has never been a study comparing diets of factory foods and real food because factory food companies would lose. As it stands, food studies help the factory food industry sell us more factory food, diets, supplements, and so on.

Another problem with studies is that few doctors bother to read them. Ask your doctor why he or she supports avoiding saturated fat and cholesterol, eating soy, eating a low-fat diet, taking statin drugs, or any other conventionally accepted doctrine that's floated today, and he or she will likely say because of studies. Okay, exactly what studies do you mean? I would venture to say that few doctors could legitimately say that they pored over the medical literature and analyzed the results of the pros and cons of the views they support.

At the same time, since the introduction of processed polyunsaturated fats there have been medical doctors and scientists who chose to stray from the status quo in search of deeper answers into the mysterious rise in heart disease.

CHAPTER 17

Finally Americans Are Told the Truth About Trans Fats

IN JULY 1971, Senator George McGovern (D-SD) announced the formation of the Select Committee on Nutrition and Human Needs, which would hold hearings on the relationship between diet and heart disease—and whose purpose was to prove that eating dietary saturated fat was as bad as cigarette smoking. McGovern declared that he would only hear testimony from those on the side of polyunsaturated vegetable oils. He did not want to hear any testimony from scientists or representatives from the dairy and meat industries who questioned the notion that eating meat, dairy products, and eggs might *not* be a contributing factor in heart disease.

Numerous scientists voiced skepticism, and presented opposing scientific papers to encourage further discussion as to the real cause of heart disease. Nevertheless, it was ultimately McGovern's committee that, by 1977—having come to nowhere near unanimous conclusions—solidified the lipid hypothesis as official policy with the issuing of the USDA's mandate to *eat less fat*.

In May 1978, Mary Enig, then a biochemistry doctoral student at the University of Maryland, was scratching her head over the McGovern report. The committee had reached their conclusions in part because of their assumptions that the increased consumption of animal fats had caused the rise in heart disease. But Enig knew that the consumption of animal fats had declined steadily, while polyunsaturated vegetable fat intake had increased. In addition, Enig was aware of numerous studies that contradicted the committee's conclusions regarding the correlation between fat intake and breast and colon cancers. She poured over the USDA data that McGovern's committee had used, and when she finished her analysis, submitted her findings to the *Journal of the Federation of American Societies for Experimental Biology.*[1]

Enig's article claimed that the McGovern report had it all wrong about the correlation between dietary fat and cancer. She offered up data that demonstrated that the use of hydrogenated polyunsaturated vegetable oils predisposed consumers to cancer, but that animal fats provided protection against cancer. She claimed that the McGovern committee's analysts manipulated the data to get the results they wanted. Her article urged immediate investigation into the dangers of trans fatty acids.

By the time Dr. Enig had reached her initial conclusions all those decades ago about saturated fats and trans fats, other researchers also understood the problems. Scientists continued to demonstrate that there was virtually no correlation between animal fat and other cholesterol-laden food intake and blood cholesterol.[2] Many studies concluded that thickening of the arterial walls is simply a natural, unavoidable process that had nothing to do with eating saturated fat and cholesterol.[3] Numerous scientists were also recognizing that total cholesterol numbers were meaningless. People with low cholesterol were more likely to have blocked arteries as those with high cholesterol.[4]

Mary Enig, Joseph Sampagna, and Mark Keeney at the University of Maryland clocked thousands of hours in the lab analyzing the trans fat content of hundreds of factory foods. The researchers found that shortenings used in cookies, chips, and baked goods contained more than 35 percent trans fat and that many baked goods and industrialized foods contained much more partially hydrogenated vegetable oil than their labels disclosed.

Enig's analyses confirmed that (at that time) the average American consumed at least 12 grams of trans fat per day. (Today Dr. Enig estimates that Americans eat, "on average 13.3 grams of trans fats per day, the typical range being between 1.6 and 38.7 grams per day. Heavy users of fast food eat far more—up to 60 grams of trans fats per day.")[5]

Enig's research concluded that trans fats interfere with the enzymes that neutralize carcinogens while increasing the enzymes that exacerbate the damage of carcinogens. Trans fats also increase (the so-called bad) LDL cholesterol and triglycerides, lower (the so-called good) HDL cholesterol. Trans fats make blood platelets sticky, interfere with insulin actions, cause aberrant cellular structures, create free radicals, and lower immune response. These factors contribute to the development of insulin resistance, Type 2 diabetes, hypertension, cancer and cardiovascular disease. Trans fatty acids lower cream volume in breast milk, are linked to low birth weight, (in men) decreased testosterone and increased levels of abnormal sperm, and (in women) can shorten gestation.[6]

Trans fats also have a deleterious effect on the brain and nervous system. The human body doesn't reject trans fatty acids as foreign but uses whatever fat it has on board to build cellular structures. And because trans fats can cross the blood brain barrier, they are incorporated into brain cell membranes and are thus linked to neurodegenerative disorders such as multiple sclerosis (MS), Parkinson's disease, and Alzheimer's disease, as well as childhood neurological disorders such as ADD, ADHD, and autism. And so if I were in my childbearing years, if I were pregnant, if I were a nursing mother or the mother of young children, I would be fearful of eating trans fats or feeding these fats and other factory fats to my children, because I would come to the logical conclusion that if the cell membranes of my baby's or child's developing brain were made of aberrant fat molecules that *things could go wrong.*

Although Dr. Enig and other researchers came to these dire conclusions about trans fats, their findings were drowned out by the overwhelming support for the lipid hypothesis, which essentially diverted attention away from the dangers of trans fats and encouraged Americans to eat more factory polyunsaturated fats. Because our medical and scientific community had endorsed polyunsaturated vegetable fats as heart healthy, promoters had already permeated our food chain with hydrogenated and partially hydrogenated fats (containing trans fats).

Since her early years as a graduate student, Dr. Enig has been a driving force in compelling the FDA to enforce the labeling of trans fats on products, which occurred on January 1, 2006. It is because of Dr. Enig that we are now aware of the dangers of trans fats and that, as of this writing, New York lawmakers have banned trans fats in restaurants and legislators in LA are considering following suit. It's a telling commentary that although Dr. Enig is currently becoming recognized for her efforts and contributions to Americans' well-being she is nowhere near the household name Betty Crocker, that fictional character that has been used for decades to give science fiction factory foods a warm and fuzzy image.

Unfortunately, for many Americans FDA labeling has been rendered ineffectual by the disclosures of that agency's ineptitude and corruption, and at the same time, many consumers have become confused and ambivalent about the FDA. It's highly likely that many food makers will continue to produce trans fat products—and that people will continue to consume those products. Even if labeling trans fats on products and banning trans fats in restaurants does make a small difference, this does nothing to hinder the marketing and sales of heat and chemical processed polyunsaturated vegetables fats that are just as much to blame for the epidemic of heart and other diseases.

Adding to consumer confusion is the fact that the medical industry and the government continue to categorize saturated fat together with trans fats as dangerous fats to avoid.

The truth may surprise you.

CHAPTER 18

Saturated Animal Fat Good, Trans Fats Bad

WHEN I WAS SEVENTEEN in 1967, I read *The Jungle*, Upton Sinclair's 1905 exposé of the grisly and unhygienic conditions in the meatpacking industry. I felt reassured that public uproar after the publication of the novel had led to the passage of the Meat Inspection Act and other food safety legislation, which I naïvely assumed had reformed the medieval slaughtering practices in the meatpacking industry. But thirty-eight years later, when I read Bob Dylan's memoir, *Chronicles, Volume One* I was stopped cold. In 1961, Dylan migrated to New York City. He talks about a friend who had worked on the kill floor of an Omaha slaughterhouse. Dylan asked his friend what it was like and he replied, "You ever heard of Auschwitz?"[1]

So why is it that we spend billions of dollars pampering our cats and dogs, and though we revile the imprisonment, torture, and brutal killing of innocent people, we accept the same treatment for the innocent animals that give us sustenance? All aspects of animal husbandry have taken a Draconian turn in the last hundred years, as the food industry has operated with single-minded focus on one goal and one goal only: To save money. This means fattening up animals as cheaply as possible in as small a space as possible.

Although we may be able to compartmentalize our angst over animal cruelty so we can continue to consume factory milk, meat, and eggs, ultimately the animals' horrible existence, garbage diet, drug intake, and gory deaths will come back to haunt us. The way an animal lives and its diet determines the nutritional value of its meat, milk, and eggs and, thus, the consumers' subsequent health. It also explains why *factory-raised* saturated fat is almost as unhealthy as trans fat.

Factory animals are tethered, stalled, or otherwise tightly confined in dark factories or pens. They stand in their own waste and often drink water contaminated with, or are fed, their own or other animals' offal.[2] To save money on feed, animals are fed municipal garbage, stale cookies, poultry "litter," chicken feathers, and restaurant plate waste.[3] Concentrated Animal Feeding Operations (CAFO) along with species-inappropriate feed, breed disease. (Species-inappropriate feed is composed of substances that the animal would not naturally eat and is not designed to digest and assimilate in a healthy way.) To treat these diseases, animals are given numerous drugs. According to cancer expert Dr. Samuel Epstein, "In the absence of effective federal regulation, the meat industry uses hundreds of animal feed additives, including antibiotics, tranquilizers, pesticides, animal drugs, artificial flavors, industrial wastes and growth-promoting hormones . . . . The hazards of U.S. meat have retrogressed from the random fecal and bacterial contamination of Upton Sinclair's *The Jungle* to the brave new world of deliberate chemicalization."[4]

Although conventional wisdom is stuck on the belief that saturated fats are as unhealthy as trans fats, saturated fats and trans fats do not necessarily belong in the same sentence. Organically raised animal fat is a naturally occurring, historically eaten fatty acid with health-giving properties. Factory animal fat is almost as deadly as trans fats, but for a different reason: Because toxins are fat-soluble, they permeate and are stored indefinitely in fat cells. When you eat factory produced animal products, you are eating all the toxins that an animal consumed or was exposed to. Most trans fatty acids are manmade aberrant molecules that destroy life. (There are naturally occurring trans fats in foods.) Because free radical oxidation generated by toxins is just as much a cause of heart disease as trans fats, you can say, "Factory-raised saturated animal fat and trans fat" in the same breath.

However, the medical community does not recognize the distinctions between organically raised saturated animal fat, factory raised saturated animal fat, and manmade trans fats, and therefore continues to summarily campaign against "saturated fat and trans fat."

Historically, humans ate fat from organically raised animals in foods like butter, whole milk, cream, eggs, and meat. It has only been since WWII that saturated animal fats have been shunned by the medical community as a factor of heart disease. But over the years, like Dr. Enig, others questioned the campaign against animal fat. In the early 1960s, George V. Mann, ScD, MD, PhD, took a team of researchers to Kenya to study the Maasai tribe who virtually lived on milk, animal blood, and meat, and found that they did not suffer from heart disease.[5]

Dr. Mann was a participating researcher in the most famous study of the causes of heart disease, "The Framingham Heart Diet."[6] This study has found no conclusive evidence that dietary fat contributes to heart disease. Dr. Mann said, "The diet-heart hypothesis has been repeatedly shown to be wrong, and yet, for complicated reasons of pride, profit, and prejudice, the hypothesis continues to be exploited by scientists, fundraising enterprises, food companies, and even governmental agencies. The public is being deceived by the greatest health scam of the century."[7]

During the mid-1980s you would have thought eggs were the spawn of Satan, but my grandma continued to refer to eggs as the perfect food. When I asked, "But Grandma, what about heart disease?" She replied in her Polish accent, "I don't know about that, honey," and fixed me a plate of eggs. She was not alone in her belief, because somewhere deep in our collective consciousness,

Americans understood that eggs are a perfect food. Still the food industry tried hard to convince us—by using studies—that real eggs were bad for our health, but that weird science eggs out of carton were healthy. And the condemnation of naturally occurring saturated fats is entrenched in our mindset. For example, in *The South Beach Diet* celebrity cardiologist cum diet doctor Arthur Agatston writes, "There is evidence now that immediately following a meal of saturated fats, there is dysfunction in the arteries, including those that supply the heart muscle with blood. As a result, the lining of the arteries (the endothelium) is predisposed to constriction and clotting. Imagine: Under the right (or rather, wrong) circumstances, eating a meal that's high in saturated fat can trigger a heart attack!"[8]

I contacted Dr. Agatston's office to obtain the study he used as "evidence" that "eating a meal that's high in saturated fat can trigger a heart attack." As it turns out, the study, "Effect of Single High Fat Meal on Endothelial Function in Healthy Subject," was published in the *American Journal of Cardiology* in 1997.[9] In this study one group was given a "high fat" meal of an Egg McMuffin, Sausage McMuffin, two hash brown patties, and a noncaffeinated beverage (something from McDonald's). The other group was fed the "low-fat" meal, which consisted of Frosted Flakes, skimmed milk, and orange juice.

I asked Dr. Enig for her opinion, and she explained that the subjects were tested for "endothelial function" by measuring the diameter change in the brachial artery after eating. Apparently there was a slight diameter change in the brachial arteries of the "high fat" eating test subjects. However, Dr. Enig said, "For years we have been hearing that high-fat foods raise so-called bad LDL cholesterol and blood pressure and therefore contribute to heart disease. But since that didn't happen in this study, the authors have declared that an inherently subjective measurement of 'endothelial function' is a better marker for heart disease. But was it saturated fat that caused the decline in endothelial function? Only 28 percent of the fat in the high-fat meal was saturated. The rest was a combination of trans fats, monounsaturated and polyunsaturated fat, any one of which, or all together are the likely culprits in the decline in endothelial function." Dr. Enig explained that the high-sugar meal did not likely contain MSG, whereas the high-fat meal did contain MSG and that the presence of MSG explained the decline in endothelial function.

To make the incendiary claim that saturated fat can trigger a heart attack, the researchers should have been able to cite other studies, said Enig. "As it becomes more and more obvious that cholesterol levels have little predictive value for heart disease—and that saturated fats in fact have little or no effect on cholesterol levels anyway—researchers are searching for other ways to demonize saturated fats."[10]

The lipid hypothesis, which has driven many Americans to fear eating saturated fats, *has never been proven.* In 1988 the U.S. Surgeon General's Office embarked on a project to write the "final and definitive" report that would once and for all put any questions about the lipid hypothesis to rest. The plan was to gather all supporting evidence, have it bound nicely, have the requisite experts review it, and then publish it with pomp and circumstance. Unfortunately, the plan did not go as smoothly as anticipated. After eleven years of active pursuit that consumed four project officers, no clear evidence could be found to prove the lipid hypothesis. The office killed the report without the pageantry.[11]

"The operative word is hypothesis," Dr. Kritchevsky told me. "The lipid hypothesis was a viable hypothesis until we learned more. The real sin here is that people [working in the field] who knew we were learning more wouldn't admit it because they were so comfortable with what was going on." (In other words, the researchers who were receiving grants from the edible oil industry.)

The balanced diet that we are talking about in this book— which will allow you to realize your genetic gifts—is comprised of the four basic food groups: protein, fats, nonstarchy vegetables, and carbohydrates. After protein, real, naturally occurring dietary fat is most important. Fatty acids make up 80 percent of our cellular structure and 70 percent of our brain. Fats are used to make neurotransmitters. Every cell membrane in your body is made up of fat. If you do not eat quality fats, your cells cannot function properly. Fats are used to make the hormones used by your endocrine system, including eicosanoids, which are the superhormones that control all other hormone production in your body.

Fats slow down the absorption of food, so that you feel satisfied and can go for longer periods of time without feeling hunger. In fact, it has been our suppression of natural fats in our diet that has greatly contributed to our national hysterical hunger. "Suppression of natural appetites, such as eating processed fats instead of natural fats, leads to weird nocturnal habits, fantasies, fetishes, bingeing, and splurging," said Dr. Enig. [12]

Fats transport fat-soluble vitamins A, D, E, and K in your system and are necessary for the conversion of carotene to vitamin A, for mineral absorption, and for numerous metabolic processes. The antioxidant vitamins E, A, and D can't be absorbed into your bloodstream without the presence of fat in your intestines. That means that, in terms of antioxidants, which scavenge the free radicals that cause oxidation, all those dry salads we ate were for naught.

Eating a variety of fats every day is important because saturated, monounsaturated, and polyunsaturated fatty acids all provide different biological properties for the smooth operation of our metabolic processes.

Saturated fats provide energy for locomotion and metabolic processes and are building blocks for cell membranes and hormones. Saturated fats strengthen your immune system, suppress production of tumors, and are necessary for your body to utilize essential fatty acids. Saturated animal fats from the meat and milk of pasture-raised, grass-fed animals contain conjugated linoleic acid (CLA), which has been shown to reduce the risk of atherosclerosis and cancer, and has the added benefit of increasing metabolic rate and burning fat. Saturated fats in organic animal products also contain enzymes (see page 155).

Saturated animal fat was not the only saturated fat to take a hit because of the lipid-hypothesis. In the mid-eighties, the American Soybean Association (ASA), eager to increase the sales of soybean oil, sent "Fat Fighter Kits" to soybean farmers instructing them to lobby to their elected officials about the dangers of tropical oils (palm, palm kernel, and coconut oil). Behind-the-scenes work by the ASA resulted in coconut oil being characterized as "poisoning America." An advertisement actually depicted a coconut as a bomb with a lighted fuse. Restaurants and factory food manufacturers switched from healthy coconut oil to heat- and chemical-processed and hydrogenated soybean oil, and movie theaters switched from popping popcorn in "artery-clogging saturated" coconut oil to hydrogenated soybean oil. The deadliest oils on the market.[13]

Drs. Eades told me, "Saturated fat, like coconut oil, has been vilified as 'artery-clogging,' but it's simply untrue. Polyunsaturated fats are easily oxidized and so we can say that they are, indeed 'artery-clogging.' But saturated fat doesn't easily oxidize so it doesn't collect in the arteries."

In *Over the Edge of the World: Magellan's Terrifying Circumnavigation of the Globe*," Laurence Bergreen writes of Magellan's fourteenth-century armada encountering tribes of healthy, beautiful, intelligent, vital, coconut-eating Pacific islanders during their voyage. Bergreen writes of the Magellan's reaction to the Philippine archipelago, "Perhaps they had found paradise . . . . Each day Magellan fed coconut milk supplied by the generous Filipinos to the sailors still suffering from scurvy." With reverence, the expedition's chronicler, Antonio Pigafetta's quill scratched out a description of the *cocho* (coconut) for all posterity to read. Bergreen writes that, "Pigafetta was so moved by the coconut's versatility that he declared, with some exaggeration, that two palm trees could sustain a family of ten for a hundred years."[14]

You have to wonder, if Pacific islanders historically ate coconuts,

coconuts, and more coconuts, why then were they so breathtakingly healthy? Hawaiian islanders historically fit that same description, and only became rotund and diseased after they eschewed their traditional diet—containing hefty amounts of coconuts—and adopted the Westernized factory food diet, including factory processed vegetable oils.[15]

Coconut oil raises HDL cholesterol. It also contains antiviral and antimicrobial properties that have been found to be effective in combatting viruses that cause influenza, measles, herpes, mononucleosis, hepatitis C, and AIDS; the fungi and yeast that result in ringworm, Candida, and thrush; parasites that cause intestinal infections such as giardiasis; as well as bacteria that cause stomach ulcers, throat infections, pneumonia, sinusitis, rheumatic fever, food-borne illnesses, urinary tract infections, meningitis, gonorrhea, and toxic shock syndrome. No wonder Magellan's scurvy suffering sailors indulged in coconut. Coconut oil is also thermogenic (fat burning—thus the gorgeous South Sea islanders). According to Dr. Enig, since allergies to coconut are caused by the proteins, the oil is probably safe for those who are allergic.[16]

In addition to cocoa butter, coconut, whole coconut milk, coconut butter and oil, other examples of healthy saturated fats are beef, butter, cheese, cream, crème fraîche, eggs, fowl fat, lamb, lard, nutmeg oil, palm kernel oil, pork, sheanut oil, sour cream, and whole milk.

Protein is your primary food group, both crucial for survival and to heal from the malnutrition that is keeping Americans fat and sick. Only protein can provide your body with the amino acids necessary to build muscle, tissues, bones, and other structures. Protein is essential for growth, repair, hormone production, immune function, and every single metabolic process in your body.

Examples of healthy proteins are pasture-raised or wild-caught beef, buffalo, chicken, duck, eggs, game, lamb, pheasant, quail, squab, and turkey, as well as wild fish or shellfish. Beef and lamb cooked rare are good sources of enzymes. *Salmonella, Listeria monocytogenes,* or *E. coli O157:H7* breed in confinement, but do not proliferate in pasture-raised animals. Never eat rare pork or chicken.

Because all fatty acids can produce free radicals when heated, meat should be cooked at a low temperature. Never eat burned or charbroiled meat.

Although the medical community has sheepishly lightened up about eggs, people still hold many misconceptions. The truth is that eggs provide us with omega-3 fatty acids as well as cholesterol, which are both necessary for life and important factors in attaining our genetic gifts. For recipes that call for raw eggs, be sure to purchase "pasture-raised" eggs. "Cage-free" does not always mean that the chickens roamed free pecking at grass, insects, larvae and earthworms. If you are in doubt, call the supplier and ask. Pasture-raised organic meats and fowl can be purchased at health food stores or online. On www.eatwild.com you can find sources for grass-fed meat from all over the country. Pasture-raised, organic eggs can be purchased at health food stores and farmers' markets. Organically raised nitrate-free ham and bacon is available at health food stores from farmers who allow their hogs to run, root, and roam.

North of Santa Barbara is cattle country where small herds scatter across the hillsides. During the seven years we lived on a ranch there, I often stopped to talk to cows that congregated near our roadside mailbox munching grass, weeds, scrub, wildflowers, brambles. They're sweet, timidly curious, with soulful, long-lashed eyes. Spring welcomes new calves that, left to their own devices, suckle their mothers until they are ridiculously too huge. I never passed these cows without pondering the plight of factory animals.

Human beings have an innate drive to survive and a primary aspect of survival is eating food. It has only been the last hundred years that people in the developed world have been completely removed from the hunting, raising, and slaughtering of animals. The stresses and strains of survival have taken on entirely new and modern challenges. We no longer have to think about, or want the added strain of thinking about how we will obtain our food.

Many animal lovers like myself struggle with the issue of eating meat. The brilliant animal scientist, Temple Grandin PhD—who has designed half of the livestock handling facilities in the United States—writes in her book *Animals in Translation: Using the Mysteries of Autism to Decode Animal Behavior*, "If I had my druthers humans would have evolved to be plant eaters, so we wouldn't have to kill other animals for food. But we didn't, and I don't see the human race converting to vegetarianism anytime soon. I've tried to eat vegetarian myself, and I haven't been able to manage it physically . . . the fact that humans evolved as both plant and meat eaters means that the vast majority of human beings are going to continue to eat both. Humans are animals too, and we do what are animal natures tell us to do."

In Charles Frazier's Civil War novel *Cold Mountain*, a wounded solider, Inman, travels perilously back home and along the way is helped and hindered by others, including a goat woman who takes him in and feeds him. Frazier writes, "A little spotted brown-and-white goat came to her and she stroked it and scratched below its neck until it folded its legs and lay down. The animal's long neck was stretched forward. The old woman scratched it close under its jaw and stroked its ears. Inman thought it a peaceful scene. He watched as she continued to scratch with her left hand and reach with her right into an apron pocket. With one motion she pulled out a short-bladed knife and cut deep into the artery below the jawline and shoved the white basin underneath to catch the leap of bright blood. The animal jerked once, then lay trembling as she continued to scratch the fur and fondle the ears. The basin filled slowly. The goat and the woman stared intently off toward the distance as if waiting for a signal."

Most animal loving meat eaters would like to know that the animals they are eating were raised and slaughtered as humanely as this little goat. Realistically, however, there is a huge difference between feeding two people and 300 million people. The sheer volume of meat necessary to feed our nation has resulted in corrupt, sloppy, inhumane practices in the meat industry first uncovered by Upton Sinclair. While Dr. Grandin has devoted her career to improving the lives and deaths of the animals we eat, one person cannot shoulder this responsibility alone.

In the film *The Last of the Mohicans*, Hawkeye is an Anglo-Saxon frontiersman who had been orphaned as a baby and adopted by the Mohican Chingachgook. The film opens with Chingachgook, his blood son, Uncas, and Hawkeye running silently through a heavily canopied forest, hunting an elk. When the elk is felled by the .59 caliber round of Hawkeye's five foot rifle, the three men kneel at the beast. In Mohican, Chingachgook speaks to the elk, "We're sorry to kill you, Brother. Forgive us. I do honor to your courage and speed, your strength."

This moving scene depicted the reverential attitude that some cultures historically held for the animals that provided them sustenance. Although many animals lovers choose to eat meat, we do have choices as to the way animals we consume are raised and killed. Today there is virtually no reason—other than protecting the shareholder profits of mega animal agribusinesses—that we cannot restore this same reverence for the animals that give us sustenance. We must care, as a nation, and we must revise the treatment of animals, or we will continue to experience the furious retribution of nature: obesity, cancer, heart disease, autoimmune conditions, infectious disease—even variant Creutzfeldt-Jakob disease—the human variant of bovine spongiform encephalopathy (BSE), which is the bovine brain-wasting disease more commonly known as "mad cow disease."

Since saving money is paramount to factory animal agribusinesses, downer cattle (cows too sick or injured to stand up) were, until 1997, slaughtered and fed to humans. When public outrage stopped that practice, these sick animals were slaughtered and ground up and fed to other factory animals (this practice was also supposedly stopped). Today a cow can still eat dried restaurant plate waste that could contain beef as well as newspaper poultry litter (chicken shit) that may also contain remnants of the cattle "meal" fed to chickens. And a cow can still eat a hog that has eaten a cow and so on. Furthermore, calves are still fed "milk replacers" made from cow blood. These practices compel herbivore—creatures that eat grass and shrubs—to be cannibals. With horrifying irony, we are now experiencing the furious backlash of nature as feeding cattle to cattle is the generally accepted theory as to how cows can become infected with BSE.

Stanley Prusiner, MD, a neurologist, won the 1997 Nobel Prize in medicine in 1997 for discovering prions, which are the malformed proteins believed to cause BSE. When infected, prions accumulate in the brain, riddling it with holes. The human variant of BSE, called variant Creutzfeldt-Jakob disease (vCJD), has been linked to consuming BSE-contaminated animal products. To date, 150 people have died from vCJD, suffering unspeakable pain as their brains liquefied.

To date, no substantive preventative measures have been taken to protect humans from contamination. Although BSE prions are supposedly harbored only in nervous system tissue such as blood, eyeballs, and brain and spinal cord tissue, these tissues have routinely entered our food supply via sloppy slaughtering practices. In 2002 the USDA issued a survey showing that approximately 35 percent of "high-risk" meat products (hot dogs, hamburgers, pizza toppings, and taco fillings) tested positive for central nervous system tissue. And although central nervous system tissue has recently been banned for sale for human consumption, slaughtering practices pretty much guarantee that all factory meat eaters have consumed products contaminated with this tissue.[17]

Although BSE prions were previously thought to be harbored in nervous system tissue, in 2004, Dr. Prusiner said, "We don't know where and how prions move through the [cow's] body before they show up in its brain."[18] So, in addition to the possibility of meat products containing BSE prions, we have to wonder about factory milk too. Since research has demonstrated that BSE prions migrate to infected organs, and infection of the udders is common in factory dairy cows, BSE prions could be harbored in the infected secretory tissue of these cows and could be passed to milk.

In the United States 35 million cattle are slaughtered each year. The USDA's current BSE surveillance program samples approximately forty thousand animals per year.[19]

In December 2003, in Washington State, the first suspected case of BSE in the United States was detected in a downer cow. In June 2005, a second case of BSE was confirmed in a downer cow in the United States. It took seven months for the USDA to disclose this fact.[20] In both instances Americans were fed the message that we needn't worry and should have every confidence in the safety of our beef.

In addition to BSE contamination, although factory animals are given numerous drugs to combat disease, they are virtually all sick and often diseased. Factory pigs suffer pneumonia, dysentery, trichinosis (parasitic infestation), and numerous other health problems, including at the time of slaughter.[21] Chickens develop cancer and other serious health problems.[22] So when we eat these animal products, we eat diseased flesh or eggs.

In addition, since factory animal products are exposed to feces, vomit, pus, and urine we are also exposed to lethal infectious organisms. According to CDC, each year food-borne diseases cause approximately 76 million illnesses, 325,000 hospitalizations, and 5,000 deaths in the United States Five pathogens account for over 90 percent of these deaths: *Salmonella* (31 percent), *Listeria monocytogenes* (28 percent), *Toxoplasma gondii* (21 percent), Norwalk-like viruses (7 percent), *Campylobacter* (5 percent), and *E. coli* (3 percent). *Escherichia coli 0157:H7* is the variant responsible for a diarrheal syndrome in which bloody discharges are so copious that death is often the result.[23]

Instead of addressing the root of this problem by closing down CAFOs and setting animals free to roam their natural habitats so that they do not become diseased and are not wallowing in bodily fluids, the USDA has initiated a campaign to irradiate all meat as a way of controlling the spread of infectious diseases. Irradiation, also known as the more innocent sounding "cold pasteurization," exposes food to nuclear radiation to render sterile the pests, eggs, larvae, and bacteria that decompose food. But it does not serve actually to remove the pest, egg, and larvae carcasses from produce, nor does it cleanse the feces, urine, pus, vomit, and tumors from the meat of slaughterhouse animals. Nuclear radiation breaks up the molecular structure of the food, creating weird science chemicals known as unique radiolytic products, which are thought to contribute to cancer and cause genetic and cellular damage. Irradiation also destroys the good bacteria and enzymes that are essential to life and rapidly disappearing from our food chain. Irradiation increases the number of free radicals in food and radically decreases antioxidant vitamins that scavenge free radicals from your body.

Although the FDA maintains that irradiation is nothing to be concerned about, numerous scientists worldwide disagree. The long-term effects of eating irradiated food are not known and have not been studied, but short-term studies link irradiated food to numerous health problems in lab animals, including premature death, fatal internal bleeding, cancer, stillbirths, mutations, organ malfunctions, and stunted growth.[24]

TV news offers up chilling new reports of Avian Flu read over news footage depicting hideously abused domestic birds. Although scientists have yet to understand how the Avian Flu originated, just seeing live birds caged by the thousands, manhandled and stuffed, live, into plastic bags to suffocate, common sense screams, *well no wonder.* Still, many people turn away, somehow believing humans can behave this way with impunity and wanting to believe we can rely on the factory food industry to supply us with nourishing food. Bill Maher cracked up his audience in his HBO stand-up special when he said, "We feed cows too sick to stand to people too fat to walk. And then you wonder why these diseases spring up. Mad cow and AIDS and ebola. You know nature, it doesn't ask a lot. It really doesn't. Don't grind up the cattle and feed them back to each other . . . not big requests."[25] This is an example of our ominously jovial "we are all in this together" attitude about our food chain. We laugh to cope, in part, because we don't believe we have alternatives.

The alternative to factory produced animal products are natural milk, meat, and eggs that come from well-treated animals, which are the same healthy historically consumed foods that produced the vibrant good health that Dr. Price documented throughout his research on indigenous peoples.

Another excellent source of protein and saturated fat is natural milk. Like saturated animal fat and polyunsaturated vegetable oils, there is much controversy and misconceptions about milk. Since the USDA's "Got Milk?" campaign, in which celebrities and luminaries—including Donna Shalala, former secretary of the U.S. Department of Health and Human Services—sport milk moustaches, millions of Americans have increased their intake of milk. To Americans, there is no other food that appears more comforting or healthy than a tall glass of frothy milk, even though studies dating from the early 1900s to the present demonstrate that factory milk is a contributing factor in the epidemic of allergies, asthma, precocious puberty, multiple sclerosis, and Type 1 diabetes, as well as degenerative diseases.[26]

CHAPTER 19

Factory Milk

ON MAY 10, 1611, a straggly band of fortune hunters watched as Sir Thomas Dale, the newly appointed governor of Jamestown, Virginia, disembarked at Jamestown Harbor. Four years earlier, the ships *Susan Constant, Godspeed,* and *Discovery* had brought these spying men, whose hopes of finding riches and a northeast water route to India had been systematically dashed by Algonquian attacks, disease, and starvation. Several ships had since arrived carrying provisions and hundreds of replacement settlers; thus the ranks of the Jamestown colonists had swelled and shrunk. Now the men observed as the ship's crew labored to bring one hundred cows to shore. Dazed and weak from the four-month sea voyage, the cows ambled into the pastures lured by tall native grasses. The arrival of milk cows spelled the beginning of prosperity in America's first permanent settlement.

Nine years later, in 1620 the Plymouth colonists arrived in Massachusetts. In the fall of 1621, the half who had survived the first year celebrated Thanksgiving on maize, seafood, and game. "Survived" being the operative word. By 1623, an observer wrote that the colonists were in "very low condition, many were ragged in aparell, and some little beter than halfe naked."[1] If not for the arrival of three heifers and a bull in March 1624 on the merchant ship *Charity*, the remaining Pilgrims would have likely perished too.

Similar accounts of milk cows saving the lives of early Americans are documented in each and every colony in sixteenth-century America. In the United States, since the early colonies, milk was a healthy, life-sustaining part of the American diet.[2] Back in the 1940s when Weston A. Price sent twenty thousand food samples back to America for analysis, he also sent milk samples, which he characterized as "the most efficient single food known."[3]

Natural milk was consumed in the United States until the War of 1812 with England, when whiskey shipments from the British West Indies abruptly halted.[4] To address this problem, distilleries sprang up, extracting alcohol from grain to produce their whiskey. Enterprising distillery owners, looking for a use for the chemically altered, acidic waste product known as "distillery slop," built dairies adjoining or in the basements of distilleries, and fed the waste product to cows. Now the cities had their whiskey and their "slop" or "swill" milk.

Distillery dairies were filthy hellholes, sullying the air with horrendous fumes. Eating steaming slop from a distillery is not the same thing to a cow as grazing in an open pasture, but cows are sweet, docile creatures that will ultimately eat anything put before them. Still cows—like humans kept in dungeons—succumbed to disease.

The unnatural swill feed lacked the life-sustaining nutrients necessary to maintain healthy metabolic processes and was foreign and toxic to bovine physiology. Thus the resulting milk lacked nutrients and was unfit for human consumption. Swill milk was doctored with starch, sugar, flour, chalk, and plaster of Paris. Milkers went about their duties with filthy hands and often came to work sick. As the swill milk business boomed, infant mortality rose, with babies dying of tuberculosis, diarrhea, typhoid, cholera, scarlet fever, and diphtheria.

In the 1860s, Louis Pasteur discovered that heating milk killed off pathogenic microorganisms that led to many infectious diseases. There were two courses of action the food industry could have taken to halt the spread of infectious diseases through swill milk; one was to clean up the filth in the dairy industry and initiate the production of pasture-fed, clean, nutrient-rich milk in the countryside to feed city dwellers. Instead, the industry continued to produce filthy milk from diseased, abused cows, and then scald the germs out of the milk.

Naturopathic physician Ron Schmid, author of *The Untold Story of Milk: Green Pastures, Contented Cows, and Raw Dairy Foods*, told me, "Given the sorry state of milk supplies in the early twentieth century, pasteurization prevented a lot of sickness and death. On the other hand, we didn't need to treat good, clean, healthy milk the same way we treated tainted, unsanitary, nutrient dead milk."[5]

What was not known in Pasteur's time is that the heat of pasteurization kills vitamin C, E, A, D_3 and B complex, diminishes calcium and other minerals, and makes them harder to absorb, as well as reducing the digestibility and lessening the nutritional value of protein. Most important, the heat of pasteurization destroys the enzymes in milk. The temperature at which substances feel too hot to touch—about 118 degrees Fahrenheit—is adequate to kill enzymes.

The ridding of enzymes from our food supply has been a major contributing factor to the downfall of American's health. Enzymes are essential to life because they are biochemical catalysts of cellular function both inside and outside of the cell. Without enzymes no biochemical activity would take place. Vitamins, minerals, and hormones cannot perform in the body without enzymes. The five thousand identified enzymes are divided into three categories. Metabolic enzymes enable all bodily processes and functions, including maintaining immune function. Digestive enzymes are manufactured in the pancreas to break down food. Enzymes in food jumpstart digestive processes when you eat.

Born in 1898, researcher Edward Howell devoted his life to

researching and promoting nutritional approaches to chronic illness. In his book *Food Enzymes for Health and Longevity*, he explained that eating foods that contain enzymes reduces the pancreas' need to produce its own digestive enzymes. If your pancreas is overtaxed during your lifetime because you are not providing your body with an adequate supply of enzymes in food, its function will decline. The length of your life depends on how fast your pancreatic enzyme-producing capacity is used up. If you place constant demand on your pancreas to produce enzymes to digest and process incoming dead food, you will die sooner than if you eat enzyme-rich food. That's why food enzymes are one key to staving off degenerative disease, slowing accelerated aging and promoting longevity. [6]

According to Dr. Schmid, although the belief took hold that we could pasteurize unhealthy milk and make it both safe to drink and healthy, the fact is that healthfulness of milk is determined by two factors: (one), the cow's diet and living conditions determine whether or not the cow is healthy; and (two), the health of the cow determines the nutritive quality of the milk.

The modern cow's diet and living conditions are not much better than a swill cow's of one hundred years ago. Modern dairy cows do not graze contentedly in pastures on farms like the precious cows I met on Dr. Schmid's farm. Today cows are housed in CAFOs where they live out their short lives tethered in stalls shoulder to shoulder in pens, standing in manure.

Modern milk cows' production is maximized by selective breeding, which has created cows with freakishly active pituitary glands that overproduce growth hormones that stimulate milk production. Selectively bred cows are highly stressed milk-producing machines that require massive amounts of species-inappropriate feed to fuel their aberrant metabolisms, as well as massive amounts of drugs to fix the health problems caused both by the feed and by the stressful environment. Milk production is further increased by 10 to 20 percent by injecting recombinant Bovine Growth Hormone (rBGH).

Confinement cows are fed soybean and grain feed, which are unnatural foods for ruminants (cud-chewing animals) that have four stomachs, designed to digest fibrous grasses, plants, and shrubs. Soybeans and grains lack the life-sustaining nutrients necessary to maintain healthy bovine metabolic processes. Grain-fed cows can become afflicted with a painful condition called subacute acidosis, requiring constant, low-level doses of antibiotics.[7] (And now we have ethanol plants springing up next to dairy farms where the corn mash byproduct is being fed to dairy cows—exactly like the swill cows of old.)

Soybeans and grains are grown with herbicides and pesticides or are genetically modified to resist pests and are grown with chemical fertilizers, which are toxic to bovine physiology and also migrate to a cow's milk. Aflatoxins are cancer-causing chemicals found in moldy grain and are secreted in the milk of grain-eating cows.[8]

Grains also cause mastitis (infection of the udders). Normal milk contains low levels of white blood cells that are shed from the secretory tissue during milking. A somatic cell count (SCC) determines whether milk contains a normal white blood cell count or a high count, signaling mastitis. An SCC level of 300,000 indicates mastitis, yet federal regulations allow the sale of milk with SCC levels of 750,000, which in simple terms means there's a lot of pus in your milk.[9] Government regulators deemed it okay as this milk will be pasteurized, and you will not be drinking live pus, but dead pus.

Because cows suffer health problems as a result of their stressful confinement and species-inappropriate diet, sixty-odd drugs are federally approved for use on dairy cows, including Penicillin G. Antimicrobial sulfonamides are suspected human carcinogens that taint milk. Antiworming agents also migrate to milk and are associated with bone marrow diseases and neurological disorders. Numerous nonapproved drugs are also used illegally. [10]

After milking this adulterated brew, pasteurization kills some of bad bacteria in milk and refrigeration keeps remaining bacteria from growing, but does not eradicate any of the contaminants; neither does ultra pasteurization although it eliminates the need for refrigeration before opening the carton, because it *sterilizes* milk.

The homogenization process breaks up butterfat globules into tiny particles, which keeps the milk "stirred up," so that the cream doesn't rise to the top, ostensibly making it more attractive to consumers. In recent years, a hypothesis has emerged suggesting that the sliced up fatty particles can abrade arterial walls, which results in attracting a protective coating of plaque. But the jury is still out on whether homogenized milk contributes to coronary artery disease. Still homogenization is for the convenience of the manufacturer. "When unhomogenized milk is transported in a tanker truck," Dr. Schmid said, "the cream rises to the top and it churns. The result is butter and buttermilk."

Modern milk suppliers are well aware of the fact that the heat of pasteurization kills vitamins and enzymes and changes the chemical composition of calcium and other minerals. Like swill milk that in the past was prettied up with chalk and other substances, today's milk is fortified with calcium and synthetic vitamins. As previously stated, Enig and Fallon point out that vitamin D_2 was yanked from our milk supply as it causes hardening of the arteries and softening of the bones. [11]

Milk suppliers can never duplicate nature's perfect ratio of nutrients and create a nutritious food by adding synthetic nutrients into weeks-old, pasteurized, denatured milk that contains high levels of contaminants and is the commingled product of thousands of cows. Like swill milk, factory milk lacks nutrients because it's produced by abused cows in mostly unsanitary conditions. Said Dr. Schmid, "The best we can expect from commercial milk is that it might support people until they begin to wear out and die at age fifty or sixty and they can go for ten or twenty years into the medical industry." [12]

So what does this milk do to us?

CHAPTER 20

Factory Milk Does a Body Bad

IN AN EPISODE of *Nip/Tuck*, Julia McNamara discovers a bloodstain in her eight-year-old daughter Annie's panties and realizes it's premenstrual spotting. To soften the blow of telling her the facts of life, Julia and a friend throw Annie a "Princess Menses" party attended by a gaggle of little girls dressed in flowing white dresses and tiaras. "She's barely out of pajamas with feet," says plastic surgeon Sean McNamara to his partner, Christian Troy. "How did this happen?"[1]

Millions of parents are asking that same question. Because today by age eight, nearly 15 percent of white girls and almost 50 percent of African-American girls experience breast development and/or pubic hair. One percent of American girls now show signs of puberty before the age of three. Nine year-old boys are experiencing penis and testicular maturation and pubic hair growth. It's only considered *precocious* puberty when a girl begins puberty earlier than seven, and a boy earlier than nine.[2]

Clearly there are many factors contributing to the rise of precocious puberty, one of which is thought to be chronic exposure to xenoestrogens, substances that have been found to mimic the actions of the hormone estrogen.

Michele L. Trankina, PhD, is a professor of biological sciences at St. Mary's University and clinical consulting nutritionist at the University of Texas Health Science Center in San Antonio. "Estrogens are hormones, which are made and used by both female and male bodies, to greater and lesser degrees," she told me. "Estrogens influence puberty, menstruation and pregnancy in women, as well as regulate the growth of bones, skin, and vital organs and tissues in both men and women."

According to Dr. Trankina, who has studied the effects of environmental xenoestrogens on our health, xenoestrogens are generated from a number of sources, including heating food in plastic; consuming fruits and vegetables grown with pesticides, herbicides, and chemical fertilizers; and consuming meat and dairy products from cows that were fed feed that contains pesticide, herbicide, and chemical fertilizer residues. "Xenoestrogens or 'estrogen mimics' bind to estrogen receptors and have essentially the same effect as natural estrogen, setting up the potential to wreck havoc on reproductive anatomy and physiology," Trankina said. "They are disruptors of endocrine function."

Dr. Trankina has suggested a link between the rise of precocious puberty and the combined influences of increased body fat and prolonged high xenoestrogen exposure. "Enhanced body fat implies reproductive readiness and signals the onset of puberty in both girls and boys. For girls, more body fat ensures that there is enough stored energy to support pregnancy and lactation. So it may be that excess body fat and exposure to estrogenic substances operate in concert to hasten puberty." Fat cells are known to produce estrogen and then continued chronic exposure to xenoestrogens "may add just enough added estrogen to exert the synergistic effect necessary to bring on puberty, much like the last drop of water causes a bucket to overflow."[3]

Since 1990, nearly 15 million new cancer cases have been diagnosed, with a new cancer diagnosed every thirty seconds. Breast, prostate, and colon cancers have risen the most dramatically in the past twenty years. One out of eight American women will develop breast cancer, and one out of nine men will develop prostate cancer. One in twenty (men and women) will develop colon cancer. Dr. Trankina links the rise in breast cancer, in part, to exposure to xenoestrogens. "Prolonged exposure to estrogen mimics can be tumor promoting." But could there also be a link between the rise of these cancers and the introduction twenty years ago of rBGH into our milk supply?

In 1980, this cheap variant of natural bovine growth hormone was created by Genentech, Inc., by inserting *E. coli* bacteria into the cow gene that creates bovine growth hormone. In 1981, Genentech sold the rights to recombinant Bovine Growth Hormone (rBGH) to Monsanto. In 1985, when Monsanto needed to conduct large-scale veterinarian trials on rBGH, the FDA approved of this study and also approved the sale of rBGH beef and milk from Monsanto's research herds and dairies to the public without disclosing the fact that the milk was obtained from rBGH treated cows. The FDA based its approval on extremely short-term (twenty-eight to ninety day) experiments in which rats were fed rBGH. Monsanto claimed the rats suffered no apparent ill effects so it was okay for humans to ingest rBGH milk. They neglected to mention details like thyroid cysts and changes to rats' prostate glands.[4]

FDA scientists who recognized the problems with the FDA approval process of Monsanto's trials were deemed potential whistle-blowers and treated with hostility, threats, and even fired.[5] Although a handful of FDA scientists resorted to anonymously protesting to Congress, the sale of rBGH meat and milk from Monsanto's research farms and ranches was ultimately green-lighted. So American families were hapless guinea pigs, consuming rBGH meat and milk.[6]

One problem couldn't be glossed over: the severe increased mastitis (infection of the udders), which required treatment with high levels of antibiotics. To address this problem, Margaret Miller, PhD, at the FDA pushed through a dramatic increase in the allowable levels of antibiotics in milk. Dairy farmers were then free to crank up antibiotic treatments of their rBGH cows and the heavily antibiotic-laced rBGH milk was then sold to an unsuspecting public.[7]

Antibiotics do not distinguish between harmful and healthy bacteria. So consuming antibiotics for long periods of time can severely disrupt the balance of your healthy intestinal bacteria, causing gastrointestinal and immune function problems as well as yeast overgrowth. Chronic antibiotic intake from milk and meat products can also result in the harmful bacteria in your body becoming resistant to the effects of prescription antibiotics.

Back in 1989, cancer expert Dr. Epstein (introduced on page 61), who is the author of the investigative journalist-oriented *Got (Genetically Engineered) Milk? The Monsanto BGH/BST Milk Wars Handbook*, was alerted to the use of rBGH by dairy farmers who came to him inquiring about consumer risks. Dr. Epstein began to analyze the scientific literature and to write about the dangers of rBGH. Although Monsanto has done everything in its power to keep the truth about rBGH from the public, Epstein has fought to reveal the truth. From time to time, he's had help from unexpected sources. "Over the last thirty years, people in agencies and industries have sent me confidential documents," he told me. "Sometimes they give me their names. Sometimes they don't."[8]

The first box containing extensive "company confidential" Monsanto files arrived anonymously, shortly after Epstein began his research into rBGH. The files detailed the extensive adverse health effects in cows treated with rBGH, including a high incidence of reproductive failure; cows injected with rBGH had much higher rates of infection and suffered from infertility, extreme weight loss, heat intolerance and lactational burnout, gastric ulcers, arthritis, and kidney and heart abnormalities. The files also documented the high level of rBGH in milk.

Although Dr. Epstein forwarded copies of these files to Congress, an investigation was launched, and Monsanto and the

FDA were charged with conspiring to manipulate critical health data, it was no more irritating than a buzzing gnat in the nostrils of Monsanto and the FDA. Ultimately cows continued to be treated with rBGH and that milk sold to the public.

By 1990, overwhelming scientific evidence demonstrated the health hazards of rBGH to both humans and cows. Incredibly, the FDA claimed "milk and meat from [rBGH] treated cows are safe and wholesome for human consumption."[9] What is true is that the injection of rBGH increases levels of a potent hormone called insulin-like growth factor-one (IGF-1), which is then passed to the cows' milk. Although natural cow's milk contains natural growth hormone—as does human breast milk—Dr. Epstein writes that rBGH milk is "supercharged with high levels of abnormally potent IGF-1, up to ten times the levels in natural milk and over ten times more potent." Worse is that when rBGH milk is pasteurized, IGF-1 increases by up to 70 percent.

When humans drink IGF-1 milk, the hormone is absorbed through the gastrointestinal tract (and infants' gastrointestinal tracts are much more permeable than adults). Because IGF-1 causes cells to divide and because IGF-1 also behaves like insulin—another growth factor—when it is absorbed into the bloodstream, it can exert rapid-cell growth on colon, breast, and prostate cells. IGF-1 also blocks the programmed self-destruction of cancer cells and enhances their growth and invasiveness. Numerous studies have demonstrated that unnatural levels of IGF-1 dramatically increases your risk of developing breast, prostate, lung, colon, and gastrointestinal cancers.[10]

Nevertheless, in February 1994, the FDA granted approval for general use of rBGH and pushed through regulatory labeling guidelines, composed by Dr. Margaret Miller and Deputy FDA Commissioner Michael Taylor. The guidelines effectively *banned* the labeling of rBGH milk as "containing rBGH" or even "rBGH free" so that consumers would not be alerted to the fact that they were consuming rBGH milk—*or even given the choice.*[11]

These public servants were not focused with single-minded passion on your health or the welfare of your children. Miller, for example, was the laboratory supervisor at Monsanto and left the biotech firm to be deputy director of human food safety at the FDA where she was still publishing papers for Monsanto when she wrote the bovine growth hormone guidelines. Taylor was the former chief counsel for the International Food Biotechnology Counsel and Monsanto. Taylor's FDA guidelines were used by his former law firm to sue dairies that dared to label their dairy products "rBGH-free."[12] After the fact, Michael Friedman, MD, who was deputy commissioner of the FDA from 1995 to 1999, went on to a position as the head of clinical research at Monsanto Co.'s GD Searle & Co. unit, which produces rBGH.[13]

Three concerned FDA scientists, Joseph Settepani, Alexander Apostolou, and Richard Burroughs, made numerous attempts to thwart the rBGH approval process but were stymied by internal intrigue, hostility, and threats. A month after the FDA approval of rBGH, they resorted to writing an anonymous letter to members of Congress. "We are afraid to speak openly about the situation because of retribution from our director, Dr. Robert Livingston," they wrote. "Dr. Livingston openly harasses anyone who states an opinion in opposition to his."[14]

Monsanto continued raking in the dough, and Americans unwittingly glugged rBGH milk. Meanwhile, by 1999, Canada banned the use of rBGH. That same year, the Codex Alimentarius Commission—the UN Food Safety agency that represents 101 nations—unanimously ruled in favor of maintaining the 1992 European moratorium on Monsanto's rBGH milk.[15]

The American Medical Association (AMA) has dismissed rBGH critics as "fringe groups." The American Cancer Society (ACS) has trivialized the link between IGF-1 and cancer, and come out in support of the use of rBGH.[16] And the FDA persists in their claims that rBGH milk is safe and wholesome. (The AMA is a partnership of physicians and professional associations dedicated to promoting the art and science of medicine and the betterment of public health, and the ACS is a national, voluntary cancer organization founded to eliminate cancer.)

Dr. Epstein added that the ACS has in the neighborhood of 340 "Excalibur industry donors" that each donate more than $100,000 per year. "Key amongst them are the techno chemical industries and agribusiness," Dr. Epstein told me. "The American Cancer Society is more interested in accumulating wealth than savings lives. Their CEOs have high salaries. They have a billion dollars of cash assets in reserves. They have major internal conflicts of interests. The National Cancer Institute and the American Cancer Society fail in their mandated responsibility to inform the public of avoidable risks of cancer." (The NCI is a government agency created for cancer research and education.)

Dr. Epstein is an outspoken critic of cancer organizations' focus on cancer drugs rather than prevention. "The National Cancer Institute's budget has increased from 200 million in 1971 to 4.6 billion today," he said. "Paralleling this increase is the increasing incidence of non-smoking cancers. Very little money is spent on preventing cancer. The overwhelming emphasis of the National Cancer Institute is producing miracle drugs that possibly increase life expectancy by a month or two."

It appears that quite a few people (including companies that make chemotherapy drugs) are making an awful lot of money from Americans' consumption of rBGH milk.

Unlike factory milk, natural milk does not contain carcinogenic contaminants. When I began researching this book, I had not had a glass of milk in ten years—something that has radically changed since I met Mark McAfee, owner of Organic Pastures in Fresno, California.

CHAPTER 21

Natural Milk to the Rescue

MARK MCAFEE GIVES the impression of being someone you could trust with your life.[1] A certified paramedic for sixteen years in Fresno, running over fourteen thousand service calls, McAfee said, "It was a constant adrenaline rush dealing with tragic life-changing events of strangers." As paramedic of the year in 1994, Mark was at the top of his game. "I said to myself, I've saved as many lives, and delivered as many babies—I want to leave it there and do something else for the rest of my life." Mark had grown up on a farm. "It was in my blood," he said. Mark and his wife, Blaine, decided to take over his father's dairy farm and manage it organically. "I took my ability to be a student and learned organic production and the clinical health benefits raw milk can bring people, which are tremendous."

Today, Organic Pastures is the only certified raw dairy in California. It produces 100 percent organic raw milk and dairy products. The dairy has 400 cows which they milk, using a Grade A approved, 60,000 pound mobile milk barn—the only one of its kind in North America. The mobile barn is moved from pasture to pasture weekly, making it possible to milk 100 cows an hour, eliminating the necessity for manure lagoons or herding the cows into concrete-floored barns for milking.

Milk is chilled to 36 degrees Fahrenheit within thirty seconds of milking. Prior to bottling, the raw milk is tested to assure it exceeds the standards of the California Department of Food and Agriculture (CDFA). (The CDFA is a state agency that works to ensure the safety and quality of food.) "The law states that milk after pasteurization must have less than 15,000 bacteria per milliliter," Mark said "Organic Pastures raw milk averages about 1,500 bacteria per milliliter. In four years of intensive testing by the CDFA, Organic Pastures' milk has never once tested positive for *Salmonella, Listeria monocytogenes* or *E. coli O157:H7.*"

Buddy, Rachel, Mousey, Mabel, and Teresa are some of the Organic Pastures' cows. To get healthy, clean milk, Mark said, "You have to care for cows like family. My wife sings to them and walks around and talks to them. The health of milk has everything to do with the way the cow is treated. You have to follow Mother Nature's blueprint. A cow would never chose to stand on concrete or next to hundreds of other cows in a big manure pile. She will go find a luscious pasture to mingle with a small group of cows and find something green to eat." Organic Pastures has kept their herds fairly small and always have the cows on a lush green environment. Cows are grazed progressively, meaning that when a pasture gets depleted, cows are moved to fresh pastures, which are irrigated year round.

Organic Pastures doesn't own, purchase, or breed selectively bred cows. A selectively bred cow could not survive in a pasture-grazing dairy, McAfee said. "Because selectively bred cows need a specialized high protein, high concentrated diet or they will waste away and die." A selectively bred cow produces up to 100 gallons of milk per day. A strictly grass-fed dairy cow produces up to a gallon and a half of milk per day. "It's about striking a balance with the organic matter cows would normally eat and added nutrition to slightly increase milk supply."

Supplementation ups milk production to 4 to 6 gallons per day. To get that slight increase in milk production, Organic Pastures cows are fed 5 pounds of organic corn and up to 25 pounds of organic alfalfa per day are added to their 30 to 40 pounds or so of pasture grass. In winter, cows are fed 5 to 10 pounds of organic hay.

In addition to Dr. Price's ten years of research on the benefits of fats such as whole, natural milk, there are numerous studies that prove the nutritional benefits of organic, raw, grass-fed milk, including those associated with vitamin D_3.[2]

In an article in *Cancer Causes and Control*, Edward Giovannucci, PhD associate professor of nutrition and epidemiology at the Harvard School of Public Health, reviewed studies that illustrated that vitamin D could prevent or slow the progression of cancer and metastasis. Unfortunately, most Americans are vitamin D deficient. Dr. Giovannucci said, "Historically, people spent a lot more time outdoors (e.g., farming). Vitamin D deficiency has become an issue with industrialization (tall buildings, indoor jobs, pollution). It is probably fair to say in some individuals, sunscreen has made matters worse. Spending most of time indoors is the main factor [in vitamin D deficiencies]. People who exercise outdoors (even walking) have higher vitamin D levels."[3]

It's not that simple to get enough vitamin D. According to Giovannucci, "To get optimal benefit from dietary intake would probably mean consuming about 2,000 international units per day. However, most vitamin D supplements provide 400 units or less. Our estimates regarding the threshold of vitamin D toxicity are unreasonably low and based on old, poorly designed studies. The average doctor will scare patients away from taking 2,000 units a day, calling that toxic. Actually it seems there is almost zero potential for vitamin D toxicity at that level."[4]

While there is no substitute for sun exposure—"One hundred glasses of milk equals twenty minutes on the beach on a sunny day," said Dr. Giovannucci, "since people tend to be low in vitamin D, any increment from the diet is helpful." Adding natural milk and dairy products to your diet can help you get that incremental supplementation of vitamin D. (Aside from natural milk and butter, vitamin D is available in egg yolks, cod liver oil, sardines, and organ meats.) Whole, raw milk contains butterfat with vitamins A and D_3 necessary for the assimilation of calcium and protein. Natural vitamin D_3 prevents autoimmune diseases such as multiple sclerosis and rheumatoid arthritis and prevents osteoporosis. Natural vitamin D_3 is also linked to improvement in mood and relieving symptoms of depression.

Butterfat is also the richest known source of conjugated linoleic acid (CLA), which, as stated earlier, reduces cancer and atherosclerosis risk, as well as increases metabolic rate and burns fat.[5]

Raw milk products also contain enzymes, without which life cannot be sustained. Because pasteurization kills enzymes, strain is put on the pancreas to produce the enzymes to digest it. Without natural enzymes in milk, lactose is indigestible for many people. Raw milk from a strictly grass-fed cow is also extremely helpful for people with gastrointestinal problems, even for people who think they are lactose intolerant because raw milk contains the lactase enzyme to help digest lactose. "My lactose intolerant patients ease raw milk into their diets to build up the enzymes to digest it," said naturopathic physician Dr. Ron Schmid. Raw milk and its by-products are also great alternatives for vegetarians as raw milk provides complete proteins.

In *Ethan Frome* by Edith Wharton, the drama of the star-crossed lovers Ethan and Mattie revolved around pickles—when Ethan's wife, Zeena, found the broken pickle dish, she immediately suspected their affair. The historical human diet contained fermented, enzymatic rich foods such as pickles, sauerkraut, live beer, whole milk, ice cream (made without heat), cream, yogurt, cheese, cottage cheese, and kefir. "Sour" and clabbered milk were eaten as digestives. Sour milk is made by allowing milk to ferment (curdle) at a warm temperature. This occurs when "good" bacterial flora such as *lactobacillus acidophilus* are present. However, pasteurization destroys the good bacterial flora. If pasteurized milk is not constantly refrigerated, undesirable lactophilic germs quickly multiply which produce acids that cause milk to putrefy. That's why you gag sour (rotten) milk into the sink after swigging out of the milk carton.

For an optimal healing approach, an enzyme-rich food should be incorporated with every meal. The easiest, of course, is a glass of natural raw milk.

Despite well-known benefits, raw milk has been unilaterally rejected by our medical community and government because it is thought to be dirty. The FDA's Web site states, "Pasteurization, since its adoption in the early 1900s, has been credited with dramatically reducing illness and death caused by contaminated milk. But today, some people are passing up pasteurized milk for what they claim is tastier and healthier 'raw milk.' Public health officials couldn't disagree more. Drinking raw (untreated) milk or eating raw milk products is 'like playing Russian roulette with your health,' says John Sheehan, director of the [FDA's] Division of Dairy and Egg Safety. 'We see a number of cases of foodborne illness every year related to the consumption of raw milk.' More than 300 people in the United States got sick from drinking raw milk or eating cheese made from raw milk in 2001, and nearly 200 became ill from these products in 2002, according to the Centers for Disease Control and Prevention [CDC]."[6]

I do not doubt that these are cases of foodborne illness connected to drinking raw milk. Not everyone is as careful as Mark McAfee and that is why he urges caution. The fact is that our food supply is dirty. Researchers estimate that 76 million illnesses, 325,000 hospitalizations, and 5,000 deaths occur in the United States every year as a result of food poisoning.[7] That said, the potential for contamination in factory meat is well documented and virtually ignored by our government. Eric Schlosser, author of *Fast Food Nation,* has written extensively about the centralization and industrialization of our food supply system, which has increased food-borne illnesses, has demonstrated how fastfood chains and agribusinesses have thwarted effective government regulation, and how federal agencies that are supposed to regulate these companies have fallen under their control.[8]

Consuming highly government regulated contaminant-free raw milk that contains nature's perfect ratio of nutrients including enzymes, which was produced by small herds of happy cows that are pasture grazed on species appropriate food, tested regularly, and milked with sanitary milking machines that transport the milk in sanitary stainless steel tanks and refrigerated trucks, strikes me as infinitely less hazardless than consuming nongovernment regulated, fecal-, vomit-, pus-, urine-, chemical-, and hormone-tainted, nutrient-lacking meat from abused confinement animals.

Allowing cows to freely roam in their natural pasture environment, munching species appropriate grass, breathing fresh air, and drinking clean water produces healthy, clean milk fit for human consumption. Healthy, clean raw milk contains beneficial flora, which inhabit your intestines, preventing disease-causing bacteria from multiplying in your body. Correspondingly, when cows are pasture grazed in clean environments, bacterial problems in the cows do not arise, do not arise as often, or are often self-corrected. In a recent study, calves that had tested positively for *E. coli* 0157:H7 were divided into two groups. One group was sequestered in a barn, and the other group was set free to graze in a pasture. During a six-month testing period, the pasture calves showed no signs of 0157:H7. Meanwhile, every barn calf tested positive.[9]

If you cannot obtain raw milk, there are many organic milk suppliers who operate humane dairies and pasture graze their cows, although all organic milk is pasteurized and often ultra pasteurized (sterilized of enzymes as well as bad and good bacteria). Keep in mind that just because milk is "organic" doesn't mean their cows were treated humanely or fed species-appropriate food. Just like the food industry–speak that has brought us factory food under the guise of "natural," the same twisted semantics are now bringing us pseudo "organic" milk.

You can find out if your state allows the sale of raw milk on www.realmilk.com. In states that have outlawed raw milk sales, it's possible to purchase a share in a cow from which you are legally allowed to share in its milk production. However, just because someone has a backyard cow doesn't mean that they are properly versed in handling raw milk. I asked Mark for some guidelines. "There are a few things to look for if a family is going to source their milk locally. I suggest looking at the standards found at www.rawusa.org. Raw milk can be very safe if given a modicum of Mother Nature's care mixed with a little testing technology."

Natural milk, meat, and eggs that come from well-treated animals are healthy historically consumed foods that produce the vibrant good health that Dr. Price documented throughout his research on indigenous peoples. On a balanced diet of real, organically produced food, including natural animal products, Americans could quell our hysterical hunger, heal from malnutrition, and thus become as tall, attractive, cheerful, robust, sexy, and fertile, and as free from mental, dental, and degenerative diseases as our genetics predispose us to be. But we have been actually discouraged from eating natural foods. The vendetta against raw milk is one example.

Then there is the larger issue of corporate agribusiness, which has gobbled up all federal farm subsidies so that small farmers and ranchers have been driven out of business and off their lands, making natural food either very hard to find or more expensive than factory food. As a result, we have been indirectly encouraged to consume the diseased, drug-and hormone-infused animal products that are produced in CAFOs by these mega corporations.

In the fall of 2006, an outbreak of the deadly strain of *E. Coli* 0157:H7 that sickened over one hundred people and killed one was linked to eating bagged spinach. This outbreak could have easily been prevented had the government cleaned up the factory cattle industry. Since factory cattle are fed soybean and grain feed, which are unnatural foods for ruminants, rather than their natural diet of grass and shrubs, they develop high levels of bacteria in their gut, including *E. Coli* which spreads to water tables of surrounding farms. The remedy for this is switching cattle from an unnatural diet of grains to a natural diet of grass and shrubs.

Immediately following this outbreak, four children were diagnosed with *E. Coli* 0157:H7, and this time the government pointed fingers at Organic Pastures. The dairy voluntarily recalled all of their milk products but was ultimately exonerated when all of their milk items tested negative for *E. Coli* 0157:H7. It seems the children were infected through other sources, and the likely culprit was undercooked factory meat.

While the government endeavors to prevent us from drinking natural milk, there are health professionals who discourage the consumption of milk in general. The standard argument is that humans are the only species to drink milk past infancy and the only species to drink the milk of other species. I have never seen back up research for those statements. Yet as I've said, I've seen 1,000-pound steers nursing from their mothers and cats and dogs lap saucers of cow and goat milk, and heard many stories about wild animals domesticated by humans and raised and nursed by family cats and dogs.

Another argument is that animal milk was not a food of hunter gatherers and thus is too "new" for modern humans to have adapted to. It's worth pondering if hunter gathers may have on occasion killed a lactating female animal and consumed the milk from the mammary glands. It seems highly likely if hunter gatherers were primarily concerned with eating as many calories per day as possible that nothing would go to waste, especially not a delicious food that required no cooking. We do know that once easy picking-food supplies began to dwindle and hunter gatherers began to dabble in domesticating plants and animals for food, that animals that produced milk were of immediate interest. According to Jared Diamond in *Guns, Germs, and Steel: The Fates of Human Societies*, a domesticated animal is defined as one whose breeding and food supply are controlled by humans. Writes Diamond, "Milked mammals include the cow, sheep, goat, horse, reindeer, water buffalo, yak, and Arabian and Bactrian camels. Those mammals thereby yield several times more calories over their lifetime than if they were just slaughtered and consumed as meat."[10] So we have to ask ourselves is ten thousand years too short of a time for humans to become adapted to a "new" food? More important, what have we done to that food? If it's natural and wholesome should we consume it?

In the game of thimblerig—also known as the shell game—a swindler uses sleight of hand to shuffle an object between three cups. The player must then guess the location of the object. But the game is always rigged to defraud. Since the year 1900, an unhealthy symbiotic relationship has developed between our medical establishment, government, the food, diet, and pharmaceutical industries, and us, their fat, sick customers. We have been encouraged to consume the profit rich products made with laboratory concocted ingredients like processed refined white sugar, refined grains, high fructose corn syrup, MSG, aspartame, industrially processed soy, and processed polyunsaturated fats, as well as factory animal products. Like shell game players, Americans believe the promises of good health, beauty, and satisfaction issued about these substances. But since these products both lack the life-sustaining nutrients necessary to maintain healthy metabolic processes and are mostly foreign and toxic to human physiology, we end up fat and sick. Lo and behold, the diet and drug industries then profit by selling us diet products and drugs.

And few seem to notice the sleight of hand.

VI

Dieting is Only Making Matters Worse

CHAPTER 22

The Malnutrition of Low-Calorie Dieting

IN GREEK MYTHOLOGY, Sisyphus was a heartless king of Corinth condemned for eternity to roll a boulder up a hill only to have it roll back down just before he reached the top. Sisyphus's plight is analogous to dieting. Because every time you diet, you fail and must diet again. The main problem with diet books, programs, systems, products, and factory-made diet foods is that the focus is on losing "weight" through starvation (dieting). But no matter how hard you try to reach a weight loss goal by starvation, you will end up failing. Although the weight-loss-by-starvation failure rate is high—we've rolled that same boulder up the hill many times—like Sisyphus, we get up and do it again.

Dieting is a modern aberration that perpetuates malnutrition. And all you have to do is turn on the TV night or day to see how much money there is to be made by keeping us fat.

A few years ago, my husband John and I stayed at a resort in the Dominican Republic. At breakfast, I watched an overweight American family at a nearby table binge on white bread rolls, Cokes, and coffee while waiting for their pancakes and syrup to arrive. Current conventional wisdom points at the volume of food people consume as the reason people are overweight and sick. If only we had better portion control. In 1960, a serving of McDonald's fries contained 200 calories; prior to this writing, a supersized portion contained 610 calories. (Morgan Spurlock's 2004 Sundance Film Festival award-winning documentary *Super Size Me,* which brought worldwide attention to the deleterious effects of eating an exclusive diet of McDonald's, shamed McDonald's into phasing out some of their supersize products.) Today diet experts urge people to eat less fast food, fewer fries, and smaller portions of factory foods. Even Dr. Phil said in his book *The Ultimate Weight Solution,* "Another way to decrease your exposure to foods you buy for your kids is to purchase these foods in smaller packages. Rather than get a jumbo sack of chips that you're likely to scarf down in one sitting, why not buy smaller single-serving sizes? With this approach, you've got automatic portion control."[1]

Are we really to believe that the vacationing family would reduce body fat and maintain a healthy weight by simply eating smaller portions of Coke, white bread rolls, and pancakes? Or as Dr. Phil suggests, smaller bags of chips?

Low-calorie dieting has been around the longest, and it makes sense intuitively. Most physicians firmly believe in the calorie in/ calorie out theory. We are told that you must restrict 3,600 calories, or 515 calories per day to lose one pound per week. Despite recent low-fat and low-carb tangents, Americans will always return to counting calories.

One hundred years ago, a hardworking man ate 6,000 to 6,500 calories and a hardworking woman ate 4,000 to 4,500 calories per day. Today an average woman needs 2,000 to 2,500 calories and an average man needs 2,500 to 2,800 calories. On the first day of the best-selling, low-calorie *South Beach Diet,* by my calculation, you're allowed 1,167 calories, which is 800 to 1,333 calories less per day than an average woman needs, and 1,333 to 1,163 less calories than the average man needs for optimal metabolic function. Still, you may be convinced that a low-calorie diet is the way to weight loss, because you have heard people say, "I lost thirty pounds on *The South Beach Diet!*" But losing weight is not the end of the story. It's what happens next that you need to consider. Because empirical evidence has demonstrated that low-calorie dieting does not work in the long term.

There are five reasons why a low-calorie diet is counterproductive to weight management. The first reason is that human beings in the twenty-first century have the same physiology as our Paleolithic ancestors. In prehistoric times food was not always plentiful. People gorged when they had food, then went without eating when food was scarce. Prehistoric human physiology evolved an "insulin-directed" fat-storage system enabling them to survive to this "feast and famine" lifestyle. The hormone insulin, which is secreted from the pancreas when food is eaten, directs nutrients into the cells. In times of famine, prehistoric humans' pancreases adjusted, so the next time they gorged during a plentiful season, their insulin secretions were higher and more food could be stored as fat.

Twenty-first century humans have this exact same fat-storage system. That means if you deprive your body of food it will perceive this deprivation as a time of famine and will adjust your insulin output so that, when you break your diet, more insulin will be secreted as a response to incoming food and more of what you eat will be stored as fat.

The second reason low-calorie dieting fails is that it slows down your metabolism, leaving you with a new metabolic set point for calorie consumption. In German concentration camps during WWII, prisoners were fed subsistence diets ranging from 600 to 1,700 calories per day (1,700 calories applied to circumstances, such as hard labor, when it was useful to keep people alive). In Vietnamese POW camps, prisoners were fed between 300 and 1,000 calories per day. Many survived by eating rats and insects. Concentration camp survivors and POWs were emaciated when the camps were liberated at the end of the wars, but survivors subsequently suffered a greater tendency toward obesity due to enforced metabolic slowdown.[2]

This is how metabolic slowdown occurs: When you eat a low-calorie diet, the meager fuel is quickly used up. Your brain needs an ongoing drip of sugar or you will lapse into a coma and die, and so it demands that you eat again. Your body keeps a ready supply of glycogen (sugar) stored in your liver and muscles to use to satisfy your brain and draw upon for fuel. But these glycogen stores are quickly used up. (Because glycogen is heavy, you can see a drop in your weight of up to ten pounds in one week.) When your glycogen stores are gone, your liver struggles to regulate the blood-sugar supply to your brain.

And so your adrenal glands work overtime to secrete the stress hormone cortisol, which breaks down bones and muscles to get the sugar (fuel) and amino acids (proteins for repair and rebuilding) that your body needs. As a protective measure to prevent catastrophic muscle and bone mass destruction, your thyroid downregulates your metabolic rate. By the time you break your low-calorie diet, you have less lean body mass and a lower metabolism (set point).

Muscle mass is the backbone of your metabolic rate. The more muscle mass you have, the higher your metabolic rate, and the less muscle mass the lower your metabolic rate. Every time you low-calorie diet, your body is a more effective fat storing machine. By simply resuming a normal diet, you will put on more weight than you lost.

Today many Americans eat a subsistence diet of less than 1,500 calories a day—even when they are not actually dieting. When they have that small bag of chips, it all goes to their butts, bellies, and thighs. Those who follow *The South Beach Diet,* after a period of time, will have an upregulated insulin response and a downregulated metabolic set point. So losing weight on a low-calorie diet is great if you want to eat that way for the rest of your life.

The third reason low-calorie diets fail is because starvation can provoke a binge response. Without adequate food, your neurotransmitters cannot replenish. To get through the day, dieters often resort to using stimulants (coffee, diet drinks, tobacco products, alcohol, OTC and prescription diet pills, as well as recreational drugs). Using stimulants may give your brain enough of a boost to resist powerful messages to EAT. But ultimately you will have to eat again and then you may binge. People who have suffered from starvation (from wartime food shortages, as prisoners of war, from being marooned or shipwrecked), or those who have imposed starvation on themselves (anorexics and volunteers in semistarvation experiments) suffer from uncontrollable urges to binge and have a greater tendency toward obesity.[3]

In one study, twenty- to thirty-three-year-old men ate 1,570 calories a day for six months (more calories than I calculated in *The South Beach Diet* meal plans). When the volunteers were then given unrestricted amounts of food, researchers noted extremely aberrant eating behaviors, such as volunteers had voracious appetites followed by large and rapid food intake; they exhibited lack of control and distress over amounts eaten; they complained of hunger despite huge meals; they believed that eating "triggered" hunger; they suffered from cravings and obsession with food, as well as secrecy and defensiveness over food; they had a new preoccupation with body shape and weight; they scavenged or ate from garbage containers; they stole, hid, hoarded food and manipulated others for food; they made bizarre mixtures of food; they ate unpalatable and inappropriate food (raw meat, scraps); they used excessive spicing and flavoring; they exhibited poor table manners (licking knives and bottle lids, collecting crumbs, gnawing at bones); they preferred to eat in isolation; they induced vomiting or ate until they vomited; they suffered self-loathing; they took drastic measures to resist binges; they relapsed into binge eating despite attempts to rehabilitate them.[4]

These behaviors are not a result of weak character but rather biological programming that is inherent in us as a survival mechanism. The experience of starvation compels us to binge in an attempt to provide our brains with fuel and our bodies with a fresh supply of nutrients necessary to heal from malnutrition.

The fourth reason low-calorie diets ultimately fail is that, although the United States is the richest country in the world, the majority of our citizens are suffering from malnutrition, especially if they are obese. Our factory food diet is viewed as a period of starvation to our bodies. Some people even attempt to *diet* on fast food and you will see these diets in magazines that target young women like *Glamour* that featured a "Fast-Food Diet" in its "Health & Food" section no less: Breakfast: McDonald's Fruit 'n Yogurt Parfait, English muffin, pack of jam: 350 calories. Lunch: Wendy's small chili, baked potato, one packet of Country Crock spread: 540 calories. Dinner: KFC Original Recipe chicken breast (no skin), large corn on the cob, baked beans: 520 calories. Total 1,410 calories.

Then there are diet factory foods such as the Special K challenge, a starvation diet that promises you will lose six pounds in two weeks by eating two bowls of their product every day—and now we have South Beach Diet cereal. Weight Watcher's, Jenny Craig, and Nutrasystem make industrialized meals that are devoid of enzymes and are otherwise nutritionally dead. These are but a few examples of the fake diet foods you can eat to perpetuate malnutrition.

A persistent state of malnutrition from eating factory food keeps Americans hysterically bingeing, obsessing, and ever seeking satiety. If you begin a low-calorie diet while in a malnourished state, you are beginning the diet with a preconditioned low metabolism, hormone imbalances, and other health issues. There's no way your body is letting go of your fat stores if your life is in danger. The reason is that we are hardwired for survival. This inherent programming to survive is the fifth reason dieting fails. Our bodies are programmed to hold onto fat cells in case we need that fat to survive in an emergency famine in the future.

In an interview on *Inside the Actors Studio*, Russell Crowe told James Lipton how bulking up forty-four pounds to play the real life tobacco industry whistle-blower Jeffrey Wigand for the movie *The Insider* ruined his metabolism for life. "I must have been clearing 235, 240, or something like that at the time. I'm only, like I said, five-eleven and a half and a bit, so that looks gigantic on me. But the one thing is my metabolism has never been the same since I did that film. Now I always have this incredible uphill battle."[5]

Crowe, who fattened up on cheeseburgers and beer, experienced an accelerated version of what many factory food–eating Americans are going through today. Getting fat on factory food bulks up fat cells, and your body does not like to let go of fat once it's onboard. Fat cells have just recently been recently recognized by the scientific community as something other than inert blobs. Fat cells are now recognized to behave like endocrine organs that secrete hormones, but scientists have yet to unlock their mysteries and how their hormones affect our metabolisms.

One clue to fat retention may lie in our factory food diet. When your body is confronted with a steady influx of toxins, those (fat soluble) toxins have to be stored away somewhere as your body cannot have toxins floating around in your bloodstream. So your body must retain fat cells as storage repositories. To convince your body that it's okay to let go of fat cells, you have to provide reassurance that there will be no more incoming poison. The more of a purist you are about eating organic, real food, the better your chances of losing fat.

I don't fault people for being obese, and I don't fault obese people for resorting to extreme measures, such as gastric bypass surgery. I fault the FDA for allowing purveyors of factory food the freedom to inundate our food supply with unhealthy, fattening, addicting substances that have created a population of neurotransmitter imbalanced, hysterically hungry people and then for allowing the diet industry to perpetuate malnutrition. When a person becomes morbidly obese there is often no turning back and they have to have some recourse or their lives are virtually over, and so some resort to gastric bypass surgery.

Obesity is a complicated problem. Fifty years ago, Adele Davis wrote, "To say that obesity is caused merely by consuming too many calories is like saying that the only cause of the American Revolution was the Boston Tea Party."[7] But it makes sense that factory food is the *primary reason* for obesity as this is the first time in history that humans have experienced this level of obesity. Often people are fat and even obese by eating the same amount of calories of factory food as thin individuals who eat real food. Sweets, soft drinks, and alcoholic beverages make up almost 25 percent of all calories eaten by Americans, 5 percent is comprised of salty snacks and fruit-flavored beverages, and 10 percent is bread, rolls, and crackers. That means 40 percent of our intake is garbage to our bodies.[8] What many Americans don't understand is that it's not the volume that is making us fat as much as it is what is actually being ingested.

I have a number of friends from foreign countries who gained weight when they came to the United States (or Canada) and ate factory food. Pedro from Brazil came to the United States as a fifteen-year-old exchange student in 1972 and gained thirty-three pounds in five months. When he returned to Brazil, he naturally lost the weight not by dieting, but by simply going back to eating the traditional Brazilian diet. John's French godson Hadrian went to college in Canada in 2003 where he lived around the corner from a McDonald's. He returned to Paris thirty pounds heavier, but lost it all and then some by simply eating the typical French diet. Fumiko from Japan came to the United States at age seventeen in 1968 to attend boarding school. She gained twenty pounds in ten months, but she too naturally lost the weight when she returned to Japan, not by dieting, but by eating the traditional real food Japanese diet. Today Fumiko is the dean of a woman's college in Tokyo. She told me, "One of my students who studied at our Boston campus gained twenty-eight and a half pounds in four months. The average weight gain among our girls who study in the United States is about nine pounds. But immediately after they return to Japan, they go back to their previous weight without dieting."

Instead of ridding our culture of factory food and providing real food abundantly, affordably, and conveniently, our government has now agreed to allow "obesity" as a Medicare diagnosis, which paves the way for more people to turn to the surgeon's scalpel in a desperate attempt to "fix" their obesity. In his book *Complications: A Surgeon's Notes on an Imperfect Science*, Atul Gawande, a surgical resident and staff writer on medicine and science for *The New Yorker* recounted a "successful" gastric bypass story in which he writes, "[The patient] was concerned about the possible long-term effects of nutritional deficiencies (for which patients are instructed to take a daily multivitamin)."[9]

Gastric bypass leaves patients with stomachs the size of a walnut. More than one bite of food initially will cause them to become violently nauseous and eating more will result in vomiting. When a person signs on for gastric bypass, it means voluntarily submitting to a procedure that will enforce starvation. In an attempt to supply the body with the nutrients it needs for 24/7/365 repair of cells, tissues and bones, and for replenishing hormones, neurotransmitters and so on, the patient is advised to take a daily multivitamin.

In a perfect world, we could take the $25–$30,000 that each gastric bypass surgery costs, and instead we'd sequester obese people in "rehab" facilities where they would get balanced meals of real food, any necessary hormone replacement, nutraceuticals (natural nutrients from plants that, when taken in specific doses, can have positive therapeutic effects), and other high-quality dietary supplements, exercise, emotional therapy, and lessons in shopping and preparing real food, so that, after one year, they would come out with balanced hormone levels, healed on the inside and out. Instead, we slice and dice their gastrointestinal track and send them home to starve to death on less factory food than they would normally eat. One year later, they are emaciated down to an acceptable weight, but God knows what has happened to their internal organs.

Anyone who is going to undergo gastric bypass would be wise to develop a relationship with a qualified clinical nutritionist who is capable of planning a nutrient dense meal plan of real food, so that starvation can be achieved in the healthiest way possible, as bizarre as that sounds.

Your doctor may tell you that all of this is nonsense, as studies on mice, rats, monkeys, and even worms and protozoa (the smallest, single-cell animal) have proven that extreme low-calorie diets extend lifespan as much as 50 percent. In humans, nutrient-dense calorie restrictive diets are believed to reduce the risk for cancer, diabetes, and atherosclerosis. Calorie restriction is said to reduce body weight, blood pressure, cholesterol, and glucose—factors that are all associated with good health and longer life. A number of hypotheses have been floated as to why calorie restriction provides greater life expectancy in studies, but so far no one knows for sure.[10]

However, problems associated with extreme calorie restriction are feeling cold, dwelling on food, including engaging in obsessive behaviors, temporary loss of energy, decreased sex drive, feeling socially isolated, and, in women, the resulting weight loss can affect fertility and increase the risk of developing osteopenia (bone loss) leading to osteoporosis, as well as loss of muscle mass.[11] These are all symptoms of malnutrition.

There's a great scene in the movie *The Truth About Cats and Dogs*, in which the thin, gorgeous Noelle muses that she doesn't know what's inside of her since she never eats anything. Most people don't give much thought about what their bodies are made out of. Eating real food has several purposes. First, your brain needs a constant drip of sugar (fuel), your body needs an ongoing supply of fats and proteins to build lean body mass on a cellular level, as well as essential amino acids, essential fatty acids, vitamins, minerals, and enzymes that are the chemical catalysts that fuel metabolic processes. People need to eat a variety of food in adequate quantity every single day to give their bodies all these necessary supplies.

Deficiencies of vitamin C (found in cabbage, kale, parsley, turnip greens, broccoli, tomatoes, citrus fruits, strawberries, and cantaloupe) result in gastrointestinal problems, slow wound and bone fracture healing, iron deficiencies, heart disease, and deficient collagen production. Without good collagen production (a structural protein), you're going to be a flabby, wrinkled mess. To have good collagen you must eat foods rich in vitamin C, every day, not just on certain "phases" of a diet program.

Deficiencies of folic acid, vitamin B_6, and vitamin B_{12} (found in oranges, green leafy vegetables, wheat germ, asparagus, broccoli, nuts) raise the level of homocysteine in your bloodstream, which leads to arterial damage and plaque that is linked to increased risk of coronary artery disease and stroke.

Deficiencies of magnesium (found in lima beans, spinach, corn, broccoli, whole grain, raisins, bananas, almonds, cashews, peanuts, walnuts, and pecans) are linked to heart disease, hypertension, diabetes, asthma, obesity, infertility, migraines, muscle pain, leg cramps and twitching, seizures, dizziness, irritability, apathy, depression, and PMS to name a few symptoms.

Deficiencies of conjugated linoleic acid (CLA), found in saturated animal fats from the meat and milk of grass-fed, pasture-raised animal increases your risk of atherosclerosis, cancer, and obesity.

These are just a few of the many health problems Americans suffer from today because they do not eat enough real food.

Because Americans' goal is weight loss, like Sisyphus who was condemned for eternity to roll a boulder up a hill only to have it roll back down just before he reached the top, the goal is eternally out of reach. Let's say you are a 200-pound woman or a 250-pound man and you need to lose 80 and 60 pounds, respectively. You can go on *The South Beach* low-cal diet and lose 30 pounds in three months. By this time your face will be hanging down around your neck and you will still need to lose 50 and 30 pounds, respectively. But can you continue eating low-calorie for more months? Now that you have lowered your caloric intake to a famine level for a substantial period of time, your body now has a higher insulin response to incoming food, a lowered metabolic set point, a biological inner drive for survival that is on red alert to hang onto fat cells, and a craving and bingeing response instigated by severe malnutrition. If you go off the diet, you will likely gain all of those pounds back and more.

If Americans would only turn to a balanced diet of real whole food, we could then achieve optimal health and body weight. Such a diet would balance our endocrine systems, heal malnutrition, ratchet up our metabolisms, calm hysterical hunger, and assure our bodies that we are not going to die so that it can let go of fat cells. In the first year, that 200-pound woman or 250-pound man may lose 2 pounds a week, but let's say they both only lose one pound a week. At the end of the year, they would weigh 148 and 198, respectively. And they would not have been suffering on a "diet." Furthermore, they will likely have exchanged 20 pounds of fat for muscle, and may not even need to lose more.

Contrary to conventional medical wisdom, there is more to good health than losing weight. If you want to live into old age thinly and happily and die a peaceful death, you will not get there by starving your body. Low-calorie dieting is not the only starvation diet. The introduction of the lipid hypothesis fifty years ago ultimately led to the low-fat diet, an extreme starvation diet.

CHAPTER 23

The Low-Fat Diet Made Us Sick

THROUGH MY INFORMAL restaurant and market research, I've learned one very important fact about Americans: We don't like to chew. Check out the way people eat their cheeseburgers, fries, and Pepsis. It's *bite, chew, chew, swallow. Bite, chew, swallow. Bite, chew, chew, swallow. Glug, glug, glug, glug.* While primitive human spent many hours every day chewing raw meat, nuts, seeds, and roots, consuming three to four hundred calories per hour, modern Americans bite, chew, chew, swallow, and glug our meals in mere minutes. According to Daniel E. Lieberman, professor of biological anthropology at Harvard University, "The size of our faces has shrunk about 12 percent since the Ice Age when humans probably spent much more time chewing harder, tougher food to get the calories they needed for survival."[1]

When the lipid hypothesis was launched in the 1950s, the message to eat less saturated fat and cholesterol turned out to be a major boon to the food industry because this message threw a monkey wrench into our community consciousness about food and set the stage for the food industry to begin making billions of dollars. Americans didn't know what to eat if they couldn't eat what they had always eaten since the dawn of humankind. First we were told that historically eaten dietary fats were unhealthy and caused disease. Then we were told to eat a low-fat, high-carbohydrate diet consisting of dry veggies, grains and fruit.

If there was ever a population less suited to a fat-free veggie diet, it was the American public. How many modern bite-chew-swallow-glug folks do you think could down bales of dry vegetables throughout the course of one day? Not many Americans choose the dry veggie diet as a lifestyle—a diet that has never been eaten by any people on the face of the earth in the history of humankind. Even vegetarian swamis in India eat ghee, which is the same deep yellow butter that nutritional researcher Dr. Price found in all the healthy primitive societies he studied.

Like all unnatural diets there are immediate and more long-term problems associated with the dry veggie/grain diet. For starters, this diet does not provide enough fat to modulate the absorption all that roughage, and people who tried this diet suffered from extreme gastrointestinal distress. In the fall of 2000, John and I spent a week at the health spa Rancho la Puerta in Tecate, Mexico. I loved the facility and treatments, but did not care for their "outstanding spa cuisine"[2] which was very bland, low-fat, high-carbohydrate food. At one point I restored to begging the cook for some fat and protein and was given a lecture about the "studies" that proved the low-fat diet prevented heart disease, a woman my size didn't need much protein, and I should take the opportunity to indulge in their healthy cuisine. I guess he meant the healthy diet that resulted in the cacophony of bodily noises in the spa's restrooms, giving new meaning to the immortal words of Ace Ventura, Pet Detective, "Do NOT go in there!"

A more serious problem with a dry veggie diet, besides the boredom, gastrointestinal distress, and all that chewing, was the fact that few people actually choose this diet of dreary, fat-free dry brown rice, dry veggies, and dry salad. Instead, Americans went for the addictively tasty carbohydrate factory foods. In fact, back when this diet was introduced, the recommended ADA breakfast for Type 2 diabetics was cold cereal, milk, banana, and orange juice—all carbohydrates. But as Americans ate more easily chewed carbohydrates (sugar), the 1970s and 1980s saw an exponential rise in obesity and disease. To address this mysterious rise in the obesity and disease, in 1992 the USDA introduced food pyramid guidelines recommending Americans radically reduce fat and increase their consumption of carbohydrates—foods like pasta and bread. The USDA advice to eat more pasta and bread was eagerly embraced by Americans, advice leading to binges on cereal, pretzels, bagels, and low-fat cookies.

Here is where the long-term problems occurred. Since carbohydrates are energy food and should be eaten in quantities that match a person's individual metabolic health and activity level, when you eat more energy than you are currently burning you will gain weight. But Americans were not given this message. They were virtually badgered into eating more carbohydrates.

The most damaging result of our radical increase in the consumption of carbohydrates was that Americans were now suffering with chronic high insulin levels. This is not a condition that creates immediate alarm. A person does not feel any different when insulin levels soar and remain elevated. But the damage occurs within, insidiously and inexorably. Chronic high insulin levels are implicated in every single degenerative disease, including Type 2 diabetes (explained below), cancer (insulin is a growth factor for cells), and heart disease (high insulin levels encourage coronary artery plaguing).[3] In fact, studies on insulin and arterial plaque date back to the 1960s. Researchers actually infused insulin into the femoral arteries of dogs and arterial plaque occurred in every dog.[4] High insulin levels are also caused by stress, dieting, caffeine, alcohol, tobacco, aspartame, steroids, sedentary lifestyle, recreational, OTC, and prescription drugs, but our focus here is sugar.

Here's how it works: Hormones are the chemical communicators between cells. For the body to function well, they must be kept at normal levels, as hormones depend on each other to do their jobs. Because all the systems of the body are interconnected, one hormonal imbalance causes another. A key hormone to keep balanced is insulin, which is secreted by the pancreas. Insulin's major function is to regulate blood sugar levels, thereby protecting the brain and other vital organs from receiving too much sugar, which damages cells. When you eat carbohydrates, they turn immediately into sugar in your system, and when too much sugar is in your bloodstream, insulin binds to insulin receptors on your cells so that they will open up and accept that extra sugar.

Years of eating too many carbohydrates mean that your cells will be clogged with sugar. When they are filled to capacity and can't fit another sugar molecule, cells reduce the number of insulin receptors so there are fewer receptors for insulin to activate. This is insulin resistance. If you live long enough, you will likely develop at least some degree of insulin resistance, which is a condition of aging. What's not normal is that elementary school children are now developing insulin resistance. The recent fashion trend of low-rise jeans (prehistorically known as hip huggers) has revealed a population of young American women with fat tummies. Today, because girls are raised on sugar, they are insulin resistant with expanding middles by the time they reach adolescence. The reason for this weight gain around the midsection is that when cells refuse to accept sugar, extra sugar in the bloodstream is diverted into fat production, and fat accumulates around the waist first.

When cells become insulin resistant, alarm bells go off in your body. Your pancreas will secrete even more insulin in an attempt to overcome this resistance. So now you have too much insulin in your bloodstream, which is called hyperinsulinemia. Your cells are being bombarded with insulin, which is like a frantic knocking, pleading to allow the excess sugar to enter. But stuffed as they are to capacity with sugar, your cells react by further reducing insulin receptors, which is increased insulin resistance.

If you continue putting too much sugar into your system until your cells have closed down all insulin receptors, the sugar has nowhere to go and remains in your bloodstream. You now have high blood sugar levels *and* high insulin levels, i.e., Type 2 diabetes, an ugly progressive disease that causes blindness, kidney disease, nerve disease (leading to amputations), heart disease, stroke and premature death.[5] Type 2 diabetes is the sixth leading cause of death in United States. In thirty years, the number of Americans with diabetes is expected to increase by 57 percent.[6] And the CDC says that if children's diets don't change, one-third of the babies born in the year 2000 will be diagnosed with Type 2 diabetes sometime in their lifetime. We now have a generation of adults who are very likely to outlive their children.[7]

Aside from those who binge to overweight or obesity on carbohydrates and consequentially suffer from chronic high insulin diseases, there are also thin people who eat very little, but everything they eat is carbohydrate. A person is a walking insulin factory who has a teeny-weenie piece of crumb cake with coffee in the morning (the no-calories-if-nibbling-while-standing-up mentality), a few bites of quiche in a white flour crust and a chocolate bon bon for lunch, and dines on one egg roll, two Dim Sum, green tea ice cream, and a fortune cookie washed down with white wine. If you are able to control your portions but those portions are mostly sugar, you are cruising the danger zone as far as chronic high insulin levels are concerned, and an insulin related disease may lurk in your future.

Contrary to the absolute science that high sugar consumption leads to insulin resistance, back in 1992 the USDA's prioritizing of foods (urging more carbohydrates) was wholeheartedly endorsed by doctors. So on top of all the carcinogenic, heart-disease causing oils that people were swigging, they dumped in loads of simple carbs into their systems. It was logical. If you can't eat eggs, meat, butter, cheese, or cream, then you have to fill your diet with something else.

Despite all evidence to the contrary, the conventional wisdom of the day was "it's the fat, not the sugar" that makes you fat. The low-fat craze morphed into the fat-free craze, which encouraged food manufacturers to remove all fat from their products and replace it with sugar. With the public becoming more confused about what to eat and what not to eat along with the rampant rise of hysterical hunger and the resultant binge eating, factory food makers understood that the market was ripe to hawk any product they could dream up. Americans went along as food makers issued their siren call with the introduction of thousands of factory food products into our marketplace—products tagged with food industry-speak pronouncements of good health, beauty, and "satisfaction." The problem was that these products contained substances that were foreign and mostly toxic to human physiology—and of course, all that sugar.

Then came the blame game. As we grew fatter and Type 2 diabetes, heart disease, and cancer were skyrocketing, the medical establishment came to the conclusion that we were not compliant enough. They hammered harder on the "no saturated fats and cholesterol" message, encouraged us to eat more carbohydrates (sugar), and frantically advised us to lose weight. But Americans could not hear any warnings about their out-of-control eating because they were crazed on carbs. The medical community beat the drum harder about our weight. But how do you break through to people you've turned into a carb addicted, binge-eaters to get them to stop at one bowl of Kellogg's "heart-smart" Special K, when they have already eaten an entire box of SnackWell's low-fat cookies?

Then there are actually people who can maintain—through superhuman willpower—a starvation diet of hot water with lemon peel and oatmeal with berries for breakfast, dry salad for lunch, and one cup of pasta with marinara sauce for dinner, accompanied by one-half cup of steamed broccoli and a small salad with a twist of lemon. These are typically the women Tom Wolfe described in his novel *Bonfire of the Vanities* as "social X rays .... They keep themselves so thin, they look like X-ray pictures .... You can see lamplight through their bones." Those who heroically restrained themselves from bingeing were disappointed to realize the low-fat diet did not produce beautiful bodies. That's because low-fat diets are typically devoid of proteins like dairy, eggs, meat, and nuts so they do not provide the building materials necessary to rebuild or create new cells that compose skin, muscles, organs, nails, hair, brain cells, and bones. Without incoming supplies, the body is forced to cannibalize its own bones and muscles to obtain the proteins necessary to keep up ongoing the rebuilding processes. (Carbohydrates are fuel; they do not supply building materials for your body to rebuild or replace cells.) If you happen to have the defiant willpower necessary to fight the biological drive to eat the food necessary for survival, you will see outward and inward manifestations of malnutrion sooner or later. In addition to developing a tubbier midsection, you may notice more cellulite taking over, along with saggy skin, thinning hair (the "pattern" balding syndrome in women), brittleness and dryness, more wrinkles, dry eyes, ridged, shredding nails, as well as heartburn, insomnia, cravings and bingeing, infertility, Type 2 diabetes, and coronary artery plaque.

A contributing factor to the wasted-away-with-a-fat-midsection look is that a diet low in protein results in diminished glucagon production, which is your body's fat burning hormone. When you eat, two hormones, glucagon and insulin, are released from your pancreas. When you eat a balanced diet of real food, these hormones are balanced. Glucagon is responsible for releasing fats from your cells to be used as fuel and building blocks within your body. Glucagon is released when you eat protein. Insulin is the fat- and nutrient-storing hormone that is released when you eat carbohydrates. The ratio between these two hormones determines whether food will be used as building materials, fuel, or stored as fat. If you eat only carbohydrates, your insulin-to-glucagon ratio will be too high, and those carbs will likely be stored as fat.

Human beings are made out of dynamic tissues that are constantly undergoing change and being replaced. This breaking-down process is essential for clearing out the old cells and cellular material (enzymes, hormones, neurotransmitters) to make room for new. The regeneration process is made possible by the fact that we eat the very same biochemicals that our bodies are inherently composed of: proteins and fats.

Of the low-fat diet, Drs. Michael and Mary Dan Eades write in *The Protein Power Lifeplan,* "Clearly the lowfat diet hasn't been the panacea that many had hoped for; in fact, it has turned out to be a dismal failure, a fact admitted publicly in 1996 by most of the world's experts in nutritional research." At the Second International Symposium on Dietary Fats and Oil Consumption in Health and Disease in April 1996, the Eades listened to nutritional researchers from numerous countries talk about the effects of fat in the human diet. They were not talking about the low-fat diet preventing heart disease but exactly the opposite. The major consensus was that the low-fat diet was a failure.[8]

In *The Cholesterol Myth: Exposing the Fallacy That Saturated Fat and Cholesterol Cause Heart Disease,* Uffe Ravnskov, MD, PhD, analyzed three hundred scientific references to disprove the nine main myths of the lipid hypothesis that had generated the low-fat diet, which are: (1) High-fat foods cause heart disease; (2) high cholesterol causes heart disease; (3) high fat foods raise blood cholesterol; (4) cholesterol blocks arteries; (5) animal studies prove the diet–heart theory; (6) lowering your cholesterol will lengthen your life; (7) polyunsaturated oils are good for you; (8) the anticholesterol campaign is based on good science; and (9) all scientists support the diet–heart theory.[9] Dr. Ravnskov, the author of more than eighty papers and letters critical of the cholesterol hypothesis, told me, "An almost endless number of scientific studies have shown that animal fat and high cholesterol are not causing heart disease. Unfortunately, these studies are ignored by the proponents of the cholesterol campaign."[10]

Science writer Gary Taubes's *New York Times Magazine* article, "What if It's All Been a Big Fat Lie?" hit the newsstands on July 7, 2002, sending shock waves through Americans' collective consciousness by questioning the validity of the low-fat diet. On December 10, 2003, when asked in an interview what made him go after the topic of the low-fat diet, Taubes, an award-winning journalist who often focuses on exposing poor and deficient science, replied, "I'd been reporting on salt and blood pressure, which is a huge controversy, and some of the people involved in that were involved in the advice to tell Americans to eat low-fat diets, and they were terrible scientists. These were some of the worst scientists I'd ever come across in my 20-odd year career of writing about controversial science."[11]

Frank Hu, MD, at the Harvard School of Public Health, has focused his research on the role of dietary and lifestyle factors in the development of obesity, Type 2 diabetes, and cardiovascular disease. Dr. Hu was an advisor to the 2005 Dietary Guidelines Advisory Committee at the HHS (mentioned on page 33). Dr. Hu told the committee that scientific evidence didn't support conventional wisdom that high fat intake leads to obesity. There is no evidence that weight loss is better with a low-fat diet, he said. In fact, Dr. Hu told the committee that new evidence demonstrated that adherence to a diet is greater, and weight loss more noticeable, if the diet allowed moderate fat intake. In Hu's opinion the exclusive focus on dietary fat has been a distraction to the efforts to control obesity.[12]

Bafflingly, the low-fat diet continues to garner support from the AHA, the CDC, the USDA, the NCI, the AMA, the ADA, and so on. Researchers continue to look for reasons for people to eat a low-fat diet. In the spring of 2005, a study was reported in the press that claimed that women who had already been treated with surgery, radiation, and/or chemotherapy could reduce their rate of breast cancer recurrence by 20 percent by following a low-fat diet.[13] Let's take a look at one of the women in the study who was assigned to a low-fat diet, to get a true picture of why the researchers were able to demonstrate this 20 percent reduction in cancer recurrence. This woman formerly ate bacon. Factory animal products contain numerous cancer-causing toxic residues. Bacon is cured with nitrates—known carcinogens. The woman in the study also said that before she went on the low-fat diet, "I slathered my sandwiches with mayonnaise." Commercial mayo is made with highly carcinogenic heat and chemical processed oils. Also, once assigned to a low-fat diet the woman made her own salad dressing. Commercial salad dressing is made with the same carcinogenic oils and contains many other toxic chemical ingredients. The woman also formerly loved cheese. Commercial cheese is made from factory milk that is contaminated with many known carcinogens. So naturally if you remove a huge load of carcinogens from a person's diet they are going to fare much better than if you continued dumping what amounts to gasoline on smoldering coals.

Less than one year after this study, a $415 million, eight-year study published in the February 2006 issue of *JAMA* found that the subjects who ate a low-fat diet had exactly the same rates of colon cancer, breast cancer, heart attacks, and strokes as the subjects who ate whatever they felt like eating. It was deemed the "Rolls Royce" of studies and the "final word" on the low-fat diet. In response, David A. Freedman, a statistician at the University of California who writes on the design and analysis of clinical trials said, "We, in the scientific community, often give strong advice based on flimsy evidence."[14]

In the decade prior to this "final word," and despite the medical communities wholehearted embracement of the low-fat diet, many Americans rebelled (due to the reasons outlined above) and decided to look elsewhere for weight loss solutions.

When cardiologist Robert Atkins published his first book, *Dr. Atkins' Diet Revolution,* in 1972, he was attacked by the AMA, which labeled his diet approach "potentially dangerous." This resulted in Congress summoning him to Washington to defend his diet. Thirty-one years and 15 million books later, the Atkins was synonymous with low-carb dieting.

CHAPTER 24

Low-Carbohydrate Dieting Was a Bust

IN SHOWTIME'S COMEDY SERIES *Weeds*, newly widowed suburban mom Nancy Botwin turns to dealing pot to help pay the bills. When she stops in to stock up at her suppliers' home, the conversation turns to cornbread. "I miss carbs," Nancy says.

A young woman filling Baggies chimes in. "My friend Heylia tried no carbs. She ate bacon and eggs for a whole month. I'm talkin' like five dozen eggs and a whole pig a day. She lost eleven pounds. That shit work."[1]

It seems like the no-carb thing is brand new, but this approach has been around for a long time. The very first low-carb diet was made popular in 1825 by French attorney Jean Anthelme Brillat-Savarin in his book *The Physiology of Taste*. In 1863, a London undertaker, William Banting, published *Letter on Corpulence* after losing fifty pounds on a low-carb diet. One hundred years later (when I was thirteen) I read about a diet that the military had been using. It was the first time I became aware of a low-carbohydrate, high-protein diet. I was mystified by the instructions: chow down on bacon, beef, and peanut butter, but absolutely avoid fruit and sweets. That was also the first time I ever heard the word "gluten." Glutens are plant proteins found in cereal grains, chiefly corn and wheat—in other words, what we commonly think of as starch. It was also the first time I heard the word "ketosis," meaning a state of starvation in which your insulin levels fall low enough to burn body fat for energy.

In 1963, a young, porky cardiologist ran across an article on low-carb dieting in the *Journal of the American Medical Association* (which may have been the same source for the military diet that I read). That cardiologist, Dr. Atkins, went on the program himself, lost weight, and subsequently wrote several bestselling books on low-carb dieting. Forty years later, his approach hit the big time, and "low-carb" and "no-carb" became catchphrases.

Studies have shown that the low-carb diet is initially more effective than a low-fat diet, but that low-carb dieters experience rebound weight gain within one year.[2] Our physiology dictates that a diet in which carbohydrates are individually modulated is the only way to reduce body fat without sacrificing health. But people are not approaching nutrition in an individualized way. People are recklessly eating zero carb diets that do not provide adequate, well-rounded nutrition. For instance, the Atkins Induction phase allows only two to three cups of vegetables every day and minuscule amounts of fruit and dairy, but many low-carb dieters decide to take extreme steps and eliminate all carbs, including veggies, fruits, and dairy. Healthy metabolic processes are dependent on adequate macronutrients (proteins, fats, and carbohydrates). But the energy supplied by these macronutrients to fuel healthy metabolic processes is released by micronutrients (vitamins, minerals, and enzymes present in plant foods, fruits, and dairy products). In other words you are not going to get the full benefit of any one food without eating it in balance with other foods.

Atkins recommends that people move on to the Maintenance Diet, which is slightly more balanced. However, Atkins reminds his readers, "Induction not only jump-starts your weight loss, it is also a convenient refuge to which you can retreat whenever you need to get off a weight loss plateau or to get back on the program after a lapse. So if you've fallen off your Lifetime Maintenance program for whatever reason, you can return to Induction."[3] That means people are going back to a diet of sub-nutritional value time and time again.

Unless great care is taken to eat grass-fed, pasture-raised animal products, Atkins followers consume excess amounts of factory animal products from diseased animals permeated with carcinogens. All this without the benefit of the antioxidants found in fruits and vegetables.

Zero carb dieters are seldom versed in how to choose healthy fats and how to avoid poison fats, and so these dieters often munch on highly toxic fats such as deep-fat–fried pork rinds and the like.

To make matters worse, most people supplement this diet with factory low-carb diet products. Before his death, Dr. Atkins sold majority shares of Atkins Nutritionals, Inc. to the tune of $500 million.[4] Atkins wannabees were in hot pursuit, unleashing a torrent of low-carb substances onto the market. In January 2004, representatives from 450 food companies including Kraft, ConAgra, and Wal-Mart, held a two-day brainstorming summit on how they could take advantage of the predicted $25 billion low-carb market.[5] Although, due to the unpalatability of low-carb foods, Atkins Nutritionals, Inc., filed for bankruptcy in the summer of 2005, factory low-carb products remain on our shelves.

Carbs are reduced in factory food products by pumping up the food's volume with soy protein and replacing sugar with sorbitol, maltitol, and lacitol, which are sugar alcohols that are promoted as having little or no impact on blood sugar levels and insulin secretion. (Some clinical nutritionists question this claim.) Sugar alcohols are molecules, like the weird science fake-fat olestra molecule, that are too big to be digested and which, like olestra, can cause gastrointestinal problems. Chemists are now hard at work trying to solve this problem by creating more science fiction sugars—like Splenda—in labs.

Splenda (sucralose), a chemically derived, chlorinated molecule, is 600 to 1,000 times sweeter than sugar with no added calories.

It was FDA approved for use in food and beverage products in 1998. Splenda has been heavily promoted in some of the most gorgeously produced and directed TV ads airing today. These ads would have us believe that Splenda will transform our dreary lives into a veritable fairyland of giddily surreal Technicolor. Splenda makers assure us that their sweetener is "Made From Sugar, So It Tastes Like Sugar." But the sugar and aspartame industries have been all over that statement in the courts, claiming false advertising, and asserting that Splenda is more like chlorine than sugar.

Just like aspartame, sucralose does not promote weight loss—and, in fact, can stimulate the appetite (see page 57). All artificial sweeteners sabotage weight loss efforts because when your tastebuds register a sweet taste, your body's natural ability to gauge food intake is flummoxed. This results in overindulging in sweet foods and beverages.[6] Your risk of obesity goes up 41 percent for every can of diet soda you drink.[7]

Testing of sucralose has demonstrated that it causes shrinkage of the thymus gland, which is crucial to your immune system, as well as enlargement of the liver and kidneys.[8] Although makers of sucralose claim it's not absorbed into the body, scientists report that 20 to 30 percent is absorbed and that it accumulates in organs and causes DNA damage in gastrointestinal organs.[9]

If you have chosen to ingest this chlorinated sugar, which happens to carry the same risks of regular old chlorine exposure—cancer, immune function malfunction, birth defects—you have to ask yourself, is it worth the risk? Serious illness changes your life forever.

"Net carbs," "net impact carbs," or "effective carbs" are arrived at by ignoring fake sugar and subtracting fiber from the total carbohydrate count. So if a product has 30 grams of carbohydrates and 16 grams of fiber, it would have 14 net grams of carbs. Factory food producers have foisted this low net carbs concept on a public eager for gluttony with impunity. The net carb concept only serves your body well when you eat *real* foods that contain fiber. For example, you can have a piece of stone ground, whole grain bread that contains 24 grams of carb and essentially cut that number in half. That is why you can eat plates of nonstarchy vegetables and count them as zero carbs.

Since none of us slimmed down on SnackWells low-fat cookies, it is not likely that we will slim down on SnackWells CarbWell Fudge Covered Grahams either. Any type of dieting is starvation to human physiology, which is designed to operate on a balanced, varied diet of real whole foods that provides enough quantity so that all the vital nutrients are onboard every single day. When you combine starvation with diet factory food, you're not going to produce a good quality human being. Going on any kind of "healthy diet" that includes factory food products is like saying you're quitting smoking while you have smoldering cigarette dangling from your lips.

Reclaiming your genetic gifts is possible if you stop dieting, stop eating factory food, and start give your body the necessary building blocks of nutrition. If you are unhealthy, you can radically improve every aspect of your health, including balancing your hormones and brain neurotransmitters in a cell-by-cell process, by eating real food.

CHAPTER 25

The Basics of a Real Food Diet

WHEN I REFER to a "real food" diet, I'm not talking about "health food." If you are old enough, you might recall the TV commercial for Post Grape Nuts in which Euell Gibbons asked, "Ever eat a pine tree? Many parts are eatable" (which was famously spoofed as, "Ever eat a picnic bench? Many parts are eatable"). A common misconception is that eating "health food" is comparable to eating a pine tree or picnic bench. Another misconception is that health food is esoteric stuff found in health food stores. In the episode of *Nip/Tuck* referenced earlier, one of Julia McNamara's friends informs her, "Health food is the new plastic surgery." Julia resolves to transform her family's eating habits and serves them Chinese mushrooms and seaweed for dinner. The kids storm off to their rooms, slamming doors.

If you go into any health food store today, you'll see that there is more than mushrooms and seaweed. But you'll also see that the health food industry is hawking products similar to those in supermarkets. The differences are that efforts are made to provide organic products or products that claim to be organic, to eliminate additives, to add a lot of soy substances, and to make health food claims on the packaging.

From ages fifteen to twenty-two, I lived in Japan, India, Sri

Lanka, Spain, and Switzerland. Right after I returned to the United States, I remember attending a birthday party, taking a bite of Duncan Hines cake, and saying, "This cake makes my mouth burn." Once you have eaten real food as I did all those years, factory food tastes science fiction-y and leaves an icky taste in your mouth. Give up factory food for a while to allow your taste buds to reboot, and you'll see what I mean.

Maybe you haven't eaten real food all your life, but you can still provide your body with the materials it needs to repair so that it can shrink down to your ideal body weight. Which doesn't necessarily mean you'll be bone thin. We've got a French postcard framed in our bathroom from 1900. The nude woman in the photograph would be considered plump today, but upon closer scrutiny, she has good muscle tone and no cellulite. In fact, she is very attractive. Being an emaciated skeleton was never considered beautiful until the mid-twentieth century. A balanced diet of real food will not result in a skin-and-bones fashion model look. The only women I've known who achieved that look were either bulimic or actual models who lived on cigarettes, candy bars, and amphetamines combined with several hours of extreme exercise per day. Eating a balanced diet of real food will, over time, produce a muscular, attractive body as your body changes on a cellular level. Your ideal body weight is a set metabolic point, and you can stay there by eating three square meals every day.

A balanced diet means eating proteins, fats, nonstarchy vegetables, and carbohydrates together, three meals a day.

By providing your body with adequate fats and proteins, your body will be able to break down and rebuild lean body mass (muscle and bone). An amplified example of the internal breaking down and building up phenomenon that continually occurs within our bodies was demonstrated by Hilary Swank when she trained four hours a day for two months to prepare for her Academy Award–winning role as female boxing champ Maggie Fitzgerald in the film *Million Dollar Baby*. Swank put on fifteen pounds of muscle prior to shooting. Because extreme training causes muscles to break down and build up in an accelerated fashion, more protein is needed for the rebuilding process. The actress (who needed to sleep nine hours every night) actually woke up in the middle of every night to down an extra protein drink to provide her body with enough supplies to keep up the accelerated rebuilding process. This is not to say that American women should—heaven forbid—"bulk up." But only that a beautiful body can be achieved by ignoring the discombobulation caused by the number on the scale and focusing more on what you look like in the mirror.

After years of extreme and public dieting and exercising, Demi Moore acknowledged her body dysmorphia, and said of her 1996 escape from Hollywood, "I'd been on a long physical run of absolutely manipulating and forcing my body. But I couldn't find that there was a peace that came with that, and when I stepped away I thought, I just have to stop. I actually stopped exercising and started to eat in a way that was very reasonable. And the amazing thing is, my body transformed closer to what I had always hoped for."[1] So we are back to moderation and balance.

Americans direly need to eat as many organic, nonstarchy vegetables as humanly possible every day to obtain the micronutrients necessary to utilize proteins and fats. Remember the bite-chew-glug folks who can down a thousand calories and hundreds of carbs in a burger, fries, and sodas in a few bites, chews, and swallows? Americans need to learn to chew. Studies prove that a fiber-rich diet is a crucial factor in weight management. Indigestible fiber was the main component in the hunter-gather diet. Hard-to-chew-and-digest raw meat, nuts, seeds, roots, and other plant materials kept primitive humans' digestive systems working overtime. (Lathering veggies in butter helps immensely with the chewing and will facilitate the assimilation of fat-soluble vitamins.) Current research points to tissue inflammation as a cause of chronic diseases, including cardiovascular disease. Both vegetables and fruits have anti-inflammatory properties.

Examples of nonstarchy vegetables are amaranth leaves, arugula, asparagus, bamboo shoots, bean sprouts, beet greens, bell peppers, broccoli, brussels sprouts, cabbage, raw carrots, cauliflower, celery, chicory greens, chives, collard greens, cucumber, dandelion greens, eggplant, endive, fennel, garlic, ginger root, green beans, hearts of palm, jicama, jalapeño peppers, kale, kohlrabi, mushrooms, mustard greens, onions, parsley, radicchio, radishes, shallots, snap beans, snow peas, spinach, summer squash, Swiss chard, turnip greens, and watercress.

Fear of carbs has become as extreme in our culture as fear of fat. In the film *The Devil Wears Prada*, Emily, fashion slave gopher to *Runway* magazine editor-in-chief Miranda Priestly, is mystified by the fact that "the fat smart girl," Andy Sachs, has scooped her to accompany Priestly to Fashion Week in Paris, lamenting "You eat carbs!" In an episode of *Dirt*, a would-be lover tries to convince Lucy Spiller of the reasons he should stay the night. "I can make pancakes from scratch," he says. "Carbs," she replies, shooting him down.[2]

But carbs are not all bad. Carbs are necessary to feel happy and not to feel hysterically hungry, as the release of the feel-good neurotransmitter serotonin is stimulated by eating carbohydrates. Yet balance is the key. Keeping meals balanced means that you will have balanced insulin levels throughout the day—and you will eliminate the risk of developing diseases associated with chronic high insulin levels. Therefore, to your balanced meals of protein, fats, and nonstarchy vegetables, add a sensible portion of carbohydrates (energy food).

How many carbs?

Although I've contributed to books that contain charts, graphs, and so on to help readers "diet," after years of working on these books and experimenting with various levels of carb intake, I am convinced that following charts and graphs is counterproductive. I once heard a shrink define neurosis as "continually making your worst fears happen." Consulting charts, graphs, and lists; keeping journals; and measuring, counting, and otherwise tracking our food intake is neurotic, and it must stop if we are to become a healthy, happy nation. We don't need how-to diet book charts to tell us that a bowl of fettuccini Alfredo has too many carbohydrates for most of us. Americans are perfectly capable of figuring out through common sense and trial and error how much energy food we need to eat.

Basic physiology dictates that weight management is determined in part by how much energy you put into your system versus how much energy you expend. Any carbohydrate, whether it's an apple or a candy bar, turns into energy (sugar) in your body, which is used as fuel. Since carbs are fuel, if you are lying in bed reading the paper, you obviously need far less fuel than someone in the third stage of an Iron Man competition. Carb levels need to increase when activity levels increase. It's common sense. If you are sedentary, you need proteins, fats, and nonstarchy vegetables to fuel ongoing metabolic processes and for internal repair, but you need very little energy food. If you are active, you need a moderate amount of carbs. If you are an extreme athlete, you can handle more carbs.

Examples of healthy, real carbohydrates are fruit, grains, legumes, nuts, seeds, sugars such as honey and molasses, milk, kefir, and yogurt, as well as starchy vegetables such as acorn squash, artichokes, beets, butternut squash, cooked or juiced carrots, corn, green peas, leeks, lima beans, okra, parsnip, potato, rutabaga, sweet potato or yam, and turnips.

Like caffeine, white sugar, cocaine, and heroin, salt is a white crystalline compound and, second to sugar, is the most seductive ingredient in factory food. Salt is used to increase the heft of a food product by binding moisture. Salt is also used to make consumers thirsty, and, like MSG, to make otherwise unpalatable fare taste good.

Still, salt is essential to life. Human blood plasma and lymphatic fluids have a composition similar to ocean water. Salt and water comprise the inorganic or mineral elements of your body and play specific roles in the functions of cells. Salt helps carry nutrients into cells and pump waste materials out. Salt helps regulate blood pressure and fluid volume, keeps the pressure balance normal in the lining of blood vessels, and is necessary for the absorption and digestion of food.

Seventy percent of supermarket salt is stripped of minerals through chemical processing; the minerals are then sold for other purposes. The stripped salt is adulterated with anticaking agents—often aluminum compounds that pose serious health risks. The FDA had synthetic iodine put into our processed salt supply some generations back to prevent goiter (enlarged thyroid). Dextrose (sugar) is added to stabilize the volatile iodine, which dyes the salt purple. To make it nice and pretty, the salt is bleached white. The resultant salt pours freely out of your saltshaker but should really only be used to melt the ice on your driveway.

Natural sea salt crystals are hand-harvested worldwide from shallow, evaporated tide pools. These salt crystals contain over eighty minerals and trace elements, including iodine. There are varied flavors in sea salt—you just have to experiment to find the ones that suit certain cuisines. A natural diet seasoned with sea salt is not likely be overkill in the sodium department.

In addition to sea salt, nonirradiated spices lend delicious flair and a distinctive edge to flavors, as well as providing antioxidants to your diet.

In the United States, for numerous reasons—our frantic lifestyles, the cheapness of factory food, and our belief that real food is deadly—we have lost the art of food. I believe that anyone, at any age, can change his or her diet, and that those changes will make a positive impact on the person's health and happiness. Even if you were raised exclusively on factory food, you can still do a complete about-face. My mother, for example, went grocery shopping once a month at the Navy commissary, so you can imagine the shelf life of the food items I grew up on. Thankfully, the desire to rekindle the art of food is slowly creeping back into our collective consciousness. And we can look to cooks like Martha

Stewart for inspiration. In her early sixties, Stewart is a stunning role model. Just looking at her luminous complexion and thick, lustrous hair, you can see the results of a lifelong diet of real food. Her approach to planning, shopping for, and preparing meals of real food is motivating, as activities surrounding eating are meant to be beautiful and pleasurable. And in the wealthiest society on earth, Americans owe it to themselves to make eating a delightful experience—every day, not just on special occasions.

In our artless food culture, people grab a bagel with cream cheese for breakfast with several cups of aspartame-dosed coffee. Lunch is a Jack-in-the-Box Bacon Cheeseburger with onion rings and a large Diet Coke. Dinner is DiGiorno pizza, an iceberg salad with Kraft Light Done Right! Ranch Dressing, washed down with Bud Lite.

Once you gain an understanding and appreciation for the art of food, your day might start with an organic spinach omelet made from pasture-raised eggs with deep orange yolks, a bowl of sweet organic strawberries, and a glass of creamy whole raw or organic milk. Coffee would be organically grown or Swiss water processed decaffeinated, with raw or organic cream. Lunch could be a fragrant mixed greens salad tossed with olive oil and rich balsamic vinegar topped with strips of naturally raised ham, quartered ripe heirloom tomatoes brought alive with a sprinkling of aromatic sea salt, followed by juicy organic watermelon chunks and cherries. Dinner might be a succulent, naturally-raised lemon- and rosemary-roasted chicken or slices of naturally raised roast beef, steamed organic asparagus spiked with herbes de Provence and drizzled with melted organic butter, crisp russet potato quarters roasted with coconut oil and seasoned with sweet paprika, sea salt, and freshly ground black pepper, a wonderfully bitter watercress salad that requires just a hint of pungent olive oil. Raw cheese and tart organic apples would be dessert. These are not hard meals to put together, as preparing delicious, gourmet meals need not be labor-intensive.

Simple two-step guidelines for achieving good health and your ideal body composition are: One, stop eating anything made of, or containing, refined white sugar, refined corn, refined grain, refined soy, refined oils, or chemicals; and two, eat organically produced meat, fish, poultry, dairy, vegetables, fruits, grains, legumes, seeds, and nuts that could (in theory) be picked, gathered, milked, hunted, or fished, and that have not undergone any processing. It is important to note that if you have been eating a starvation diet of factory food, like say, Special K for breakfast, a Zone power bar for lunch, and Lean Cuisine for dinner, then you will need to introduce real food and slowly build up your intake, so as not to shock your body into storage mode.

The pop diet culture is now pushing snacking as a way to "balance blood sugar," but unless you suffer from hypoglycemia, Type 2 diabetes, or are otherwise ill, you do not need to snack regularly. The American diet always comprised three square meals a day until the food industry inundated our environment with factory snack products. Historically, people didn't snack. Rather, they ate meals and came to the table hungry. Eating-a-meal, going-hungry, eating-a-meal, and going-hungry is a microcosm of human experience prior to 1900. This gave their systems a chance to assimilate food from the previous meal before more food entered and for all their hormones to complete their processes. This is different than gorging and starving, which is the prehistoric feast-and-famine phenomenon that resulted in higher fat storage after each binge. That said, there are times when we cannot get to the next meal soon enough. But that doesn't mean we should eat a Snickers or even a Balance Bar.

Factory food makers have reacted to the public outcry over supersizing by making 100-calorie "snack" packs—from which they are making a killing (literally). In 2006 alone, factory food companies introduced forty-two new 100-calorie snacks to the market. Whether you eat a little or a lot of poison, it must be first processed by your liver and then, because poison is fat soluble, those toxic little 100-calorie snack packs are going to end up in storage repositories on your butt. The factory snack packs, in addition to being laced with poisons (MSG, high fructose corn syrup, colored dyes, preservatives, and so on), are also generally made up of genetically modified, highly processed wheat flour— i.e., carbohydrates.

An optimal meal or snack should contain, in this order: protein, fat, and a small amount of carbohydrate. With a little thought you can dream up all kinds of interesting snacks that fit this model: peanut butter with apple quarters; raw cheese with a handful of walnuts and a couple of dried figs; a leftover chicken breast with a cut-up bell pepper; tuna fish salad with grapes and cucumber slices; hummus with carrot sticks; deviled eggs and a few raisins. By opening your horizons while shopping, you'll discover delicious foods to snack on.

America is a nation of night eaters who complain about not feeling hungry in the morning. But everyone needs to eat a good breakfast. In *French Women Don't Get Fat,* the spring breakfast "*Menu du Jour*" is yogurt, cereal with strawberries, a slice of whole-wheat or multigrain bread, and coffee or tea. This meal plan of all sugar and stimulants might not wreak too much havoc on someone who has eaten relatively well his or her entire life and has balanced brain neurotransmitters. But for the average sugar-addicted, neurotransmitter-imbalanced, hysterically hungry American, this breakfast would guarantee binge eating later that morning. Eating a protein-based breakfast of real food sets your inner thermostat for the rest of the day, and bestows your body with the building materials for ongoing metabolic repair and building processes.

On the contrary, skipping breakfast or eating sugar tells your body it's famine time and your inner thermostat must ratchet down. Sumo wrestlers gain their massive girth by skipping breakfast, eating lunch after they train, taking a four-hour nap, eating dinner, and going to bed. Not feeling hungry in the morning is an obstacle that can only be overcome by forcing yourself to eat a big protein breakfast as soon as you get up.

One hundred years of eating factory food products and the further malnutrition caused by low-calorie, low-fat, and low-carb dieting has created a society that is obese, disease ridden, and on a trajectory toward ugly death. So now that we're fat and sick, we're sold on miracles in a bottle—snake oil supplements and drugs.

VII

Miracles in a Bottle, Snake Oil Supplements, and Drugs

CHAPTER 26

That @*#!& Stress is Making Us Fat!

On December 23, 2003, I was driving along the Pacific Coast Highway in Santa Barbara, station surfing on my car radio, when a voice broke through the static. It was Greg Cynaumon, a "psychologist," exclaiming, "Lose thirty pounds before Christmas!"

Madison Avenue has promoted just such dubious claims in annoying advertisements for so long that, like most Americans, I no longer flinch when I hear ads like that. This time, I paid attention. The ad was playing on Laura Schlessinger's show. Schlessinger is a trusted radio talk show host famous for her Old Testament moral standards, who happens to have a degree in physiology from Columbia University and surely knows that no pill alone could cause a weight loss of thirty pounds in *two days*, two weeks, or for that matter, ever.

The ads for CortiSlim claimed that persistently elevated levels of cortisol are the underlying cause of weight gain and that CortiSlim controls cortisol levels, balances blood glucose levels, reduces cravings, and increases metabolism, thereby burning the fat around "your tummy, thighs and stomach." While the CortiSlim Web site provided a description of an unpublished study by CortiSlim creator Shawn Talbott, PhD, no evidence of the effectiveness of reducing or modulating cortisol levels by CortiSlim or any other herbal remedies, botanical formulation, or supplement for weight loss has ever been published in peer-reviewed medical journals.[1]

Christmas came and went, but Greg Cynaumon persisted. CortiSlim TV ads ran so repetitively that I could not hit the mute button fast enough. "I'm Dr. Greg Cynaumon, and no offense to casual dieters, but if you only want to lose five to ten pounds, then CortiSlim is not for you. CortiSlim is the weight loss capsule created by my associate, Dr. Talbott, for people who are disgusted with diets and quickly want to lose fifteen pounds or more." This particular TV ad ended with Cynaumon holding up a bottle of CortiSlim and smirking. You could almost read his thoughts: *Ka-ching!* Because he knew that millions of Americans were sprawled out on the couch in front of the TV with fists buried to the wrists in bowls of caramel corn. And he knew that thousands of those people would decide then and there to try that CortiSlim stuff, because Greg Cynaumon's a doctor, and so sincere. Cynaumon was right. Countless people logged onto the Internet or called the 800 number, and ordered one-month supplies of CortiSlim for $49.95. What a relief to know that second-day mail was going to bring a magic bullet to solve all of their weight problems.

The CortiSlim claim that stress-induced cortisol production leads to midsection fat accumulation is *true*. When you're stressed out, your adrenal glands secrete adrenaline in response to dramatic, acute stress (like getting into a car wreck) and cortisol in response to every day stress (like working too late). Your adrenals secrete numerous other hormones, but our focus is these two. One primary objective of these hormones is to supply your brain and body with the sugar (fuel) necessary to deal with this stress. Adrenaline releases glycogen that's stored in your liver and muscles for emergency use. And cortisol actually breaks down your lean muscle mass to convert it into more sugar. Now that you've got a dump of sugar into your bloodstream, your pancreas secretes insulin, which stores any unused sugar away into cells. After years of pounding stress, your cells will be stuffed to capacity. As you read earlier, when cells cannot accept one more sugar molecule, they reduce the number of insulin receptors so there are fewer receptors for insulin to activate. This is insulin resistance. One hallmark of insulin resistance is weight gain around the middle, because, though it may strike us as an unfair mistake of nature, fat stored as a result of insulin resistance is hoarded around the waist first.

Our autonomic or unconscious nervous system, which regulates metabolic processes, is divided into the sympathetic and the parasympathetic nervous systems. During the day we're predominantly in the sympathetic state—which is appropriate, because our bodies need the operational metabolic processes that take place during this time.

The parasympathetic mode, which occurs predominantly at night, counteracts the sympathetic mode by turning on the repair processes such as making new cells, membranes, tissues, enzymes, hormones, and neurotransmitters (thus appropriately referred to as "beauty sleep"). In times past, humans didn't necessarily sleep uninterrupted all night long, largely due to problems such as threats to safety, vermin, smelly chamber pots, crowded conditions, hunger, and other irritants.[2] Today we have creature comforts, which allow for some sleep. When it gets dark, our systems could hypothetically change rhythm from daytime work (sympathetic) to nighttime rest (parasympathetic). But this is not the reality. Our circadian rhythms are shattered by overwork and jet travel. We overuse stimulants and indulge in other adrenal assaults that keep our bodies in a constant state of sympathetic dominance. So, while we have the allowances to sleep, these other factors have resulted in epidemic insomnia. And all this pounding stress is taking a toll. One of the major signs that we are not allowing our bodies to spend enough time in the parasympathetic mode is the spare tires we are lugging.

The solution to reducing the accumulation of stress-induced midsection body fat is to lower our cortisol and insulin levels, which will reverse insulin resistance (i.e., empty fat cells). This can only be accomplished by overhauling our lifestyles, not by popping a pill. One of the pluses of achieving overall health is that your body will shrink down to its natural body weight. Maximum health is accomplished by not eating factory food, eating a balanced diet of real food, reducing stress, cutting down on or quitting all stimulants (caffeine, tobacco), drinking only moderately (giving up alcohol until you lose the fat), quitting recreational drugs and any *unnecessary* OTC and prescription drugs, avoiding toxic exposure and drinking plenty of water to flush poisons from your system, indulging in mind-clearing playtime, going to bed as early as possible (preferably by ten), and getting eight hours of rest, as well as taking hormone replacement if you need it.

Although this is a book about food, there is one more vital ingredient to achieving maxium health. Americans need to stop making excuses for not exercising and get on with it. A lot of busy people make time for exercise, and we can look to their examples to figure out how they manage their time. It's only very recently in history that humans have huddled near their fossil-fuel-burning heat sources sniffing Glade Tropical Mist Plug-Ins instead of having to brave the winter elements. There are any number of health clubs, fitness DVDs, and home gyms, not to mention companies that make effective all weather clothing and rain gear so that we can now exercise outside in inclement weather.

In the spring of 2004, two new CortiSlim commercials came out, one featuring Greg Cynaumon and the other with his "associate" Shawn Talbott. This time they began the ads saying, "Lose forty pounds in thirty days? I don't think so!" Er, no, just thirty pounds before Christmas . . . .

On July 12, 2004, a nationwide class action suit was filed against the makers of CortiSlim, charging them with making invalid and unsubstantiated weight loss claims. On August 19, 2004, the FDA sent a warning letter to the makers of CortiSlim for making unsubstantiated claims. On October 5, 2004, the Federal Trade Commission (FTC) filed a compliant against the makers of

CortiSlim in the U.S. District Court in Los Angeles for deceptive and false advertising, marketing, and sales of CortiSlim. (The FTC is a government agency set up to prevent fraudulent, deceptive, and unfair business practices.)

By the fall of 2004, Cynaumon (who has been accused of buying his doctorate from Sierra University, a correspondence degree–mill that was ultimately shut down by the state of California[3]) had become "Dr. Greg" and CortiSlim ads continued on radio and TV, conspicuously omitting all the quick weight loss promises. By the winter of 2005, the tone of the commercials had entirely changed from the miracle-in-a-bottle mentality to a familial, completely full of it invitation to join the "CortiSlim lifestyle." "Dr. Greg Cynaumon here to encourage you to turn your frustration into motivation. A healthy change to the CortiSlim lifestyle of diet, exercise, and CortiSlim can reshape your future and that's the *resolution solution.* [Emphasis mine.] Buy CortiSlim at your favorite store or call the number on your screen. Go ahead, get your hopes up. Get excited. And get into the CortiSlim lifestyle."

Then, without warning, we experienced a merciful, albeit brief, respite from the CortiSlim camp. Just when we thought it was safe to turn on the TV, who do we see? None other than Shawn Talbott, spouting a new angle about stress eating and cortisol, and actually offering to send us "free" CortiSlim. The announcer on this particular ad invited viewers to "be part of television history." This ad was brought to us courtesy of a $4.5 million settlement to the FTC. The lesson: If you have enough money, you can continue spouting rubbish to the public.

In early 2004, two class action suits were filed against the makers of another weight loss supplement, TrimSpa, alleging violations of California and New York's false and misleading advertising business practice laws. On February 9, 2004, Anna Nicole Smith, the product's spokesperson, appeared on *Larry King Live* in what could only be viewed as the paradoxical spokespitch of the century. "Our guest is Anna Nicole Smith," Larry King said. "Last time I saw Anna was at the Kentucky Derby last year. And boy, you sure look different now. She credits the diet pill TrimSpa for the loss. She's now a paid spokesperson for that pill. How did you and that pill come together?"

"Well, actually," Anna Nicole Smith drawled, "I took the pill first, before they approached me, so that's kind of weird. And I was taking the pill for a little bit, and then, weird enough, they contacted Howard, my lawyer, and they wanted me to be their spokesmodel for TrimSpa. So I was, like, okay."

Prior to her death on February 8, 2007—due to an accidental prescription drug overdose—the sixty-nine-pounds-lighter Anna Nicole Smith appeared in magazines advertisements and on the TrimSpa Web site cavorting with a creepy guy under the tag line "Be Envied." But should we envy anyone who takes TrimSpa?

TrimSpa contains the African plant hoodia gorgonii. Within hoodia is an active molecule that has shown to have appetite-suppressing properties in rats. However, as hoodia is extremely difficult to grow, takes six years to mature and has been depleted, hoodia is not currently available to diet pill manufacturers. Researchers found that synthesizing the active ingredient created damaging liver side effects. And so as naturally occurring hoodia is virtually impossible to obtain, we can safely assue that all products claiming to contain hoodia are counterfeit. What risks are associated with fake hoodia substances are anyone's guess.[4]

TrimSpa originally contained the natural stimulant ephedra, which is extracted from the Chinese herb ma huang. Ephedra was restricted by the FDA after being linked to over 150 deaths related to cardiac arrest.

So-called "natural" stimulants such as green tea, ma huang, and guarana cannot be used with impunity just because they are natural. Ma huang is a very good example of the diet industry's abuse of a useful therapeutic Chinese herb. Henry Han, OMD, my coauthor on *Ancient Herbs, Modern Medicine: Improving Your Health by Combining Chinese Herbal Medicine and Western Medicine*, told me,

"My teacher, Song Tian Bing taught us, 'Ma huang has energy like a wild untamed horse, so you never want to relinquish control. Don't ever forget when you use ma huang that you saddle it so that you have the reins.'"

Stimulants keep your body in a state of sympathetic dominance by mimicking and magnifying the actions of adrenaline, which revs cellular functions. You think faster. Your heart beats faster. But the human body isn't meant to be in a state of sympathetic overdrive. Stimulant users will eventually begin to feel agitated. Although most people do not enjoy the pounding heart and jittery nerves, they get hooked on stimulants by the initial good feelings and keep going back for more. People in later stages of burnout reach for stimulants in a vain attempt to re-create that initial boost of energy and momentary lift in mood. (The stimulant rush is caused by the same outpouring of insulin and the resultant dump of feel good neurotransmitters in your brain that you get from eating sugar, which we reviewed on page 18.)

After the FDA ruling against the use of ephedra, TrimSpa was reformulated. A daily dose of TrimSpa now packs 1,050 milligrams of caffeine.

In America we have a skewed definition of "drug users." Since the passage of the Harrison Act on December 1914 that banned nonmedical use of cocaine (which previously provided Coca-Cola with its "medicinal benefits"), our judicial system has come down hard on reprobate users of illegal drugs. Thousands of dopers rot in prisons at taxpayers' expense. After 9/11, John Ashcroft instigated marijuana raids on "drug users," who incidentally happened to be dying from AIDS and cancer. You may not think of yourself as a drug user. Like a friend of mine said, "I've never tried drugs." Really? Well, try going without your coffee tomorrow, then let me know if you want to issue a revised statement.

People are unaware of how much caffeine they ingest daily since caffeine is the only drug that is widely added to the food supply, and manufacturers can add caffeine to any food or beverage without disclosing the dosage. The majority of Americans are frothing at the mouth from dehydration, and we seek to slake this thirst by drinking dehydrating caffeinated drinks like Starbucks Breakfast Blend, which packs 327 milligrams of caffeine, Diet Coke at 47 milligrams of caffeine per can, and other newly introduced caffeinated drinks like Shock, which boasts "Sleep is overrated" and contains 200 milligrams of caffeine.

When you jump start your heart with caffeine, the odorless, slightly bitter alkaloid is rapidly absorbed in the digestive tract and diffuses into nearly all of your tissues. Using caffeine keeps your body in a heightened state of sympathetic dominance with your adrenals overproducing stress hormones so that your body cannot rest. Like all drugs, caffeine provokes the desire to consume more and more as your addiction drags on.

Ultimately your adrenals will become fatigued and that is why many people who used to be able to "diet" by drinking coffee eventually find themselves fatigued, unable to get the same jolt from more and more coffee. Caffeine does so many bad things that space here does not allow your basic A-to-Z list. Suffice it to say, caffeine use is linked to heart disease, cancer, ulcers, urinary and prostate problems in men, and accelerated aging, infertility, fetal loss, spontaneous abortion, and fetal growth retardation, anxiety, sleeplessness, addiction, and withdrawal symptoms in children, among other problems.[5]

I understand that asking Americans to stop drinking coffee is tantamount to asking skid row alkies to give up beer. I also don't think that people should give up everything they love. In nature, animals forage for nuts and berries to get high on. It's ridiculous to demand that people live completely chaste lives of deprivation. But if caffeine is controlling you and destroying your health, and you want to cut down or quit, it's important to note that that quitting cold turkey halts the demand on your adrenals too suddenly, and you will experience withdrawal symptoms, including headache, fatigue, lethargy, muscle pain and an overall nasty mood.[6] It's best to wean yourself slowly. Decaffeinated coffee still contains significant amounts of caffeine, and all but Swiss water-processed decaffeinated coffee is decaffeinated with methylene chloride, a carcinogen, which you then ingest with your decreased caffeine.[7]

The best drink, of course, is clean, fluoride- and chlorine-free spring water. The human body is 75 percent water. Optimal is eight to ten 8-ounce glasses of water per day.

All stimulants stress your body and lead to adrenal disaster both by causing the release of adrenaline and by mimicking and exaggerating the actions of adrenaline. This eventually results in depleting your adrenal reserve, which will lead to anxiety, mood roller coaster, and insomnia. In addition to damaging your adrenals, using stimulants also taxes and depletes your body's balancing and calming neurotransmitters, which creates the potential for panic attacks—something that is not very pretty, if pretty is what you're after. However, if you would rather be dead than fat, you can always buy Emagrece Sim, better known as the Brazilian Diet Pill, online that contains the extremely dangerous cocktail of Fenproporex (a stimulant that is converted in the body to amphetamine), Librium (a sedating hypnotic drug to counteract the jitters), and Prozac (to make you feel better about ruining your health).

Many Americans are willing to saddle up a wild horse and relinquish the reins when it comes to using stimulants to lose weight. Never was George Bernard Shaw so correct in saying, "Youth is wasted on the young" as when it comes to young people resorting to extreme diet measures in an attempt to lose or maintain extremely low body weight. Taking natural stimulants, guzzling coffee and diet drinks, taking "metabolism enhancers," fat burners, appetite suppressants, carb blockers, fat blockers, smoking cigarettes, vomiting, taking laxatives, or using steroids, human growth hormone, and thyroid replacement outside of the care of a physician erodes the beauty or good looks with which a person is born.

The diet industry focuses solely on thinness. But there are many thin people walking around who are disasters on the inside, whose bodies do not have adequate building materials to replenish existing cellular structures or make new ones. Without the necessary building blocks of nutrition, bones weaken, endocrine systems falter, brain neurotransmitters become off-kilter, and ultimately organ function begins to flag. Outward manifestations of internal disaster can be seen in dull and thinning hair, brittle nails, dry skin, wrinkles and skin disorders and an overall lackluster appearance—all of which the beauty industry capitalizes on with a myriad of preparations to apply to the outside.

Americans idealize youth and beauty, but the fact is that many if not most Americans are on an accelerated aging path. Imagine the forces of nature young American men and women would be if they stopped eating all factory food, never used stimulants or other diet products, and ate balanced diets of real food. Right now, there are not many forces of nature walking around. Instead, ironically the drive to be beautiful in this country has caused people to inflict dire ugliness upon themselves. It begins with young girls kicking back diet pills with their diet drinks and, if they can keep up with the extreme dieting measures necessary to remain bone thin, it ends with chronically ill middle-aged, emaciated, hormone depleted insomniacs sucking up coffee and cigarettes (or if they are "health-minded" hot water with lemon peel) to dampen their hunger pains so they don't have to eat. Then there are the "failures"—the majority of people who indulge in chronic dieting using diet aids—those who blimp out due to the factors we talked about earlier.

Diet pills are a classic example of the type of products people desperately cling to after being fattened up on factory food. Therefore, although on March 26, 2004, the FDA sent a letter to VitaMaker.com warning the company to stop making false and misleading claims about TrimSpa Carb Blocker and TrimSpa Fat Blocker, people were still wasting $39.95 on a fifteen-day supply of TrimSpa X32 or a ten-day supply of CarbSpa or LipoSan Ultra. It remains to be see what impact, if any, Anna Nicole Smith's death will have on this company.

In addition to stimulant diet pills, there are the diet supplements that fall into the category of "let's just make up science as we go along." TV psychologist Phil McGraw's Shape Up! supplements provide an example of exploitation of fat people. These supplements were supposedly formulated for two body types: Apple-bodies notoriously carry fat as paunches, while Pear-bodies pack fat around hips, butt, and thighs. One of Dr. Phil's specially designed supplements supposedly helped Apples "metabolize carbohydrates," whatever that meant, and another purportedly promoted fat metabolism and increased the Pear-body's ability to burn calories. Adding the "Intensifier" was promoted to take weight management efforts to the next level. Taking either Apple or Pear along with the Intensifier cost consumers $120 per month.

The supplement labels claimed, "These products contain scientifically researched levels of ingredients that can help you change your behavior to take control of your weight." But there were no scientific studies to back up the claim that Apple and Pear bodies need different nutrients to lose body fat. Jules Hirsch, MD, a nutrition and obesity researcher and professor emeritus at Rockefeller University, called Dr. Phil's claims, "gibberish." A leading expert in nutrition policy, Dr. Kelly D. Brownell, author of the aforementioned *Food Fight,* referred to the supplements as "a recipe for making money."[8] It was a great marketing ploy until an FTC investigation and a class action suit brought on by dissatisfied customers compelled McGraw's company to stop marketing the products.[9] And in fake news anchor Stephen Colbert's immortal words, after Oprah "bitch slapped" James Frey for his revisionist memoir *A Million Little Pieces,* Jon Stewart remarked, "Don't you think it's going to be one entertaining hour of television when Oprah realizes that Dr. Phil is full of shit?"[10]

With Americans spending $15.2 billion per year on diet products, the makers of miracles in a bottle rake in so much money that they can't be stopped by consumer class action lawsuits, warning letters from the FDA, or legal action by the FTC. With the astronomical success of CortiSlim (note Americans are not slimmer), the sales of diet pills have reached a feverish pitch on TV, targeting everyone from testosteronized teenage boys to matron-phobic menopausal women by trotting out remarkable before and after testimonials, attractively no-nonsense Ivy League doctor-spokespitchers, and incredible free offers for products that can be summed up as X-TREMEBS4U. And if you are so inert that you can't even get off the couch to walk your dog, you can now give the pathetically fat creature Slentrol, diet pill approved by the FDA in early 2007 (note that there are no fat animals in nature).

Diet pills are not the only pills that are being foisted on the American public eager to see magical weight loss results by doing, as the diet pill Propolene claimed, "nothing" but "taking a pill." Because fat is not our only problem.

CHAPTER 27

Snake Oil Supplements

THE AMERICAN DIET is foreign and toxic to human physiology. We exacerbate this nutrient drain by dieting and popping diet pills. And so we are falling apart from the inside out. All you have to do is turn on the TV to understand that Americans do not look or feel as well as they could.

Enter the makers of miracles-in-a-bottle—for which we spend an additional $19 billion per year—like the medicinally, futuristic-sounding, once-a-day botanical cure-alls made by Berkeley Premium Nutraceuticals. According to their TV ads, with *just one daily pill* of Avlimil, Enzyte, Altovis, Ogöplex, Rogisen, Rovicid, Dromias, Numovil, Nuproxi, Pinadol, Rudofil, or Suvaril, at a monthly cost of between $29.95 and $34.99, your life will be balanced (if female), you will have natural enhancement and orgasmic intensification (if male), and both sexes will overcome fatigue, stave off macular degeneration and experience enhanced night vision, enjoy better heart health, sleep well, fight memory decline, have youthful skin, fight stress, live comfortably and manage your weight.

As if, but still.

In 1994, the U.S. Congress passed the Dietary Supplement Health and Education Act, which classified botanical and herbal supplements as food. Manufacturers of dietary supplements do not have to demonstrate that their products are safe nor are they required to report adverse affects to the FDA. They do not even have to demonstrate that their products are effective. They can insinuate on labeling that their product improves or supports or gives balance to or any number of quasi claims as long as they don't say "cures."

That said, according to Mike Katke, cofounder of Metagenics, (formulator and manufacturer of premium-quality nutritional products), the FDA does regulate the manufacturing of nutraceuticals and dietary supplements. "There are regulations as to what ingredients can be included or not included, potency, accuracy of labeling, standards for manufacturing and so on," Katke told me. "The FDA monitors compliance too, but not adequately. The FDA visits manufacturers periodically to determine whether or not we are operating up to the regulations, and there is a state FDA as well that also regulates and checks up on manufacturers. The problem is that they don't have the manpower or budget to keep up with everybody."[1]

Because a natural substance cannot be patented, pharmaceutical companies have no incentive to research the benefits of vitamins, minerals, and herbs. If a company were to spend millions of dollars researching natural substances, and found that certain natural supplements were superior to drugs, companies could not recoup their research costs in the spectacular fashion they have become accustomed to with drugs.

Still, there are companies like Metagenics that choose to do their own research, and these companies are supplying top-grade supplements to the market. Since the FDA has done such a poor job of monitoring drugs and food additives, it would not serve consumers for the FDA to regulate supplement manufacturers. If this were to happen, multinational drug corporations would likely inundate the market with inferior products while the small top-quality supplement manufacturers would get bogged down in fees and regulatory expenses so that their supplements would become economically unobtainable to the average consumer. The best way to force inferior products and snake oil out of the marketplace is to not buy them.

Nutraceuticals and dietary supplements are important today as we have more toxins, stress, and less nutritive soil than in times past. But contrary to the claims of the Greg Cynaumons, Berkeley Nutraceuticals, and other exploiters of desperate Americans, nutraceuticals and supplements alone can't make you healthy, thin, sleep better, and improve your sex life. They can only help you go the last fraction of the distance after you have addressed the most important factors of good health. We should get the bulk of our nutrition from real food. Supplements are *supplemental*. Too many people gobble handfuls of supplements arbitrarily without having a clue what they are taking. Worse, they are taking synthetic supplements. Ever notice how teeny tiny those vitamin pills are? The synthetic nutrients are compacted into hard little bullets that are cheap for manufacturers to make and easy for lazy consumers to swallow. The nutrients in those hard little pebbles are virtually inaccessible to the absorptive surfaces of your digestive system. Quality supplements are loosely packed, bioavailable tablets and capsules.

According to naturopathic physician Ron Schmid, "Cheap supplements are made with synthetic versions of nutrients and a host of toxic fillers and additives. Quality supplements are made with absolutely no additives and contain only pure nutrients." Dietary supplement makers that produce hypoallergenic, high-quality supplements—Dr. Ron's Ultra-Pure, Metagenics, Body Wise, and Thorne Research, among others—are more expensive than health food store brands and considerably more expensive than supermarket, drugstore and Big Box brands. However, you get a more bang for your buck if you take fewer high quality, pure supplements.

By consulting a qualified health practitioner to determine what is right for you, you maximize the effectiveness of your protocol, do not end up wasting money on junk supplements, and do not put money into the coffers of junk supplement businesses.

For those who don't have access to sound nutritional counsel, I asked naturopathic doctor Dr. Ron Schmid and clinical nutritionist Dr. Kayla Daniel for simple guidelines. "Take a couple of tablespoons daily of top quality, unrefined cod liver oil–the closest thing to a magic remedy that I've seen in twenty-five years of practice. Dr. Schmid told me store brands have had most of the vitamins removed. What you want is the real thing, old-fashioned pure cod liver oil." Dr. Kayla Daniel agreed, "There are many misconceptions about good sources of omega-3. Flax oil is high in omega-3s but does not contain readymade EPA and DHA fatty acids, which are needed for hormonal and brain health. Theoretically, our bodies can make the conversion from omega-3s to EPA and DHA but in practice most of us cannot. Although fish oils contain the valuable EPA and DHA, I prefer cod liver oil, especially one that is naturally high in vitamins A and D. Cod liver oil has been the key to healing for many of my clients, may of whom where either on flax or fish oils before coming to me."[2]

As for what else to take, Dr. Schmid said, "Complement [cod liver oil] with a top-quality, additive-free multivitamin that includes antioxidants, and a calcium formula made with hydroxyapatite calcium from grass-fed, organically-raised animals. These three supplements provide a base of critical nutrients that will go a long way toward solving medical problems and staying healthy and vibrant."[3]

If you want to go the extra distance, Dr. Schmid also recommends Activator-X, the deep yellow butter produced by grass-eating cows, that is consumed now more as a "supplement" than a food. "Activator-X was found by Dr. Weston Price to work synergistically with full-vitamin cod liver oil to enhance mineral metabolism and immunity," he said.

Useless supplements are not the only pills that Americans are reaching for today. Since the time of Louis Pasteur, when medicine turned away from nutrition as standard care and embraced drugs as the primary modality in the practice of medicine, Americans have become convinced that drugs are the answer to *curing* illness. However, a new trend in medicine has arisen recently: using drugs to *prevent* disease.

CHAPTER 28

Drug Pushers

IN THE LAST TWO decades, pharmaceutical companies have begun advertising on TV. The phenomenon started slowly, but has built to a truly alarming frequency as more people have become have become ill or are at risk for disease, and as drug companies recognized an opportunity to compete for our business. Drug ads typically focus our attention on our *hopes,* for which they sell us *quality of life,* and our *terror,* for which they sell us *hope.* We know what cancer centers to go to should we be diagnosed with cancer and what drugs to take to prepare for chemotherapy. We've learned that our cholesterol comes from food and from Grandma Rose and all about the cholesterol-lowering drugs which pharmaceutical companies are making $60 billion per year, and will soon have doctors prescribing to *children.* To treat our Type 2 diabetes we are reassured by ads like the ones with BB King grinning happily even though he has a life-threatening illness. It's comforting to know that our insulin and/or glucose modulating medications can be delivered right to our doors by that nice man, Wilfred Brimley.

While watching an episode of *Law and Order: Special Victims Unit,* in which Detective Elliot Stabler was taking an anti-HIV drug protocol after saving someone's life and being exposed to HIV, it occurred to me that I should make it perfectly clear that this isn't a drug-bashing book. Still, we must be cognizant of the fact that when it comes to taking drugs, you always get a two-fer. First you get the benefit of the drug, though not always. Allen Roses, MD, geneticist for the world's largest pharmaceutical corporation GlaxoSmithKline, said that 90 percent of drugs only work in 30 to 50 percent of people.[1] Even if you do get the purported benefit, *all* drugs have side effects, sometimes multiple potentially life-threatening side effects. Nevertheless, I think we can all agree that drugs have their place and can be beneficial, even lifesaving, when used judiciously.

What I'm talking about is that the food industry has made us fat and sick, dieting has failed, and now the drug industry is selling us drugs that are making us even sicker. There are many such drugs that do not need to be taken, and in fact, are either exacerbating our problems, creating new health problems, or the condition they are supposedly addressing could be easily corrected by stopping eating all factory food and eating real food, and by using alternative or natural healing or preventative approaches.

Unfortunately, Americans are bewildered about so-called "alternative" approaches outside of conventional medicine.

For example, bioidentical HRT (which we talked about briefly back in chapter 9) is an example of a controversial "natural" therapy that is confounding many doctors and menopausal women today. Suzanne Somers is an outspoken advocate of bioidentical hormone replacement. However, in the winter of 2006 Somers was taken to task on *Larry King Live* by a panel of doctors for including a bioidentical hormone protocol from an unaccredited "independent researcher" in her book *Ageless*. The protocol in question is designed to cycle women through estrogen and progesterone levels that match the hormone levels of a twenty-year-old woman. In other words, high estrogen and high progesterone. Instead of discussing the pros and cons of bioidentical hormones, the panel was reduced to a catfight, leaving Somers unable to get a word in edgewise and making room for a consultant to pharmaceutical companies to step in and discredit bioidentical hormones. He referred to the panel as "a cult" and went on to claim that there was no difference between synthetic Premarin Provera and bioidentical hormones. He maintained, "The physicians [who prescribe bioidentical HRT] are selling promises, silver bullets against aging with barely a nanoshred of evidence."[2]

David R. Allen, MD of the Longevity Medical Center in Los Angeles, has spent thirty years researching holistic treatment methods and is an advocate of bioidentical HRT. He said of this *Larry King Live* show, "In the late 1800s naturopathic medicine was the medicine of choice of the intelligencia in the United States. Then conflict developed between the high dose advocates and low dose advocates. Rather than have a reasoned discussion of the benefits of naturopathic medicine, the two camps were at each other's throats. Ultimately naturopathic medicine was dismissed by the conventional medical community."

The food, diet, and drug industries have fought hard to convince us that synthetic is as good—or better—than nature. When it comes to HRT millions of women disagree, but millions more continue to be confused. And advocates of natural HRT like Suzanne Somers run headfirst into the financial interests of pharmaceutical corporations.

Because Americans are confused about natural alternatives the drug industry has successfully convinced millions of people to medicate themselves and their children when often there is a natural, safe alternative. Brain neurotransmitter imbalance is a prime example of a condition that could be corrected by stopping eating all factory food and eating real food, and by using alternative or natural healing or preventative approaches. Millions of American children suffering from ADD and ADHD are medicated to enable them to function in school and in society. Family schedules are disrupted by stressful, expensive shrink appointments. Nothing's worked so far—but FYI, drug companies aren't really bothered by little failures like a few million kids.

In fact, if drug companies have learned one thing from the

sale of ADD and ADHD drugs, it is that medicating children is extremely lucrative. Incredibly, the largest growing market for antidepressant drugs is the age group between *infant to five-year-old*.[3] This is truly the most illustrative example of what I'm talking about in this book: As baby gestates, instead of eating real food which provides the crucial amino acids, essential fatty acids, cholesterol and other nutrients humans need to for fully developed brain development and neurotransmitter production, Mommy eats sugar and chemicalized garbage. As a result, baby begins his life with a lesser brain than he could have had, is deprived of mother's milk, fed antinutritious soy juice, and is then weaned on sugar and industrialized junk.

When neurotransmitter-imbalanced baby starts showing understandable signs of going haywire, he's given antidepressant drugs. And baby could possibly be among the 2 to 3 percent of children taking antidepressants who suffer from suicidal thoughts or behavior as a result of taking these drugs. Tarek A. Hammad, an FDA analyst who conducted a review of selective serotonin reuptake inhibitors (SSRIs) and other antidepressants in the fall of 2004, said that this outcome "is beyond the suicidality as a result of the disease being treated."[4]

FDA employee and Vioxx whistle-blower, Dr. David Graham said, "In early 2004, SSRI antidepressants and suicidal behavior was a big safety issue. The FDA suppressed a report written by a colleague of mine in drug safety and had prevented him from presenting this information in an advisory committee meeting. That information leaked to the media, embarrassing the FDA because it had been caught suppressing very important information—that most antidepressants don't work for treating children."[5]

Drug companies are also not all that upset when neurotransmitter-imbalanced children grow up to be brain neurotransmitter imbalanced adults. Lonely men and women who self-medicate with binges on FDA-approved, caffeinated, high fructose corn syrup sodas, baked goods, ice cream, and other factory products, then take FDA-approved SSRIs and other antidepressant medications in an attempt to dredge up a modicum of interest in life, as well as a shred of self-control and self-esteem. In 2003, 145 million prescriptions were written for antidepressant drugs, constituting about half of our population.

The dopamine reuptake inhibitor Wellbutrin XL's television ad features hysterically happy people riding horseback while the narrator slips in these deadly tidbits of information: "There is a risk of seizure when taking Wellbutrin XL, so don't use if you've had a seizure or eating disorder, or if you abruptly stop using alcohol or sedatives. Don't take with MAOIs or medicines that contain bupropion. When used with a nicotine patch or alone, there is a risk of increased blood pressure, sometimes severe. To reduce risk of serious side effects, tell your doctor if you have liver or kidney problems. Other side effects may include weight loss, dry mouth, nausea, difficulty sleeping, dizziness, or sore throat." The makers of Wellbutrin XL apparently think that the deal clincher is that there's supposedly a low risk of "sexual side effects." Yay! We can have sex while our liver slowly deteriorates.

On June 24, 2005, Tom Cruise appeared on NBC's *Today Show* to promote his film *War of the Worlds*, but quickly segued into a passionate discourse against antidepressant drugs. It began when host Matt Lauer mentioned the fact that Cruise had criticized Brooke Shields in a TV interview on *Access Hollywood* for taking antidepressants to treat her suicidal postpartum depression. Cruise, a member of the Church of Scientology, described psychiatry as a pseudoscience and said that people should turn to exercise and supplements rather than taking drugs to treat psychiatric problems. "I'm saying that drugs aren't the answer," Cruise argued. "These drugs are very dangerous. They're mind-altering, anti-psychotic drugs. And there are ways of doing it without that so that we don't end up in a brave new world."[6]

A week later, July 1, 2005, the FDA issued a public health advisory regarding the link between increased risk of suicidal tendencies in adults taking antidepressants, but this got virtually no press.[7]

In the meantime, Cruise was eviscerated by much of the media. Mike Duffy from the *Hollywood Reporter* summed up the general consensus: "We're seeing Tom Cruise gone wild and it's not pretty." Other reporters suggested that his stance against antidepressants and psychiatry would alienate fans.[8] The *New York Times* supported Cruise's behavior as a refreshing departure from publicist controlled, scripted happy talk.[9]

Clinical nutritionist Carol Simontacchi thought that, Scientology aside, Cruise made a valid point. "We're medicating without a good sound reason for doing so," said Simontacchi.[10] "We're just stuffing pills into our people without understanding their issues. The problem with the medical community is that they don't look at the body as a whole unit. You give them a symptom and they have a pill to solve the problem. They don't look at the underlying biochemistry. There's a whole list of possible biochemical influences that could be driving a person toward depression so why not look at that first?"

Ideally, Simontacchi said, a person would be evaluated for hypothyroidism, adrenal exhaustion, and female sex hormone imbalances, among other factors that could be causing their depression. When it comes to diet, Simontacchi, who treats people with depression with diet and amino acid supplementation, said there are many influences of the diet on depression. "Doctors do not evaluate patients' diets to understand whether or not the fundamental building blocks of neurotransmitters are being provided through nutrition. They don't evaluate whether patients are suffering from low blood sugar as a result of a high sugar diet. Food allergies, magnesium deficiency, zinc deficiency, B complex deficiency, fatty acid deficiency, or yeast overgrowth are all factors in depression. We're approaching a very frightening new world where we medicate against everything. The amount of money that is spent on advertising to the general public to medicate us even further is scary as heck."

Tom Cruise subsequently paid a visit to Brooke Shields to personally apologize for using her as an example but did not change his position on drugs, and I have to say that I mostly agree with him. Of course there are new mothers who suffer from life-threatening postpartum depression, the extreme example being Andrea Yates, whose postpartum depression ambushed her into a psychosis so dark that it compelled her to drown her five children. People with deep depression and especially psychosis can be spared a comparable tragedy by being offered a temporary lifeline of antidepressants. But for the millions of others who are not likely to experience a psychotic break due to their depression, there are options to taking drugs.

Logically one would think of starting by eliminating high fructose corn syrup altogether from our diet, as a diet of HFCS results in brain neurotransmitters imbalances. Yet, as Op-Ed columnist Nicholas D. Kristof writes, "Imagine if Al Qaeda had resolved to attack us not with conventional chemical weapons but by slipping large amounts of high-fructose corn syrup into our food supply. That would finally rouse us to action—but in fact it's pretty much what we're doing to ourselves."[11]

Another idea would be to use a "natural" remedy for depression. In the standard (albeit cruel) test of the efficacy of antidepressant drugs referred to as a "forced swim," rat subjects are tested to compare how long it takes for them to stop swimming (i.e., "give up") when given antidepressants as compared with rats that were not given antidepressants. Researchers at a Harvard affiliated hospital found that rats respond to omega-3—as in cod liver oil—the same way they respond to antidepressant drugs.[12]

Remember back in chapter 3 when we talked about the association between neurotransmitter imbalance and violence? A recent dietary experiment conducted in a maximum security institution for young offenders, demonstrated that essential fatty acids can also calm violent tendencies. More than two hundred inmates took part in a double-blind, randomized, placebo-controlled study.

Those given multivitamin, mineral, and fatty-acid supplements, as found in cod liver oil, experienced a 25 percent drop in antisocial behavior and a 35 percent stay of violent incidents. Among the placebo group, there was no change.[13]

What if our surgeon general got on TV and urged Americans to stop eating all high fructose corn syrup and to take cod liver oil daily and to give it to their children? What if he said, "I have something very important to tell you if you or your children are sad, depressed, aggressively acting out, or are suffering from other symptoms of neurological imbalance. Healthy brain neurotransmitters are dependent on the food you eat. When you eat food, your body uses it to fuel your brain, rebuild cells and tissues, and make the brain neurotransmitters you need to feel good. Since all that factory food you've been eating and feeding your children is not real food, your brain hasn't been getting the nutrients it needs to make neurotransmitters. That could be why you and your kids feel terrible all the time. One solution would be to stop eating all factory food and to eat real food!"

As we talked about earlier, aside from a natural food diet, there are alternatives to drugs for many conditions. Neurofeedback therapy, for example (which retrains brain wave patterns), has forty years of research behind it and can be used to safely treat numerous neurological problems from ADD to insomnia to schizophrenia.[14] If you are interested in learning more about neurofeedback you can log onto www.isnr.org.

But since insurance companies and doctors are mostly dismissive of neurofeedback therapy and other noninvasive, safe, and effective approaches to neurological disorders, the factory food and drug companies are free to march on, hand in hand all the way to the bank—with FDA approval—as Americans get sicker.

Speaking of sex. Many Americans felt that Bill Clinton deserved to be impeached from the office of the president of the United States because he lied about a dalliance in the Oval Office. Many parents were incensed that they had to explain to their children what "oral sex" meant. Today, just a few short years later, there's no discussion about the fact that children are learning from the TV ads of pharmaceutical companies that men who take impotence medications should seek medical attention *if their erections last more than four hours.*

Let's take a closer look at this issue because it represents the reprehensible levels that drug companies will stoop to get us to buy their drugs. In the last decade or so, pharmaceutical companies have branded the human condition. The purpose of branding is to cultivate and maintain a loyal customer base. These days without branding it is virtually impossible to market a product. Branding begins with identification. The drug industry would like you to feel identified with disease. And so the drug industry, which is intent on convincing us that we are diseased and that the "cure" is their drugs, brands our sicknesses with acronyms. The list of conditions that have been abbreviated and woven into the daily weave of our lives is now endless. One "disease" that has become alarmingly familiar has been branded with the acronym ED, for *Erectile Dysfunction.*

The term "erectile dysfunction" is a frightening, insulting, degrading, and humiliating condemnation for any man. And the cloying way this "disease" is presented on TV commercials would make any man feel like a mouse. It would make any man willing to do whatever it took to restore his manhood. Even if it meant taking pills that could cause blindness and erections that last over four hours.

Way back in 1954, Adele Davis wrote in *Let's Eat Right to Keep Fit,* "Studies of men in prison camps, of the conscientious objectors in the starvation experiments at the University of Minnesota, and of numerous clinical investigations show that libido decreases or disappears when the nutrition is inadequate."[15] And in his book, *A Brief History of Everything,* philosopher Ken Wilbur writes, "It appears that testosterone basically has two, and only two, major drives: fuck it or kill it." Now both the connection between inadequate nutrition and libido and the relationship between sex hormones and male drives take us back to Francis Pottenger's cats. Fed nutrient dead-diets, the females were she-devils, and the males, meek and cringing. Could we find some similarities in men and women who eat nutrient-dead diets? Yet instead of focusing on providing adequate nutrition for endocrine glands to produce the sex hormones necessary for a healthy libido, men take Viagra, Cialis, and Levitra (giving new meaning to the adage "love is blind.").

Although the pharmaceutical industry has not yet developed a sex drug for women, the hack supplement industry has jumped right in to sell women on hopeful-sounding female sexual function restoratives like Zestra Feminine Arousal Fluid. The reality is that the ability to engage in artificially induced sexual performance does nothing to repair our flagging endocrine systems. But as we continue on our accelerated aging path toward ugly death, at least we can still do it once in a while.

One commercial for ED tells men that high blood pressure and Type 2 diabetes are conditions that could result in ED. The commercial does not tell men that there are ways of dealing with high blood pressure and Type 2 diabetes, like not eating that KFC bowl of industrialized mashed potatoes, chemicalized sweet corn, deep fried factory chicken, classic glurk gravy, and factory cheese. The commercial does not say, "Hey, if you get some exercise, eat real food, stop taking all of our drugs, you'll feel like having sex." Okay, if you are a man or woman over fifty you might choose to take a physiologic dose of bioidentical HRT but that is due to a natural decline in hormones; it is not because you are "diseased."

Gastrointestinal problems are a multibillion dollar source of revenue for the drug industry. These problems could mostly be resolved by stopping eating all factory food and eating only real food. Comedian Bill Maher said it best in his 2005 HBO stand-up special: "Last year we passed in our Congress this giant Medicare entitlement prescription drug bill . . . . And it's going to cost literally trillions and trillions of dollars. And why they were debating this, nobody ever stood up and said, 'Excuse me, but why are we so sick? Why do even older people need this amount of drugs?' Could it be because we eat like Caligula? You know the top five of those prescription drugs that are so popular, they're all antacids, antibloating medicines, digestive aides, all things to put out the fire in our stomach from the poison that we call lunch. Folks, it's the food. I know that people hate to hear that. But when you look at those ads on the evening news at night, people farting and burping and bloating, it's all shit trying to get out of you. Take a hint . . . . You're not going to die from secondhand smoke, or SARS, or monkey pox. It's the food. The call is coming from inside the house. The killer is not West Nile or Avian Flu or shark attacks. It's the Buffalo wings. It's the aspartame and the NutraSweet, and the red dye number two and the high fructose corn syrup and the MSG and the chlorine and whatever shit is in special sauce."[16]

Ads on the tube for gastrointestinal medications invariably feature people eating pizza, fast food chili, and other glop made up of that very same special sauce Maher referred to.

Then there are those who get the call from inside the house, but suffer from chronic all-systems lockdown which they seek to break through by consuming all sorts of truly repugnant sounding OTCs such as X-LAX, Rite-Aid Col-Rite Stool Softener, and Metamucil, when a couple of tablespoons of flavored cod liver oil every day would do the trick nicely.

Tissue inflammation is culprit behind the pain that causes people to seek out prescriptions for Cox-2 inhibitors. Cod liver oil contains omega-3 fatty acids, which are used to make hormones that control inflammation. In addition to taking cod liver oil, eating anti-inflammatory foods such as cold water fish (mackerel, salmon, sardines, and tuna) and their oils, flaxseeds (in moderation), walnuts, and organically fed, range-free eggs seems like a less life-threatening approach than taking pills that have already been proven to cause damage to the heart.

Would you be surprised to learn that, despite alarming statistics, osteoporosis is really a very rare condition? Embroidered statistics have been brought to us courtesy of drug companies who have redefined the testing of low bone mineral density. As it turns out, the measure of your bone mineral density (BMD) is only one of many factors that determine the risk of bone fragility. The reality is that everyone will naturally lose bone density as part of normal aging and all bones, no matter how dense, will break if smacked hard enough. But the new standards in testing have made it nearly impossible for anyone over fifty to have a "normal" diagnosis.[17] Thus we of a certain age are scared silly about falling down, fracturing a hip, and dying a horrible death. Or we are panicked about developing a dowager's hump from spinal compression (vertebral fractures).

The new BMD statistics commercials and print ads for FDA-approved osteoporosis drugs sell us on medications that have grab a bag of side effects and contraindications. Drugs like Actonel, which claims to "help fight fracture," carry the warning, "You should not take Actonel if you have low blood calcium, have severe kidney disease, or *cannot sit or stand for thirty minutes.* [Emphasis mine.] Stop taking Actonel and tell your doctor if you experience difficult or painful swallowing, chest pain, or severe or continuing heartburn, as these may be signs of serious upper digestive problems. Side effects are generally mild or moderate and may include back or joint pain, stomach pain or upset, or constipation."

Fosamax is another nasty drug that dramatically increases the risk of stomach ulcers when taken with the arthritis drug Naprosyn.[18] Joseph Mercola, MD, who hosts the alternative website www.mercola.com writes, "Fosamax is in the same chemical class (phosphonate) that is used in the cleaners used to remove soap scum from your bath tub." Fosamax has also been linked to osteonecrosis (bone death) of the jaw.[19]

Bones are living tissues that are constantly breaking down and rebuilding in order to maintain structural integrity. Bones are like tubes that are made of and filled with protein and hardened by calcium. It's the hardening of this protein that makes bone solid. The osteoclast cells break down and eliminate old bone, and then osteoblast cells lay down new bone matrix, which is made up of collagen. Collagen, a protein, is the structure of bone. After the bone matrix is laid down, hormones direct calcium to be laid down on top of the protein. This new bone matrix is thus calcified.

When Fosamax kills osteoclast cells, bones get denser temporarily, but in time, bones weaken because the natural process of breaking down and building up has been disrupted. And disrupting normal bone metabolism spells less bone formation and increased bone breakdown, which ultimately results in osteopenia (less bone) and then osteoporosis (fracture).[20]

Whether Fosamax has reduced hip fractures by even one percent has been disputed.[21]

Unlike a teaching skeleton that can hang pretty much indefinitely in a classroom, a fifty-year-old woman does not have the same skeleton that she had when she was thirty. Every single cell has been broken down and replaced numerous times. And does anyone really believe that her skeleton can be replaced with enriched cereal, Tums, Fosamax, Actonel, or, the once-a-month "bone builder" Boniva? It's common sense that living tissue can only be replaced by eating the same biochemicals that make up bones.

In a perfect world, the surgeon general would be on TV urging Americans to prevent osteopenia—the thinning of bones that results in osteoporosis—by using bioidentical HRT (if that is your choice), quitting the use of stimulants, quitting smoking, exercising more—especially outside in the sun to obtain vitamin D—abstaining from factory food, and, instead, eating real foods that provide adequate protein, fat, calcium, and other minerals, vitamins, and enzymes.

There are many other examples of drugs that are making matters worse, but the most classic are the cholesterol-lowering drugs. Because of the lipid hypothesis, the subsequent low-fat diet, and the accompanying science fiction fats that launched the epidemic of heart disease, drug companies are now cleaning up selling us these drugs.

On January 4, 2004, when the highly-touted guidelines for

preventing heart disease and stroke in women were issued by the AHA, there was not one mention that women should stop eating hydrogenated and partially hydrogenated polyunsaturated vegetable oils, chemical- and heat-treated polyunsaturated vegetable oils, refined white flour, refined white sugar, high fructose corn syrup, MSG, aspartame, factory-produced animal products and other factory substances. No, just eat "heart healthy" (i.e., a low-fat, low-cholesterol diet) and have a piece of Fudgy Chocolate Walnut Pie and a bowl of Lucky Charms, and, of course, take cholesterol-lowering medication.

For over fifty years we've had hammered into our heads the misconception that total cholesterol numbers are the number-one indicator of our risk of a heart attack. The fear of cholesterol is so entrenched in our culture that it is likely here to stay. On June 9, 2005, Ben Stiller accepted his MTV Movie Award for "Best Villain" for his role as a menacing gym owner in the movie *Dodgeball*. In his acceptance speech, Stiller lampooned Hollywood celebrities' tradition of speaking out for causes by segueing into a shtick about cholesterol. "Take a look at this fella," he said, holding up an egg. "He's killed more people than all the Hollywood bad guys combined. Crush cholesterol now!" Yolk and shell splashed over the podium.

Numerous studies have demonstrated that high cholesterol is not a risk factor for women, that women with high cholesterol live longer than women with low cholesterol, and that it's more dangerous for women to have low cholesterol than high. People who suffer from heart disease sometimes have elevated blood cholesterol numbers, but not everyone who has elevated blood cholesterol numbers develops heart disease. Everyone with heart disease does not have elevated blood cholesterol numbers. In fact, most people with heart disease do not have elevated blood cholesterol.[22]

Study after study has proven that your cholesterol number, regardless if it is high or not, is not an indication of risk or lack of risk for heart disease.[23] Dr. Enig told me, "Blood cholesterol levels between 200 and 240 mg/dl are normal. These levels have always been normal. In older women, serum cholesterol levels greatly above these numbers are also quite normal, and in fact they have been shown to be associated with longevity. Since 1984, however, in the United States and other parts of the western world, these normal numbers have been treated as if they were an indication of a disease in progress or a potential for disease in the future."[24]

Dr. Enig maintains that cholesterol in the blood is a good thing. "The official advice to lower serum cholesterol levels has brought about numerous supplements with the attached claim that consuming them will lower cholesterol. This further supports the myth of cholesterol as an undesirable component of body and diet. In fact, the body uses cholesterol to repair and to protect. When improvement to the health of the body brought about by good changes in lifestyle or diet results in a lowering of serum cholesterol, it can be counted as an example of the body no longer needing the extra circulating cholesterol. The repair has been accomplished."[25]

Cholesterol is a waxy alcohol that maintains the structure of every single cell in your body. In fact, every cell in your body makes its own cholesterol and your liver manufactures it day and night. Your body has a system of checks and balances so that it will always have enough cholesterol to keep up the ongoing repair and replenishing of your body on a cellular level.

Cholesterol and triglycerides, which are water insoluble, are packaged into water-soluble lipo-proteins so they can float through your watery bloodstream. Your total cholesterol is arrived at by adding together the three different cholesterol-carrying lipoproteins: high density lipoproteins (HDLs), low density lipoproteins (LDLs), and very low density lipoproteins (VLDLs). HDLs, LDLs, and VLDLs are delivery vehicles that take cholesterol and triglycerides to and fro within your body via your bloodstream. They have been labeled good and bad, but each lipoprotein actually has a healthy purpose in your body.

HDLs are said to be "good" lipoproteins because they recycle cholesterol back to the liver. LDLs carry cholesterol from the liver to your cells for use as raw material. LDLs are labeled "bad" because they can get damaged en route and end up as deposits of cholesterol in your artery walls. Damage occurs to LDL lipoproteins by oxidation caused by free radicals.

Another way LDLs get damaged is from excess blood sugar, which "caramelizes" LDL lipoproteins, similar to dunking an apple into a bubbling cauldron of caramel. In addition to coating LDLs, this candy coating also builds up on your cells and arteries. By not eating sugary and high carbohydrate factory food and eating a balanced diet of whole real food, you will protect your LDLs.

VLDLs carry triglycerides (fat) throughout your body for use as energy. Since HDLs and VLDLs levels are like kids on a teeter-totter, if your eating and lifestyle habits raise your HDLs you are going to see your VLDLs go down proportionately, and vice versa.

Since HDLs, LDLs, and VLDLs all perform different functions, adding them up to arrive at a total cholesterol number does not tell you anything one way or another. Nevertheless, the food, diet, and drug industries have made billions of dollars on cholesterol-lowering measures such as "heart healthy" food products, lab tests, and so on. The drug industry would also like each and every adult—(*and now children*)—to take cholesterol-lowering drugs even though study after study has concluded that atherosclerosis increases in patients whose cholesterol is decreased by more than 60 mg/dl and that atherosclerosis worsens just as fast or faster when cholesterol levels go down as when cholesterol levels go up, that people with low cholesterol levels suffer from just as much atherosclerosis as people with high cholesterol levels, and that lowering cholesterol levels increases your risk of dying from violence or suicide.[26]

If you don't eat enough cholesterol to sustain your body's need for cholesterol, your body sees this deprivation as a time of famine and activates the enzyme HMG-CoA Reductase in your liver, which overproduces cholesterol out of the carbohydrates you eat. Cholesterol-lowering drugs work by switching off this enzyme.

Switching off HMG-CoA Reductase means that your body may not be getting the cholesterol it needs for important ongoing building and replenishing.

In the spring of 2004, a study that compared high doses of Lipitor (made by Pfizer) with less potent Pravachol (made by Bristol-Myers Squibb, which sponsored the trial) showed that patients taking Lipitor were significantly less likely to have heart attacks or to require bypass surgery or angioplasty. Lipitor was shown to halt plaque growth; Pravachol was shown to only slow plaque growth.[27]

I asked Drs. Eades to weigh in. "The study showed only very modest benefit [0.6 percent reduction in occurrence rate of heart attack in five years] at an enormous cost. One hundred and sixty-five healthy people would, over a period of five years, have to spend $1.2 million purchasing Lipitor to extend the life of one person by five years. Statins don't come without side effects, some of which are merely debilitating, some of which are lethal. Although the statin class of drugs do indeed lower cholesterol, a number of recent studies have begun to dispel the notion that elevated cholesterol is even a player in the development of heart disease. Moreover, if lowering cholesterol is the point, a recent study of modern hunter-gatherers shows that these groups naturally maintained LDL levels below the magic 100, without benefit of statins, simply by following a healthy meat-based diet, higher in protein, lower in carbohydrate and replete with good fats. Our advice: eat real food, save the money you'd spend on statins, and don't risk the possibility of serious side effects."[28]

With the top selling cholesterol drug, Lipitor ($2.2 billion in sales in 2005), due to lose patent protection in 2011, Pfizer was motivated to pull out all the stops in researching a new patentable drug. But on December 4, 2006, after spending $800 million on research, Pfizer was compelled by the FDA to halt clinical trials on its star heart-disease drug torcetrapib after documenting an increase in deaths and heart problems in the test subjects. Torcetrapib was supposed to increase HDLs, so-called "good" cholesterol.[29] This failure will not stop the industry from pursuing other angles.

Factory food makers are married to drug manufacturers in two important ways: First, factory foods make people sick, thus the need for drugs. And second, factory foods and drugs are both purchased by individuals who are convinced that what they are doing is healthy. In addition to eating "healthful" factory substances approved by the FDA, the AMA, and the AHA, we are now convinced that Americans are heart attacks waiting to happen, and to prevent a heart attack from occurring we must take cholesterol-lowering drugs. If the $60 billion per year cholesterol lowering drugs we are taking are so effective, why are Americans still dropping from heart disease?

What is really sad is that people are now programmed into thinking that they can continue eating factory food substances as long as they take drugs. Moreover, many people are deathly afraid of the real food diet that would save them from developing the maladies that are causing them to take prescribed drugs in the first place. These are the people who look askance at a rib eye steak and real butter but admit to being on a perilous cocktail of drugs, including statins, antidepressants, and impotence drugs. Americans have become so acculturated to drugs that having a medicine cabinent full of drugs is normal.

In the Fox drama *House*, each episode follows Dr. House, a Vicodin addicted, brilliant, but acerbic diagnostician, and his three interns as they misdiagnose a patient, prescribing a toxic dose of some drug. Invariably the experiment causes life-threatening and often unspeakable side effects before the lightbulb comes on for House, allowing him to save the patient's life with another drug.

Philip Roth's novel *Everyman* explores the remorse of a man whose philandering and hedonistic obsessions had left him bereft of meaning and companionship in his golden years. Along the way he suffers one cardiac event/surgery after the next. A background cast of characters are by turns decimated by drugs. One is laid low by chemotheraphy, one has a stroke from taking a risky migraine drug, and another's back pain cannot be allievated by pain pills so she gobbles enough to do herself in. Since drugs, drugs, drugs, and more drugs (and their side effects) are perfectly natural for us, drugs are thus a likely backdrop for "everyman's" story.

Meanwhile, our anti-real food, socially acceptable pharmacutical (but *not* recreational!) drug mentality, perpetuated by organizations like the American Heart Association—"the most respected source for health and nutrition"—is killing Americans.

It's important to note that stress can temporarily cause your cholesterol numbers to skyrocket—so if you are stressed out about having high cholesterol the day that you have your labs drawn, the number that comes back is likely not going to be an accurate account of what is really going on with your cholesterol. Nevertheless, it's not any one lipoprotein number or the total cholesterol number that should scare you. And the emphasis on your genetics is just another unnessary (and frightening) detour. A genetic predisposition does not automatically mean that you are doomed. There is more and more evidence that heart disease is caused by a constellation of factors related to eating and lifestyle habits.

Deficiencies of B vitamins in the diet (folic acid, vitamin B_6, and vitamin B_{12}) raise the level of an amino acid called homocysteine in the bloodstream. When elevated, homocysteine has been found to cause arterial damage and plaquing. You can reduce your risk by eating foods rich in vitamin B, or by taking quality vitamin B supplements. Foods high in folic acid are brewers' yeast, oranges, green leafy vegetables, wheat germ, asparagus, broccoli, nuts. Foods high in vitamin B_6 are whole grains, meats, fish, poultry, nuts, and brewers' yeast. And foods high in vitamin B_{12} are meat, fish, poultry, eggs, and dairy.

Prolonged high insulin levels, as we talked about earlier, encourage coronary artery plaquing. Factors that keep insulin in a prolonged high state are reviewed on page 259.

It is now understood that inflammation is a major risk factor of heart disease. Normal inflammation is part of the immune reaction that helps your body to heal from injury. When the immune system refuses to turn off, inflammation can result in a relatively small arterial plaque ballooning and blocking the passage to the heart causing heart attack (heart muscle death). Why are we so inflamed? Could the gallons of coffee and Diet Coke have something to do with it? The cocktails of OTCs and prescription drugs? Sitting on our butts, watching TV, while eating carbs and transfats? An anti-inflammatory diet includes fish (small so you are not getting a biweekly dose of mercury), wheat germ and walnuts, a few fresh flaxseeds (from time to time), healthy oils (reviewed on page 124); and any brightly colored vegetable or fruit all contain anti-inflammatory properties.

Chapters 14 through 18 explained the relationship between chemical- and heat-processed polyunsaturated fats (trans fats and free radicals) and heart disease. I would venture to say if these fats had never entered our food chain we would not be discussing heart disease today.

I Googled the word "healing" and got 53,800,000 results; on Amazon it was 93,200,000. In the past several decades, Americans have turned their attention toward preventative measures and healing because our instincts are telling us that we are sick on a deep level. Although we may not be conscious of it, the repercussions of our individual ill health manifest in the collective ill health of our society as a whole. For example, if a child does not do well in school because he or she suffers from neurotransmitter imbalances, it ultimately affects society as a whole for the span of that child's life.

Modern medicine discarded nutrition along with the focus on disease prevention. Instead, the focus has been on treating disease after it occurs, primarily with drugs. Unfortunately, more recently the focus has shifted to *preventing* disease with drugs. However, you cannot hit one health issue with a sledgehammer and expect to feel and be well because all drugs impact your body's homeostasis. Whenever the body perceives an abnormal state, its coordinated adaptive responses attempt to return it back to homeostasis, or the status quo.

When the baby boomers started aging, antiaging medicine began to emerge which focused on nondrug, preventative modalities such as balanced nutrition, stress reduction, hormone replacement therapy (HRT), nutraceuticals/dietary supplements, and exercise. Antiaging medicine is generally viewed by mainstream medicine as a vanity driven, fringy, wayward cousin to real medicine. But lo and behold, as a result of the advances in antiaging medicine, another branch of preventative medicine sprang up, spearheaded by enlightened physicians and clinical nutritionists who broke ranks from the traditional dietitian mentality of old—those dietitians who planned the Ensure-cornflakes-coffee hospital meals described earlier. These nutritionists and physicians are developing a new medical approach based on the philosophy that many health problems (including obesity) can be resolved or at least significantly helped by this same protocol.

This new frontier in medicine takes us back to Hippocrates, who focused on the effects of food, occupation, and environment in the development of disease. Today's new breed of health practitioners understands that seeking to balance the entire body is the key to optimal wellness. And the primary factor in overall balance is keeping or bringing hormone levels into balance.

People tend to think of menopausal women in connection with hormone imbalance. But as you now understand, many diseases such as Type 2 diabetes, heart disease, and some cancers are the result of prolonged high insulin levels caused by eating too much sugar, eating a low-fat diet, stress, dieting, drinking too much caffeine and alcohol, using tobacco, ingesting aspartame, using steroids, having a sedentary lifestyle, using recreational drugs, and taking too many OTC and prescription drugs. Stress, sugar, and stimulants have resulted in adrenal imbalances (what we call burnout). Overeating goitrogenic (thyroid inhibiting) foods like soy, as well as chemical exposure, has resulted in a rise in hypothyroidism. Children who were raised on sugar, soy, and chemicals are medicated for depression and other neurological disorders, which are imbalances of brain neurotransmitters. Factory food-eating men and women are going into early andropause and menopause. And twenty-something women—raised on factory food, diets, and drugs—have estrogen levels comparable to menopausal women.

When your body's various systems (endocrine, immune, neurological, and so on) are not operating at capacity, there are health consequences. If you are fat and unhealthy, it is guaranteed that your endocrine system is not operating as smoothly as it could and that you have some type of hormonal imbalance, whether it is insulin, sex hormones, melatonin, thyroid, cortisol, or other.

This does not mean that you should rush out and self-medicate.

I have heard DHEA mentioned on TV as "an over-the-counter supplement." However, DHEA—like all other hormones—needs to be modulated by a qualified hormone specialist according to laboratory blood draws and symptoms. DHEA supplementation can result in facial hair on women. This is just one example of irresponsible medical commentary we get from TV and other media sources that gets people going off on tangents with over-the-counter hormone replacement (and other supplementation). Since all systems of the body are interconnected and hormones are the chemical messengers, it stands to reason that we would want to be hypercareful about the hormones we take.

If you're overweight and sick, your first course of action should be to attempt to rebalance your endocrine system by stopping eating all factory food and eating only real food. Then if you still suffer from symptoms of hormone imbalance—or if you are over the age of say, forty—you may choose to use some form of HRT.

It's important to find a qualified practitioner who you feel in sync with, who can prescribe HRT and monitor your results and symptoms.

The examples in this chapter of "preventative" drugs demonstrate how industry has clutched American consumers in a death grip of an unhealthy symbiotic relationship in which they are fattened up on factory food and "treated" for subsequent obesity and disease with diets and drugs. And to keep us in this relationship, these industries use wooing, denial, ridicule, and threats.

VIII

Wooing, Denial, Ridicule, and Threats . . . And Why We Buy Into Them

CHAPTER 29

Wooing, Denial, Ridicule, and Threats

IN 1968, at age eighteen, I was swept into the mass exodus of the love generation overland from Europe through Turkey, Iran, Pakistan and Afghanistan, to India and Ceylon (now Sri Lanka). In the jungle in Ceylon I met my lifelong friend Jitka Gunaratna, then a Czechoslovakian expatriate, fishing with a safety pin and a shred of coconut. It was less than a year after the infamous Prague Spring and Jitka, who had been in Czechoslovakia during the Russian invasion, was still reeling from that horrible event. As we ate her fish, she cried and reiterated the story to me.

Twenty-five years later, Jitka visited me in Santa Barbara, where I caught her in front of the TV watching a chemical company ad about caring for some bird. "You're not crying, are you?" I asked her.

"Well, I see this advertisement on CNN International and I find it so touching," she sniffed. "I always cry."

"Jitka," I said darkly, "aren't you the little Czech girl who also cried when Russian tanks rolled over your fellow citizens in the Wenceslas Square in Prague in 1968, and cried again when that Communist regime decimated your country?"

"Uh-huh," she admitted, smiling sheepishly as she wiped away a tear.

"*You,* of all people, should understand the meaning of *propaganda.*"

"But it's so heartwarming," she insisted. "Those birds."

Propaganda works. In fact, an insidious campaign of extremely effective propaganda using wooing, denial, ridicule, and threats has enslaved Americans to factory food and ensnared us in an unhealthy symbiotic relationship with the medical establishment, government, and industries.

Back in 1966, when Professor Timothy Leary was launching himself as a psychedelic visionary, a media savvy friend gave him some advice: "The key to your work is advertising. You're promoting a product. The new and improved accelerated brain. You must use the most current tactics for arousing consumer interest. Associate LSD with all the good things that the brain can produce—beauty, fun, philosophic wonder, religious revelation, increased intelligence, mystical romance. Word of mouth from satisfied consumers will help, but get your rock and roll friends to write jingles about the brain."[1]

Okay, this sounds vaguely familiar if you look at the first tactic used to get us to eat, diet, and take drugs—it involves wooing through all of the above mentioned strategies. For example, Americans are infatuated with celebrities. They are beautiful, fun, sexy, romantic. You could even say their images provoke philosophic wonder and religious revelation (to some). And so they are used prolifically to woo us into consuming products. But the reality is that professional athletes, movie stars, celebrities, and musicians do not know what is best for us just because they are on an athletic field or court, on TV, in a movie, or on a musical stage. Historically, actors, athletes, buffoons, fools, jesters, singers, musicians, jugglers, and other entertainers were societal outcasts, only tolerated to the extent that they could amuse and entertain. Today, however, even though these people earn obscene amounts of money in their professions, they are paid extra obscene amounts of money to woo us into eating industrialized food with promises of good health, beauty, fitness, and satisfaction. Recent examples are Jessica Simpson and Queen Latifah for Pizza Hut, Paris Hilton for Carl's Jr., and Mary-Kate Olsen—fresh out of a treatment facility for an eating disorder—paid to endorse McDonald's Happy Meals (in France, no less). Coca-Cola, as of this writing, celebrated winning the global marketing rights for the *Harry Potter and the Sorcerer's Stone*, a franchise estimated at $75 million, paid to the author J. K. Rowling, who is already worth *one billion dollars*. Factory food makers spend a fortune licensing cartoon heroes to woo kids into eating sugar.

On October 16, 2006, Disney announced that they were going to begin restricting licensing agreements with their cartoon characters on food products targeted at children. As soon as current licensing agreements run out in 2008 they will curtail their licensing on some products and will begin to endorse "healthy" food. So we are back to the issue of what is healthy? Banning trans-fats from all foods is a good thing. But restricting "fats" unilaterally for children is not healthy; children need abundant fat and cholesterol to develop their young brains. It appears that corporations consider a "healthy" meal to be a salad of greens grown with chemical fertilizers near cattle factories that are the harbingers of *E. Coli* 0157:H7 bacteria doused in salad dressing containing free radical vegetable oils, MSG, and various chemicals.

Aside from celebrities (human or otherwise), there is blatant seduction with Denny's breakfast ads that air on prime time TV, wooing us with powdered sugared French toast and oozing syrup so that's we're psychologically primed to go to Denny's A-sap in the A.M.

An attractively housewife-ish actress woos us into believing the preposterous claim that the Enova blend of (unhealthy) canola and soy oils is so healthy that "less of it is stored in the body as fat."

Product manufacturers twist science to woo us into eating their products. General Mills claims that "studies show whole grain is good for the heart," to promote the sales of Cinnamon Toast

Crunch, Golden Grahams, Lucky Charms, Cocoa Puffs, Trix, and so on. This mangling of science takes extreme forms such as the Glucerna candy bars and shakes that are pitched to a population of diabetics in danger of going blind and suffering amputations as "smart nutrition for people with diabetes." Their Web site, "Diabetics Health Connection," assures diabetics that "the unique blend of slowly digested carbs in Glucerna Bars and Shakes are clinically shown to help manage blood sugar, so enjoy Glucerna and take control of your diabetes."[2]

Denial comes with statements issued by companies that claim their products' efficacy, safety, or health benefits are backed up by voluminous scientific research, which upon closer scrutiny was paid for by the industries intent on making profits on these products.

Denial comes from the government and food companies that refuse to admit that industrialized products are not the same as natural food. A prime example is the attempt to tarnish the meaning of the word "organic."

By the mid–1990s many Americans had caught the scent of an ill wind blowing in our food industry. In an effort to protect themselves and their children, they joined the organic food movement, shopping in more expensive "health food" stores and local farmer's markets. But the food industry's goal is to render the term "organic" as meaningless as the word "natural" has been since the recipe for granola got away from that hippie girl way back when.

Organic labeling for dairy products, for example, generally means that the product is free of antibiotic, herbicide, pesticide, growth hormone, chemical fertilizer, and genetically modified organism residues, and that animals have "outdoor access" to pastures and are fed one hundred percent organic feed. But as it turns out "organic feed" does not necessary mean that the animals are fed a species-appropriate diet or that they spend all their time, or even a majority of their time, or any time at all, in the pasture, even though the nutritional value of the milk crucially depends on these factors.

Horizon Organic Dairy (owned by Dean, the largest milk supplier in the United States) controls 70 percent of the organic retail market in the United States, offering a full line of "certified organic dairy products."[3] Their own labeling declares that their milk is ultra pasteurized (sterilized). Numerous watchdog agencies have reported that Horizons has circumvented the organic regulations and that their cows are not pasture grazed, but rather kept in dry lots.

This example rocks the organic food movement's dreams of supporting small, local farmers and of treating animals humanely and the environment responsibly in the process of producing the highest quality food for human beings. Unless monitored by consumers, these dreams could be obliterated as the multibillion dollar dominating corporations charge in with their wallets open and with lax standards about animal caretaking and human nutrition. The newly-purchased operations are likely to evolve into exactly the kind of monster commercial industries that organically-minded consumers are trying to escape.

In May 2004 the *New York Times* reported, "Federal standards for what foods can be called organic might have seemed like the final word on the issue when they went into effect two years ago. But the Agriculture Department's interpretation of the laws governing the National Organic Program has fed a fierce debate on what should be allowed in such products." The article went on to explain that the Agriculture Department had recently issued a "clarification of the standards," which allowed antibiotics in dairy cows.

Senator Patrick Leahy (D-VT), "the father of national organic standards," immediately asked Agriculture Secretary Ann M. Veneman to rescind these directives and to seek public comment before making these and other changes to organic standards. In response, Barbara Robinson, the deputy administrator of Agricultural Marketing Services, which is in charge of the National Organic Program, said that the department *was not creating new rules but was only seeking to clarify existing regulations.* For that reason, they didn't have to seek public comment or consult with the National Organic Standards Board, which is an expert advisory group that, by law, establishes standards.

The bottom line was that the government was seeking to blur the lines between adulterated foods and organically grown foods—but to innocently deny they were doing so.

Governmental attempts to dilute the meaning of organic and deny there is any problem are being made on behalf of mega industrialists such as Dean Foods, Smucker's, and Kraft that are intent on making cheap, noxious factory fare and passing it off as nourishing. In October 2005, the Agricultural Appropriations Conference Committee—a Congressional subcommittee—granted "organic" manufacturers the right to use synthetic ingredients in the processing of their wares, an act in direct defiance of the 1990 Organic Foods Production Act, which established consistent standards for the term organic. The stealth tactics of Congress benefits corporations, taints the integrity of all organic products, and sets back the growth of small farmers and ranchers who supply real organic food. Thus, although alternative farmers have sacrificed for thirty-five years to provide a growing demand for organic food, today you may regularly be eating a pretend organic or certified organic factory product that defies the true ideology behind these terms.

Martin E. O'Conner, the chief of the standardization branch of the U.S. Department of Agriculture, has some bizarre ideas about the definition of "grass-fed" meat. Now that the term grass fed has become a buzz-term, organic eating Americans have come to assume grass fed to mean "meat from organically raised animals that roamed contentedly on pastures."

But O'Conner would like to change that definition to "animals that are kept in feedlots and fed 'forage,' i.e., legumes and soybeans." In other words, if Conner has his way animals that have never so much as seen a blade of grass in the pasture and that are pumped up on hormones and antibiotics will be slaughtered and their meat labeled "grass fed."[4]

Another example of denial that industrialized food is not the same as real food is the USDA's dairy "checkoff" program, which requires farmers and ranchers to pay for generic advertising aimed at boosting industry sales.

Joseph and Brenda Cochran and their fourteen children own and operate a third-going-on-fourth-generation family farm in Westfield, Pennsylvania. The USDA collects a mandatory fee of fifteen cents per hundred pounds of milk from dairy farmers like the Cochrans to pay for checkoff programs such as the popular "Got Milk?" campaign. But the Cochran family didn't want to continue contributing to a campaign that was not being straight with the public.

"The checkoff system treats all milk the same and that's simply not the case," Joe told me. "People who graze cows have a different type of milk. Some dairies treat their cows with growth hormones. The milk that comes out of those cows is different from our milk. The advertising fund takes money from us and puts it into a generic fund that gives consumers a sense that there's really no difference. This type of advertising does not give the consumer enough information to make informed choices."

Although these milk suppliers did not endorse the governments "Got Milk?" campaign, they were forced to take legal action to be released from contributing to it. Supported by the Center for Individual Freedom in Alexandria, Virginia, on April 2, 2002, the Cochrans filed suit against the government seeking to end the payments that were costing the family business up to $4,200 per year. The Cochran's suit maintained that the First Amendment granted them the right to speak *and* the right to remain silent. After two long years of legal wrangling, on March 5, 2004, the court ruled, by unanimous decision, that the dairy checkoff was unconstitutional under the First Amendment.[5]

This story illustrates the government denial that there is any difference between milk produced by ill treated, sick, unhappy cows in factories and pure, healthy, natural, organic milk produced by pasture grazing, happy cows.

The totally science fiction fat olestra is another example of denial. Although Procter & Gamble admitted that there were some problems with the interference of vitamin E absorption and that olestra caused anal leakage, on January 24, 1996, the FDA approved olestra for use in chips, crackers, and tortilla chips with one caveat: Products had to carry a label that stated, "This product contains olestra. Olestra may cause abdominal cramping and loose stools. Olestra inhibits the absorption of some vitamins and other nutrients. Vitamins A, D, E and K have been added." I personally can't wrap my mind around putting anything in my mouth that has a warning label bearing the word "stool," but apparently that didn't stop people from eating olestra.

Indeed, olestra snack products were off and running (as it were). A year later, more than one thousand reports of adverse reactions to olestra products were submitted to the FDA, and this appeared to represent only a small fraction of the people sickened by products containing olestra.

When the FDA held advisory committee meetings to review the safety and labeling of olestra, Procter & Gamble argued that complaining consumers could not prove that it was olestra that was causing fecal incontinence, projectile vomiting, projectile bowel movements and diarrhea, cramping, bleeding, and yellow-orange oil in toilet bowls and in underwear—symptoms so severe in some consumers they required hospitalization, surgery, and colonoscopies.

By 2000, the FDA had received twenty thousand negative reports about olestra.[6] Yet, in August 2003, the FDA ruled to no longer require companies that manufactured products containing olestra to put warning labels on their products.[7] So despite poopy panties and the risk of serious health problems, people still eat products containing olestra like Proctor & Gamble Fat-Free Pringles, PepsiCo Inc.'s Wow! Chips, and UTZ Yes! Potato Chips.[8]

On March 15, 2004, Eric Peoples, a thirty-two –year- old former factory worker at the Gilster-Mary Lee Corporate microwave popcorn plant in Jasper, Missouri, was the first of thirty workers with lung disease to be awarded $20 million in compensatory personal injury damages. The jury ruled against International Flavors and Fragrances, Inc., and its subsidiary Bush Boake Allen, Inc., the manufacturers of the chemical in the butter flavoring diacetyl, which is used in butter-flavored microwave popcorn. Diacetyl, currently being studied by the Environmental Protection Agency (EPA), a government agency founded to protect human health and the environment), is believed to cause lung damage when its vapors are inhaled. The jury didn't need to get the EPA report before they ruled against the chemical manufacturers. When the microwave popcorn verdict broke, media reports claimed that "health officials" insisted that making and eating microwave popcorn at home is perfectly safe.

Deny. Deny. Deny. It works.

In abusive relationships, when wooing and denial fail, abusers often turn to ridicule. If you, as a patient, stray from the standard of care in medicine, you will likely be faced with a certain amount of ridicule—especially if you stray from the standard of nutritional care. For example, if you go to a doctor complaining of symptoms you believe were caused by aspartame, you will likely be ridiculed. Excitotoxin expert Dr. Russell Blaylock maintains that if a physician sees a child who has had a seizure, it isn't likely to be connected to the use of aspartame because physicians are not generally aware of the research on excitotoxins. "They'll just tell the mother, 'Well, I don't know how that could be related—something you drank when you were pregnant.'"[9]

If you eat saturated animal fat and your doctor finds out, you will likely be ridiculed. If you have high cholesterol and refuse statin drugs, your doctor may "dismiss" you as a patient. Until very recently, if you came out against soy, you were more than likely going to be labeled as a kook. Remember Dr. Weil who used the very loaded word "paranoia" to describe the reasonable questioning of the introduction of new, often industrially processed food into our food culture?

In the November 29, 2004, issue of the *New Yorker,* Frederick Kaufman writes, "In a Hell's Kitchen basement, the other day, Manhattan's first shipment of raw milk—unpasteurized, unlicensed, unhomogenized, and illegally transported across state lines—was delivered to the grateful, if wary, members of a private raw-milk coven."[10] Every traditional culture from the beginning of humankind has eaten real food, and many consumed raw milk products. Today, Americans who want to consume pure raw, grass-fed, enzyme-rich milk that contains nature's perfect ratio of nutrients are characterized as fringy fanatics.

Apropos of a discussion on health care reform, Nicholas D. Kristof writes, "Raising cigarette taxes saved far more American lives, for example, than any army of neurologists ever could. In the same spirit, I'd like to see a French-fry tax. And imagine the health gains if we banned potato chips and soda from schools."[11] Instead, on March 10, 2004, the House of Representatives approved legislation called the "Personal Responsibility in Food Consumption Act," which bars suing industrialized food restaurants for making people fat. The bill was championed by Republicans, supported by the Bush administration White House, 221 Republicans, 55 Democrats, the National Restaurant Association, and the National Federation of Independent Businesses.

The chief sponsor of the so-called "Cheeseburger bill," Representative Ric Keller (R-FL) said, "The food industry is under attack and in the crosshairs of the same trial lawyers who went after big tobacco." But in fact, in the same week, the government issued a report that obesity-related illnesses were soon to surpass tobacco related illnesses as the number one preventable cause of death in United States. Correct me if I'm wrong, but no one in the public sector is crying crocodile tears over tobacco companies having to cough up (pardon the image) what is justly due to smokers who have suffered as a result of tobacco CEOs' cover-ups about the health hazards of smoking.

Nevertheless, the Bush White House, an administration

notoriously obsessed with protecting the profits of corporate business, issued a statement that "food manufacturers and sellers should not be held liable for injury because of a person's consumption of legal, *unadulterated food* and a person's weight gain or obesity" (Emphasis mine). Representative F. James Sensenbrenner Jr. (R–WI), chairman of the Judiciary Committee, charmingly remarked, "This bill says, 'Don't run off and file a lawsuit if you are fat.' It says, 'Look in the mirror because you're the one to blame.'"[12]

Despite foes such as Representative Bob Filner (D–CA) who asserted, "Congress is headed in the wrong direction with this bill, which removes any and all incentives for the food industry to improve the healthfulness of their products,"[13] on October 19, 2005, the Cheeseburger bill was passed a second time by the House of Representatives. Representative Lamar Smith (R–TX) gloated, "We should not encourage lawsuits that blame others for our own choices and could bankrupt an entire industry."[14] The bill stalled out the first time in the Senate, and only time will tell what will happen next time around.

When wooing, denial, and ridicule fail, then there are personally targeted threats for those who dare to face off with the food industry.

In the late 1980s London Greenpeace passed out leaflets entitled "What's Wrong with McDonald's? Everything They Don't Want You to Know" accusing McDonald's of exploiting food producers in developing countries, children, and employees, destroying rain forests, producing unhealthy food, and torturing and murdering animals. McDonald's sued for libel. Two Greenpeacers, Helen Steel and Dave Morris, known as "The McLibel Two," were compelled by lack of funds to act as their own defense in what was the longest, most complex, most expensive civil trial in Britain's history. McDonald's spent $15 million pursuing two people whose combined incomes were $12,000 per year. Although Justice Rodger Bell found evidence to support some, but not all, of the fact sheet's claims, he ultimately ruled against the defendants. Steel and Morris were ordered to pay £40,000 to McDonald's in libel damages (about $66,000 at that time). Ultimately, McDonald's dropped the claim and limped away, humiliated by the press, with the entire world alerted to the toxic nature of their industrialized food.[15]

This is but one example of how questioning industry standards can land you in an expensive, protracted lawsuit with a huge damages award and even criminal sanctions. "Don't mess with us because we're dangerous" is the message.

Listen carefully and you will recognize threats in print ads, TV commercials, and newscasts. Back in 1970, Fleishmann's threatened American parents with the question, "Should an eight-year old worry about cholesterol?"[16] Since that time there have been no end to the threats of impending heart disease that coerce Americans into eating an ever expanding array of deadly factory food with the promise of "lowering your cholesterol." These threats can take on a saccharine tone, "You already know Honey Nut Cheerios is packed with an irresistible honey sweet taste, but did you also know the soluble fiber from whole grain oats in Honey Nut Cheerios makes it irresistible for your heart? As part of a heart healthy eating plan, Honey Nut Cheerios can help lower your cholesterol. This is great news for you, your family and your heart!"[17] This one truly falls under the rubric of "gag me with a spoon."

The makers of Plavix claim it "helps keep blood platelets from sticking together and forming clots," and goes for a chilling boogeyman approach in threatening former victims with, "You don't want another heart attack or another stroke to sneak up on you."

The barrage of cholesterol-lowering drug ads tell us that the industry is making a killing on these drugs, otherwise it could not afford the millions of dollars it takes to produce and air TV ads. The makers of Crestor decided to take a lighthearted, endearing tone in threatening our lives. One ad's annoying narration was actually delivered in pseudo Dr. Seuss verse; another featured an actor who is not-really-a-doctor-but-played-one-on-TV. "Crestor's not for everyone," the actor reassured, "including people with liver disease and women who are nursing or may become pregnant. A simple blood test is needed to check for liver problems. Tell your doctor . . . if you experience muscle pain or weakness because they may be a sign of serious side effects." It's a revealing commentary that drug companies' baloney has worn us down to the point where we are so inured to the possibility of drug side effects that we would consider for even a fleeting moment to take something that might cause *severe liver damage.*

Print ads for Actonel, a prescription osteoporosis medication, threaten, "If your grandmother had osteoporosis, you could, too." In Nexium TV ads, a sincere actor threatens gastric reflux suffers, "If left untreated, your condition could get worse." The print ad for the once-a-day asthma inhaler, Singulair, warns, "If you use your fast-acting inhaler for symptoms more than twice a week, talk to your doctor, because your asthma may not be under control."

Today thirteen states—Alabama, Arizona, Florida, Georgia, Idaho, Louisiana, Mississippi, North Dakota, Ohio, Oklahoma, South Dakota, Texas, and Colorado—have passed "veggie libel" laws, which have made it illegal to question the safety of our food supply.

Now that you are aware, I'm sure you will recognize other examples of wooing, denial, ridicule, and threats from industry, the medical community, and from our government. Wooing, denial, ridicule, and threats create an effective fog machine to keep you distracted from what you are putting into your mouth.

In addition to these abusive tactics that keep us ensnared in the unhealthy symbiotic relationship with that evil axis of industry, the ominously jovial "we are all in this together" mentality we talked about way back in the Introduction is also a vital contributing factor to keeping us comfy in the status quo.

CHAPTER 30

We Are All in This Together

IN THE 1980s I was living in Los Angeles and would occasionally swing by Randy's Donuts on West Manchester Boulevard. Because of the familiar enormous donut on top of the donut shop, Randy's is often used by filmmakers in montages to establish the location as LA. One morning both of the owners were at the pick-up window. "I have a love/hate relationship with you," I said as I accepted my donut bag. "What do you mean?" asked one owner. "She loves me, and she hates you," quipped the other. I laughed. Of course, I meant the donuts.

Americans joke and laugh off the fact that our factory food diet is damaging our health. Everyone else is eating it, so it must be okay. Ha. Ha. In fact, it's socially acceptable to eat an unnatural, disease-causing diet.

Americans have a what-me-worry attitude about our increasing obesity problem. In fact, in his summer 2005 HBO comedy special, Bill Maher had his audience rolling in the aisle when he said, "In 1900, the average woman's shoe size was four. In 1980, it was seven. Now it's nine. We are evolving into a completely new species with webbed feet to support our massive girth."[1]

The media plays a huge role in our acceptance of factory

food, diets, and drugs. Today all bad news is delivered by bubbly newscasters. Terribly wrong nutritional advice is presented by these same trustworthy messengers. Many nutritional experts, fearing being pegged as fringy, kooky, or downers, soften their messages to the point of practically siding with the food, diet, and drug industries.

We are the most highly evolved capitalistic, mercenary society to ever walk the face of the earth. So every detail of copy on every factory food package, has been scrutinized, analyzed, test marketed, and reviewed to arrive at an image and message that is most likely to hook you into succumbing to your addiction. Madison Avenue refers to consumers as the lowest common denominator, and Madison Avenueites make it their business to know all the personas currently in vogue so they can best target our egos. If you want to be perceived as a cool, popular kid, sexy, brainy, a good parent, he-man, cave-man, manly-man, master of the universe, there are products that will appeal to your sense of self.

Consumers are no longer targeted with quaint print-ads and TV commercials. Susan Linn, EdD, associate director of the Media Center of Judge Baker Children's Center, instructor in psychiatry at Harvard Medical School and author of *Consuming Kids: The Hostile Takeover Of Childhood*, said, "Comparing the marketing of today with the marketing of yesteryear is like comparing a BB gun to a smart bomb."[2] Companies use product licensing, promotions and contests, co-branding (like Coca-Cola Barbie), program-length commercials, advergaming (putting products into computer games) and kiosks, carts, and vending machines in schools. They infiltrate our minds subtly with product placements, which play perfectly into our ominously jovial "we are all in this together" mentality about what we eat and drink.

TV executives have one goal: to get companies to buy commercial time during their programming. Companies have one goal, and that is to get you to spend money on their products. It's part of the symbiotic relationship. David Chase, the creator *of The*

Sopranos said, "The function of an hour drama is to reassure the American people that it's OK to go out and buy stuff. It's all about flattering the audience and making them feel as if all the authority figures have our best interests at heart."[3]

In addition to the advertising that keeps us eating factory food, celebrity doctors contribute to our "we are all are in this together" mentality with books, pills, diet systems, TV shows, products, infomercials, and so on that make us feel all chummy about our obesity problem. Because doctors wield a lot of influence, some doctors are looking for ways to capitalize on their credentials beyond practicing medicine. For example, Dr. Agatston, author of *The South Beach Diet,* is now developing factory food products for Kraft. Dean Ornish, MD, founder of the Preventative Medicine Research Institute and author of five bestselling books on the low-fat diet, including *Dr. Dean Ornish's Program for Reversing Heart Disease: The Only System Scientifically Proven to Reverse Heart Disease without Drugs or Surgery*, is a paid consultant to the McDonald's Corporation, PepsiCo and ConAgra Foods. Kenneth H. Cooper, MD, the "father of aerobics" and author of numerous books on the merits of exercise beginning with *Aerobics*, profits by allowing his name to accompany "health tips" on packages of Frito-Lay's baked chips.[4] Then there are doctors in the diet business to make money who don't care one bit about you or the quality of your life. As one bestselling diet doctor told me, "The more I charge, the more people want to see me."

Over the past few decades, celebrities have gained such elevated status in our society that what they say is gold. And it doesn't take much to achieve celebrity status these days. Even those glossy-lipped, thin, beautiful, diet soda–drinking girls are perceived as celebrities in our society. I mean, they got on television, didn't they? They must be, like, actresses or something. One of the top publicists in the country told me, "You can't launch a book or product anymore without a celebrity endorsement. The morning TV shows won't even talk to you unless you have a celebrity attached to your project.

It doesn't even have to be an actual star. It can be as insignificant as some celebrity's hairdresser or ex-personal assistant. But it has to be someone who the public perceives as having celebrity status. If you've got a celebrity, you can sell anything to the public." For many consumers, a celebrity or even a quasi-celebrity's word is even more credible than a doctor's. Factory food makers bank on the fact that the American public is so insecure, naïve, and gullible that we will take the word of someone who's combed some famous person's hair about something as important as what we're putting in our mouths and into the mouths of our children.

The food industry also capitalizes on our addiction to the high we get from combining scandal, stimulants, and sugar (i.e., sugary products, alcohol, caffeinated beverages, and refined carbs, like chips). While there are no published, peer-reviewed studies that demonstrate that mixing scandal, sugar, and stimulants is fatally addicting, millions of Americans habitually sit in front of the TV being entertained by other people's intimate secrets while they eat hideously injurious substances in an attempt to make themselves feel better. In Jane Fonda's autobiography *My Life So Far*, she explores how her need to be physically perfect developed into an addictive eating disorder. She writes, "Psychologist Marion Woodman says, 'An addiction is anything we do to avoid hearing the messages that body and soul are trying to send us.'"[6]

Our nation is possessed by celebrity voyeurism. Every detail of these people's lives is now up for grabs. It's natural for us to examine the lives of spokespeople to see whether or not they are walking their talk. But what's not useful is that media meddling has resulted in our society losing the ability to distinguish between entertainment and personal tragedy. For example, in the past there have been health advocates who died relatively young, after which the media posthumously ridiculed their health crusades. Adele Davis, for instance, fought valiantly over fifty years ago to get Americans to stop eating factory food, but died at age seventy of cancer. Her platform was then trivialized. Jim Fixx, a long-distance runner and author of *The Complete Book of Running*, died at age fifty-two of a heart attack while out on his routine ten-mile run. His ideals about jogging were then scoffed at. Euell Gibbons, "the father of modern wild foods" and author of books like *Euell Gibbon's Handbook of Edible Wild Plants*, died in at age sixty-five of a heart attack. His belief in the power of natural foods was then dismissed.

In the immortal words of John Lennon, "Life is what happens to you when you're busy making other plans." Even when a person does everything right, cancer and other diseases can still rear their ugly heads. But the goal of avoiding disease and an ugly death doesn't seem remotely worth trying for when you are demoralized, deflated, and defeated. So again, there's that siren song calling you to the frozen factory food section of the supermarket.

The public has come to expect tantalizing real people stories attached to any nonfiction enterprise. Case histories can take the form of "before and after" fat stories, they can illustrate how well such-and-such health or diet approach works, or they can infuse drama with tragic sagas of suffering. A well-known health book writer recently e-mailed me about her struggles to get a very important book into the public eye. "I met with producers from *20/20*, *Dateline*, National Public Radio, *Good Morning America*, *The View*, etc. in NYC and they told me flat out that they would be very interested in airing [my book], but only if I can get some of the parents [in the case histories] to go public, show their faces on TV, cry in public about their [tragedies]." In other words, the important message her book had to offer was not enough. Real life pathos was necessary to sell it.

The expectation that we are entitled to be entertained by peeping in on, discussing, and judging strangers' goings on and suffering is likely to continue to be force-fed to us by the media, because scandal sells advertising and advertisers know that scandal goes very well with sugar and stimulants. It's the high that keeps us numb.

Indeed, many Americans are anesthetized to anything but the screaming of their own pain. Many Americans are numbly gorging on chemicalized factory food in a demoralized, deflated, and defeated state, laughing it all off. And when we are in this neurotransmitter-depleted state, companies can release their seductive siren call to us with promises of health, beauty, and satisfaction. All we have to do is eat, drink, or swallow their products—and go back for more.

Exacerbating our problem is that a prolonged use of stimulants, sugar, and chemicals also makes us dumb. As we saw in chapter 3, the dumbing down of America is due in part to the fact that millions of American brains are not getting the real food necessary for healthy brain formation and development, but instead are being malformed by the use of sugar, stimulants, and chemicals. This numb and dumbed-down contingency is a captive audience for prurient and freakish news, talk, reality, and makeover shows wherein companies air ads for their products.

Americans bear such enormous burdens that we have been compelled into our "we are all in this together" mentality as a coping mechanism. First we have the obvious problems we've discussed above, such as the ubiquitous mind controlling messages that seduce us into indulging in the abundance of factory junk in our food supply. Then, even when we want to eat real food, we cannot even locate a source for real food in all-poison-sandwiches-all-the-time situations such as when driving on the interstate, airplanes, hospitals, or entertainment venues such as zoos, theme parks, movie theaters, sports arenas, and so on. Compounding these problems is the fact that we have virtually no one in places of power taking our side. Instead we are told that what we are "personally responsible" for what we eat and what we feed our children. Never are we as justified to retreat into our "we all in this together" cocoon as when this personal responsibility bull is foisted on us.

A recent newspaper banner read: "A report raises the possibility that ads contribute to obesity in children; the industry begs to differ." The article went on to say, "Madison Avenue was challenged again yesterday over the way it markets food to children, as a new report was released suggesting that advertising contributes to childhood obesity. The report, by the Henry J. Kaiser Family Foundation, summarized existing studies on obesity and the media like television, video games and movies that capture children's attention. Although it endorsed no solutions, it did discuss possible policy changes, like regulating or reducing food advertising aimed at children."[7]

The article said that advertisers disagreed with the report and felt it was up to parents to "accept responsibility for their children's health." "We want kids to buy our products," said Steven Rotter, chairman of the Rotter Group in New York, an agency that specializes in marketing to children. "But Mom and Dad, if your kid is eating too much and eating the wrong stuff, don't let them have it." I was incredulous, so I called Mr. Rotter up and said, "I'm writing a book on the American diet and I read your article and I thought it was kind of harsh. I wanted to know if you wanted to revise your position." Mr. Rotter, as it turns out, is the father of three children who doesn't believe that sugar is poisonous. He maintains that, "Most advertising doesn't work" (a disclosure his clients might be interested in), that kids "shouldn't be allowed in supermarkets," that "we live in a generation of parents who blame everyone else," and that calling advertising to children brainwashing is "silly."[8]

Indeed, the factory food industry has taken this defensive "personal responsibility" stand against arguments that it is wrecking American's health. They argue that (one) the responsibility is on individuals for being overweight, (two) the factory food industry is only responding to consumer demand by supplying us with factory food, and (three) free enterprise allows them carte blanche to market as they see fit—and any impingement would be an assault on their freedom.[9]

In *Food Politics,* Dr. Nestle, the expert in nutrition policy who was introduced in chapter 4, writes, "Food companies—just like companies that sell cigarettes, pharmaceuticals, or any other commodity—routinely place the needs of stockholders over considerations of public health. This conclusion may not surprise anyone who follows the political scene, but I had heard few discussions of its significance among my professional colleagues, despite its evident implications. Food companies will make and market any product that sells, regardless of its nutritional value or its effect on health. In this regard, food companies hardly differ from cigarette companies. They lobby Congress to eliminate regulations perceived as unfavorable; they press federal regulatory agencies not to enforce such regulations; and when they don't like regulatory decisions, they file lawsuits. Like cigarette companies, food companies co-opt food and nutrition experts by supporting professional organizations and research, and they expand sales by marketing directly to children, members of minority groups, and people in developing countries—whether or not the products are likely to improve people's diets."[10]

When the U.S. surgeon general finally got around to acknowledging that cigarette smoking is bad for our health, cigarette advertising was banned from TV and cigarette smoking advertising directed toward children was ultimately banned, including, for example, the Camel cigarette cartoon character whose image was designed to target children. But today it's still perfectly okay, *even cute,* for Ronald McDonald to peddle poisonous, extremely fattening, and addicting factory food to children (and precious when he visits them in hospitals). Then when children grow up with compulsive eating problems, we have weighty legislation as the Cheeseburger bill that is supposedly for our own good as it will help these fattened-up-on-fast-food adults be more responsible.

America was built on great and innovative ideas. People should make money on their ventures. But writers, celebrities, doctors, or anyone else who presents a health message to the American public through books, TV, newspapers, radio, or the Internet have the responsibility to be accurate, truthful and, most of all, rabidly focused on improving the quality of Americans' lives. We can't continue to make excuses about our free market system when people are dying on the vine. If a writer, celebrity, doctor, or food supplier is not part of the solution, then he or she or it is part of the problem. And those who are part of the solution must be committed to ending the trickery and seduction that leads people to eat factory food, and must not be contributors to the exploitation of those people once they get fat and sick.

Dr. Phil has been unapologetic from the onset about his foray into the nutritional food and supplement market. When asked about his Shape Up! products in an interview, he replied that he didn't consider endorsing these products to be a commercial venture because proceeds would go to a charitable foundation (though he didn't elaborate). "I think it's a good product," he said, "and I'm doing it for a really good reason and purpose, although if I was doing it for a commercial—as a brand extension of my own—I wouldn't apologize for that either."[11] I'm confused—I thought that if you have your grinning thumbs-up photograph plastered all over a product line that millions of people see and buy, then that is a brand extension.

We'll never know if Dr. Phil would have gotten hip to the fact that he was eroding the credibility of his brand and alienating his faithful by endorsing his so-called "nutritional" bars, supplements, and other such products if his hand hadn't been forced by the FTC and by the class action suit. He has since broken off with CSA Nutraceuticals and given the www.shapeup.com Web site the heave-ho. It appeared that Dr. Phil was concerned about restoring the credibility of his brand so he could continue to exploit fat people with other weight loss products designed to inspire affable "we are all in this together" camaraderie, including complete nonsequiturs like (I am not kidding) "I Love Dr. Phil" T-shirts (up to size 3X), photo coffee mugs, and baseball caps.

Once we have determined that the makers of factory food, diet products, and drugs probably do not have our best interest in mind, we can begin to revise our "we are all in this together" mentality. The next step is to fully examine and come to terms with our own culpability. One area in which Americans are not scoring very high marks is in the feeding of their children. The following chapter requires guts to read. If you're willing to face off with your own accountability, please read on.

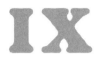

IX

The Home Front

CHAPTeR 31

Change Begins at Home

MOBY DICK'S ON CAPE COD, Massachusetts, like many New England restaurants, serves up fried seafood, but they also have fresh lobster, coleslaw, grilled fish, and salads. On one beautiful summer afternoon at Moby Dick's, John and I sat across from a mother, father, and teenage son who appeared to weigh in at 200, 250, and 350 to 400 pounds,, respectively. They ordered fried seafood, fries, milk shakes and ice cream sundaes. This family also had an adorable ten-year old boy who was about 150 pounds, a boy who was condemned by virtue of the family he was born into to become a binge eater, to possibly reach 400 pounds like his brother, and likely to die young from a heart attack or complications of Type 2 diabetes.

In the year 1900, only 5 percent of Americans were obese. Today, an estimated 129.6 million Americans are overweight (10 percent over normal weight), another 60 million are obese (30 percent over normal weight), and 10 to 15 million are morbidly obese (50 to 100 percent over normal weight or 100 or more pounds over normal weight). Today, 68 percent of us are fat or obese.

Acceptance of fat has changed dramatically in the past three decades. In the film *Midnight Express*, the true story of American drug trafficker Billy Hayes who was imprisoned in Istanbul's infamously brutal Sagmalicar prison, the fat twin sons of the Turkish head guard Hamidou represent the juxtaposition of Hamidou's brutalization of Billy and his allegiance toward his own. Back in 1978, when the boys first come on screen, the reaction to the sight of them was both shocking and sickening, first that they were so fat and second knowing that the boys were safe and protected, eating baklava by the pound, as Billy starved, forsaken by his government and victimized by Hamidou. Today we see fat kids onscreen too, but they are cast merely to represent normal kids in movies and TV commercials.

While visiting South Beach, Florida, John and I got up at five A.M. to catch an early flight. From our third floor hotel window, I watched a full-on gang fight on the street below with a policeman brandishing a gun, the arrival of several police cruisers, a chase, and a bust. I had never seen anything like that before in real life, and the violence was disturbing. But what struck me was that—although I hadn't previously equated "tubby" with "tough"—some of the homies were fat.

Another time we were in the Phoenix, Arizona, airport waiting for a flight, sitting across from a Burger King, where I watched enormous people lumber in and out of that establishment. What impressed me about that experience was that some of the obese people were with other obese people, but many were alone.

Although being overweight today is the norm, it is not yet socially acceptable to be obese. In a study that asked college students who they would be the least inclined to marry, an embezzler, cocaine user, ex-mental patient, shoplifter, sexually promiscuous person, communist, blind person, atheist, marijuana user, or obese person, the students said they would rather marry (in this order) an embezzler, cocaine user, shoplifter, or blind person before they would marry an obese person.[1] Children who were shown pictures of children in a wheelchair, missing a limb, on crutches, facially disfigured, or obese, said they were least likely to play with the fat child.[2] Obesity is the last acceptable area of discrimination, and obese adults are discriminated against in many areas of life including every stage of the employment cycle (selection, placement, compensation, promotion, discipline, and discharge). Overweight people are even stereotyped as emotionally impaired, socially handicapped, and as possessing negative personality traits. They get paid less money.[3]

The fact is that children of overweight/obese parents are more likely to be overweight/obese.[4] And once a child is overweight, he or she is likely stay that way for the rest of his or her life.[5]

Although obesity often condemns people to less than happy lives, our society accepts that a child born into a family of binge eaters will likely become a binge eater as well, and we shrug. Oh well. Sad, isn't it? And to make matters worse, our medical community has labeled this pattern "genetics." Most doctors and most people cling to the belief that genes make people obese. *Genes—not behavior.* Everyone in my family is overweight. My genes are working against me. Type 2 diabetes runs in my family. Oh I see, genes give people Type 2 diabetes, not the fact that by the time the little boy from Cape Cod was ten years old, he had eaten *1,200 pounds of sugar,* give or take several hundred pounds. This is not even counting the hundreds of pounds of other carbohydrates, like cereal, toaster pastries, chips, french fries, candy, cookies, cake, pie, pastry, donuts, bread, pizza, pasta, waffles, pancakes, muffins, and cornbread that American families typically eat. If a family feeds their children huge quantities of sugar/carbohydrates/factory food over the prolonged period of their childhoods, that is not genetics, that is behavioral programming that creates the conditioned response we talked about way back in chapter 3.

When people feed children Fruit Loops, Happy Meals, Spaghettios, or Cheetos, they do so with impunity. But if people gave their children heroin they would be considered abusive parents, and their children would be taken away from them. Fortunately, our government does not see addicting children to sugar and factory food in the same light as addicting them to heroin, or millions of American families would be torn asunder.

It is becoming more common to hear heartrending stories of

children and obesity in the news. Like the three-year-old British girl who weighed in at 83.6 pounds when she died of congestive heart failure, and the thirteen-year- old California girl whose 680 pound bedsore ridden body was found nude on her mother's living room floor, instigating a five day trial wherein the mother was acquitted of felony child abuse.[6] And as these types of tragedies occur more frequently, there may be legal repercussions for the parents.

Then there is the completely bizarre American concept of "kid food." On one of my research outings, I went shopping at Star Market in Boston. At the checkout I stood in line behind an overweight, early thirties father and his chubby, two-year-old son. The man spent $200 on a head of iceberg lettuce and three plums. I'm exaggerating. He only spent three dollars on a head of iceberg lettuce and three plums. The other $197 were spent on Austin Zoo Animal Crackers, Nabisco Barnum's Animals Crackersice cream, Kraft Handi-Snacks, Teddy Graham Bearwiches, Elfin Magic Iced Apple Cinnamon Bars, Keebler Journey Peanut Butter with Fudge Chunks, Nestle Nesquik Chocolate Flavored Milk Mix, and other cartoon-emblazoned kid food products. It was all I could do not to grab the man and plead, "Please buy some food for your son!"

In *The Ultimate Weight Solution,* when Dr. Phil urged his readers to "begin today to reprogram your environment and set yourself up for success," he went on to say, "Okay, I suspect that right now you're thinking, 'Well, that sounds fine and good, but there are foods I need to keep around for my kids. They aren't fat. Why should they suffer?' Dr. Phil suggests designating a "specific cabinet" in your kitchen for kid food such as "pizza, brownies, potato chips and all the rest."[7] This is supposed to protect you from temptation but allow your kids to eat that garbage. In other words, a major role model, bestselling diet doctor tells us that *not feeding* kids poisonous substances would cause them to "suffer." Have you ever noticed that these so-called kid foods are the most processed, chemicalized and sugar-laden foods on the market? Can you imagine feeding that stuff to your dog? Heavens no! "People food" isn't good for dogs! In other words, in our society's ominously jovial "we are all in this together" mentality about factory food, we will feed "kid food" to kids, *but not to our dogs*. In conversations about nutrition, I've heard parents say, "We just go to McDonald's for a treat." A treat? Why don't you just take the kids down to the local Home Depot. They have some nice blocks of maple syrup–infused with rat bait. I know the dogs love 'em.

You might be saying, "But my Dakota won't eat anything healthy. All he likes is pizza." But let's say that pizza makers listed Drano as a pizza ingredient. Would you still feed Dakota pizza? Of course not! Drano's poison! But many pizzas contain partially hydrogenated fat (trans fats). Sodium hydroxide (i.e., lye, an ingredient in Drano and Easy Off) and phosphoric acid (a chemical used in bathroom cleaners) are both used to process vegetable oils before they are hydrogenated.[8]

I do not have children and am aware that the obstacles parents face today are formidable; however, I have yet to understand how parents can feed their children sugar and then sit in the dentist's waiting room strumming through magazines listening to the whine of the dentist drill excavating cavities from their kids' teeth. And then (according to my dentist) greet their shell-shocked children with rewards of candy bars.

In the movie *Deceived*, Adrienne (Goldie Hawn) is so frustrated with parents who are kowtowing to their little girl who has taken a priceless ancient Egyptian necklace to play dress up with that she blurts, "Oh, for Christ sake isn't anyone in charge around here?" before grabbing the necklace off the girl's teddy bear. The line got a lot of laughs because we all recognized the obsequious parental behavior. Consider this scenario that we have all witnessed in restaurants: A mother, father, and their four-year-old son sit down to eat, and the waitress comes to take their order. "Honey bunny," asks the mommy, "want the macaroni and cheese with chips?" To the waitress, "He'll have the macaroni dinner." The waitress writes it down.

"I don't want it!" the kid whines.

"What do you want then, precious? How 'bout the hot dog and fries?" To the waitress, "Change that to the hot dog." The waitress writes it down.

"Noooo," the kid whimpers, squirming in his seat.

"Hmm, well don't the pancakes with chocolate chips sound yummy?"

The kid nods.

"Make that the pancakes instead." The waitress writes it down.

"I want another Coke," the kid bellyaches.

To the waitress, cloyingly now because everyone's nerves are tautly stretched, "Could you please bring another Coke when you have a sec?"

"I want it now!" the kid screeches.

"Listen mister, I'm going to take you outside if you don't lower your voice."

The order comes. The kid takes one look at the pancakes. "I don't want it!"

"What's the matter, honey, you don't like the nice pancakes?"

"I want *french fries.*"

The father takes the boy's plate. "I'll eat it."

The mother pleads, "Could you please bring the hot dog dinner?"

So it goes. I'm sitting there thinking about my mother's (sorry, Mom) unappetizingly overcooked pot roast, mashed potatoes, and peas that I sat and ate at least once a week for my entire childhood, whether I liked it or not. Someone needs to be in charge when it comes to selecting the foods that kids *learn* to like. In Japan kids eat the slimiest, strangest, most godawful looking stuff, with chopsticks no less. In India, toddlers eat eyeball-melting curries with their fingers. Millions of children over the world happily dine on insects. I have seen children in France refuse an offer of dessert at the end of a meal. Tastes for food are established in childhood—some experts say as early as three years old. That explains why Indian babies can munch on chili peppers that would send us to the ER, why German children will eat liver, Finnish children will eat stinky dried fish, and French children will eat green vegetables like candy.

Here in the United States kids eat pretty much nothing but "kid food," and they get fat. The logical response is to put him or her on a diet, though I can't tell you how many tragic stories I've heard that have started with the sentence, "When I was eight, my mother took me to Weight Watchers." Since the 1970s, obesity in adolescents has increased by 75 percent. Researchers have found that, "The very act of starting any diet increases the risk of eating disorders in adolescent girls." Obsessions with body image, low self-esteem, depression and suicide, and sudden cardiac death resulting from extreme weight loss practices are increasingly common with teenagers.[9] The practices of dieting, fasting, extreme exercise, taking diet pills, bingeing, vomiting, and using laxatives will soon creep from high school and college to elementary school-age children if parents do not intervene. Starvation and vomiting both result in a pleasurable release of the endorphins, which are our neurotransmitter equivalent to heroin, and if your child gets hooked on the pleasure associated with starvation and vomiting, you will have a much more difficult challenge on your hands in getting them to stop these behaviors.

On the other hand, studies demonstrate that kids can learn how to eat a healthy diet and will be much less likely to be overweight or obese if their parents provide them access to healthy foods and provide kids with role models to emulate by developing good habits themselves.[10] In other words, no matter how old your children are and how programmed they are, you can still begin to teach them that factory food erodes health and that real food will give their bodies and brains the building blocks of nutrition so that they can fully realize their genetic gifts—and their dreams. In addition to talking to your kids, you can form your children's lifelong attitudes about food by what you put on the table, what is in the refrigerator, what you order, or allow them to order in restaurants.

So it's a hassle to take along your own freshly prepared real food when you are, say, getting away from home. But when you are in poisonous food situations it's even more important to set an example to your children that you will not accept what is being foisted on you by the food industry just because it's more convenient. That you will go the extra step necessary to put real food into your body and into the bodies of your children will make concrete impressions on your children.

Remember the advertising executive whose career was hawking noxious products to children who told me that kids "shouldn't be allowed in supermarkets"? Since our environment is permeated with cartoon festooned junk, keeping kids out of supermarkets is not going to shelter them from these images and the messages they sear onto impressionable minds. How trusting are kids? In the 1950s and 60s there was a zany kids' program on TV, *The Soupy Sales Show*. On one show Soupy (Milton Supman) gazed with his doggie eyes into camera and suggested that kids sneak into their sleeping parent's bedrooms and extract from their wallets and purses all the little green pieces of paper and send them to him at Channel 5 in New York. Allegedly he received $80,000 from his fans, which his producer insisted was mostly Monopoly money. Soupy got in lots of hot water for that prank. But the point here is that kids are *innocent*. Right now kids are getting mostly one side of the story about factory food—what advertisers want them to hear.

Just as parents warn children not to get into strangers' cars, not to fall for lost puppy stories, or accept candy from strangers, parents might consider warning their children that Ronald McDonald, Tony the Tiger, Pokemon, Scooby-Doo, SpongeBob SquarePants, and all the other predatory characters that hawk poisonous factory food substances are only posing as nice. They are bad characters who trick and hurt children. Sound too scary? Well so are Type 2 diabetes, rotten teeth, attention deficit disorder, and obesity.

Bill Clinton has teamed up with the AHA to create the Clinton/ American Heart Association Initiative in an attempt to halt childhood obesity in the United States by the year 2010. The initiative includes "working with the food and restaurant industry to improve the quality and portion size of food products and to develop marketing and promotion strategies that support change within the industry."[11] As you now understand, the changes the food and restaurant industry need to make are extensive. Having children eat smaller bags of carcinogenic fries and fewer cheeseburgers made from factory raised, diseased, hormonal, carcinogenic beef or fewer bowls of Berry Burst Cheerios and other garbage bearing the AHA heart-check mark is not going to put a dent in our childhood obesity problem.

Another example of trading one poison for another is the campaign to rid schools of sodas containing high fructose corn syrup. After years of protest, the American Beverage Association is now working with schools to remove sugary soft drinks in vending machines, and instead providing diet sodas and other "healthier" choices: caffeine, aspartame, and Splenda will remain readily available to the developing brains of America.[12]

Removing all factory food from our food chain and feeding children real food that fosters brain health would be a step in the right direction. Neurotransmitter balance is of the utmost importance in halting the hysterical hunger, craving, and bingeing cycles that condition children to knee jerk react to every stressful situation by eating catastrophic and fattening substances. Remember the analogy of creating the best quality grape—or the best quality human being? Americans are not going to create the best quality human beings out of our children unless we provide them with healthy *real food.*

Instead of stigmatizing overweight kids as outsiders ("the fat one on a diet"), positive change can occur by changing your eating habits as a family from factory food to real food. Then we will make healthy, life-lasting impressions and quality human beings.

Of course you will need to rid your kitchen of all factory food and replace it with real food, and you will need to strap on the old apron and prepare meals for your family. But really, what choice do you have?

Conclusion

What Thomas Jefferson Would Have Done

ON MARCH 2, 1962, the C57D ship from the Forbidden Planet landed on Earth. Terrified humans fled as nine-foot tall Kanamits emerged with threatening eyes floating from within enormously bulbous cranial cavities. Tensions eased when Mr. Chambers deciphered the title of a book the aliens had brought along; it was *To Serve Man*. While military decoders attempted to unscramble the text of the book, the human race became convinced that the Kanamits were *nice*. Their mission was humanitarian—to end all wars. As the Kanamits prepared humans for the journey back to the Forbidden Planet, and Chambers joined a long line of people filing into the C57D ship, his assistant, who had been mulling over the alien book, arrived, crying out, "It's a cookbook!"

Rod Serling's creepy story is analogous to what's happening in the United States today. There is definitely a signpost up ahead because many Americans have blindly fallen into lock step with the innocently nice food, diet, and drug industries only to realize too late that their lives are in serious jeopardy. Millions of Americans have obesity, chronic illness, autoimmune conditions, neurological disorders, and degenerative disease in their futures. In the next twenty years, new and scarier diseases will develop as a result of our prolonged ingestion of chemicalized food. As the incubation period for variant Creutzfeldt-Jakob (mad cow) disease is believed to be up to forty years, some day, millions of Americans may even develop vCJD and suffer agonizing brain meltdowns and death. Although these fates could befall you or me, or one of our loved ones, most of us do not give these possibilities more than a fleeting thought. Meanwhile our government is not taking the appropriate steps to protect or warn us about the dangers of factory food. The collective blinders we have on about our diet call to mind a quote from Vice President Al Gore in his book *Earth in the Balance: Ecology and the Human Spirit*, "The assumption that important things remain the same and don't move is a common source of opposition to discomfiting new ideas."

But things do change. Bad things can happen to people who eat unnatural substances for the prolonged period of their lifetime. Although I was only able to cover a few poisonous substances in this book, our food supply is also permeated with colored dyes, preservatives, miscellaneous and sundry chemicals and flavorings, and numerous other substances than can harm humans. Americans are in denial about the health hazards posed by factory foods. This denial is manifested both in our ominously jovial "we are all in this together" attitude about our factory food diet and in our belief in our government's assurances that they have public interest in mind. The truth is that to date we have not had a single president committed to fighting the food businesses that are greatly contributing to the epidemic of obesity and disease. Instead, we hear empty statements of concern about "health care reform" from elected officials as they sit down to expensive meals with the very CEOs whose factory food products are killing us, only to reach compromises so these businesses won't lose profits.

Even as scandal after scandal is revealed in Washington, too many Americans maintain a laissez-faire attitude about the fact that a handful of rich and powerful men and women are controlling our government. Back in chapter 7 we talked about the fact that we can't really call the industrializing of our food supply a "conspiracy." But that doesn't mean that we shouldn't be terrified about what is happening in our government today and that we should ignore our government's role in the industrialization of our food chain. It is safe to say that there is no longer *any* voice of the common person in government, especially when it comes to what we are putting in our mouths and into the mouths of our children. As Pulitzer Prize–winning journalist Carl Bernstein told Larry King on February 19, 2006, "The legislative system and the Congress and the state legislature is subject only to money."[1] And so while the rich and powerful elected government officials get richer they write rules that allow food industrialists to produce and market poisonous food with government sanctioned subsidies and propaganda.

However, as industry CEOs, the White House, and Congress trample on the Jeffersonian ideal of the family farm with utter disregard for human health and welfare, the treatment of animals and stewardship of our environment, we as individuals do have recourse. Today Americans with no money to speak of have the power to revive Jefferson's ideal of the family farm as the backbone of American democracy.

When I was a child, there was a pugnacious cartoon character who was always picking up an oversized black telephone and shouting into the receiver, "*Buy low, sell high!*" Without having an MBA from an Ivy League business school, we understand the golden rule of business: produce a product or service at the lowest possible cost and sell it at the highest cost the market will bear. But how does a business know what the market will buy in the first place? *Demand.* Demand is the single avenue Americans have to change our food supply and restore the Jeffersonian family farm landscape of America. If Americans boycotted supermarkets and demanded humanely produced, organic, environmentally responsible food, we would ultimately get these foods just as abundantly, affordably, and conveniently as we are getting cruelty-produced, toxic, environmentally damaging food today—

because whenever there is a demand there are businesses that spring up to meet that demand.

When it comes to meat, milk, and eggs, we have three choices. One is to continue to support the industrialized agribusinesses whose practices harm the environment, animals, and humans. Another choice is to become vegetarians, although I don't see this as a realistic expectation for most Americans. Or we can choose to support small farmers and ranchers who practice humane and healthy animal husbandry and who produce animal products that contribute to human health and to the health of the environment. It is important to note that one cannot claim to be an environmentalist while eating foods that are bad for the environment.

Since the year 1900, small farmers and ranchers have been engaged in a literal fight to the death with our government and corporate agribusinesses as mega industrialized food corporations with their government subsidies have driven millions of nonsubsidized family farmers and ranchers out of business. In his book, *Crimes Against Nature: How George W. Bush and His Corporate Pals Are Plundering the Country and Hijacking Our Democracy*, Robert F. Kennedy Jr. argues that the disappearance of the traditional family farm is not inevitable and its demise has little to do with market forces. Kennedy writes, "It is the direct consequence of government polices deliberately designed to favor agribusiness over traditional farmers. For 300 years, this country's family farmers produced more than enough beef, pork and chicken for American consumers and export markets. They used traditional techniques of animal husbandry, recycling their manure to fertilize the soil to grow feed crops. They were proud stewards of their land and generally raised their animals in a humane manner. Study after study shows that these small operations are far more efficient than the giant farm factories. But agribusiness has used its political and financial clout to eliminate agricultural markets, seize federal subsidies, and flout environmental laws to gain competitive advantage."[2]

Seventeenth-century philosopher René Descartes said that

animals were mindless machines that did not feel. Today we have a "moral values" White House with these same Cartesian attitudes toward animals and a moral barometer that measures virtue in the profits of corporate agribusinesses rather than in the health and welfare of its citizens. Treating animals with kindness was lost in the McDonaldization of America as corporations and the White House joined forces with a single-minded, self-interested profit mentality. This new entity (the White House and corporations) works together to shelter corporate agribusinesses so that they do not have to lose profits by reforming their cruel animal practices—even though these practices pose dire risks to human health and welfare as well as the environment. Like Gordon Gekko in the 1987 movie *Wall Street*, this new entity's creed is "Greed is good."

But we can still act alone to reform agribusiness, without government support. Today there are more and more small ranchers who are eschewing the cruel mega-agribusiness methods of animal husbandry and going back to the humane and healthy practice of traditional animal husbandry.

We can also support small farmers who produce organic fruits, vegetables, nuts, seeds, legumes, and grains. On December 3, 2004, Tommy Thompson resigned from his cabinet post as secretary of the U.S. Department of Health and Human Services. "For the life of me, I cannot understand why the terrorists have not attacked our food supply because it is so easy to do," he remarked as he bid us adieu. Thompson was referring to the dangers involved with food imports.[3] In 2005, the United States was expected to consume more imported than domestically grown food. In addition to the threat of tampering by terrorists, consumers have no clue how their food is grown in foreign countries. One of many examples of the potential dangers of foreign grown food is the use of the insecticide dichloro-diphenyl-trichloroethane (DDT) on produce. This potent carcinogen and xenoestrogen is banned for use in the United States, but it is still manufactured here and sold to the foreign countries that grow our food. But again, Americans would not have to worry about the safety of their food if they purchased locally grown food from small organic farmers.

I have been told that suggesting people buy organic, especially "out there" food items like raw milk, is "elitist." And I couldn't agree more. It's shameful that in our prosperous country you have to be wealthy to afford real food. It's disgraceful that hurricane Katrina victims were given military Meals Ready to Eat rations that are so artificial that they can withstand a 1,250 foot drop from a helicopter, temperatures from minus 60 to 120 degrees Fahrenheit, and have a minimum three-year shelf life. The only way to lower prices of organic foods—and to pave the way for all fifty states to allow the sale of raw milk—is for those who can afford organic food and live in states where the sale of raw milk is allowed is to make a commitment to buy and consume these real foods. When there is enough demand, prices will come down. Then someday we may see real, organically produced food in food banks for the poor on news footage at Christmas and Thanksgiving instead of the canned, boxed, and otherwise noxious stuff they are typically forced to accept as "charity."

I have often heard people complain about the price of real food (including myself). In *Fast Food Nation,* Eric Schlosser writes, "Americans now spend more money on fast food than on higher education, personal computers, computer software, or new cars. They spend more on fast food than on movies, books, magazines, newspapers, videos, and recorded music—combined."[4] Fifty years ago, Americans spent one-fifth of their disposable incomes on food, with one-fifth of that expense going to eating out. Today, Americans spend one-tenth of their disposable incomes on food, with one-half of that expense going to eating out.[5] So it appears that at least some Americans have enough money to buy real food if we wanted to.

The United States spends $117 billion a year on medical expenses related to obesity. These expenditures have doubled since 1980. The reality is that if you don't want to spend the money to buy real food, and you keep eating science fiction goods, you would be wise to create a matching fund to cover doctors' bills, drugs, surgeries, chemotherapy, radiation, wheelchairs, colostomy bags, in-home nursing, or hospice care, and the mortuary, and funeral. Even if factory food is currently cheaper than organically grown real food, the health problems we will ultimately suffer from by saving a few pennies now will most certainly be regretted later. In the immortal words of my grandma, Stella, "Saving pennies and spending dollars!" Consuming certified organic foods that are produced in an environmentally responsible way is an immediate expense that provides enduring, positive quality of life effects.

Organic foods are whole, nongenetically modified, nonirradiated foods that can (theoretically) be picked, gathered, milked, hunted, or fished from a natural, clean environment and within natural conditions. True organic foods do not contain additives or poisons or synthetic processing residues, and have not been subjected to any harmful processing. Therefore a box of cereal cannot reasonably be called organic. Milk from cows kept in dry lots and fed species unnatural feed is not really organic. Meat from cattle that were fed an unnatural diet cannot be called "grass fed." You must seek out the true among the counterfeit organic in your daily hunt for sustenance.

And we also need to be vigilant about the introduction of pretend healthy food into our food chain. In May 2004, Mike Roberts, ceremoniously introduced the "Happy Meal for Adults." The meal consisted of a "premium" salad with or without a chicken breast, Newman's Own dressing, a bottle of water, and a toy step-o-meter. With that success, in the June 2005 issue of *Vanity Fair*, McDonald's spent a fortune on an oversized, pop-out-fold-out thingamajigger print ad for their new Fruit & Walnut Salad. The ad copy read, "i don't know who loves this salad more. me? or my fork? wow, McDonald's has really done it with their new Fruit & Walnut Salad. it's just what a girl wants. a heavenly combination of fresh, crisp apples . . . juicy, seedless grapes . . . creamy, low-fat yogurt and sweet candied walnuts. and the best part? it's perfect for breakfast, lunch or snacktime. so I can get a 'fruit buzz' . . .

whenever. finally, fresh fruit is at McDonald's! i don't think it gets any better than that."

Shall we agree to disagree? Because I personally know I can do infinitely better than ingesting pesticide/fungicide ridden apples and grapes, low-fat yogurt concocted from sugar, and pasteurized factory milk that contains toxic contaminants, along with candied walnuts that have been fried up in toxic polyunsaturated vegetable oil and are permeated with sugar and enhanced with "natural" and "artificial" flavors—additives, which as you may recall, frequently contain MSG.[6] Clearly McDonald's upper management deemed this pretend healthy salad a cutting edge response to consumer demand for more healthy food. But McDonald's pretend healthy meals are not what I am talking about when I say real food. Real food is organically grown and hasn't undergone any chemical processing.

As I said in the Introduction, there is a division of the classes occurring in our country that is not necessarily about money, but about personal choice. This country is rife with wealthy people who have private planes and numerous homes yet eat the same diet as an out-of-work-tool-and-die-maker: pizza, diet drinks, fast food, and so on. They also have that tool-and-die-maker's HMO health care of statin drugs, antidepressants, and impotence drugs. The only difference is the rich can afford the best cardiologists to crack open their chests when that diet catches up to them.

But it doesn't have to be that way for rich or poor in America.

I would venture to say that Washington, Jefferson, and other early Americans would've been horrified that twenty-first-century Americans are factory food, diet, and drug addicts, and they would rightly conclude that if we do not turn away from the deadly factory foods, diets, and drugs that are making us obese and killing us off, America will not remain the greatest nation on earth. Throughout history powerful nations have been felled by ignoring their obvious signs of weakness.

We are fighting a socially accepted foe that is destroying the potential of our youth, ruining the productive years of American adults, and leading us to illness and ugly death. But I believe Americans have the grit to prevail against the wooing, denial, ridicule, and threats that have kept us eating poison, dieting, and taking drugs.

Although America missed its opportunity for utopia, and we are now poised upon a precarious precipice, one of our culture's greatest attributes is that we love a comeback story. It's not too late for America to become the utopia it was meant to be—individual by individual. Like the Pilgrims, colonial revolutionary Americans, and pioneers of the West, my hope is that Americans will rebel against the tyranny that's kept us blinded to the industries that are profiting at the expense of our health, reject the industrialized food diet offered to us by the powerful elite, break out of the bubble that has kept us hysterically hungry, fat, and sick, and begin to forge new dietary paths by eating real food. This one simple change would allow us to achieve and enjoy our genetic gifts and would drastically reduce the number of patients who are now flocking to obesity clinics, ERs, and shrinks' offices.

Rejecting the socially acceptable industrialized food diet is challenging. As we discussed earlier, there are many strikes against us with powerful forces, influences and obstacles assisting us in resisting doing what we know we need to do.

Each one of us must conquer our resistance to change. We must face off every single day with the resistance that makes us want to succumb to the seductive siren call of the food, diet, and drug industries. We must fight both our own resistance and these powerful forces as individuals, as families, as communities. But what else is worth fighting for, if not your health and happiness, especially for your children?

It's the American way.

Notes

CHAPTER 1

1. Nicholas D. Kristof, "Health Care? Ask Cuba," *New York Times*, January 12, 2005, p. A-21.
2. Burkhard Bilger, "The Height Gap: Why Europeans Are Getting Taller and Americans Aren't," *The New Yorker*, June 3, 2004. Web site: http://mailman1.u.washington.edu/ pipermail/pophealth/2004-April/000855.html. Accessed October 27, 2005; John Komlos, "Anthropometric History: What Is It?" *OAH Magazine of History 6* (spring 1992). Web site: http://www.oah.org/pubs/magazine/communication/komlos.html. Accessed July 4, 2004; E-mail from John Komlos, July 1, 2004, 12:08 P.M.
3. "Depression in Children and Adolescents." Child Development Institute Web site: http:// childdevelopmentinfo.com/disorders/depression_in_children_and_teens.htm. Accessed November 4, 2004; "ADHD—A Public Health Perspective." Web site: http://www.cdc. gov. Accessed October 31, 2004; Bill Sardi, "How to Quell the Rising Rate of Autism." Web site: http://www.knowledgeofhealth.com/pdfs/autism.pdf. Accessed November 1, 2004.
4. Adele Davis, *Let's Eat Right to Keep Fit: The Practical Guide to Nutrition Designed to Help You Achieve Good Health through Proper Diet* (New York: Harcourt, Brace, 1954), p. 256.
5. World Health Organization. "Social Determinants of Health: the Solid Facts." 2nd edition (2003): p. 26.

CHAPTER 2

1. Mary Enig, *Know Your Fats: The Complete Primer for Understanding the Nutrition of Fats, Oils and Cholesterol* (Silver Spring, Maryland: Bethesda Press, 2000), p. 249.
2. Mira B. Irons, "Cholesterol in Childhood: Friend or Foe?" Pediatric Research 56 (2004): 679–681.
3. Nadia Bennis-Taleb, "A Low-Protein Isocaloric Diet during Gestation Affects Brain

Development and Alters Permanently Cerebral Cortex Blood Vessels in Rat Offspring," *Journal of Nutrition* 129 (1999): 1613–1619; W. Prasad, "Maternal Protein Deficiency in Rats: Effects on Central Nervous System Gangliosides and Their Catabolizing Enzymes in the Offspring," *Lipids* 26 no. 7 (July 1991): 553–556.

4. Weston A. Price, *Nutrition and Physical Degeneration*. 6th ed. (La Mesa, CA: Price-Pottenger Nutrition Foundation, 1939–2003); Maureen Mulhern-White, "Brain Power Starts in the Womb: DHA: An Omega-3 Fatty Acid that's Critical for Brain Development." Web site: http://www.wholehealthmd.com/hk/articles/view/1,1471,950,00.html. Accessed October 31, 2005; Gerard Hornstra, "Essential Fatty Acids in Mothers and Their Neonates," *American Journal of Clinical Nutrition* 71 no. 5 (May 2000): 1262S–1269S; Guoyao Wu, et al., "Maternal Dietary Protein Deficiency Decreases Amino Acid Concentrations in Fetal Plasma and Allantoic Fluid of Pigs," *Journal of Nutrition* 128 no. 5 (May 1998): 894–902; Alan Parkinson, et al., "Elevated Concentrations of Plasma Omega-3 Polyunsaturated Fatty Acids Among Alaskan Eskimos," *American Journal of Clinical Nutrition* 59 (1994): 384–388; Monique D. M. Al, Adriana C. van Houwelingen, and Gerard Hornstra, "Long-Chain Polyunsaturated Fatty Acids, Pregnancy, and Pregnancy Outcome," *American Journal of Clinical Nutrition* 71 no. 1 (January 2000): 285S–291S.

5. R. J. Wurtman, J. J. Wurtman, "Brain Serotonin, Carbohydrate-Craving, Obesity and Depression," *Obesity Research*, 3 Suppl. 4 (1995): 477S–480S.

6. Lisa W. Foderaro, "These Days, the College Bowl Is Filled with Milk and Cereal," *New York Times*, November 14, 2004, front page.

7. Ken C. Winters, "Adolescent Brain Development and Drug Abuse," *A Special Report Commissioned by the Treatment Research Institute* (November 2004): 1.

8. Michael Eades and Mary Dan Eades, *The Protein Power Lifeplan: A New Comprehensive Blueprint for Optimal Health* (New York: Warner Books, 2000), 3–4.

9. Adele Davis, *Let's Eat Right to Keep Fit: The Practical Guide to Nutrition Designed to Help You Achieve Good Health through Proper Diet* (New York: Harcourt, Brace, 1954), 107.

10. Mary Enig and Sally Fallon, *Eat Fat, Lose Fat: Three Delicious, Science-Based Coconut Diets* (New York: Hudson Street Press, 2005), 90; "Cereals Production: From Grain Flour to Crunchy Delight." Web site: http://www.buhlergroup.com/19889EN.htm?grp=60. Accessed October 30, 2005; "Canine Nutrition." Web site: http://www.pamperedpawswimspa.com/html/canine_nutrition.html. Accessed October 30, 2005.

11. Web site: http://www.nutri-grain.com/nutrigrain.htm. Accessed July 23, 2004.

12. Russell L. Blaylock, *Excitotoxins: The Taste That Kills* (Santa Fe, NM: Health Press, 1977), 255–256; Ruth Winter, *A Consumer's Dictionary of Food Additives* (New York: Three Rivers Press, 1999), 210, 405, 136, 216; Kaayla T. Daniel, *The Whole Soy Story: The Dark Side of America's Favorite Health Food* (Washington, DC: New Trends, 2005), 69.

13. Lance Armstrong, *It's Not about the Bike: My Journey Back to Life* (New York: Putnam, 2000), 28–29.

CHAPTER 3

1. Web site: http://www.shapeup.com/Products.aspx. Accessed February 16, 2004; "Class Action Sought for 'Dr. Phil' Diet Suit," Web site: http://www.cnn.com/2005/LAW/10/04/dr.phil/. Accessed November 5, 2005.

2. Sherri Day, "Dr. Phil, Medicine Man," *New York Times*, October 27, 2003, Media.

3. Betsy Schiffman, "The Doctor is Out." Web site: http://www.forbes.com/2004/03/05/cx_bs_0305movers.html. Accessed October 27, 2005.

4. Phil McGraw, *The Ultimate Weight Solution: The 7 Keys to Weight Loss Freedom* (New York:

Free Press, 2003), 108, 119.

5. Karen Ritchie, "Why Doctors Don't Listen." Web site: http://www.cancerlynx.com/doctorlisten.html. Accessed October 30, 2005.

6. Ralph Selitzer, *The Dairy Industry in America* (New York: Dairy & Ice Cream Field, 1976), 37.

7. Bureau of Justice Statistics. Web site: http://www.ojp.usdoj.gov/bjs/correct.htm. Accessed June 27, 2005.

8. Fox Butterfield, "Epilogue from 'All God's Children: The Bosket Family and the American Tradition of Violence'" (1995). Web site: http://www.pbs.org/wgbh/pages/frontline/shows/little/readings/butterfieldepi.html. Accessed June 27, 2005.

CHAPTER 4

1. Web site: http://www.americanheart.org. Accessed February 3, 2004.

2. Ibid.

3. "What Certification Means." Web site: http://www.americanheart.org/presenter.jhtml?identifier=4973. Accessed November 6, 2005.

4. E-mail from Scott Murphy, scott.murphy@heart.org, July 15, 2004, 4:07 P.M.

5. Web site: http://www.americanheart.org. Accessed March 10, 2004.

6. Web site: http://www.americanheart.org/foodcertification/. Accessed March 10, 2004.

7. "The Food Pyramid Scheme," *New York Times*, September 1, 2004, Editorial; Web site: http://www.health.gov/dietaryguidelines/dga2005/document/. Accessed February 23, 2005.

8. Editorial, "The Fat of the Land," *New York Times*, February 2, 2004, A-24.

9. Kelly D. Brownell and Marion Nestle, "The Sweet and Lowdown on Sugar," *New York Times*, January 23, 2004, A-25.

10. "White House Takes Aim at Obesity." Web site: http://www.cnn.com. Accessed September 17, 2004.

11. Web site: http://www.washingtonpost.com. Accessed September 17, 2004.

12. Erik R. Olson, et al., "Inhibition of Cardiac Fibroblast Proliferation and Myofibroblast Differentiation by Resveratrol," *American Journal of Physiology Heart Circirculatory Physiology* 288 (2005): H1131–H1138; Jian-Gang Zou, et al., "Effect of Red Wine and Wine Polyphenol Resveratrol on Endothelial Function in Hypercholesterolemic Rabbits," *International Journal of Molecular Medicine,* 11 no. 3 (2003): 317–320.

CHAPTER 5

1. E-mail from John Olney, June 18, 2004, 6:24 P.M.

2. E-mail from Russell Blaylock, March 28, 2005, 12:45 P.M.

3. Ibid.

4. Russell L. Blaylock, *Excitotoxins: The Taste That Kills* (Santa Fe, M: Health Press, 1977), 255–256.

5. Ibid., 45.

6. E-mail from Russell Blaylock, March 28, 2005, 12:45 P.M.

7. *Sweet Misery: A Poisoned World*, Sound and Fury Productions (2001): VHS.

8. E-mail from Russell Blaylock, March 28, 2005, 12:45 P.M.

CHAPTER 6

1. E-mail from Russell Blaylock, August 23, 2005, 11:23 A.M.

2. www.dorway.com.

3. *Brown Book: War and Nazi Criminals in West Germany* (Dresden, Germany: National Council of the National Front of Democratic Germany Documentation Centre of the State Archives Administration of the German Democratic Republic, 1965), 33–34; Dan J. Forrestal, *Faith, Hope & $5,000* (New York: Simon and Schuster, 1977), 149, 159–161; Erik Olson and Elliot Negin, "EPA Reverses Ban on Testing Pesticides on Human Subjects," National Resources Defense Council, Press Release, November 28, 2001. Web site: http://www.nrdc.org/media/pressReleases/011128a.asp. Accessed December 17, 2005.

4. *Adverse Effects of Aspartame-January '86 through December '90, 167 Citations* (National Institutes of Health, U.S. Department of Health and Human Services, National Library of Medicine pamphlet, 1991).

5. Morando Soffritti, et al., "Aspartame Induces Lymphomas and Leukaemias in Rats," *European Journal of Oncology* 10, no. 2 (2005): 107–116; H. J. Roberts, "Does Aspartame Cause Human Brain Cancer?" *Journal of Advancement in Medicine* 4, no. 4 (Winter 1991): 232–240; C. Orange, "Effects of Aspartame on College Student Memory and Learning," *College Student Journal,* 32, no. 1 (1998): 87–92; J. A. Konen, et al., "Perceived Memory Impairment in Aspartame Users," Presented at the Society for Neuroscience 30th Annual Meeting, November 6, 2000; Ralph G. Walton, "Adverse Reactions to Aspartame: Double-Blind Challenge in Patients from a Vulnerable Population," *Biological Psychiatry,* 34 (1993): 13–17; H. J. Roberts, "Reactions Attributed to Aspartame-Containing Products: 551 Cases," *Journal of Applied Nutrition* 40 (1988): 85–94.

6. J. W. Olney, et al., "Increasing Brain Tumor Rates: Is There a Link to Aspartame?" *Journal of Neuropathology and Experimental Neurology* 55, no. 11 (November 1996): 1115–1123.

7. Russell L. Blaylock, *Excitotoxins: The Taste That Kills,* (Santa Fe, NM: Health Press, 1977), 214.

8. E-mail from Russell Blaylock, March 28, 2005, 12:45 P.M.

9. *60 Minutes*, "How Sweet Is It?" (December 29, 1996); J. W. Olney, et al., "Increasing Brain Tumor Rates: Is There A Link to Aspartame?" *Journal of Neuropathology and Experimental Neurology* 55, no.11 (1996): 1115–1123.

10. Morando Soffritti, et al., "First Experimental Demonstration of the Mutlipotential Carcinogenic Effects of Aspartame Administered in the Feed to Sprague-Dawley Rats," *Environmental Health Perspectives* 114, no. 3 (March 2006): 379–385.

11. Russell L. Blaylock, *Excitotoxins: The Taste That Kills* (Santa Fe, NM: Health Press, 1977) 213.

12. R. J. Wurtman, "Neurochemical Changes Following High-Dose Aspartame with Dietary Carbohydrates," *New England Journal of Medicine* 309, no. 7 (August 18, 1983): correspondence.

13. H. J. Roberts, *Aspartame (Nutrasweet®) Is It Safe?* (Philadelphia, PA: Charles Press, 1990), 49, 142–144, 148–150; H. J. Roberts, "The Hazards of Very-low-calorie Dieting," *American Journal of Clinical Nutrition* 41 (1985): 171–172; J. E. Blundell and A. J. Hill, "Paradoxical Effects of an Intense Sweetener (Aspartame) on Appetite," *The Lancet* 1 (1986): 1092–1093.

14. 1986 American Cancer Society, "Medical Self-Care."

15. J. W. Olney, "Brain Lesions, Obesity, and Other Disturbances in Mice Treated with Monosodium Glutamate," *Science* 165 (1969): 719–721; John Olney, "Trying to Get Glutamate Out of Baby Food," Citation Classic, Current Contents, *Clinical Medicine* 18, no. 34 (1990): 20; Jack L. Samuels, "The Obesity Epidemic: Should We Believe What We Read and Hear?" Web site: http://www.westonaprice.org/msg/msgobesity.html. Accessed November 7, 2005; J. W. Olney, "Toxic Effects of Glutamate and Related Amino Acids on

the Developing Central Nervous System," *Inheritable Disorders of Amino Acid Metabolism* (New York: John Wiley, 1974).

16. "Carbohydrate Addiction." Web site: http://www.americanheart.org/presenter. jhtml?identifier=4467. Accessed December 1, 2005; J. Barua, and A. Bal, "Emerging Facts About Aspartame" *Journal Of The Diabetic Association Of India* 35, no. 4 (1995): 92–107.

17. J. D. Smith, et al., "Relief of Fibromyalgia Symptoms Following Discontinuation of Dietary Excitotoxins," *Annals of Pharmacotherapy* 35, no. 6 (2001): 702–706; Rapid Responses to Editorials: Joseph M Mercola, "Aspartame Can Damage Your Health," John P. Briffa, "It's Not Just Misleading Web Sites That the Public Should Be Protected From," Dr. Janet S. Hull, "Aspartame Dangers ARE Real," John P. Briffa, "What Aspartame Has in Common with Any Artificial Sweetener ('Natural' or Not) in Effects on Health," *British Medical Journal* 329 (2004): 755–756; L. Kovatsi, and M. Tsouggas, "The Effect of Oral Aspartame Administration on the Balance of Magnesium in the Rat," *Magnesium Research* 3 (September 14, 2001): 189–194; L. C. Newman, and R. B. Lipton, "Migraine MLT-down: An Unusual Presentation of Migraine in Patients with Aspartame-Triggered Headaches," *Headache* 41, no. 9 (2001): 899–901. B. Christian, et al., "Chronic Aspartame Affects Maze Performance, Brain Cholinergic Receptors and Na+, K+-ATPase in Rats," *Pharmacology, Biochemistry and Behavior* 78, no. 1 (2004): 121–127. Daniel DeNoon, "Rat Study Links Aspartame to Cancer." Web site: http://www.medscape.com/viewarticle/509619. Accessed November 7, 2005.

CHAPTER 7

1. Statement by Michael Friedman, MD, Deputy Commissioner for Operations, Food and Drug Administration, Department of Health and Human Services, before the subcommittee on human resources and intergovernmental relations committee on government reform and oversight, U.S. House of Representative,. May 10, 1996. Web site: http://www.fda.gov/ola/1996/foodbor.html. Accessed October 24, 2005.

2. Federal Food, Drug, and Cosmetic Act. Web site: http://www.fda.gov/opacom/laws/fdcact/fdcact1.htm. Accessed October 24, 2005; FDA Backgrounder. Printed October 1991. Web site: http://www.geocities.com/HotSprings/2455/bak-msg.html. Accessed October 24, 2005.

3. M. M. Wolf, D. R. Lichtenstein and G. Singh, "Gastrointestinal Toxicity of Nonsteroidal Anti-inflammatory Drugs," *New England Journal of Medicine* 340 (1999): 1888–1899.

4. "FDA Implicated in Conflict of Interest for Manufacturers of COX-2 Inhibitor Drugs," *Validation Times.* Web site: http://www.fdainfo.com/vtonlinepages/valtimesweb041105.htm. Accessed July 2, 2005.

5. Gardiner Harris and Alex Berenson, "10 Voters on Panel Backing Pain Pills Had Industry Ties," *New York Times*, February 25, 2005: A-1.

6. Alex Berenson, "Evidence in Vioxx Suits Shows Intervention by Merck Officials," *New York Times*, April 24, 2005: National.

7. Alex Berenson, "Jury calls Merck Liable in Death of Man on Vioxx," *New York Times*, August 20, 2005: Health—Chronology; Associated Press, "Vioxx Trial Loss Raises Merck Strategy Questions," April 6, 2006. Web site: http://www.msnbc.msn.comb/ld/12173094/. Accessed Jan. 5, 2007.

8. Interview: Dr. David Graham, "Prescription Drug Alert: Millions at Risk from Serious and Possibly Deadly Side Effects," *Crusader* (June/July 2005): 1–8.

9. Deborah Franklin, "Poisonings from a Popular Pain Reliever are Rising," *New York Times*, November 29, 2005. Web site: http://wwwnytimes.com/2005/11/29/health/29cons.

html?incamp=article_popula&pagewanted=print; John G. O'Grady, "Broadening the view of acetaminophen hepatotoxicity," *Hepatology* 42, no. 6 (2005): 1252–1254.

10. Robert F. Kennedy Jr., "Deadly Immunity." Web site: http://www.rollingstone.com/politics/story/_/id/7395411, posted June 20. Accessed June 27, 2005.

11. Telephone interview with Samuel Epstein, December 21, 2004.

12. *San Francisco Chronicle*, January 2, 1970. Web site: http://www.advancedhealthplan.com/fdafraud.html. Accessed November 8, 2005.

13. Michael Culbert, *Medical Armageddon* (San Diego, CA: C and C Communications, 1997), 333–334.

14. Donald G. McNeil, Jr. "Review Finds Scientists with Ties to Companies," *New York Times*, July 15, 2005: A-15; Meredith Wadman, "One in Three Scientists Confesses to Having Sinned," *Nature* 435 (June 9, 2005): 718–719.

15. *Sweet Misery: A Poisoned World*, Sound and Fury Productions (2001): VHS.

16. "Artificial Sweeteners: No Calories…Sweet!" *FDA Consumer Magazine* (July-August 2006). Web site: http://www.fda.gov/fdac/features/2006/406_sweeteners.html. Accessed March 18. 2007.

17. Jason Lazarou, Bruce H. Pomeranz, and Paul N. Corey, "Incidence of Adverse Drug Reactions in Hospitalized Patients," Journal of the American Medical Association 279, no. 15 (April 15, 1998): 1200–1205; "Study: Drug Reactions Kill an Estimated 100,000 a Year." Web site: http://www.cnn.com/HEALTH/9804/14/drug.reaction/. Accessed Dec. 1, 2005; Brenda C. Coleman, "Prescription Drug Reactions Kill More Than 100,000 a Year." Web site: http://www.pathlights.com/nr_encyclopedia/hn041598.htm. Accessed Dec. 1, 2005.

18. L. Tollefson, "Monitoring Adverse Reactions to Food Additives in the U.S. Food and Drug Administration," *Regulatory Toxicology and Pharmacology* 8, no.4 (December 1988): 438–446.

19. E-mail from Russell Blaylock, March 28, 2005, 12:45 P.M.

CHAPTER 8

1. E-mail from Christine Northrup, July 21, 2004, 3:13 P.M.

2. E-mail from Bradley Willcox, August 23, 2004, 8:45 P.M.

3. Web site: http://www.drweil.com. Accessed June 13, 2004.

4. E-mail from Kaayla Daniel, August 16, 2004, 2:52 P.M.

5. Interested readers can take a look at pro and con research in the "Report on Phytoestrogens and Health" by the British governments Committee on Toxicity at: Web site: http://www.food.gov.uk/multimedia/pdfs/phytoreport0503. Accessed November 10, 2005.

6. Russell L. Blaylock, *Excitotoxins: The Taste That Kills* (Santa Fe, NM: Health Press, 1977), 220; Web site: http://www.westonaprice.org. Accessed March 14, 2005; Kaayla T. Daniel, *The Whole Soy Story: The Dark Side of America's Favorite Health Food* (Washington, DC: New Trends, 2005).

7. "FDA Scientists Questions Soy Safety—But Where Is GM Testing?" Web site: http://www.netlink.de/gen/Zeitung/2000/000609.html. Accessed November 10, 2005.

8. FDA Talk Paper, "FDA Approves New Health Claim for Soy Protein and Coronary Heart Disease." Web site: http://www.fda.gov/bbs/topics/ANSWERS/ANS00980.html. Accessed June 20, 2004.

CHAPTER 9

1. Kaayla T. Daniel, *The Whole Soy Story: The Dark Side of America's Favorite Health Food*

(Washington, DC: New Trends, 2005), 295–310, 331–356.

2. Ibid., 363; M. Penotti, et al., "Effect of Soy-Derived Isoflavones on Hot Flashes, Endometrial Thickness and the Pulsatility Index of the Uterine and Cerebral Arteries," *Fertility and Sterility* 79, no. 5 (2003): 1112–1117; E. Nikander, et al., "A Randomized Placebo-Controlled Crossover Trial with Phytoestrogens in Treatment of Menopause in Breast Cancer Patients," *Obstetrics and Gynecology* 101, no.6 (2003): 1213–1120; J. L. Balk, et al., "A Pilot Study of the Effects of Phytoestrogen Supplementation on Postmenopausal Endometrium," *Journal of the Society of Gynecological Investigation* 9, no. 4 (2002): 238–242; D. Kotsopoulous, et al, "The Effects of Soy Protein Containing Phytoestrogens on Menopausal Symptoms in Postmenopausal Women," *Climacteric* 3, no. 3 (2000): 161–167; L. J. Lu, J. A. Tice, and F. L. Bellino, "Phytoestrogens and Healthy Aging: Gaps in Knowledge," Workshop Report. *Menopause* 8, no. 3 (2001): 157–170; Editorial notes from Dr. Daniel on manuscript (September 2005).

3. E-mail from Kaayla Daniel, August 16, 2004, 2:52 P.M.

4. Marian Burros, "Eating Well: Doubts Cloud Rosy News on Soy," *New York Times*, January 26, 2000: Dining In, Dining Out/Style Desk.

5. Telephone interview with Earl Mindell, June 28, 2004.

6. Telephone interview with Clare Hasler, June 28, 2004, 4:00 P.M.

7. Mike Fitzpatrick, "Soy Formulas and the Effects of Isoflavones on the Thyroid," *New Zealand Medical Journal* 113 (February 11, 2000): 24.

CHAPTER 10

1. E-mail from Bradley Willcox, August 23, 2004, 8:45 P.M.

2. E-mail from Kaayla Daniel, December 18, 2005, 6:22 P.M.

3. E-mail from David Zava, June 22, 2004, 6:35 A.M.

4. Pearl S. Buck, *The Good Earth* (New York: Washington Square Press, 1931), 109.

5. Web sites: http://www.accesseonline.com/printstoryb.php?type=travel&id=3, http://www.clearspring.co.uk/pages/site/products/macro/info1.htm, http://www.hi-net.zaq.ne.jp/yossy/global_education/example/note.html, http://en.wikipedia.org/wiki/Japanese_cuisine, http://www.members.tripod.com/~Doc_In_The_Kitchen/japan, Accessed November 11, 2005.

6. Kaayla T. Daniel, *The Whole Soy Story: The Dark Side of America's Favorite Health Food* (Washington, DC: New Trends, 2005), 53.

CHAPTER 11

1. Jeffrey M. Smith, *Seeds of Deception: Exposing Industry and Government Lies about the Safety of the Genetically Engineered Foods You're Eating* (Fairfield, IA: Yes! Books, 2002), 1.

2. Anonymous, "Health risks of genetically modified foods," *Lancet*, 353, no. 9167 (1999): 181.

3. Michael Crichton, *Prey* (New York: Avon Books, 2002), xiii–xiv.

4. Kaayla T. Daniel, *The Whole Soy Story: The Dark Side of America's Favorite Health Food* (Washington, DC: New Trends, 2005), 113, 115.

5. J. J. Rackis, M. R. Gumbmann, and I. E. Liener, "The USDA Trypsin Inhibitor Study. I. Background, Objectives, and Procedural Details," *Plant Foods for Human Nutrition* (Formerly *Qualitas Plantarum*) *(Historical Archive)*, 35, no. 3 (September 1985): 213–242; "Evaluation of the Health Aspects of Soy Protein Isolates as Food Ingredients," Prepared for FDA by Life Sciences Research Office, *Federation of American Societies for Experimental Biology*, 1979, 9650 Rockville Pike, Bethesda, MD 20014, Contract No. FDA 223–75–

2004; Kaayla T. Daniel, *The Whole Soy Story: The Dark Side of America's Favorite Health Food* (Washington, DC: New Trends, 2004), 93, 260, 266.

6. Kaayla T. Daniel, *The Whole Soy Story: The Dark Side of America's Favorite Health Food* (Washington, DC: New Trends, 2004), 95.

7. E-mail from Carol Simontacchi, June 16, 2004, 8:44 A.M.

8. Mary Enig and Sally Fallon, *Eat Fat, Lose Fat: Three Delicious, Science-Based Coconut Diets* (New York: Hudson Street Press, 2005), 97, 99.

9. Joanne K. Tobacman, "Review of Harmful Gastrointestinal Effects of Carrageenan in Animal Experiments," *Environmental Health Perspectives*, 109, no. 10 (October 2001) 983–994.

10. Russell L. Blaylock, "Rebuttal to Seriously Confused Soy Enthusiast." Web site: http://www.mercola.com/2005/apr/6/rebuttal.htm. Accessed November 11, 2005.

11. Kaayla Daniel, "Soy Milk Implicated in Sudden Deaths of Twins," News Release. E-mail from Kaayla Daniel, October 27, 2005, 7:02 A.M.

12. Web site: http://www.drweil.com/u/QA/QA326575/. Accessed May 9, 2005.

13. Kaayla T. Daniel, *The Whole Soy Story: The Dark Side of America's Favorite Health Food* (Washington, DC: New Trends, 2005), 307; Francine Grodstein, Richard Mayeux, and Meir J. Stampfer, "Tofu and Cognitive Function: Food for Thought," *Journal of the American College of Nutrition,* 19, no. 2 (2000): 207–209.

CHAPTER 12

1. Cases courtesy of Kaayla Daniel. All names and identifying characteristics have been changed.

2. V. Beral, et al., "Breast Cancer and Breastfeeding: Collaborative Reanalysis of Individual Data from 47 Epidemiological Studies in 30 Countries, Including 50,302 Women with Breast Cancer and 96,973 Women without the Disease." *Lancet,* 360, (2002): 187–195.

3. Carol Simontacchi, *The Crazy Makers: How the Food Industry is Destroying Our Brains and Harming Our Children* (New York: Tarcher, 2000), 62.

4. C. Garza, et al., "Special properties of human milk," *Clinical Perinatology*, 14, no. 1 (March 1987): 11–32; Carol L Wagner, "Human Milk and Lactation." Web site: http://www.emedicine.com/ped/topic2594.htm#section~biochemistry_of_human_milk. Accessed November 16, 2005.

5. Sheila Innis, "Essential Fatty Acids in Growth and Development," *Progress in Lipid Research*, 30, no. 1 (1991), 66–67.

6. Mary Enig, *Know Your Fats: The Complete Primer for Understanding the Nutrition of Fats, Oils, and Cholesterol* (Silver Spring, MD: Bethesda Press, 2000), 186.

7. Kaayla T. Daniel, *The Whole Soy Story: The Dark Side of America's Favorite Health Food* (Washington, DC: New Trends, 2005), 144.

8. David Goodman, "Manganese Madness," *Wise Traditions.* Web site: http://www.westonaprice.org/soy/manganese.html. Accessed March 27, 2005.

9. Retha R. Newbold, et al., "Uterine Adenocarcinoma in Mice Treated Neonatally with Genistein," Cancer Research, 61 (June 1, 2001): 4325–4328; D. R. Doerge, "Goitrogenic and Estrogenic Activity of Soy Isoflavones," *Environmental Health Perspectives,* 110, Suppl. 3 (June 2002): 349–353; C.Y. Hsieh, et al. "Estrogenic Effects of Genistein on the Growth of Estrogen Receptor Positive Human Breast Cancer (MCF7) Cells in Vitro and in Vivo," *Cancer Research,* 58 (September 1, 1998): 3833; Gabe Mirkin, "Soy Causes Cancer?" Web site: http://www.drmirkin.com/nutrition/9288.html. Accessed November 16, 2005. Joseph Mercola, "Newest Research On Why You Should Avoid Soy," Website: http://

www.mercola.com/article/soy/avoid_soy2.htm. Accessed November 16, 2005.

10. P. Fort, et al., "Breast and Soy-formula Feedings in Early Infancy and the Prevalence of Autoimmune Thyroid Disease in Children," *Journal of the American College of Nutrition*, 9, no.2 (April 1990): 164–167; Y. Ishizuki, et al., "The Effects on the Thyroid Gland of Soybeans Administered Experimentally in Healthy Subjects," *Nippon Naibunpi Gakkai Zasshi*, 67, no. 5 (May 20, 1991): 622–629; M. Fitzpatrick, "Soy Formulas and the Effects of Isoflavones on the Thyroid," *New Zealand Medical Journal*, 113 (2000): 234–235. Web site: http://www.soyonlineservice.co.nz/04thyroid.htm. Accessed November 17, 2005.

11. Mary G. Enig. From a summary of a presentation given on May 25, 2001, at the 8th International Symposium of the Institute for Preventive Medicine in Vancouver, Canada. Web site: http://www.westonaprice.org/soy/soy_controversy.html. Accessed November 17, 2005; Katherine M. Flynn, et al., "Effects of Genistein Exposure on Sexually Dimorphic Behaviors in Rats," *Toxicological Sciences*. 55 (2000): 311–319; Amy B. Wisniewski, et al., "Exposure to Genistein during Gestation and Lactation Demasculinizes the Reproductive System in Rats," *Journal of Urology* 169, no. 4 (April 2003): 1582–1586; P. Fort, et al. "Breast Feeding and Insulin-dependent Diabetes Mellitus in Children," *Journal of the American College of Nutrition* 5 (1986): 439–441.

12. Wendy Jefferson, Retha Newbold, Elizabeth Padilla-Banks, and Melissa Pepling, "Neonatal Genistein Treatment Alters Ovarian Differentiation in the Mouse: Inhibition of Oocyte Nest Breakdown and Increased Oocyte Survival," *Biology of Reproduction* 74, no. 1 (2006): 161–168; E-mail from Kaayla Daniel, January 11, 2006, 7:00 P.M.

13. Telephone interview with Clare Hasler, June 28, 2004, 4:00 P.M.

CHAPTER 14

1. Ginanne Brownell, "Can't Buy Me Lard," *Newsweek*, December 6, 2004: 10.

2. Weston A. Price, *Nutrition and Physical Degeneration*, 6th ed. (La Mesa, CA: Price-Pottenger Nutrition Foundation, 1939–2003), 5.

3. Ron Schmid, "Raw Milk–History, Health Benefits and Distortions," *Medical Veritas* 1 (2004): 278–286; "Dr. Francis M. Pottenger, Jr., MD." Web site: http://www.price-pottenger.org/pottenger.htm. Accessed November 18, 2005.

4. Ancel Keys, "Atherosclerosis: A Problem in Newer Public Health," *Journal of Mount Sinai Hospital* 20 (1953): 118–139.

5. Uffe Ravnskov, *The Cholesterol Myth: Exposing the Fallacy That Saturated Fat and Cholesterol Cause Heart Disease* (Washington, DC: New Trends, 2000), 101.

6. Uffe Ravnskov,http://qjmed.oxfordjournals.org/cgi/content/full/95/6/ - FN1 "Is Atherosclerosis Caused by High Cholesterol?" *QJM: Monthly Journal of the Association of Physicians* 95 (2002): 397–403.

7. Uffe Ravnskov, *The Cholesterol Myth: Exposing the Fallacy That Saturated Fat and Cholesterol Cause Heart Disease* (Washington, DC: New Trends, 2000), 122–123.

8. Telephone interviews with David Kritchevsky, January and March 2004.

CHAPTER 15

1. Stephanie Saul, "Gimme an Rx! Cheerleaders Pep Up Drug Sales," *New York Times*, November 28, 2005. Web site: http://www.nytimes.com/2005/11/28/business/28cheer.html?th&emc=th.

2. Marion Nestle, *Food Politics: How the Food Industry Influences Nutrition and Health* (Los Angeles: University of California Press, 2002), 117, 113–114.

3. Donald G. McNeil Jr., "Review Cites Ethical Lapses By Scientists," *New York Times*, July

15, 2005: A-15.

CHAPTER 16

1. Stephanie Saul, "Gimme an Rx! Cheerleaders Pep Up Drug Sales," *New York Times*, November 28, 2005. Web site: http://www.nytimes.com/2005/11/28/business/28cheer. html?th&emc=th.

2. Marion Nestle, *Food Politics: How the Food Industry Influences Nutrition and Health* (Los Angeles: University of California Press, 2002), 117, 113–114.

3. Donald G. McNeil Jr., "Review Cites Ethical Lapses By Scientists," *New York Times*, July 15, 2005: A-15.

CHAPTER 17

1. M. G. Enig, et al., "Dietary Fat and Cancer Trends: A Critique," *Federation Proceedings* 37, no. 9 (July 1978): 2215–2220; Mary Enig and Sally Fallon, "The Oiling of America." Web site: http://www.westonaprice.org/knowyourfats/oiling.html#enig. Accessed October 23, 2005.

2. Edward R. Pinckney and Cathey Pinckney, *The Cholesterol Controversy* (Los Angeles: Sherbourne Press, 1973), 127–131.

3. Mary Enig and Sally Fallon, "The Oiling of America," *Nexus Magazine* 6, no. 1–2 (February–March 1999) (December 1998–January 1999).

4. Uffe Ravnskov, *The Cholesterol Myth: Exposing the Fallacy that Saturated Fat and Cholesterol Cause Heart Disease* (Washington, DC: New Trends, 2000), 23.

5. Email from Mary Enig, August 15, 2004, 3:49 P.M.

6. Mary Enig, *Trans Fatty Acids in the Food Supply: A Comprehensive Report Covering 60 Years of Research,* 2nd ed. (Silver Spring, MD: Enig Associates, 1995), 4–8; Mary Enig, *Know Your Fats: The Complete Primer for Understanding the Nutrition of Fats, Oils and Cholesterol* (Silver Spring, MD.: Bethesda Press, 2000): 86.

CHAPTER 18

1. Bob Dylan, *Chronicles, Volume One,* (New York: Simon & Schuster, 2004), 27.

2. John Robbins, *Diet for a New America: How Your Food Choices Affect Your Health, Happiness, and the Future of Life on Earth* (Tiburon, CA: H. J. Kramer, 1987), 113–118.

3. Jo Robinson, "Grass-Fed Basics." Web site: http://www.eatwild.com/Grass-Fed%20Basics. pdf. Accessed November 21, 2005.

4. Samuel S. Epstein, "The Chemical Jungle: Today's Beef Industry," *International Journal of Health Services* 20, no. 2 (1990): 277–280.

5. G. V. Mann, R. D. Shaffer, and H. H. Sandstead, "Cardiovascular Disease in the Masai," *Journal of Atherosclerosis Research* 4 (1964):289–312.

6. Web site: http://www.framingham.com/heart/. Accessed May 13, 2004.

7. Web site: http://www.xetex.com/diabetes/Lipid_Hypothesis.html. Accessed May 13, 2004.

8. Arthur Agaston, *The South Beach Diet: The Delicious, Doctor-Designed, Foolproof Plan for Fast and Healthy Weight Loss* (New York: Rodale 2003), 21–22.

9. Email from Gerry Casanova, August 19, 2005, 10:15 A.M.; R. A. Vogel, "Effect of Single High Fat Meal on Endothelial Function in Healthy Subject," *American Journal of Cardiology* 79, no. 3 (February 1, 1997): 350–54.

10. Email from Sally Fallon, October 19, 2005, 10:55 A.M.; *Wise Traditions,* Website: http://www.westonaprice.org. Accessed Fall 2005.

11. Gary Taubes, "Nutrition: The Soft Science of Dietary Fat," Science 291 (2001): 2536–2545; Uffe Ravnskov, *The Cholesterol Myth: Exposing the Fallacy that Saturated Fat and Cholesterol Cause Heart Disease* (Washington, DC: New Trends, 2000), 46–47.

12. Telephone conversation with Mary Enig, Summer 2000.

13. Bruce Fife, *The Healing Miracles of Coconut Oil* (Colorado Springs, CO: Piccadilly Books, 2001), 27–28.

14. Laurence Bergreen, *Over the Edge of the World: Magellan's Terrifying Circumnavigation of the Globe* (New York: Perennial, 2003), 240–241.

15. Bruce Fife, *The Healing Miracles of Coconut Oil* (Colorado Springs, CO: Piccadilly Books, 2001), 15.

16. Mary G. Enig, "Lauric Oils as Antimicrobial Agents: Theory of Effect, Scientific Rationale, and Dietary Applications as Adjunct Nutritional Support for HIV-infected Individuals in Nutrients and Foods in AIDS," ed. R. R. Watson (Boca Raton, FL: CRC Press, (1998), 81–97; Bruce Fife, *The Healing Miracles of Coconut Oil* (Colorado Springs, CO: Piccadilly Books, 2001), 162.

17. United States General Accounting Office. GAO Report to Congressional Requesters. January 2002, MAD COW DISEASE: Improvements in the Animal Feed Ban and Other Regulatory Areas Would Strengthen U.S. Prevention Efforts. GAO-02-183; Michael Greger, "The Return of Mad Cow." Web site: http://www.counterpunch.org/greger05232003. html. Accessed November 27, 2005; USDA, Food Safety and Inspection Service, "USDA Begins Sampling Program for Advanced Meat Recovery Systems," News Release, March 3, 2002. Web site: http://www.fsis.usda.gov/OA/news/2003/amrsampling.htm. Accessed November 27, 2005.

18. Sandra Blakeslee, "Jumble of Tests May Slow Mad Cow Solution," *New York Times*, January 4, 2004: 10. Sandra Blakeslee, "Study Finds Broader Reach for Mad Cow Proteins," *New York Times*, January 21, 2005: A-18.

19. Web site: http://www.downbound.com/categary_s/56.htm. Accessed June 26, 2005; Donald G. McNeil Jr., "Mad Cow Case Confirmed; U.S. Testing Will Change," *New York Times*, June 25, 2005: 7; USDA Animal and Plant Health Inspection Service, "Bovine Spongiform Encephalopathy (BSE) Ongoing Surveillance Plan," July 20, 2006: 6, 8; USDA's BSE Surveillance Efforts (Factsheet). Web site: http://www.aphis.usda.gov/publications/animal_health/content/printable_version/fs_BSE_ongoing_vs.pdf. Accessed Jan. 23, 2007.

20. Donald G. McNeil Jr., "Testing Changes Ordered after U.S. Mad Cow Case," *New York Times*, June 25, 2005: 7; Donald G. McNeil Jr. and Alexei Barrionuevo, "For Months, Agriculture Department Delayed Announcing Result of Mad Cow Test," *New York Times*, June 26, 2005. Web site: http://www.nytimes.com/2005/06/26/national/26beef. html?ei=5070&en=0542e3793fdae07f&ex=1133240400&pagewanted=print. Accessed November 27, 2005.

21. John Robbins, *Diet for a New America: How Your Food Choices Affect Your Health, Happiness, and the Future of Life on Earth* (Tiburon, CA: H. J. Kramer, 1987), 73–96.

22. Ibid., 52–72.

23. Paul S. Mead, et al, "Food-Related Illness and Death in the United States," *Emerging Infectious Diseases Journal* 5, no. 5 (September–October 1999); F. Angulo, et al., "Determining the Burden of Human Illness from Foodborne Diseases: CDC's Emerging Infectious Disease Program Foodborne Disease Active Surveillance Network (FoodNet)." Web site: http://www.cdc.gov/foodnet/pub/publications/1998/angulo_1998p.pdf. Accessed November 27, 2005. "New Data on Incidence of Food-Borne Illness

and Death in the United States," *Safefood News* 4, no. 1 (Fall 1999). Web site: http://www. colostate.edu/Orgs/safefood/NEWSLTR/v4n1s01.html. Accessed November 30, 2004.

24. "Potential Health Hazards of Food Irradiation. Verbatim Excerpts from Expert Testimony." Web site: http://www.ccnr.org/food_irradiation.html. Accessed November 28, 2005; "Food Irradiation Q & A's." Web site: http://www.citizen.org/cmep/foodsafety/food_ irrad/articles.cfm?ID=12341. Accessed March 30, 2005; "Frequently Asked Questions about Food Irradiation." Web site: http://www.organicconsumers.org/irradlink.html . Accessed March 30, 2005.

25. Bill Maher, HBO Stand-Up Special, "'I'm Swiss': and other Treasonous Statements," July 30, 2005, 10:00 P.M.

26. References can be found on http://www.realmilk.com/indexpage.html and http:// www.eatwild.com/references.html.

CHAPTER 19

1. Ralph Seltzer, *The Dairy Industry in America* (New York: Dairy & Ice Cream Field, 1976), 3–8, 22–39.

2. Rose Marie Williams, "Environmental Issues: What's Milk Got?" Web site: http://www. townsendletter.com/Oct_2002/milk1002.htm. Accessed November 28, 2005.

3. Weston A. Price, *Nutrition and Physical Degeneration*. 6th ed. (La Mesa, CA: Price-Pottenger Nutrition Foundation, 1939–2003), 385.

4. Ron Schmid, *The Untold Story of Milk* (Washington, DC: New Trends, 2003), 32–37.

5. Interview with Ron Schmid, November 14, 2004.

6. Edward Howell, *Food Enzymes for Health and Longevity 2nd Edition* (Twin Lakes, WI: Lotus Press, 1994), 17–21.

7. F. Diez-Gonzalez, T. R. Callaway, et al., "Grain Feeding and the Dissemination of Acid-resistant Escherichia Coli from Cattle," *Science* 281, no. 5383 (1998): 1666–1668.

8. Elaine F. Weiss, "Thwarting Cancer Before it Strikes," *Johns Hopkins Magazine*, April 2000. Web site: http:// www.jhu.edu/~jhumag/0400web/48.html. Accessed November 18, 2004.

9. Ron Schmid, *The Untold Story of Milk*, (Washington, DC: New Trends, 2003), 203–204.

10. Ibid., 193–229.

11. Mary Enig and Sally Fallon, *Eat Fat, Lose Fat: Three Delicious, Science-Based Coconut Diets* (New York: Hudson Street Press, 2005), 97, 99.

12. Interview with Ron Schmid, November 14, 2004.

CHAPTER 20

1. *Nip/Tuck*, episode titled "Mrs. Grubman," FX; July 13, 2004.

2. Marcia Herman-Giddens, et al., "Secondary Sexual Characteristics and Menses in Young Girls Seen in Office Practice: A Study from the Pediatric Research in Office Settings Network," *Pediatrics* 99, no. 4 (April 1997): 505–512; Marcia Herman-Giddens, et al., "Secondary Sexual Characteristics in Boys," *Archives of Pediatrics & Adolescent Medicine* 155 (Sept 2001): 1022–28. Sandra Cabot, "Toxins in Food and the Environment." Web site: http://www.liverdoctor.com. Accessed November 29, 2004.; Lindsey Tanner, "Study Pointing to Earlier Puberty in Boys." Web site: http:// www.mindfully.org. Accessed November 29, 2004.

3. Phone call with Michele L. Trankina, December 2, 2004, fax, December 3, 2004, e-mail, December 9, 2004; "The Hazards of Environmental Estrogens." Web site: http://www.

worldandi.com. Accessed December 1, 2004.

4. Peter Montague, "Milk Controversy Spills into Canada." Web site: http://www.garynull. com/Documents/erf/milk_controversy_spills_into_can.htm. Accessed November 28, 2005.

5. Jeffrey M. Smith, *Seeds of Deception: Exposing Industry and Government Lies About the Safety of the Genetically Engineered Foods You're Eating* (Fairfield, IA: Yes! Books, 2003), 79–81.

6. Samuel S. Epstein, *Got (Genetically Engineered) Milk?: The Monsanto BGH/BST Milk Wars Handbook* (New York: Seven Stories Press, 2001), 69; "Monsanto's Genetically Modified Milk Ruled Unsafe by the United Nations," Press release: *PR Newswire* (August 18, 1999); Telephone interview with Dr. Epstein (December 21, 2004); Samuel S. Epstein, *Got (Genetically Engineered) Milk?: The Monsanto BGH/BST Milk Wars Handbook* (New York: Seven Stories Press, 2001), 79–80.

7. "The Tainted Milk Moustache—How Monsanto and the FDA Spoiled a Staple Food," reprinted from *Alternative Medicine Digest* (January 1999). Web site: http:// www.afpafitness. com/articles/MilkMustache.htm. Accessed December 20, 2004.

8. "A New Study Warns Of Breast Cancer And Colon Cancer Risks From rBGH Milk," report on press conference by Cancer Prevention Coalition in Washington, DC (January 23, 1996); "Monsanto's Biosynthetic Milk Poses Risks of Prostate Cancer, Besides Other Cancers," Press release: *PR Newswire* (March 15, 1998); "Monsanto's Hormonal Milk Poses Serious Risks of Breast Cancer, Besides Other Cancers," Press release: *PR Newswire* (June 21, 1998); S. E. Hankinson, et al, "Circulating Concentrations of Insulin-like Growth Factor 1 and Risk of Breast Cancer," *Lancet* 351, no. 93113 (1998): 1393–1396; "Potential Public Health Hazards of Biosynthetic Milk Hormones," report by Dr. Samuel S. Epstein. *International Journal of Health Services* 20, no.1 (1990): 73–84.

9. Samuel Epstein, "FDA Is Ignoring Dangers of Bovine Growth Hormone," Letter to the editor of *Austin American Statesman* (June 2, 1990).

10. S. E. Hankinson, et al, "Circulating concentrations of insulin-like growth factor 1 and risk of breast cancer," *Lancet* 351, no. 93113 (1998): 1393–1396; June Chan et al, "Plasma Insulin-Like Growth Factor-1 [IGF-1] and Prostate Cancer Risk: A Prospective Study," *Science* 279 (January 23, 1998): 563–566; R. Torris, et al, "Time Course of Fenretinide-induced Modulation of Circulating Insulin-like Growth Factor (IGF)-1, IGF-II and IGFBP-3 in a bladder cancer chemo-prevention trial," *International Journal of Cancer*, Vol. 87 No. 4 (August 2000): pp. 601–605.

11. Food and Drug Administration, "Interim Guidance on the Voluntary Labeling of Milk and Milk Products from Cows that Have Not Been Treated with Recombinant Bovine Somatotropin," *Federal Register* 59, no. 28 (1994): 6279–6280; Samuel S. Epstein, "Unlabeled Milk From Cows Treated With Biosynthetic Growth Hormones: A Case of Regulatory Abdication," *International Journal of Health Services* 26, no. 1 (1996): 173–185.

12. Jeffrey M. Smith, *Seeds of Deception: Exposing Industry and Government Lies About the Safety of the Genetically Engineered Foods You're Eating* (Fairfield, IA: Yes! Books, 2003), 82–83.

13. *The Agribusiness Examiner*, Issue #38 (June 17, 1999). Website: http:// www.electricarrow. com/CARP/agbiz/agex-38.html. Accessed December 20, 2004; "The Tainted Milk Moustache—How Monsanto and the FDA Spoiled a Staple Food," reprinted from *Alternative Medicine Digest* (January 1999). Web site: http:// www.afpafitness.com/articles/ MilkMustache.htm. Accessed December 20, 2004; Web site: http://www.rockefeller.edu/ lectures/friedman112700.html. Accessed February 21, 2005.

14. Jeffrey M. Smith, *Seeds of Deception: Exposing Industry and Government Lies About the Safety*

of the Genetically Engineered Foods You're Eating (Fairfield, IA:Yes! Books, 2003), 81.

15. Samuel S. Epstein, *Got (Genetically Engineered) Milk?: The Monsanto BGH/BST Milk Wars Handbook* (New York: Seven Stories Press, 2001), 66; "Monsanto's Genetically Modified Milk Ruled Unsafe by the United Nations," Press release: *PR Newswire* (August 18, 1999).

16. Samuel S. Epstein, *Got (Genetically Engineered) Milk?: The Monsanto BGH/BST Milk Wars Handbook* (New York: Seven Stories Press, 2001), 460–490.

CHAPTER 21

1. Telephone interview with Mark McAfee, December 6, 2004.

2. T.R. Dhiman, et al.,"Conjugated Linoleic Acid Content of Milk from Cows Fed Different Diets," *Journal of Dairy Science* 82 (1999): 2146–56; S. K. Searles, et al., "Vitamin E, Vitamin A, and Carotene Contents of Alberta Butter." *Journal of Diary Science* 53, no. 2 (1999): 150–154; S. K. Jensen, "Quantitative Secretion and Maximal Secretion Capacity of Retinol, Beta-carotene and Alpha-tocopherol into Cows' Milk." *Journal of Dairy Research* 66, no. 4 (1999): 511–522; S. Banni, et al., "Conjugated Linoleic Acid-Enriched Butter Fat Alters Mammary Gland Morphogenesis and Reduces Cancer Risk in Rats." *Journal of Nutrition* 129, no.12 (1999): 2135–2142; Burton P. Koonsvitsky, et al., "Olestra Affects Serum Concentrations of Alpha-Tocopherol and Carotenoids" Journal of Nutrition 127, no. 8 (August 1997): 1636S-1645S; E. S. Ford, and Anne Sowell, "Serum Alpha-tocopherol Status in the United States Population: Findings from the Third National Health and Nutrition Examination Survey." American Journal of Epidemiology 150 (August 1, 1999): 290–300; G. Jahreis, et al., "Conjugated Linoleic Acid in Milk Fat: High Variation Depending on Production System." *Nutrition Research* 17, no. 9 (1997): 1479–1484.

3. E-mail from Ed Giovannucci, October 6, 2005, 10:31 A.M.

4. Craig Lambert, "Solar Tonic: Too Much Sunscreen?" *Harvard Magazine* 108, no. 1 (September–October 2005): 12.

5. C. Ip, et al., "Conjugated Linoleic Acid. A Powerful Anti-carcinogen from Animal Fat Sources," *Cancer* 74, no. 3 suppl, (1994): 1050–1054; A. Aro, et al., "Inverse Association Between Dietary and Serum Conjugated Linoleic Acid and Risk of Breast Cancer in Postmenopausal Women," *Nutrition and Cancer* 38, no. 2 (2000): 151–7; Z. Wu, L. D. Satter, and M. W. Pariza, "Paddocks containing red clover compared with all grass paddocks support high CLA levels in milk," U.S. Dairy Forage Research Center (1997).

6. Linda Bren "Got Milk? Make Sure It's Pasteurized." Web site: http://www.fda.gov/fdac/features/2004/504_milk.html. Accessed November 30, 2004.

7. Paul S. Mead, et al., "Food-Related Illness and Death in the United States," *Emerging Infectious Diseases* 5, no. 5 (September–October 1999): 607.

8. Eric Schlosser, *Fast Food Nation: The Dark Side of the American Meal* (New York: Perennial, 2002).

9. M. E. Jonsson, et al., "Persistence of Verocytotoxin-Producing Escherichia Coli 0157: H7 in Calves Kept on Pasture and in Calves Kept Indoor," *International Journal of Food Microbiology* 66, no. 1–2 (2001): 55–61.

10. Jared Diamond, *Guns, Germs, and Steel: The Fates of Human Societies* (New York: Norton 1999), 88.

CHAPTER 22

1. Phil McGraw, *The Ultimate Weight Solution: The 7 Keys to Weight Loss Freedom* (New York: Free Press, 2003), 120.

2. U.S. Dept. of Health, Education, and Welfare, *Obesity and Health*. (Washington, DC: U.S. DHEW, PHS Publication No. 1485, 1966).

3. A. Favaro, F. C. Rodella, and P. Santonastaso, "Binge Eating and Eating Attitudes among Nazi Concentration Camp Survivors," *Psychological Medicine* 30, no. 2 (March 2000): 463–466; M. M. Hagan, R. H. Whitworth, and D. E. Moss, "Semistarvation-Associated Eating Behaviors among College Binge Eaters: A Preliminary Description and Assessment Scale—Statistical Data Included," *Behavioral Medicine* (Fall 1999). Web site: http://www.findarticles.com/p/articles/mi_m0GDQ/is_3_25/ai_58669772. Accessed October 28, 2005.

4. M. M. Hagan, R. H. Whitworth, and D. E. Moss, "Semistarvation-Associated Eating Behaviors among College Binge Eaters: A Preliminary Description and Assessment Scale—Statistical Data Included," *Behavioral Medicine* (Fall 1999). Web site: http://www.findarticles.com/p/articles/mi_m0GDQ/is_3_25/ai_58669772. Accessed October 28, 2005.

5. *Inside the Actor's Studio*, Bravo, September 2, 2004, 1:00 A.M.

6. "Welcome to Diets FAQ." Website: http://www.dietsfaq.com/. Accessed December 13, 2005; "Why Diets Don't Work: The Myths that Make Us Massive." Web site: http://www.refityourself.com/refit/healthtopics_article5.html. Accessed December 13, 2005.

7. Adele Davis, *Let's Eat Right to Keep Fit* (New York: Harcourt, Brace, 1954), 246.

8. Gladys Block, "Foods Contributing to Energy Intake in the US: Data from NHANES III and NHANES 1999–2000," *Journal of Food Composition and Analysis,* 17, no. 3–4 (June–August 2000): 439–447.

9. Atul Gawande, *Complications: A Surgeon's Notes on an Imperfect Science* (New York: Metropolitan Books, 2002), 183.

10. Joseph M. Dhahbi, et al., "Temporal Linkage between the Phenotypic and Genomic Responses to Caloric Restriction," *Proceedings of the National Academy of Sciences* 101, no. 15 (April 13, 2004): 5524–5529; "Calorie Restriction Reduces Risk of MI, Stroke and Diabetes," *Native American Cancer Research*. Web site: http://natamcancer.org/page29.html. Accessed June 10, 2005.

11. Scott LaFee, "Eating Less May Mean a Longer Life if You Can Stand the Hunger Pangs," *San Diego Union Tribune*, November 24, 2004. Web site: http://www.signonsandiego.com/uniontrib/20041124/news_lz1c24cr.html. Accessed June 9, 2005; Kim Pierce, "Disciplined and Dedicated, They Eat Light for a Long Life," *The Dallas Morning News.* Web site: http://www.imminst.org/forum/index.php?s=&act=ST&f=69&t=4701. Accessed June 9, 2005.

CHAPTER 23

1. E-mail from Daniel E. Lieberman, February 24, 2006, 1:53 A.M.

2. Web site: http://www.spamagazine.com/new/advertorials/lapuerta.asp. Accessed April 1, 2005.

3. S. Gallistl, et al., "Insulin is an Independent Correlate of Plasma Homocysteine Levels in Obese Children and Adolescents," *Diabetes Care* 23, no. 9 (2000): 1348–1352; D. S. Michaud, et al., "Dietary Sugar, Glycemic Load, and Pancreatic Cancer Risk in a Prospective Study," *Journal of the National Cancer Institute* 94, no. 17 (September 4, 2002): 1293–1300; Anu Kareinen, et al., "Cardiovascular Risk Factors Associated With Insulin Resistance Cluster in Families With Early-Onset Coronary Heart Disease," Arteriosclerosis, Thrombosis, and Vascular Biology 21, no. 8 (August 2001): 1346–1352; Gerald Reaven, "Insulin Resistance, Hypertension, and Coronary Heart Disease," *Journal of Clinical Hypertension* 5, no. 4 (2003):

269–274.

4. Robert W. Stout, "Insulin and Atheroma 20-year Perspective," *Diabetes Care* 13, no. 6 (June 1990): 631.

5. Web site: http://www.cdc.gov/nchs/fastats/diabetes.htm. Accessed June 2, 2004; Web site: http://www.diabetes-tests.com/Diabetes_Facts.html. Accessed June 2, 2004; K. Gu, C. C. Cowie, and M. I. Harris, "Mortality in Adults with and without Diabetes in a National Cohort of the U.S. Population," *Diabetes Care* 21 (1998): 1138–1145, 1971–1993; Centers for Disease Control and Prevention National Diabetes fact sheet: general information and national estimates on diabetes in the United States (2002). Atlanta, GA: U.S. Department of Health and Human Services, Centers for Disease Control and Prevention (2003). Web site: http://www.diabetes.org/diabetes-statistics/national-diabetes-fact-sheet.jsp. Accessed June 2, 2004.

6. Patricia Reaney, "Obesity/Diabetes Could Hit Life Expectancy: Experts." *Reuters Health Information* (2004). Web site: http://www.lap-band-surgery.org/obesity.cfm/39715398/ Obesity/diabetes-could-hit-life-expectancy-experts/index.html. Accessed December 5, 2005.

7. Ibid.

8. Michael R. Eades and Mary Dan Eades, *The Protein Power Lifeplan* (New York: Warner Books, 2000), xix-xx.

9. Uffe Ravnskov, *The Cholesterol Myth: Exposing the Fallacy that Saturated Fat and Cholesterol Cause Heart Disease* (Washington, DC: New Trends, 2000).

10. E-mail from Uffe Ravnskov, November 5, 2005, 12:57 P.M.

11. Web site: http://www.pbs.org/wgbh/pages/frontline/shows/diet/etc/synopsis.html. Accessed July 5, 2004.

12. "Dietary Guidelines Advisory Committee Meeting Meeting Summary." Web site: www. health.gov/dietaryguidelines/ dga2005/dgac012004minutes.pdf. Accessed April 9, 2005.

13. Gina Kolata and Lawrence K. Altman, "Study of Breast Cancer Patients Finds Benefit in Low-Fat Diets," *New York Times*, May 17, 2005: Health.

14. Gina Kolata, "Low-Fat Diet Does Not Cut Health Risks, Study Finds," *New York Times*, February 8, 2006. Web site: http://www.nytimes.com/2006/02/08/health/08fat.html? ex=1140066000&en=4eb4d476df0744a2&ei=5070; Howard, et al., "Low-Fat Dietary Pattern and Risk of Cardiovascular Disease: The Women's Health Initiative Randomized Controlled Dietary Modification Trial," *JAMA* Vol. 295 No. 6 (Feb. 8, 2006): pp. 655–666. Ross L. Prentice, et al., "Low-Fat Dietary Pattern and Risk of Invasive Modification Trial," *Journal of the American Medical Association* 295, no. 6 (February 8, 2006): 629–642; Shirley A. A. Beresford, "Low-Fat Dietary Pattern and Risk of Colorectal Modification Trial," *Journal of the American Medical Association* 295, no. 6 (February 8, 2006): 643–654.

CHAPTER 24

1. *Weeds*, pilot episode titled "You Can't Miss the Bear," Showtime, August 7, 2005.

2. Frederick F. Samaha, et al., "A Low-Carbohydrate as Compared with a Low-Fat Diet in Severe Obesity," *New England Journal of Medicine* 348, no. 21 (May 22, 2003): 2074–2081; D. L. Katz, "Competing Dietary Claims for Weight Loss: Finding the Forest through Truculent Trees," *Annual Review of Public Health* 26 (2005): 61–88.

3. Robert C. Atkins, *Dr. Atkins' New Diet Revolution* (New York: Quill, 2002), 215.

4. "UK Food Agonises Over Atkins." Web site: http://www.telegraph.co.uk/money/main. jhtml?xml=/money/2004/01/04/ccdiet04.xml; Atkins Launching Education Campaign to Improve Steak and Bacon Image." Web site: http://www.medicalnewstoday.com/index.

php?newsid=7400. Accessed June 13, 2004.

5. Kate Zernike and Marion Burros, "Low-Carb Boom Isn't Just for Dieters Anymore," *New York Times*, February 19, 2004: A-16.

6. T. L. Davidson and S. E. Swithers, "Pavlovian Approach to the Problem of Obesity." *International Journal of Obesity* 28, no. 7 (2004): 933–935.

7. Daniel DeNoon, "Drink More Diet Soda, Gain More Weight?" Web site: http://www. webmd.com/content/article/107/108476.htm. Accessed January 5, 2006.

8. Andy Coghlan, "Shrunken Glands Spark Sweetener Controversy," *New Scientist* 1796 (November 23, 1991).

9. B. A. John, S. G. Wood, and D. R. Hawkins, "The Pharmacokinetics and Metabolism of Sucralose in the Mouse," *Food Chemical Toxicology* 38, Suppl. 2 (2000): S107-S110; Y. F. Sasaki, et al., "The Comet Assay with 8 Mouse Organs: Results with 39 Currently Used Food Additives," *Mutation Research* 519, no. 1–2 (August 26, 2002): 103–119.

CHAPTER 25

1. Krista Smith, "Demi Gloss," *Vanity Fair*, February 2007: 256.

2. Dirt, episode titled "Blogan," FX; January 9, 2007.

CHAPTER 26

1. Web site: http://www.cortislim.com/. Accessed March 18, 2007.

2. Roger Ekirch, *At Day's Close: Night in Times Past*, (New York: W.W. Norton, 2005).

3. Roy Riverburg, "This Diet Pill Contains Saturated Advertising." Web site: http://medialit. med.sc.edu/diet_pill_contains_ads.htm. Accessed August 21, 2005; "Greg Cynaumon's Study Doesn't Exist." Web site: http://lizditz.typepad.com/i_speak_of_dreams/2004/06/ greg_cynaumons_.html. Accessed August 21, 2005.

4. Robyn Dixon, "Hoodia Fever Takes a Toll on Rare Plant," *Los Angeles Times*, December 26, 2006; Jay Rath, "New Drug Tempting Dieters, but Experts Debate Hoodia's Merits," *Wisconsin State Journal*, September 5, 2005: D-1; Joan Morris, "Little Research Behind Claims that Hoodia is Safe, Effective for Losing Weight," *Seattle Times*, March 9, 2006; Jasjit Bindra, "A Popular Pill's Hidden Danger," *New York Times*, April 26, 2005.

5. Ottar Nygard, et al., "Coffee Consumption and Plasma Total Homocysteine: The Hordaland Homocystein Study," *American Journal of Clinical Nutrition* 65, no. 1 (1997): 136–143; C. K. Stanton and R. H. Gray, "Effects of Caffeine Consumption on Delayed Conception," *American Journal of Epidemiology* 142, no. 12 (1995): 1322; Claire Infante-Rivard, et al., "Fetal Loss Associated with Caffeine Intake Before and During Pregnancy," *Journal of the American Medical Association* 270 (December 22/29, 1993): 2940–2943; Mark A. Klebanoff, et al., "Maternal Serum Paraxanthine, a Caffeine Metabolite, and the Risk of Spontaneous Abortion," *New England Journal of Medicine* 341, no. 22 (November 25, 1999): 1639–1644; Stephen Cherniske, *Caffeine Blues* (New York: Warner Books, 1998), 7.

6. Diane Welland. "As Caffeine Controversy Rages on, What's a Coffee Lover to Do?" *Environmental Nutrition* 19 (1996): 1.

7. "Decaffeinating Coffee." Web site: http://www.hi-tm.com/Facts&tips/Decaf.html. Accessed December 7, 2005; R. G. Liteplo, G. W. Long and M. E. Meek, "Relevance of Carinogenicity Bioassays in Mice in Assessing Potential Health Risks Associated with Exposure to Methylene Chloride," *Human and Experimental Toxicology* 17, no.2 (February 1998): 84–87; E. Lynge, A. Anttila, and K. Hemminki, "Organic Solvents and Cancer," *Cancer Causes and Control* 8, no.3 (May 1997): 406–419.

8. Marian Burros and Sherri Day, "Doubt Cast on Food Supplements for Weight Control,"

New York Times, October 27, 2003: Media. Web site: http://www.nytimes.com. Accessed May 16, 2005.

9. "Dr. Phil McGraw Facing Class-Action Suit." Web site: http://www.casewatch.org/civil/drphil/classactioncomplaint.shtml. Accessed December 30. 2005.

10. *The Colbert Report.* January 30, 2006; *The Daily Show with Jon Stewart.* January 30, 2006.

CHAPTER 27

1. E-mail from Mike Katke, February 7, 2004, 11:00 A.M.

2. E-mail from Kaayla Daniel, February 5, 2007, 7:46 A.M.

3. E-mail from Ron Schmid, September 11, 2005, 5:55 A.M.

CHAPTER 28

1. Sultan Muhammad, "Business with Disease: The Scourge of Prescription Drugs," FinalCall. com News. Web site: http://www.finalcall.com/artman/publish/article_1255.shtml. Accessed October 30, 2005.

2. *Larry King Live*, November 15, 2006. Web site: http://transcripts.cnn.com/TRANSCRIPTS/0611/15/lkl.01.html. Accessed January 3, 2006.

3. Kelly Patricia O'Meara, "Diagnosing Infants with Depression." Web site: http://www.antidepressantsfacts.com/2004–05–03-infants-depression-antideps.htm. Accessed May 9, 2005.

4. Shankar Vedantam, "FDA Confirms Antidepressants Raise Children's Suicide Risk," *Washington Post*, September 14, 2004: A-1.

5. "The FDA Exposed: An Interview with Dr. David Graham, the Vioxx Whistleblower." Web site: http://www.newstarget.com/z011401.html. Accessed December 8, 2005.

6. Associated Press, "Cruise Clashes With Lauer on 'Today' Show," (June 24, 2005). Web site: http://www.miami.com/mid/miamiherald/entertainment/11980135.htm. Accessed June 24, 2005; Web site: http://www.drudgereport.com/flash3tc.htm. Accessed June 26, 2005.

7. Michael Smith, "Final Word May Not Come for a Year." Web site: http://www.webmd.com/content/biography/7/40428.htm. Accessed July 1, 2006.

8. "Tom Cruise Spars with Lauer on 'Today' Show." Web site: http://www.ctv.ca/servlet/ArticleNews/story/CTVNews/20050624/cruise_lauer_050624?s_name=&no_ads=. Accessed June 26, 2005.

9. Alessandra Stanley, "Talk Show Rarity: A True Believer's Candor," *New York Times*, June 25, 2005: A-15.

10. Telephone interview with Carol Simontacchi, June 27, 2005.

11. Nicholas D. Kristof, "Mike Huckabee Lost 110 Pounds. Ask Him How," *New York Times* January 29, 2006: 17.

12. William A. Carlezon, et al., "Antidepressant-like Effects of Uridine and Omega-3 Fatty Acids Are Potentiated by Combined Treatment in Rats," *Biological Psychiatry* 57, no. 4 (February 15, 2005): 343–350.

13. C. B. Gesch, et al., "Influence of Supplementary Vitamins, Minerals and Essential Fatty Acids on the Antisocial Behaviour of Young Adult Prisoners," British Journal of Psychiatry 181 (2002): 22–28; S. J. Schoenthaler, and I. D. Bier, "The Effect of Vitamin-Mineral Supplementation on Juvenile Delinquency among American Schoolchildren: A Randomized, Double-blind Placebo-controlled Trial," *Journal of Alternative Complementary Medicine* 6, no. 1 (2000): 7–17; France Bellisle, "Effects of Diet on Behaviour and Cognition in Children," *British Journal of Nutrition* 92, no. 0S2 (October 2004): S227-S232.

14. Web site: http://www.isnr.org/nfbarch/nbiblio.htm.

15. Adele Davis, *Let's Eat Right to Keep Fit* (New York: Harcourt, Brace, 1954), 249.

16. Bill Maher, HBO Stand-Up Special, "'I'm Swiss': and other Treasonous Statements," July 30, 2005, 7:00 P.M.

17. Gillian Sanson, *The Myth of Osteoporosis: What Every Woman Should Know About Creating Bone Health* (Ann Arbor, MI: MCD Century Publications, 2003). Web site: http://www.findarticles.com/p/articles/mi_m0ISW/is_245/ai_111496966. Accessed December 21, 2005.

18. David Y. Graham, and Hoda M. Malaty, "Alendronate and Naproxen Are Synergistic for Development of Gastric Ulcers," Archives of Internal Medicine 161, no. 1 (2001): 107–110.

19. S. L. Ruggiero, et al., "Osteonecrosis of the Jaws Associated with the Use of Bisphosphonates: A Review of 63 Cases," *Journal of Oral and Maxillofacial Surgery* 62, no. 5. (May 2004): 527–34.

20. C. V. Odvina, et al., "Severely Suppressed Bone Turnover: A Potential Complication of Alendronate Therapy," *Journal of Clinical Endocrinology and Metabolism* 90, no. 3 (March 2005): 1294–1301.

21. G. Sanson, "The Myth of Osteoporosis." Web site: http://www.healthyskepticism.org/library/ref.php?id=1166. Accessed December 20, 2005.

22. Uffe Ravnskov, *The Cholesterol Myth: Exposing the Fallacy that Saturated Fat and Cholesterol Cause Heart Disease* (Washington, DC: New Trends, 2000), 206, 2, 61.

23. Ibid. Web site: http://www.ravnskov.nu/cholesterol.htm. Accessed August 13, 2004.

24. E-mail from Mary Enig, Aug.ust 15, 2004, 3:49 P.M.

25. E-mail from Mary Enig, August 15, 2004, 3:49 P.M.

26. Uffe Ravnskov, *The Cholesterol Myth: Exposing the Fallacy that Saturated Fat and Cholesterol Cause Heart Disease* (Washington, DC: New Trends, 2000): 130–131, 135, 238–239.

27. Gina Kolata, "New Conclusions on Cholesterol: Study Sees Gain for Heart in Levels Kept Very Low," *New York Times* March 9, 2004: front page.

28. E-mail from Michael and Mary Dan Eades, July 5, 2004, 4 P.M.; Loren Cordain, et al., "Origins and Evolution of the Western Diet: Health Implications for the 21st Century," *American Journal of Clinical Nutrition* 81, no. 2 (February 2005): 341–354.

29. Aaron Smith, "Heart Drug Pulled, Pfizer Tumbles," CNNMoney.com, December 4, 2006. Web site: http://money.cnn.com/2006/12/04/news/companies/pfizer_stock/index.htm. Accessed January 5, 2007.

CHAPTER 29

1. Louis Menand, "Acid Redux: The Life and High Times of Timothy Leary," *The New Yorker*, June 26, 2006, 79.

2. Web site: http://www.diabeteshealthconnection.com/products/nutrition/glucerna/index.aspx. Accessed March 3, 2006.

3. "Horizon Organic, Now Dean Foods, Threatens Livelihood of Organic Farmers." Web site: http://www.organicconsumers.org/organic/horizon_farmers.cfm. Accessed November 30, 2004; Web site: http://www.horizonorganic. Accessed November 30, 2004.

4. Marion Burros, "Grass-Fed Rule Angers Farmers," *New York Times*, July 26, 2006: 79.

5. Telephone interview with Joe and Brenda Cochran, December 10, 2004.

6. " New Olestra Complaints Bring Total Close To 20,000—More Than All Other Food Additive Complaints In History Combined." Web site: http://www.cspinet.org/new/olestrapr_041602.html. Accessed March 20, 2004.

7. Brad Dorfman, "Companies Putting Olestra in Chips Can Remove Diarrhea Warnings,"

Reuters, August 1, 2003. Web site: http://www.organicconsumers.org/foodsafety/olestra. cfm. Accessed October 28, 2005.

8. Web site: http://www.olean.com/products/snacks.html. Accessed March 20, 2004.

9. *Sweet Misery: A Poisoned World*, Sound and Fury Productions (2001). VHS.

10. Frederick Kaufman, "Contraband: Psst! Got Milk?" *The New Yorker*, November 29, 2004: 62.

11. Nicholas D. Kristof, "Medicine's Sticker Shock," *New York Times*, October 2, 2005. Web site: http://select.nytimes.com/2005/10/02/opinion/02kristof.html?&emc=etal/. Accessed October 17, 2005.

12. Carl Hulse, "Vote in House Offers a Shield for Restaurants in Obesity Suits," *New York Times*, March 11, 2004: front page.

13. Todd Zwillich, "House Passes 'Cheeseburger' Bill." Web site: http://www.cbsnews.com/ stories/2005/10/19/health/webmd/printable956858.shtml. Accessed Dec. 12, 2005.

14. Ibid.

15. John Vidal, *McLibel: Burger Culture on Trial* (New York: New Press, 1997).

16. Edward R. Pinckney and Cathey Pinckney, *The Cholesterol Controversy* (Los Angeles: Sherbourne Press, 1973), 4, 63.

17. Web site: http://www.honeynutcheerios.com. Accessed March 17, 2005.

CHAPTER 30

1. Bill Maher, HBO Stand-Up Special, "'I'm Swiss': and other Treasonous Statements," July 30, 2005, 7:00 P.M.

2. Karen Kersting, "Marketing Encourages Teens to Tie Brand Choices to Personal Identity." Web site: http://thestressoflife.com/marketing_encourages_teens_to_ti.htm. Accessed December 12, 2005.

3. Dan DeLuca, "Maestros of Misconduct: Creeps We Love to Envy." *Santa Barbara News Press*, March 22, 2004: D-3.

4. Melanie Warner, "Is a Trip to McDonald's Just What the Doctor Ordered?" *New York Times*, May 2, 2005. Web site: http://query.nytimes.com/gst/health/article-page.html?res=9C0DE2 D61E31F931A35756C0A9639C8B63. Accessed July 8, 2005.

5. Mike Falcon, "Marilu Henner Rounds up Soy Benefits," *USA Today*. Web site: http:// www.usatoday.com/news/health/spotlight/2001–05–02-henner-soy.htm. Accessed June 5, 2005.

6. Jane Fonda, *My Life So Far*, (New York: Random House, 2005): 85.

7. Nat Ives, "A Report Raises the Possibility That Ads Contribute to Obesity in Children; The Industry Begs to Differ," *New York Times*, February 25, 2004): C-3.

8. Telephone interview with Steven Rotter, May 18, 2004, 1:10 P.M.

9. Kelly Brownell and Marion Nestle, "Are You Responsible for Your Own Weight?" *Time*, June 7, 2004: 113; Kelly D. Brownell, *Food Fight: The Inside Story of the Food Industry, America's Obesity Crisis and What We Can Do about It* (New York: Contemporary Books, 2004), 48–51.

10. Marion Nestle, *Food Politics* (Berkeley, Los Angeles, London: University of California Press, 2002), viii.

11. Sherri Day, "Dr. Phil, Medicine Man," *New York Times*, October 27, 2003\. Web site: http://www.nytimes.com. Accessed May 16, 2005.

CHAPTER 31

1. Lilka Woodward Areton, "Factors in the Sexual Satisfaction Of Obese Women in Relationships," *Electronic Journal of Human Sexuality* 5 (January 15, 2002). Web site: http://www.ejhs.org/volume5/Areton/03Background.htm. Accessed October 28, 2005.

2. Norman Goodman, et al., "Variant Reactions to Physical Disabilities," *American Sociological Review* 28 (1963): 429–435.

3. M. Roehling. "Weight-Based Discrimination in Employment: Psychological and Legal Aspects," *Personnel Psychology* 52 (1999): 969–1016.

4. R. C. Whitaker, et al., "Predicting Obesity in Young Adulthood from Childhood and Parental Obesity," *New England Journal of Medicine* 337, no. 13 (1997): 869–873.

5. M. S. Treuth, N. F. Butte, and J. D. Sorkin, "Predictors of Body Fat Gain in Non-obese Girls with a Familial Predisposition to Obesity," *American Journal of Clinical Nutrition* 78, no. 6 (December 2003): 1051–2.

6. "Three-year-old Dies From Obesity," *BBC News,* May 27, 2004. Web site: http://newsvote.bbc.co.uk/mpapps/pagetools/print/news.bbc.co.uk/1/hi/health/3752597.stm. Accessed October 28, 2005; Susan Reed, "Obese Girl's Mother Guilty of Misdemeanor Child Abuse," *U.S. News,* January 9, 1998. Web site: http://www.cnn.com/US/9801/09/obese.abuse/. Accessed October 28, 2005.

7. Phil McGraw, *The Ultimate Weight Solution: The 7 Keys to Weight Loss Freedom* (New York: Free Press, 2003), 119.

8. KeShun Liu, *Soybeans Chemistry, Technology and Utilization* (New York: Springer, 1997), 297–347.

9. Allison Daee, et al., "Psychologic and Physiologic Effects of Dieting in Adolescents" *Southern Medical Journal* 95, no. 9 (2002): 1032–1041.

10. Sally Squires, "Teaching Kids To Eat Well." Web site: http://www.washingtonpost.com/wp-dyn/content/article/2005/06/06/AR2005060601671.html. Accessed October 29, 2005; "The Dietary Intervention Study in Children (DISC)." Web site: http://www.nhlbi.nih.gov/resources/deca/agreements/disc.pdf. Accessed October 29, 2005.

11. Web site: http://www.clintonfoundation.org/050305-feature-wjc-aha-healthier-generation-initiative1.htm. Accessed August 6, 2005.

12. "Bottlers Want to Limit School Soft Drinks." Web site: http://www.cnn.com/2005/HEALTH/diet.fitness/08/17/soda.in.school.ap/index.html. Accessed August 17, 2005.

INDEX

HOW TO TAKE
GOOD PICTURES

HOW TO TAKE
GOOD PICTURES

Copyright © 1981, 1982 by Eastman Kodak Company

Library of Congress Catalog Number: 81-66172
ISBN 0-345-33900-2

Manufactured in the United States of America
34th Edition (Revised), 1982 Printing

9 8

CONTRIBUTORS

Eastman Kodak Company, Author
    Martin L. Taylor, Text and Editorial Coordination
    Donald S. Buck, Photography
    Neil Montanus, Photography
    William M. Czamanske, Photography
    Robert Brink, Production

Mark Hobson, Photography
Tom Beelmann, Photography
William Paris, Photo Research and Art Direction
Quarto Marketing Ltd., Design
Roger Pring and Christopher Meehan, Designers
Ken Diamond, Design Assistant
Dan Marciano, Revision Design Coordinator

4

Table of Contents

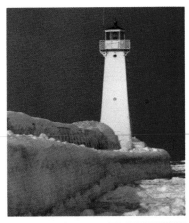

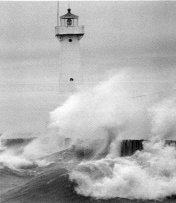

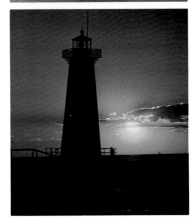

INTRODUCTION

Photography offers a twofold thrill to picture-takers. There's the delight in the event that you are planning to capture, and there's the pleasure in reviewing the pictures days, weeks, or even years later. With a little confidence in your knowledge, skill, and experience, you'll find that arranging or discovering a photogenic scene provides great satisfaction. Pictures are reminders, keys to the past—even bits of history, personal or documentary. They also express your moods, impressions, and feelings of the moment—visible statements of a very personal art.

How to Take Good Pictures will help you improve your pictures with any kind of camera. The advice on the following pages will familiarize you with many basic elements and techniques of photography. And as you become better acquainted with the principles of successful picture-taking, you'll feel more confidence in your own results.

How to Take Good Pictures gives instruction with pictures, rather than with columns of number- and formula-laden text. In this step-by-step primer, words serve to emphasize or clarify the messages offered by the illustrations. The book begins with basic ideas for picture improvement and moves on to advanced concepts. Start with the Ten Top Techniques for Better Pictures on the next 8 pages. Then, either read on in sequence or turn to those sections that interest you the most.

Keeping a ready camera and searching for the best viewpoint can pay rich rewards, as in this view of Mont St. Michel. Notice how the peaceful grazing sheep help to establish distance relationships. Muted light from cloudy skies gives a special mood.

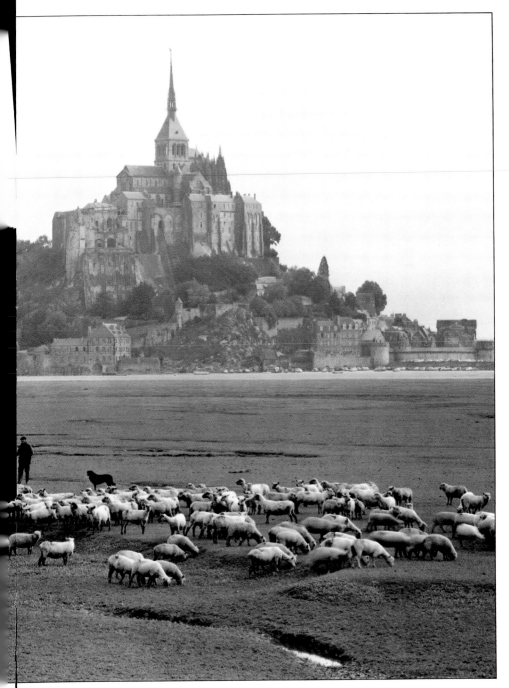

THE TEN TOP TECHNIQUES FOR BETTER PICTURES

(If you read no further, these ideas will give your picture-taking a dramatic improvement.)

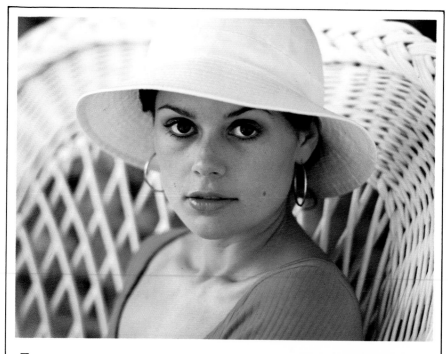

1

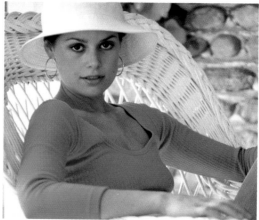

Move close to your subject. Whether it is a New England church, the Matterhorn, or a child with ice cream, get close enough so that you see only the most important elements in the viewfinder. Failure to observe this simple guideline accounts for more unsuccessful pictures than any other photo mistake.

2

Make sure that your automatic or manually adjustable camera is adjusted to give correct exposure. If your pictures are too light or too dark, check the camera manual and the film instructions. Remember to set the film speed—ISO (ASA) or ISO (DIN)—on most automatic cameras and sometimes the shutter speed or the aperture. On a manually operated camera, set the film speed, shutter speed, and aperture.

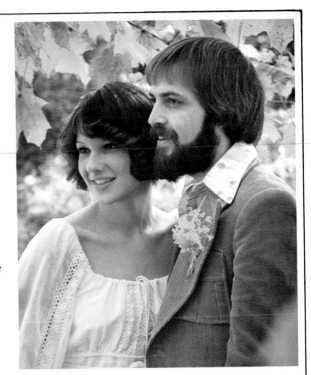

Correct exposure

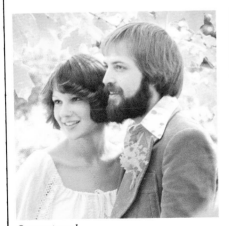

Overexposed

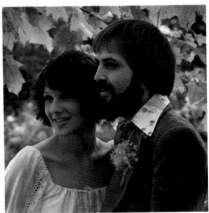

Underexposed

3

Carefully observe both background and foreground in your viewfinder before you take the picture. Clutter or confusing elements tend to dilute the strength of your subject. Keep your pictures as simple as possible.

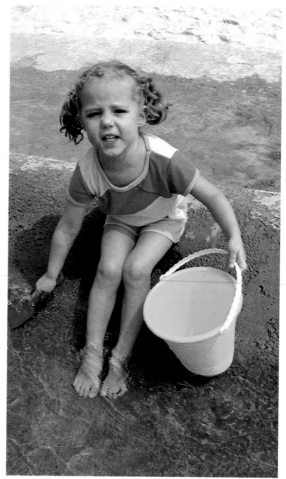

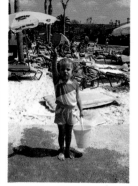

Cluttered background   *Simple background*

4

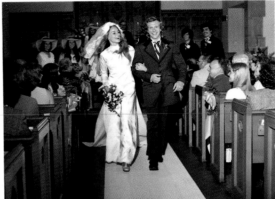

Correctly exposed flash pictures must be made within the flash-to-subject distance range for snapshot cameras. For automatic or manually adjustable cameras, the distance determines any adjustments to be made.

Flash is for dark places.

5

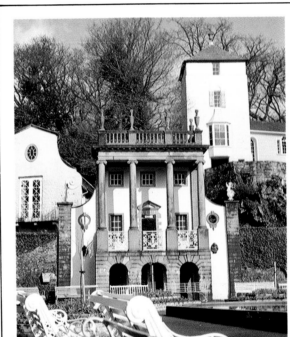

Hold your camera steady. Shaky hands or punching the shutter-release button may give you fuzzy pictures. Brace the camera with both hands against your forehead and smoothly press the shutter release.

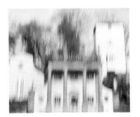

Steady camera, sharp pictures.

Shaky camera, fuzzy pictures.

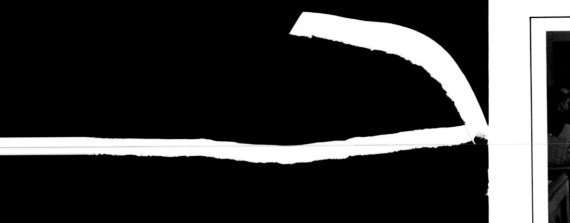

6

Become thoroughly familiar with your camera. Read the instruction manual carefully so that you'll be comfortable making adjustments under a wide variety of conditions. As you read the manual, keep your camera in hand for reference.

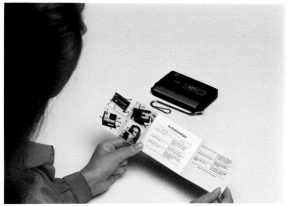

Read your camera manual thoroughly.

7

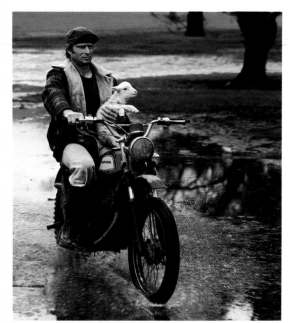

Set your subject slightly off-center. When shown dead-center in a picture, your subject may appear static and rather dull. Experiment to see where different subjects look best. Some cameras take square pictures and others take rectangular ones. If your camera takes rectangular pictures, you can get both horizontal and vertical pictures by holding the camera flat or on end.

Try putting your subject off center.

8

Rather than posing people in a starchy,

engage them in a natural, absorbing activity so eyes off you and the *~~mera. When people ? doing something familiar, their bodies and faces will relax.* posed, of course, but the *picture-taker found a way to draw their attention and commemorate a holiday*

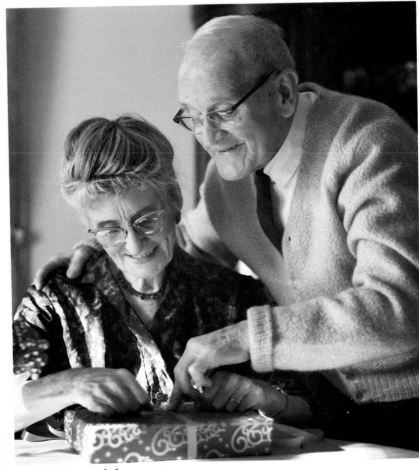

Keep people occupied.

9

Watch the direction of light in your scene. People tend to squint in bright, direct light and the dark shadows are often unattractive. Light from the side or from behind your subject may be more effective than light from the front. Picture-taking in the shade or on an overcast day may be better, too, if it is possible with your camera.

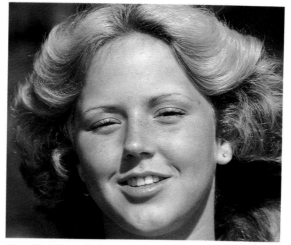

Frontlighting—light from the front

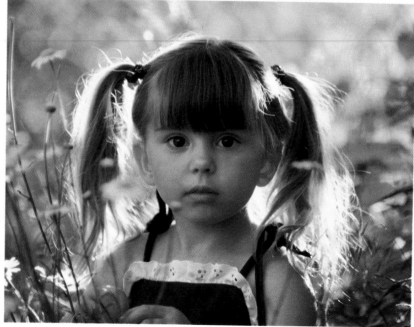

Backlighting—light from behind

10

*Take plenty of pictures.
Every professional
knows that the
potential for success
rises with the number
of pictures taken.
Compared with some of
the rare scenes you'll
encounter film is far*

opportunity.

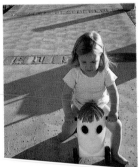

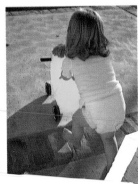

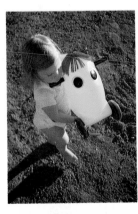

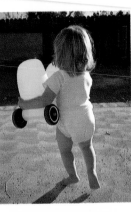

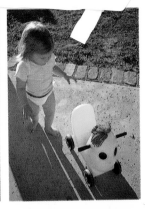

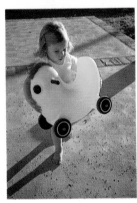

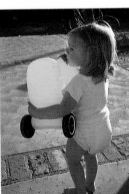

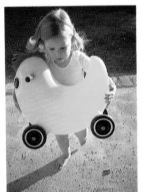

OPERATING YOUR CAMERA

TYPES OF CAMERAS

All cameras provide the same function—to allow a measured quantity of light to strike film. The light makes an image on the film and you get a picture. If you have an instant camera and film, you get a finished print from the camera. If you have a conventional camera that takes black-and-white, color negative, or color slide film, the film is usually processed by a photofinisher. You get slides or prints and negatives.

In this book, we'll discuss the use of several camera types: disc, instant, cartridge-loading, and 35 mm. These cameras all work in basically the same way. Their layout may be slightly different, but the controls perform similar functions. In the next few pages, we'll provide a thumbnail sketch of each camera type, including its assets and its operating procedures. Since some cameras are more complex than others, we'll devote more space to them for greater clarity.

We'll be showing and describing some current cameras in this section. No matter what camera you have, you'll want to refer to the instruction manual for specific information on loading and operating procedures. Kodak can furnish a replacement manual for a recent Kodak camera if your manual has disappeared. The same may be true with other manufacturers. Try your photo dealer if information for your camera is unavailable. Dealers are familiar with many cameras and should be happy to help.

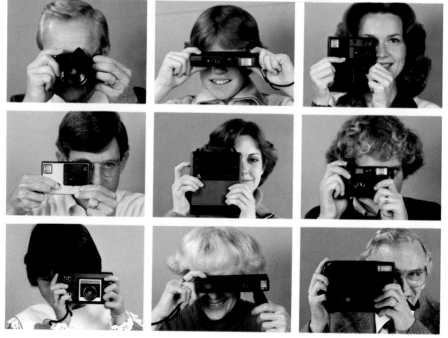

KODAK DISC CAMERAS

Dramatic gains in photo technology give a dynamic go-anywhere, do-anything capability to the attractive new KODAK Disc Cameras and Film. A sensitive computer adjusts the exposure settings and provides flash when necessary. A built-in motor advances the high-speed film disc. And battery energy powers all camera functions. With its compact size and reasonable price, the KODAK Disc Camera can be your constant companion. Sophisticated engineering will allow you to capture almost any situation with aim-and-snap simplicity.

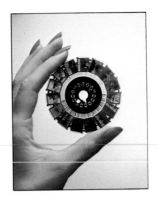

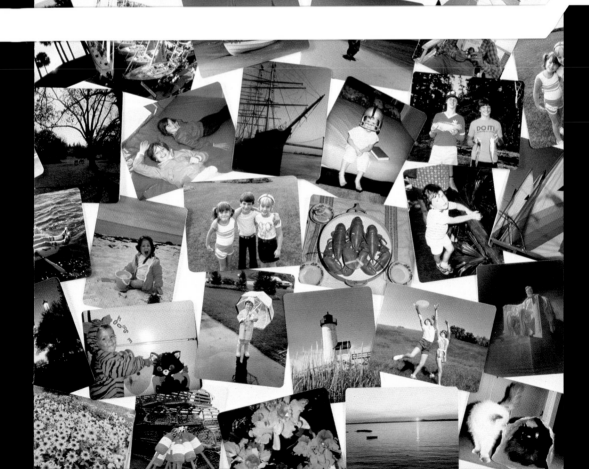

OPERATING DISC CAMERAS

Because KODAK Disc Cameras determine their own adjustments, you need only load the camera and snap the shutter. On some advanced models, you can choose a close-up lens. The KODAK Disc 8000 Camera provides a switch for the self-timer and rapid sequence functions.

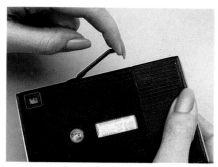

1. When a disc shows "x" in the frame window, lift the disc door lever.

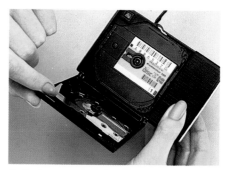

2. Swing open the disc door and remove the exposed disc film.

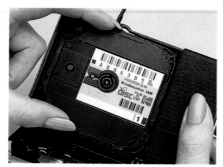

3. Unwrap a new disc film and insert it— it fits only one way.

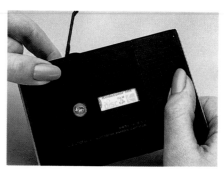

4. Close the disc door until seated— then push the door lever down to lock.

Use the close-up lens selector on advanced models for subjects in a 1½-4 foot range. The normal position of the lens is marked with a ⌂, the close-up position with a ♟.

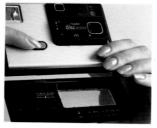

With a KODAK Disc 8000 Camera, set the switch at the left of the nameplate to the top position for a rapid sequence of pictures—at the bottom to activate the self-timer. The middle position allows normal operation.

MOTORIZED FILM ADVANCE

All KODAK Disc Cameras feature automatic film advance, powered by an electric motor. This motorized advance allows you to record more than a single glimpse of an activity. Keep your eye to the viewfinder to follow your subject and take a series of pictures that show a complete short story. The KODAK Disc 8000 Camera offers a rapid sequence feature that takes as many as three pictures a second in bright daylight to capture faster action.

Top row: Document a chain of events with the automatic film advance of any KODAK Disc Camera.

Bottom rows: By setting the rapid sequence switch on the KODAK Disc 8000 Camera, you can shoot surprisingly fast action.

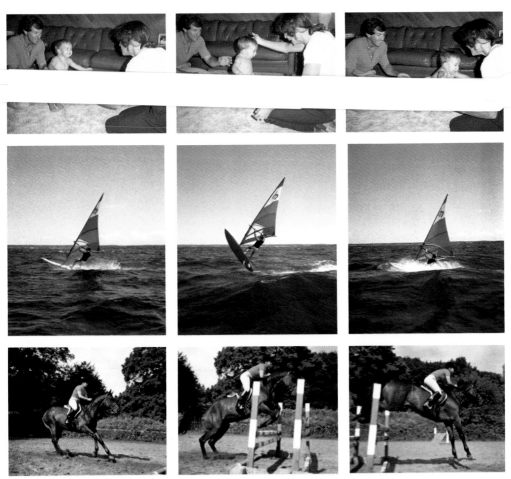

19

EXPOSURE FLEXIBILITY

KODAK Disc Cameras can take bright, well-exposed pictures in a wide variety of lighting conditions. Directed by an intelligently programmed computer, the camera's exposure controls will give you great photos in sunlight, gloomy overcast, bright interiors, and a host of other situations. And, if it's too dark, the flash will fire automatically to brighten your main subject. The result—a freedom to photograph almost anything you see.

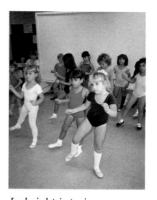

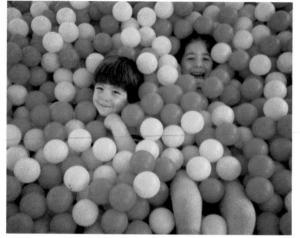

In bright interiors, your KODAK Disc Camera will preserve the mood by taking excellent pictures with the natural light that exists in the scene, as the pictures above and at left illustrate. In darker conditions, as in all the pictures at right, the flash will assist to brighten nearby subjects.

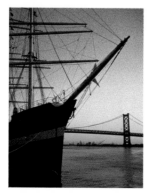

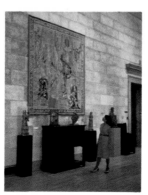

Early in the morning, late in the evening, under stormy skies, in museums, or at brightly lighted entertainment, your KODAK Disc Camera will capture more scenes than you ever thought possible.

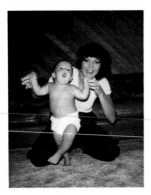
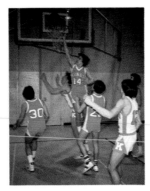
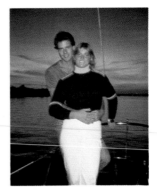

~~~~~~~~~~ ELECTRONIC FLASH

Camera fires the ~~~
release. You won't have to wait long, either—the recycle time is very short. The brief intensity of electronic flash will stop action. The range of good exposure is extraordinary, and there are many possibilities for using the flash when the ambient light is adequate but dull. Dim interiors, deep shade outdoors, and backlighted subjects early or late in the day are typical situations when your flash will make a bright picture in a drab situation.

*At top left the always alert
~~~~ ~f ~ KODAK Disc.*

The center and right photos illustrate how the flash and the low-light capability complement each other by giving brightly lighted foreground subjects against still-visible interesting backgrounds.

Notice at right how the flash illuminated the girls in the dark foreground to provide an attractive lighting balance with the bright doorway.

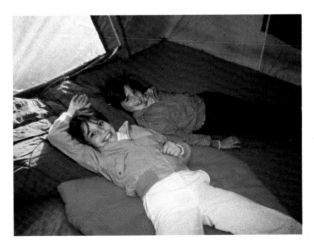

CLOSE-UPS

Every KODAK Disc Camera will take sharp pictures in a broad range of distance—from 4 feet to infinity. But for small subjects the KODAK Disc 6000 and 8000 Cameras offer an auxiliary close-up lens that will help you get big images at close distances. By sliding the close-up lens lever into position, you can move as close as 18 inches or as far as 4 feet.

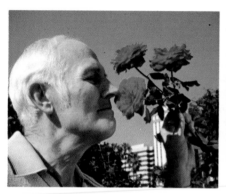 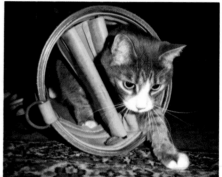

SELF-TIMER ON THE *KODAK* DISC 8000 CAMERA

Here's an opportunity for the photographer to be photographed. In addition to all its other features, the KODAK Disc 8000 Camera boasts a shutter release delay that allows you ten seconds to join the group in the picture. Make sure to leave room for yourself when you compose the scene.

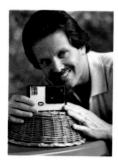 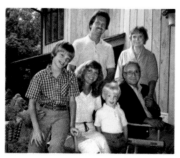

Pull the camera cover back for support and place the camera on a convenient surface. Compose the picture in the viewfinder. Set the self-timer switch, press the shutter release, and get into position. A red light will flash and the camera will beep until the picture is taken.

DISPLAY YOUR DISC PICTURES

You'll be proud of the pictures you take with your KODAK Disc Camera. Show it by keeping your best results visible. Some outstanding ones deserve to be enlarged and framed or placed prominently in an album. Good storytelling snapshots should be the historical core of your album collection. And there are other ways to display your efforts that appear on pages 112-114.

Incidentally, the numbers on the back of each print offer an excellent basis for organizing your photos. The first number (in brackets) is the individual negative number. The longer number at right is the unique disc number that you can see on the disc negative. If you label the outside of each processing envelope with the disc number, it will be

brackets will tell the photofinisher which picture you want.

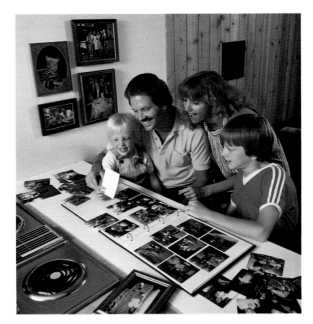

Taking care of your pictures will help them last longer. Although you'll find ideas for safekeeping on page 115, please review these tips for proper treatment and handling of pictures taken with KODAK Disc Cameras. Keep disc film, exposed and unexposed, out of hot, humid places and out of direct sunlight. Use the cardboard protector to send your disc film in for processing. When the finished package returns, keep the negative safe in its cardboard envelope. And never touch it except by the edges.

INSTANT CAMERAS

Most instant cameras are delightfully easy to use. Flash operation differs from model to model, and a few models may need to be focused, but generally there is little to learn and less to fuss with.

Advantages Instant cameras are great when you want to see your pictures right away. Parties and gatherings of all types are natural situations. Travel and vacations are fun with instant cameras, because you can send instant prints instead of postcards. Anyone with children will appreciate the instant results when taking pictures of youthful antics. The kids love them.

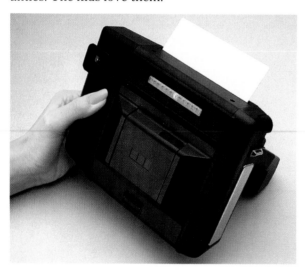

The beauty of instant photography lies in the complete picture that arrives only minutes after you snap the shutter. Share exciting photos with friends, party guests, travel acquaintances, and amused family members. Send prints to penpals and relatives. Get even more mileage from your instant efforts when you order copyprints or enlargements from your photofinisher.

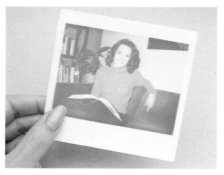
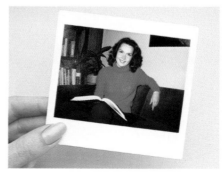

OPERATION

KODAK Instant Cameras are easy to operate. You'll want to know how to load your camera, how to make any adjustments, and how to operate the flash. Let's start with unloading/loading.

Unloading/Loading

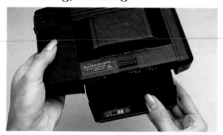

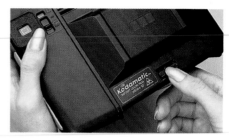

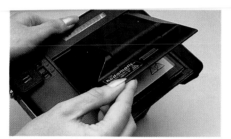

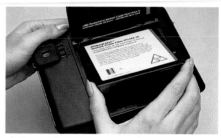

3. Open the door and remove the spent film container. Unwrap the new one.

4. Insert the container, blue stripe to blue stripe or orange stripe to orange stripe.*

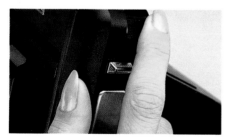

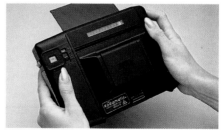

5. Close the door and press the shutter release.

6. Allow the protective black covering to eject. You're ready to take pictures.

*Older KODAK Instant Cameras use orange stripe film—the new KODAMATIC™ Instant Cameras use blue stripe film. Do not mix them except in emergencies. Check your camera manual.

25

Flash

When there's not enough light for your instant camera, you can use flash for nearby subjects— usually in a range from 4 to 12 feet. Your camera manual will give the exact distance. Most KODAMATIC Instant Cameras have a built-in electronic flash that fires for each picture regardless of the ambient lighting to help all your subjects. In a place where flash is prohibited, you can turn the flash off. Older instant cameras may have built-in flash or will accept flash devices such as flipflash or accessory electronic flash units. Newer models may have a built-in electronic flash. With electronic flash, always wait for the ready light to glow or blink before taking a picture.

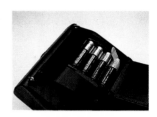

Although batteries in KODAMATIC Instant Cameras may last 2 years, you'll have to replace those in older Kodak models more often. Follow instructions in the manual.

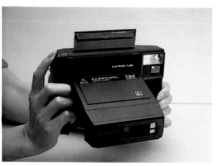

Most KODAMATIC Instant Cameras have automatic built-in electronic flash units.

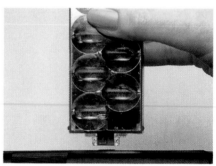

Older or less expensive instant cameras accept flash devices such as flipflash.

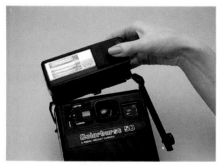

Many cameras that accept flash devices also accept accessory electronic flash units.

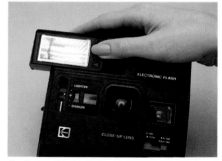

Activate the built-in electronic flash in an older camera by sliding it to the side.

Adjustments

KODAK Instant Cameras automatically set camera exposure for the lighting conditions, and most KODAMATIC Instant Cameras fire the built-in flash to improve every picture. If, however, a red light appears in the viewfinder of your KODAK Instant Camera, use flash.

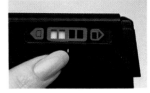

If a print is a little too dark or light, use the *lighten/darken* control to correct your next print.

If a picture looks too dark or light, adjust the lighten/darken control to improve the next picture.

Some models have a lens that requires focusing. You may have to estimate the distance and set the focusing control or focus with the help of visual aids in the viewfinder. On others, you can make an adjustment to take close-up pictures.

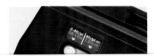

Special Conditions

come out best if allowed to develop in the shade.

In extremely cold weather, keep the cameras as warm as possible. For best results, place a developing print in an inside, warm pocket as soon as it leaves the camera.

Set the close-up lens on advanced models for subjects as close as 2 feet.

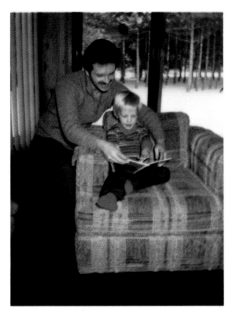

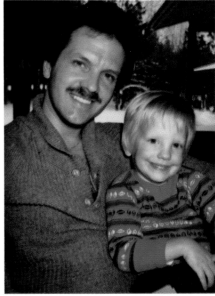

CARTRIDGE-LOADING CAMERAS

Cartridge-loading cameras are among the simplest to operate of all conventional film cameras. Loading is easy, and there are few if any adjustments to be made.

The small, 110-size cartridge fits in pocket cameras. The larger 126 cartridge fits in the familiar KODAK INSTAMATIC ® cameras.

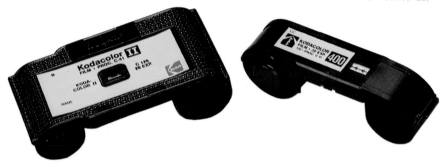

Advantages Cartridge-loading cameras—particularly the 110 size—are small and lightweight so that they're easy to pack around. Although you have to send the film to be processed, you will have a great variety of processing services available. Print quality is superb in most situations and the cost of the camera is usually fairly low.

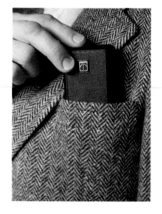

The simplest of all cartridge-loading cameras give the greatest ease of operation. There is nothing to do except load the film and snap a picture. You can take pictures on sunny days or hazy days outdoors, or use flash for nearby subjects when the light is dim.

More advanced models, which naturally cost more, may adapt to a wider range of lighting conditions. Not only can you take pictures in bright conditions, but you can also take pictures under heavy overcast or in the shade. Some cameras even allow you to take pictures without flash in the typical light of your home.

Operation Picture-taking with a cartridge-loading camera is easy and fun. Loading is usually the first step. Let's take a look. (Again, we'll first show unloading in case your camera contains a completely exposed cartridge of film and your instruction manual has disappeared.)

Unloading

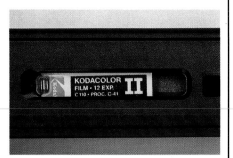

When you see an empty cartridge in the window of a 110 or 126 camera, it's time to unload.

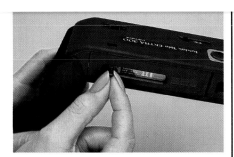

Open the film-compartment door by sliding or depressing the latch and swing the door open.

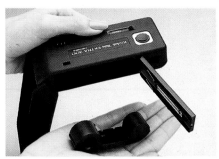

Drop the cartridge into your hand.

Loading

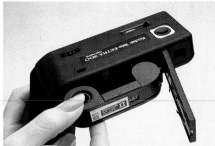

Insert the new cartridge—it fits only one way. Close the film-compartment door and lock the latch, if necessary.

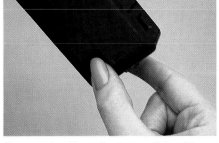

Operate the film advance until it will go no farther.

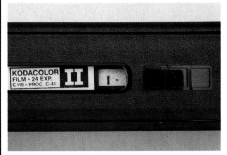

Number "1" will appear in the window—you're ready to take pictures.

29

Flash

Flash is easy with cartridge-loading cameras. Some cameras have built-in electronic flash. Others need to have a flash device inserted. Attachable electronic flash units are usually available, as well as disposable devices such as flipflash, magicubes, or flashcubes. With a camera that has a built-in or attachable electronic flash, you merely turn on the flash and wait for the ready light to glow. Then you're ready to take a picture. After you've taken a picture, you must wait for the light to glow again before you take the next picture.

All electronic flash units work on batteries. Replace the batteries as soon as the time required for the ready light to glow between pictures exceeds the number of seconds suggested in the instruction manual.

Adjustments

There are few adjustments to be made. Sophisticated cartridge-loading cameras have automatic exposure meters that set the camera for the prevailing light conditions. Less sophisticated models give excellent pictures within a narrower lighting range.

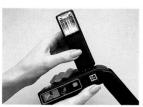

Many cartridge-loading cameras accept an accessory electronic flash unit.

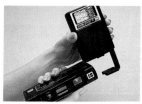

Insert it into the slot that accepts accessory flash devices.

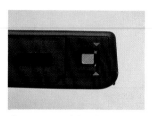

A new cartridge-loading camera may have an automatic electronic flash unit built-in.

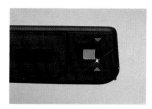

When the camera senses a dark scene, the red light will come on. The green light comes on when the flash is ready.

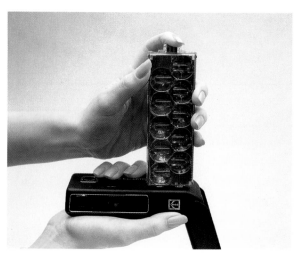

Some cartridge-loading cameras have a focusing control. You focus by estimating the distance between you and the subject and making the appropriate setting. Or you move the focusing control and watch for the sharp focus indicator in the viewfinder.

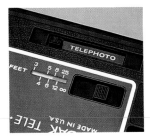

Film

Cartridge-loading cameras accept films for color and black-and-white prints and color slides. Kodak offers color films with different sensitivity to light. A sensitive or high-speed film will let you take pictures in darker conditions than with a less

On some cartridge-loading cameras you may focus the camera with a lever on top of the camera. Some cameras require that you

eras using 110 cartridges.)

others, you'll see a focusing cue in the viewfinder.

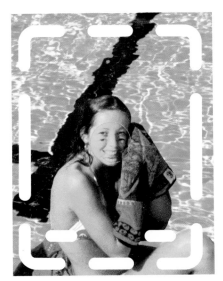

When you look at a subject in the viewfinder of a focusing camera, the center spot may show two images side by side. If you snap the shutter, the resulting picture may be fuzzy.

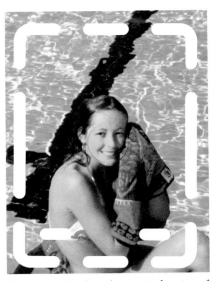

By moving the focusing control on top of the camera, you align the two images in the center of the viewfinder, and the entire scene will appear sharp. The resulting picture should also be sharp.

31

35 mm CAMERAS

There are dozens of current 35 mm cameras, and probably hundreds of older cameras. They fall into two basic groups—reflex and rangefinder. Rangefinder cameras are smaller, less expensive, and somewhat less flexible than the reflex variety. Many reflex cameras can be fitted with a warehouse of accessories that will give every photographic effect imaginable.

These cameras usually cost more than instant-print or cartridge-loading cameras because they're quite a bit more capable. For the extra cost, you get the capability to take pictures more precisely in a wide range of lighting conditions. The combination of manual or automatic exposure control, a selection of shutter speeds and apertures, and a great variety of general and special-purpose films allow you to photograph whatever you choose and in almost any circumstance.

To keep things simple, we'll divide 35 mm cameras into two groups, reflex and rangefinder. Many non-reflex cameras do not have rangefinder focusing, but share most other features with true rangefinder cameras.

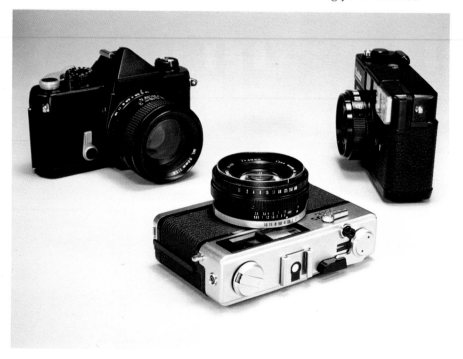

Operation Operating a 35 mm camera requires a bit of understanding for best results. We'll give enough basic information in this section to get you started with your 35 mm camera. For a better understanding of how photography works, and how such information applies to you and your 35 mm camera, turn to page 126. That section of the book will clarify questions about settings. There's also information on flash, filters, and other subjects that will help you make better pictures in a variety of situations.

The obvious place to start our description of 35 mm operation is with film loading. (A camera that hasn't been used recently may have exposed film

Rangefinder cameras are typically automated so that you merely load film into the camera, set the film speed, focus (although some cameras have automatic focusing), and take a picture. Many reflex cameras are completely automatic and with others you adjust one element of the exposure setting so that the camera can make the

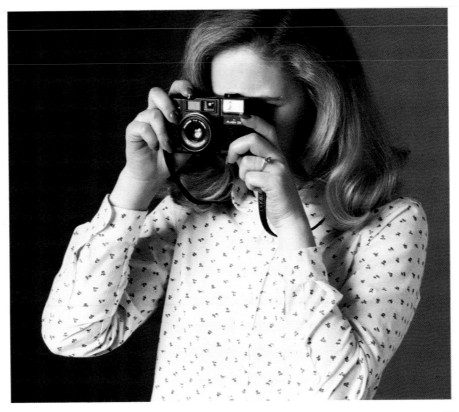

Unloading 35 mm Cameras

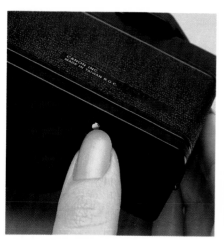

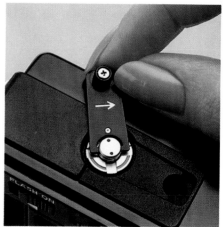

If your camera has made the last exposure on a magazine of film, depress the film-advance release button on the bottom of the camera.

Pull out the rewind lever, and turn it in the direction indicated until you feel no more resistance.

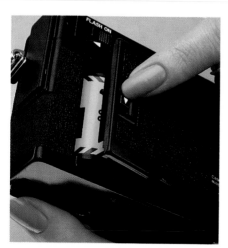

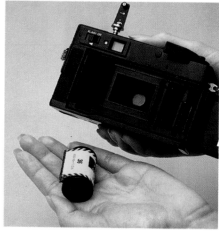

Open the film-compartment door by sliding a latch on the back or side of the camera or by pulling up the rewind lever.

Remove the film magazine by pulling up the rewind lever, if necessary, and dropping the magazine in your hand.

Loading 35 mm Cameras

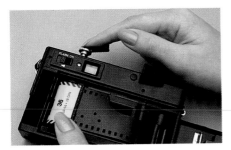

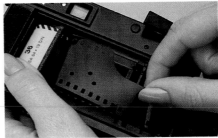

*Insert a new film
magazine into the film*

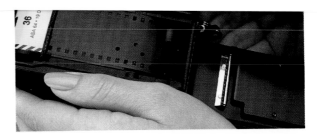

*the bottom. Press the
rewind lever down to lock
the magazine in position.
Hook a sprocket hole into
the film take-up spool.
Advance the film until
both sets of sprocket holes
are riding on the sprockets.*

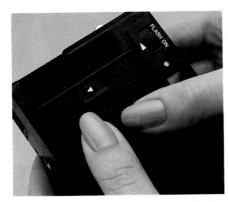

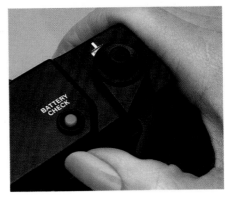

*Close the film-compartment door so that
it snaps shut.*

*Advance the film and snap the shutter
several times until the number "1"
shows in the film-counting window.*

35

Exposure with Automatic and Semi-Automatic Cameras

All automatic 35 mm cameras and cameras with built-in exposure meters have one exposure adjustment in common—the film-speed setting. When you load a roll of film into the camera, always check the film-speed setting and reset it, if necessary. Many new rangefinder cameras make all the other exposure adjustments themselves without any help from you. With some rangefinder models and many reflex cameras, you set either aperture or shutter speed—the camera then measures the light on the scene and makes the other setting.

You're expected to understand the reasons for choosing one setting over another. You may not understand now, but you want to get out and begin taking pictures. You can learn as you go along. At this point, we'll give you enough information to start taking good pictures, but for a fuller enjoyment of your camera, read the sections on exposure and depth of field starting on page 136.

Shutter-Speed Preferred If your camera is shutter-speed preferred, you choose the shutter speed and the camera chooses the aperture. A general

Note: If the film speed selector on your camera cannot register a very high-speed film such as ISO (ASA) 1000, compensate by setting it to 500 for this instance and using the next faster shutter speed or the next smaller aperture. For an automatic camera with an exposure compensation dial, set the film speed selector to 500 and the compensation dial to 1 stop less exposure.

Set the film speed of the film you're using on the film-speed selector.

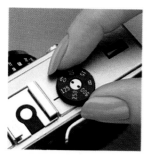

A shutter speed of 1/125 second (125 on the shutter speed dial) is excellent for general picture-taking with a medium-speed film.

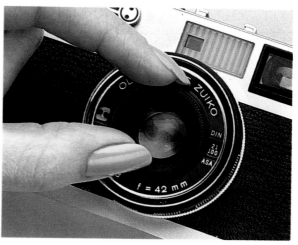

shutter speed for most daylight conditions is 1/125 second, represented by the number 125 on the shutter speed dial. When you're photographing a moving subject in fairly bright light, try 1/250 second (250 on the shutter speed dial). In case the lighting conditions get so dim that you can't take a picture, try a shutter speed of 1/30 second (30).

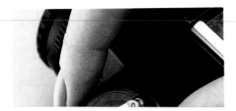 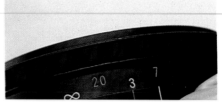

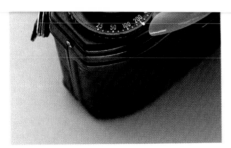 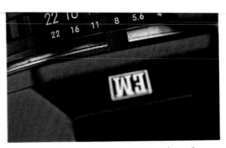

Aperture Preferred If your automatic camera is aperture preferred, you choose the aperture and the camera chooses the shutter speed. For most daylight picture-taking with a general-purpose film [ISO (ASA) 64–200], you can set the aperture ring to *f*/8 and expect fine results. If the light becomes substantially dimmer, use larger apertures. (The larger the aperture, the smaller the number—*f*/4 might be a good choice for a dark day with an ISO (ASA) 64–200 speed film.) In very dark surroundings, use the largest aperture available. At the beach or on snow in bright sunlight, use a small aperture such as *f*/16.

An aperture-preferred automatic camera requires that you set the aperture; the camera sets the shutter speed for the lighting conditions. First, make sure that the correct film speed is set on the camera. Then, set the aperture. A good aperture for general picture-taking is f/8.

37

Manual Cameras

Many 35 mm cameras are not automatic. Most are quite simple to operate. The majority have built-in exposure meters that help you make appropriate settings for the lighting conditions and for the film you're using.

Some cameras give you exposure information in the viewfinder. You may see the shutter speed set on the camera and the aperture set on the lens. Visual cues such as a set of LEDs or LCDs or a needle in a bracket will tell you when the settings will give good exposure. When the meter is turned on, the viewfinder display becomes active. Adjusting either the shutter speed dial or the lens aperture ring, or both, will center the needle in its bracket or light the correct LED or LCD.

Older cameras may have the visual cues on the outside of the camera. You point the camera at the subject and adjust the camera until the cue—usually a needle—is centered in the bracket. The meter window is often found on top of the camera. You read the suggested shutter speed and aperture settings from this window and transfer the information to the shutter speed dial and the lens aperture ring.

There are cameras that are completely manual—there is no built-in meter. You may have a separate, handheld meter that will help you determine the settings for a well-exposed picture. With most meters you merely aim the meter at the subject, turn on the meter, and read the recommended settings from the meter dial. You may have to transfer a value indicated by the meter needle to a scale that will show you all the possible exposure combinations of shutter speed and lens aperture.

No matter what kind of exposure meter you're using, two things are critical—setting the correct film speed on the meter and operating it according to the manufacturer's instructions. Write the manufacturer for instructions, if you don't have them, or ask your photo dealer for help.

Instructions *For an adjustable camera with no exposure meter or if the meter is not working, try the exposure combinations listed at right. In each box the bold combination is the most logical choice. Other combinations are listed for your convenience. (See pages 136-143.) For darker conditions, refer to the existing light exposure table on page 165. Shutter speeds slower than 1/30 second have not been included because they require steady camera support, such as a tripod. Notice that film speed varies the combinations of settings shown in the table. Film is available for 35 mm cameras in different sensitivities or speeds. High- or very high-speed film—ISO (ASA) 250-1250—is for dim lighting conditions. Other, less sensitive films are best in normal lighting.*

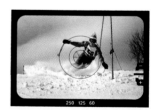

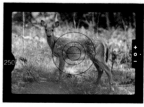

Outdoor Daylight Exposure Settings for a Manual Camera

Film Speed ISO (ASA)	Light Conditions				
	Bright or Hazy Sun on Light Sand or Snow	Bright or Hazy Sun (Distinct Shadows)	Weak Hazy Sun (Soft Shadows)	Cloudy Bright (No Shadows)	Open Shade or Heavy Overcast
25–32	1/125, f/11 1/60, f/16 1/30, f/22 1/250, f/8 1/500, f/5.6 1/1000, f/4	1/125, f/8 1/60, f/11 1/30, f/16 1/250, f/5.6 1/500, f/4 1/1000, f/2.8	1/125, f/5.6 1/60, f/8 1/30, f/11 1/250, f/4 1/500, f/2.8 1/1000, f/2	1/125, f/4 1/60, f/5.6 1/30, f/8 1/250, f/2.8 1/500, f/2 1/1000, f/1.4	1/60, f/4 1/30, f/5.6 1/125, f/2.8 1/250, f/2 1/500, f/1.4
64 100*– color negative	1/125, f/16 1/60, f/22 1/250, f/11 1/500, f/8 1/1000, f/5.6	1/125, f/11 1/60, f/16 1/30, f/22 1/250, f/8 1/500, f/5.6 1/1000, f/4	1/125, f/8 1/60, f/11 1/30, f/16 1/250, f/5.6 1/500, f/4 1/1000, f/2.8	1/125, f/5.6 1/60, f/8 1/30, f/11 1/250, f/4 1/500, f/2.8 1/1000, f/2	1/125, f/4 1/60, f/5.6 1/30, f/8 1/250, f/2.8 1/500, f/2 1/1000, f/1.4
color negative	1/1000, f/8	1/500, f/8 1/1000, f/5.6	1/250, f/8 1/500, f/5.6 1/1000, f/4	1/250, f/5.6 1/500, f/4 1/1000, f/2.8	1/250, f/4 1/500, f/2.8 1/1000, f/2
200 400*– color negative	1/500, f/16 1/250, f/22 1/1000, f/11	1/500, f/11 1/125, f/22 1/250, f/16 1/1000, f/8	1/250, f/11 1/125, f/16 1/60, f/22 1/500, f/8 1/1000, f/5.6	1/250, f/8 1/125, f/11 1/60, f/16 1/30, f/22 1/500, f/5.6 1/1000, f/4	1/250, f/5.6 1/125, f/8 1/60, f/11 1/30, f/16 1/500, f/4 1/1000, f/2.8
400	1/1000, f/16 1/500, f/22	1/500, f/16 1/250, f/22 1/1000, f/11	1/500, f/11 1/250, f/16 1/125, f/22 1/1000, f/8	1/500, f/8 1/250, f/11 1/125, f/16 1/60, f/22 1/1000, f/5.6	1/500, f/5.6 1/250, f/8 1/125, f/11 1/60, f/16 1/30, f/22 1/1000, f/4
1000– color negative	1/1000, f/22	1/1000, f/16 1/500, f/22	1/1000, f/11 1/500, f/16 1/250, f/22	1/1000, f/8 1/500, f/11 1/250, f/16 1/125, f/22	1/1000, f/5.6 1/500, f/8 1/250, f/11 1/125, f/16 1/60, f/22

Note: Shutter speeds are in seconds. Exposure settings in heavy type indicate suggested settings for general use.

*Since these color negative films tolerate moderate overexposure, the values in the table above are designed for maximum exposure latitude. Slide films, however, must be exposed accurately.

Focusing

If you have a completely automatic camera, either rangefinder or reflex, you need only focus the camera to take a picture. There are generally two systems for focusing. With the simpler, you estimate the distance between you and your subject and set that distance in feet or as indicated by the appropriate symbol on the camera lens. More advanced systems allow you to view the subject through the viewfinder and turn the focusing ring on the lens until a visual cue tells you that the lens is focused. Since focusing varies from camera to camera, it's wise to consult your instruction manual. Some cameras now have an automatic focusing device that does all the work for you. You point the camera at your subject, press the shutter release, and you've taken a sharp picture.

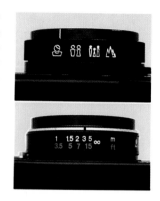

Flash

Electronic flash is the most common source of portable light with 35 mm cameras. It is convenient and compact and provides a way for you to take pictures when there isn't enough light.

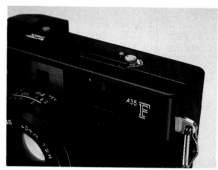

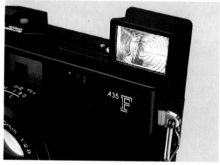

Many rangefinder cameras have a small electronic flash unit built into the camera. To take a flash picture you extend the flash unit and turn it on. When the ready light glows, you take a picture. You must wait for the ready light to glow again before taking the next picture. Occasionally, you will have to replace the separate batteries that power the flash. You can tell that the batteries are ready for retirement when the ready light takes

Many nonreflex cameras have a built-in electronic flash unit. Slide or depress a switch to turn it on. For a sharp, correctly exposed picture, set the camera-to-subject distance on the lens. When the orange ready light glows, you're ready to take a picture.

longer to glow than the instruction manual recommends. Although focusing the camera on your subject sets the camera for flash exposure, check the manual for the flash range that will give you good pictures.

Other rangefinder and reflex cameras are equipped so that you can attach an auxiliary flash unit. A shoe on the top of the camera will accept the foot of most flash units. The first step is to insert the flash unit into the shoe. If the accessory shoe and flash foot are "hot" (check the camera instruction manual), all the necessary electrical connections have been made by inserting the flash unit. If the flash shoe or foot isn't hot, you make the electrical connection with a small cord (the PC cord) usually supplied with the flash unit. Plug the cord into the flash and into the correct socket on the camera and you're in business. Set the camera shutter speed as

Newer cameras usually have an electrically wired accessory shoe on top of the camera. When you slide a similarly wired flash unit into the shoe, all the electrical connections are established. Older cameras or older flash units may require the use of a small cord that comes with the flash unit to make the connection.

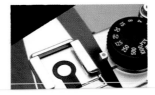

chronization setting for electronic flash would be 1/60 or 1/125 second.

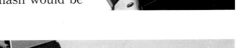

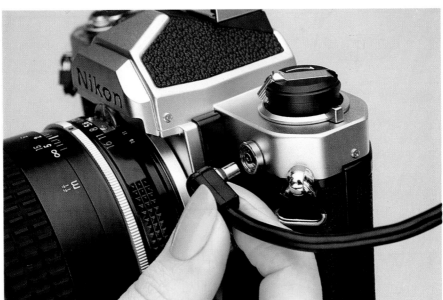

Flash Exposure

Setting the aperture depends on the flash-to-subject distance. Generally, there are three systems for choosing the aperture, which we'll discuss in more detail in the "Flash" section of the book, page 152—self-quenching automatic, dedicated, and manual. Self-quenching automatic means that the flash unit has a sensor that shuts off the flash when enough light has reached the subject. First, you set the film speed on the flash unit. Then choose an aperture/distance-range mode and set the recommended aperture on the camera for that mode. To take a picture, you focus, make sure that the subject is in the distance range for that flash mode, and snap the shutter.

Automatic flash units require that you set the film speed on the calculator on the back of the flash unit. Then choose an automatic flash mode for the distances you'll be photographing. Here we chose the yellow mode. Set the aperture—f/8 in this case—recommended by the flash unit. Make sure that the distance between flash and subject falls within the automatic flash range— 1.6 to 8.5 feet in this case.

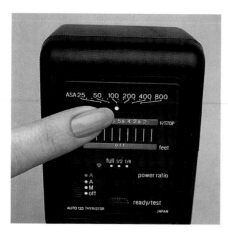

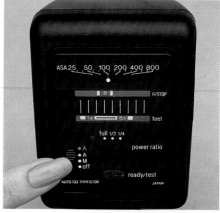

Dedicated flash systems differ, but the idea is generally the same. A sensor in the camera (not on the flash) determines when enough light has reached the film, and then shuts off the power in the flash unit. Since these systems vary, you'll want to pay careful attention to the instructions. Some rangefinder cameras allow you to set the guide number of the flash (a number found in the flash instruction manual that describes the power of the unit with a specific film) on the camera. When you set the camera to a flash mode, you select the aperture by focusing the camera.

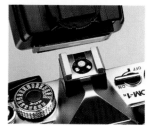

A dedicated flash and camera system will establish all connections when the flash is attached.

42

Manual flash is easier to talk about but takes a few more steps to perform. When the flash is all connected to the camera, you set the film speed on the flash calculator, and focus on the subject. Refer to the distance scale on the lens barrel for the camera-to-subject distance. Then apply that distance to the flash calculator. The aperture number will appear across from the distance. Set the lens aperture and take a picture.

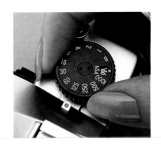

Set the recommended flash shutter speed on the camera. Then set the film speed on the flash calculator dial. Focus on your subject. The flash-to-subject distance will appear on the lens distance scale. Apply that distance to the flash

calculator. Here it is 10 feet. The recommended aperture setting, here, between f/5.6 and f/8, will appear across from the flash-to-subject distance. Set the recommended aperture on the lens-aperture ring.

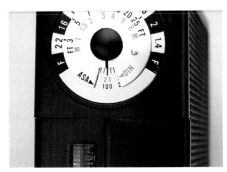

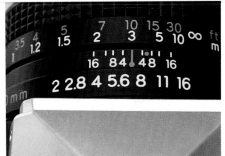

Electronic flash units work on either rechargeable batteries or disposable batteries. When the recycle times get longer than recommended by the flash manual, replace or recharge the batteries. For more important flash battery information, refer to page 157.

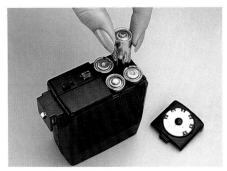

Note: *If the film-speed dial won't register the 1000-speed film you're using, set it to 500 and select a lens opening one stop smaller than indicated.*

43

CAMERA HANDLING

Proper camera handling may be one of the most important contributions to good pictures. We have a number of tips to help you improve the way you take pictures.

Holding the Camera Steady

Start taking sharp pictures by holding the camera steady. Stand comfortably balanced with your legs slightly apart. Grip the camera, one hand on each side, and gently press your elbows into your side. If you've been exerting—walking up a mountain trail, for example—let your breathing resume a slow, steady pace before taking a picture.

Pressing the Shutter Release

Slowly press the shutter-release button until the camera takes a picture. This will give you a better chance at sharp pictures and help you maintain good composition.

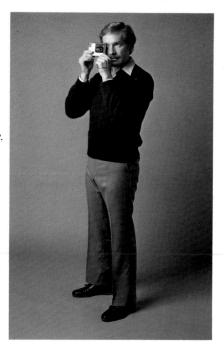

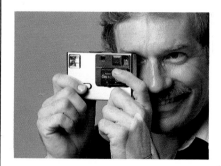

Keeping the Lens Clear

One common problem is arranging a beautiful scene in the viewfinder only to discover later that a finger, the camera strap, part of the camera case, or even the lens cap covered the lens while you took a picture. Make it a practice to clear the lens area of obstructions before taking the picture.

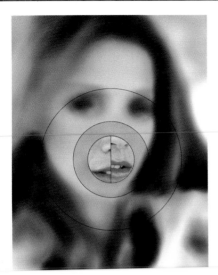
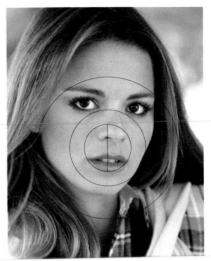

Focusing

There are three typical focusing operations. The simplest is choosing one of several symbols on the distance scale on the lens that corresponds to the approximate distance between you and your subject. Or, you set the camera-to-subject distance in feet or metres.

Some cameras have a rangefinder coupled to the lens. To focus, you turn the lens focusing ring until the two images in the center of the viewfinder coincide. You can also set the calculated distance in feet or metres on the lens distance scale.

With automatic focusing, thoroughly digest the information in the camera instruction manual.

In a single-lens-reflex camera you can see when the lens is focused because you see the same image the lens sees. There are a number of aids to help you, usually found in the center portion of the viewfinder.

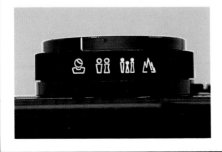
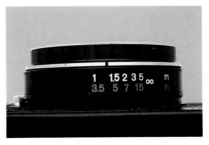

Using the Viewfinder

In some camera viewfinders, the picture area is defined by a bright rectangle or square. Other camera viewfinders use the entire viewfinder. Check your instruction manual to get the important elements of the scene into your picture.

When you see foreground litter or a confusing background in the viewfinder, choose another position. Horizons should be level.

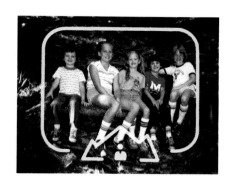

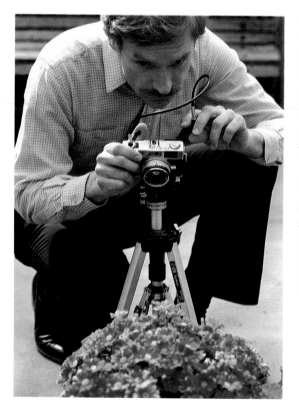

Camera Support

Many automatic and adjustable cameras will operate at shutter speeds slower than 1/30 second. At these slow speeds, even your steadiest position, grip, and release may jiggle the camera and result in blurred pictures. Lean against a tree or wall or rest the camera on a table or rock. A tripod will give the most reliable steady support. A cable release will remove your shaky hands from the camera.

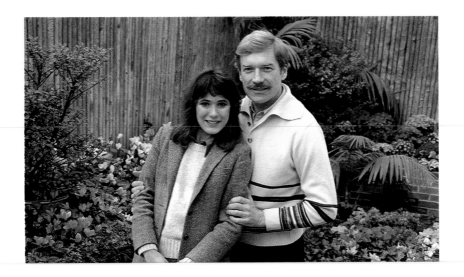

Using the Self-Timer

The self-timer is handy when you want to include yourself in the picture. Set the timer, press the shutter release, and position yourself in the picture. You'll have between 8 and 12 seconds to get there. When you're arranging the picture in the viewfinder, leave room for yourself. Place your camera on a solid support such as a table, fence post, rock, or tripod.

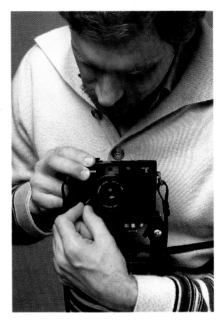

FILM

Film is available in different sizes for different cameras. Check your camera instruction manual for the correct size film. And, choose film for the kind of pictures you want—color prints, color slides, or black-and-white prints.

Films are also available for some cameras with different speeds, or sensitivities to light. High- or very high-speed films are very sensitive. You might use them in dim light. There are also slower films that are good for very sharp pictures in bright light. You'll probably want to use a medium-speed film for most picture-taking.

The speed is identified by ISO, ASA, or DIN numbers. (These letters stand for different standard-setting organizations. ISO (DIN) values are common in Europe while ISO (ASA) values are used in the US and England.) A medium-speed film

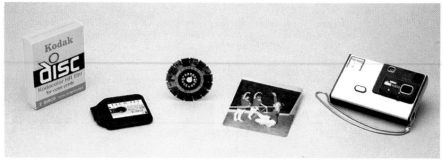

Disc-size box   enclosure   negative   print   camera

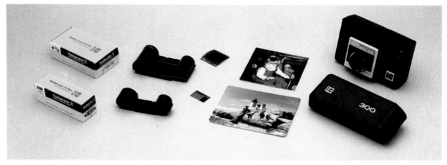

| *126-size* | *box* | *cartridge* | *negative* | *print* | *camera* |
| *110-size* | *box* | *cartridge* | *negative* | *print* | *camera* |

might have an ISO (ASA) rating of 64 to 200. High-speed film would be 250 to 640; very high-speed film 800-1250, and a low-speed film 50 or less.

Most films are manufactured to give pictures in daylight. Others, however, are designed to give pictures with correct color appearance when used with artificial light sources—household bulbs (tungsten) or photographic lights. See pages 134 and 168-169 for more information about these films.

There is an expiration date on most film packaging. Film, like food, can go bad from aging and may yield pictures of inferior quality. Check the date when you buy new film, and don't forget the film in your camera. Take the pictures and get them processed quickly. Film doesn't like extreme heat or humidity, either. Keep it out of direct sunlight and other hotspots.

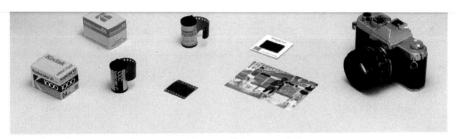

135-size   box   magazines   negative   slide   print   camera

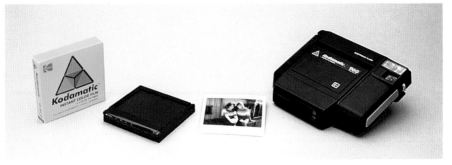

Instant   box   film container   print   camera

PEOPLE

When you photograph people—friends and family or interesting strangers—you want them to look their best. Portray them naturally. Show some of the unique traits that distinguish them from the rest of the crowd. Spend a moment considering what important characteristics identify the people close to you. It might be helpful to suggest expressions, clothing, props, and activities that will encourage the real people to emerge from behind the snapshot smile-masks.

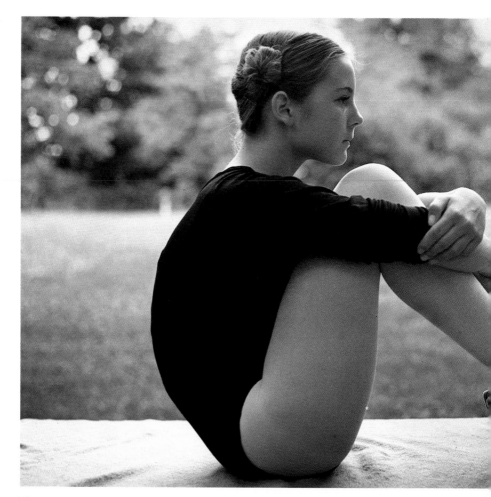

Direction of light

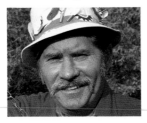
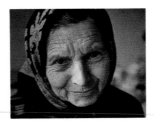
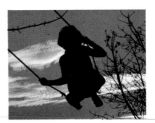

Frontlighting   *Sidelighting*   *Backlighting*

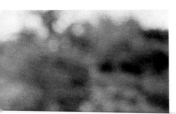

OUTDOORS

Light—its direction and intensity—is all-important in your outdoor portraits. Direct sunlight can illuminate a subject from one of three directions. *Frontlighting* is harsh, usually causing a person to squint, and often making heavy shadows on the

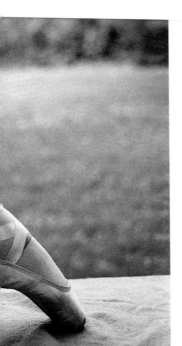

al. *Backlighting* will give a silhouette when the camera is adjusted for a sunlight exposure; it can give a gentle appearance, however, when the camera is adjusted to record the subject's most important features. (Backlighting can fool an automatic camera. See page 142.)

There are two ways to cope with direct, bright sunlight from any direction. One way is to place a piece of white cardboard in a position to reflect some light into the shadow areas. Almost anything in a light, neutral tone will do—bedsheets, a newspaper, towels, a white wall, or even a sidewalk.

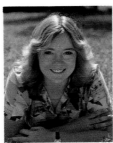
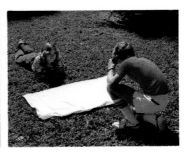

51

Fill-in Flash

Fill-in flash can brighten dark shadows in outdoor pictures. A camera that has built-in flash or that takes disposable flash devices provides easy flash fill. Position your subject near the maximum distance recommended by the camera manual and take a flash picture.

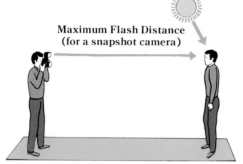

Maximum Flash Distance
(for a snapshot camera)

Using Flash in Daylight

If you have an adjustable or automatic camera that accepts an accessory flash, perform all the usual steps to take a flash picture (see pages 40 and 152-157). Set the camera for the sunlighted situation, but select a shutter speed that will synchronize with the flash—generally 1/60 or 1/125 second. A medium- or slow-speed film may be helpful. Then position your subject at a distance that will require more flash power than your flash unit can provide. You want the flash to fill the shadows subtly, not overpower the sunlight. See pages 160-161 for more on fill-in flash.

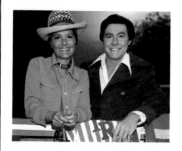

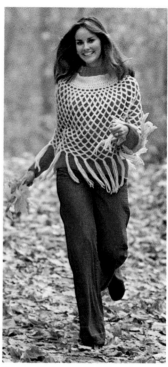

Overcast sky

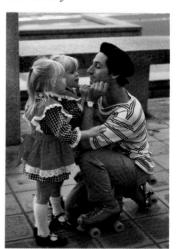

From above

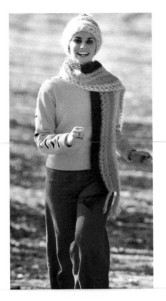

Another way is to use a flash unit on your camera to add a little brightness to the shadows. Photograph your subject from a distance where the flash provides a little less than half the light necessary for proper exposure. (See pages 160-161 for more information on flash-fill exposure.)

Light shade or overcast skies give more appealing pictures of people than direct sunlight. You'll get open, easy expressions without dark shadows. Since there's less light in these conditions, an automatic camera will automatically give more exposure. With a manual camera you'll have to make the necessary adjustment. (See pages 136-143.)

You can subtly change a person's appearance by changing the camera angle. A person photographed from above, a high angle, seems smaller and less important than someone photographed from below, a low camera angle. When the camera

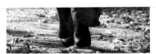

graphed at eye level. Be careful that an unusual camera angle doesn't distort your subject.

Direct sunlight

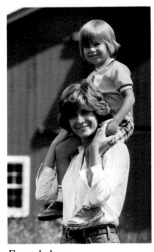

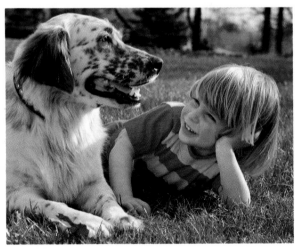

From below   *At eye level*

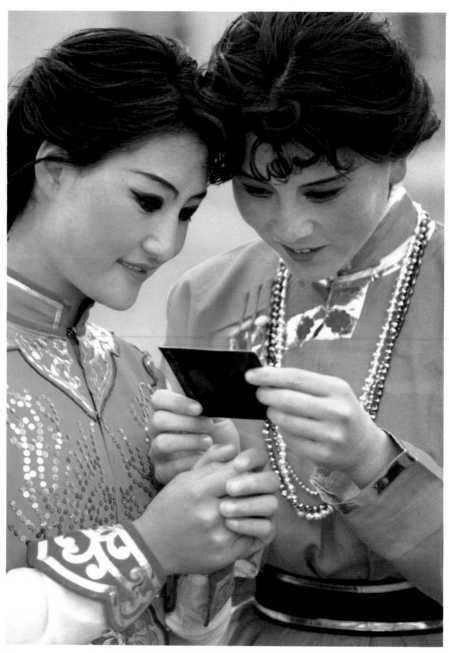

People wear natural expressions when they're occupied.

Look through the viewfinder at the entire scene. Make sure that no clutter in the background or foreground interferes with your view of the subject. Move in close to the person—close enough to keep only the essential features in the picture. (If using fill-in flash, move in only as far as good exposure will permit.) Another way to keep foreground and background simple is to change camera position and angle until you see exactly what you want in the viewfinder. You can also control depth of field so that the person is sharp and the rest of the scene is blurred. (See page 144.)

People wear natural expressions when they're comfortable. Try to have your subjects in relaxed positions—leaning against something or seated. When people have something to occupy their hands and attention, you'll get authentic portraits. Make sure your model is wearing clothing he or she finds appropriate and that is acceptable to your

Depth of field

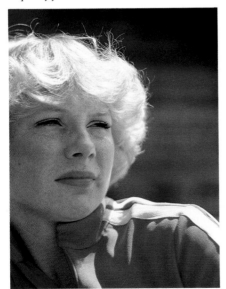

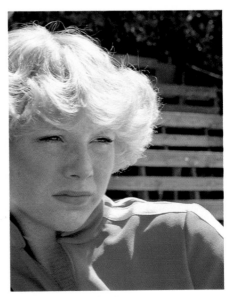

Large aperture—f/2

Small aperture—f/22

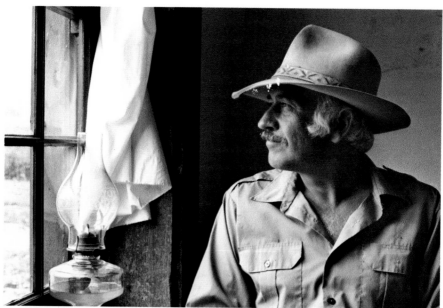

Window light

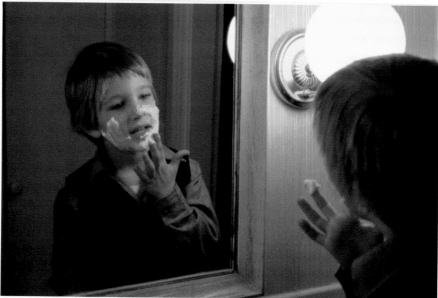

Tungsten light

INDOORS

Most of the outdoor guidelines apply to making effective portraits indoors. You want people to be comfortable, relaxed, and to appear in pictures as they do in day-to-day life. Seated comfortably in a pleasant spot with an attractive, simple background is one answer. An alternative is to engage your subject in an activity that is interesting, familiar, and appropriate, such as a hobby or sport.

Again, lighting is important. You'll find four possible sources for indoor light: existing light from outdoors shining through a window or a door, artificial light given by tungsten or fluorescent bulbs, flash, and strong tungsten bulbs in reflectors called photolamps. (See next page.)

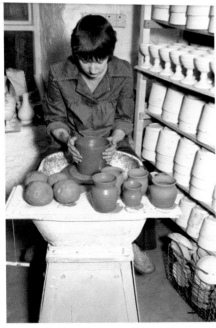

Flash

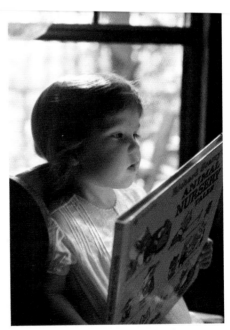

Window light reflected from book

Existing Light The existing light* looks best, of course, whether it's from the outdoors or from artificial sources such as household lamps. If you use light from the outside, move your subject close to a window or doorway, positioned so that lighting on the face is even and so that your picture will not include much of the bright window or doorway. The bright area could fool an exposure meter or automatic camera into underexposing the subject's face. A reflector can brighten the shadows caused by light from a single direction.

Taking pictures by household lamps requires high- or very high-speed film [ISO (ASA) 250–1250], slow shutter speeds (1/60 second or less) and wide apertures (f/2.8 or larger) because normal home lighting is much dimmer than daylight

Using Photolamps

Create effective lighting with photolamps. Bulbs and reflectors are sold by photo, hardware, and electrical dealers. One lamp, reflecting off a wall, will give a pleasing portrait. Three lamps give many lighting possibilities. Using an exposure meter or an automatic camera should give good exposure.

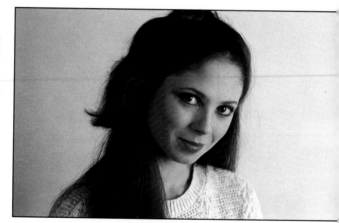

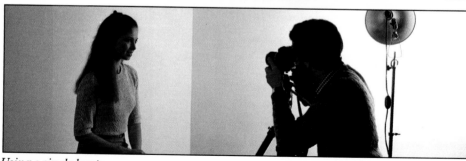

Using a single lamp.

outdoors. Pose people near bright light sources, but don't include those lights in your picture. Try to have the lighting as even as possible on the person's face. When the lighting is extremely dim and you need a shutter speed slower than 1/30 second, mount your camera on a steady support such as a tripod for sharp pictures.

Tungsten bulbs give a different color light from daylight. Use a high-speed film designed for tungsten light or use daylight film with an 80A filter attached to the camera lens†. In fluorescent light, also a different color from daylight, use daylight film and a CC30M filter†. Otherwise, your pictures may have a greenish tint. If you use KODACOLOR VR1000, VR400, or 400 Films for color prints, you can expect good results without a filter.

*See pages 162-165 for more on existing light.
†See pages 166-177 for more on filters.

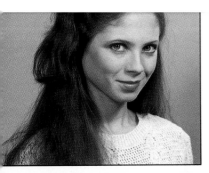

Using An Exposure Meter

about setting the camera for unusual lighting conditions. These cameras generally have a built-in exposure meter that either gives you advice on how to set the camera yourself or makes the adjustments for you. Older adjustable cameras may not have a built-in meter. If yours doesn't, you may know how to operate a handheld meter.

The best advice for using any meter, built-in or handheld, is to make a reading as close as possible to the subject, excluding the meter or camera shadow. Make your settings as the meter indicates from the close-up position. If the camera is automatic, there is usually some way to override the automatic setting feature in unusual exposure situations. Take a meter reading close to the subject and then back off to your preferred camera position. Adjust the camera manually to keep the exposure settings recommended by the meter at the close position. For a better understanding of exposure, see pages 136–143. For better understanding of how your particular camera operates, check the instruction manual.

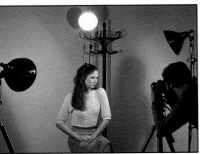

Three lamps.

Flash Flash, of course, is one of the most popular sources for light in dark places. Electronic flash units are available for most cameras, and the cost per flash is very low. Many units are automatic within certain distance ranges, allowing sufficient exposure without further adjustment. As with photolamps, a single flash will provide enough

Flash Pictures

Flash photography is easy with nearly any camera. Most snapshot cameras are equipped for an attachable flash device such as a flip-flash or an accessory electronic flash unit. Some snapshot cameras have built-in electronic flash. Attach and/or turn on the flash device or unit; make sure that your subject is in the flash distance range, and take a picture. Allow the ready light on an electronic flash unit to glow before you take the next picture.

With 35 mm cameras that have built-in flash, you turn the flash on, focus the camera if necessary, and take a picture. Adjustable or automatic cameras that accept accessory flash units may require some adjustment. Some dedicated systems may need to have a particular aperture set on the camera. More sophisticated dedicated systems may need other settings.

Automatic, self-quenching flash units operate in several distance ranges at different aperture settings, depending on film speed. Determine the typical distance you'll be photographing, and choose the appropriate mode on the flash unit. The unit usually requires a specific aperture setting for each flash mode.

With a manual flash you set the film speed on the calculator on the back of the flash unit, then focus on the subject. Look at the lens distance scale to find out camera-to-subject distance. Refer to the flash calculator dial and find the aperture to set on your camera—it will be approximately across from the camera-to-subject distance. There's a lot more to know about flash photography with automatic and adjustable cameras. See pages 152-161 for more information.

Using Flash

The most important guide for successful flash photography is to keep within the flash range. For snapshot cameras, the range might be 4 to 12 feet. With more advanced flash, the range may vary. Check the instruction manual for your camera and flash.

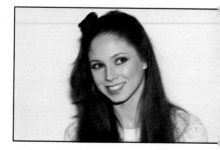

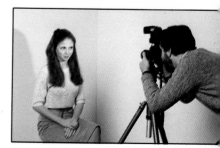

Direct flash

light, but it may be rather harsh. Bounce the flash off a light, neutral-color wall, ceiling, or white card for a softer light more suitable for portraiture. Flash exposure depends on flash-to-subject distance. For more information on flash exposure and bounce flash, refer to pages 154-159.

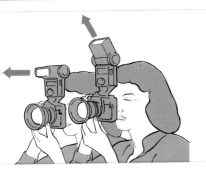

Bounce Flash

Bouncing the flash off a ceiling or wall softens the harsh effect common to direct flash. It's easy with most cameras that accept accessory electronic flash units.

Some sensor-automatic electronic flash units will function automatically when you tilt the flash head toward the bounce surface. The sensor must remain aimed at your subject. Use the automatic mode that requires the largest lens aperture (smallest number), and stay well within the maximum flash range. Automatic

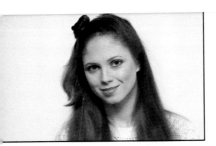

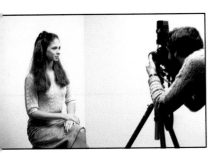

With a manual electronic flash unit or with one that has a fixed (non-tilting) flash head, you must remove the flash from the camera. You'll be able to connect flash and camera with a special electrical cord (PC-cord), sold by photo dealers. Make settings as follows. Determine the approximate distance that the flash will travel from flash to bounce surface to subject and use that distance to find the corresponding lens aperture on the flash calculator. Increase the recommended lens aperture by 2 *f*-stops and you have a good starting point for successful bounce flash exposure.

An effective bounce surface should be light-toned and neutral colored to reflect as much light as possible and to give natural color appearance. Make sure to aim the flash at a point midway between you and the subject so that the lighting will be even.

Bounced flash

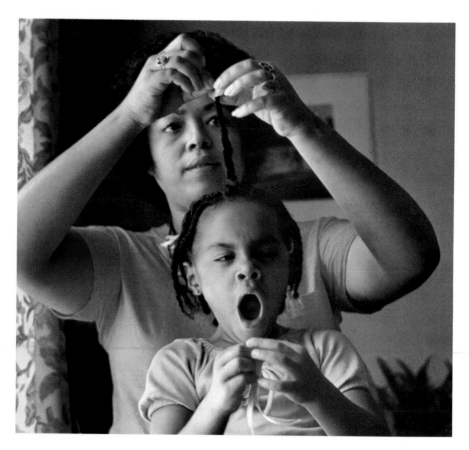

CANDID PICTURES

The word candid applies to family holiday celebrations as well as to stalking an interesting character on your travels. Your challenge is to photograph people in a natural atmosphere without calling attention to yourself. The reward is capturing the genuine emotions and expressions that give real clues to character.

There are two approaches to candid photography. One is to immerse yourself in whatever is going on, wait until the participants lose interest in you and resume their activity, and then start taking pictures. You can get totally natural, unselfconscious expressions—real slice-of-life material.

The other way is to find an unobtrusive position where you can remain unnoticed and take your pictures from a distance. Unless you use a camera that accepts auxiliary telephoto lenses, your subjects may appear a bit too distant. A normal or wide-angle lens such as that found on most snapshot or automatic cameras, actually helps you get good results when you're in the middle of the action as described at left.

It may be helpful to preset your focus and use a small aperture, a fast shutter speed, and a fast film. This way you can concentrate on your subjects rather than divert attention to your adjustments.

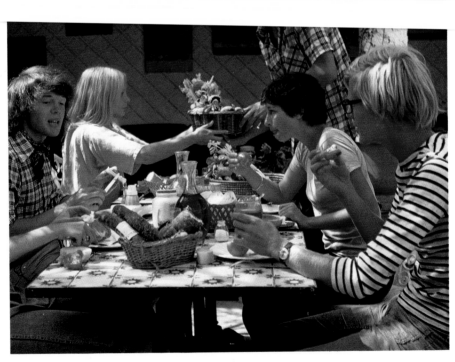

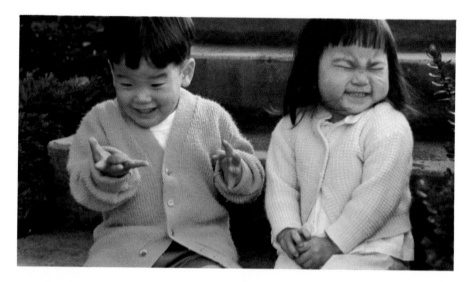

CHILDREN

Children resemble adults in many ways, except that they're smaller and faster. Because they're smaller you must move closer to get a full-sized image in your picture. You'll also have to get down for an eye-level view. Children behave more naturally when the photographer is on their level.

Because they're so fast, you'll want to take the following precautions. Use a fast shutter speed— 1/250 second or faster, if possible. Use flash indoors to capture the movement. Don't ask for poses or antics until you're completely ready to shoot. Use a high-speed film that will allow you a small aperture for maximum depth of field. (See page 144 for more information about depth of field.) The greater the range in acceptably sharp focus, the better chance you'll have to get sharp pictures of a quick youngster. Needless to say, if you have a game or some activity prearranged in a certain location, you should have all the time you need to take fine pictures while the child is occupied.

Most children have soft, clear skin that doesn't improve with harsh shadows. Backlighting, shady spots, and overcast days will portray any child's smooth complexion.

Above
A child's discovery can provide memorable pictures. Make sure to move close. Get down for a better view of the activity and the expressions. Be ready for one or more special moments.

Right
The soft light from a shaded window gently illuminates the subtle tones of a child's skin. Because such a scene is fairly dim, consider a high-speed film for sharp pictures.

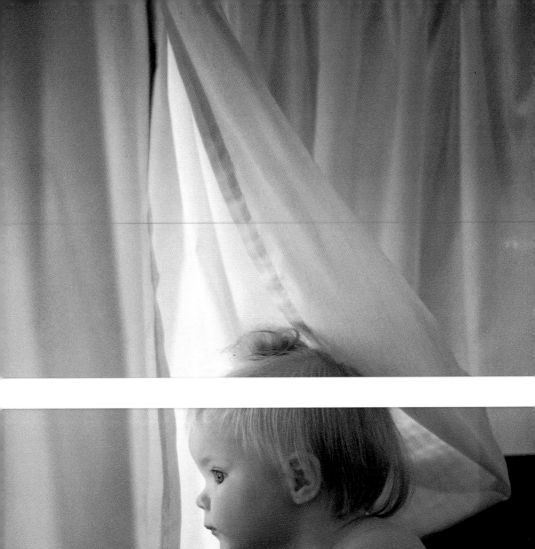
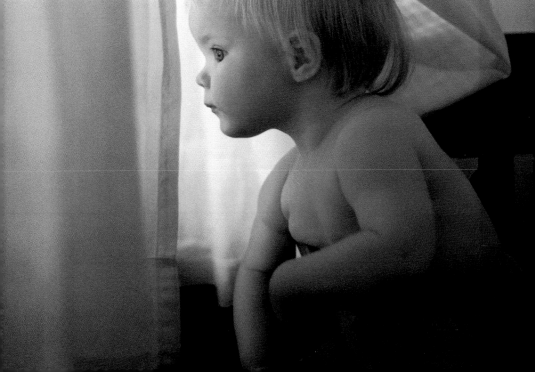

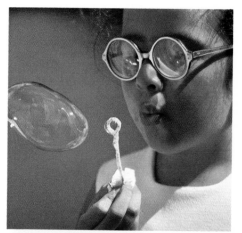

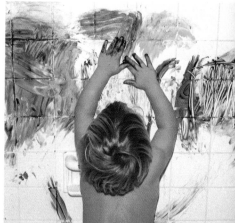

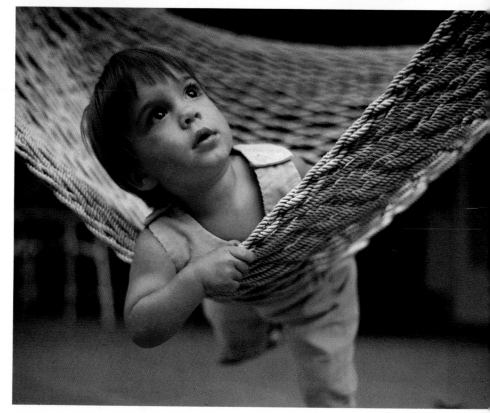

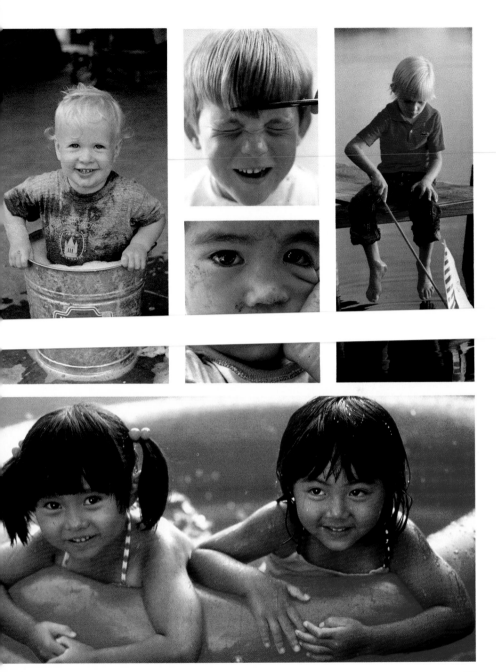

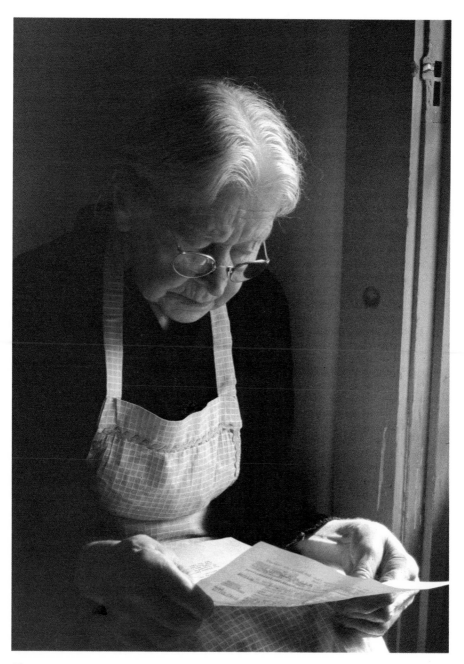

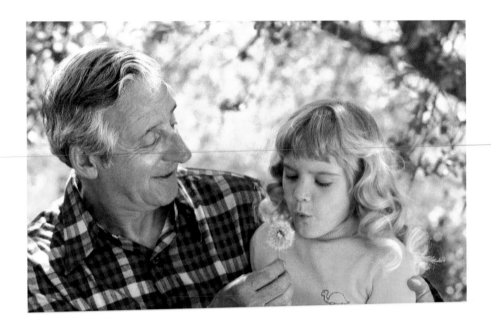

ELDERLY

A flattering portrait calls for soft, even lighting that will play down wrinkles and/or other complexion irregularities. Such a portrait might be made outdoors in the shade or on an overcast day or indoors with indirect light from outside. Bounce flash provides another possibility. Your subject will be more relaxed and comfortable if involved in one of his or her typical activities, and you'll get more natural expressions. Remember, keep the picture simple by avoiding or removing objects that will clutter or distract.

On the other hand, if you want to emphasize character displayed in a weather-beaten face or in gnarled hands, you will want strong directional lighting to give shape to the lines and to enhance the texture. Sidelighting can be very effective for this, and it needn't be terribly harsh. Too strong a light will cause so much contrast that you'll lose the fine gradations between highlight and shadow.

WEDDINGS

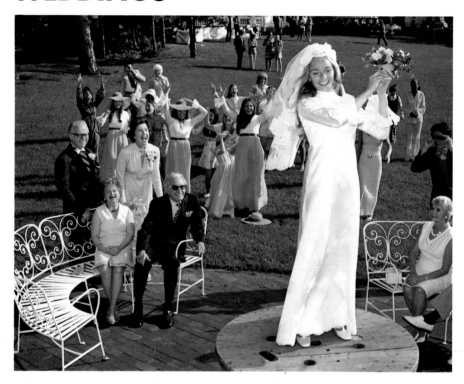

The volume of emotion at a wedding is usually far greater than at any other occasion. To the amateur photographer this is doubly important. First, you'll see more potential pictures than you can probably take. Second, the pictures you do take can have a rich significance in the years to come.

Since everyone wants to have a good time, including the photographer, try to plan ahead. Figure out what activities you want to record and ask the bride for a timetable and a list of locations. Check to see if you can take pictures in the church—particularly if you plan to use flash. If you feel strongly about planning, visit the locations beforehand to choose picture-taking spots and to choose what films you'll want (if there's a possibility of taking existing-light photos).

The next important step is to anticipate possible activity spots before a crowd gathers. This way

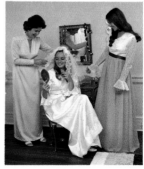

Getting ready.

70

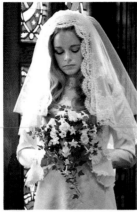

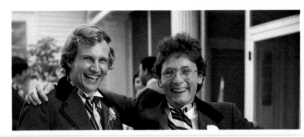

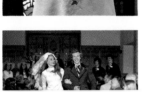

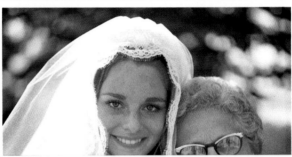

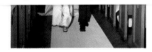

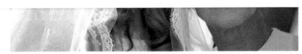

you'll have the best vantage points. Take plenty of pictures. If you think you missed the most dramatic moment of the cake cutting, for instance, persuade the couple to do it again. Incidentally, let the professional photographer cover the wedding without interference. Professionals are fast and decisive and usually will allow you plenty of opportunity to get great shots.

One advantage you'll have is knowing some of the family and guests. Watch the live wires of the crowd for delightful candid snapshots. These informal pictures you'll take of people and happenings between the main events will be treasured by all concerned, particularly the bride and groom. In fact, you can give a very nice after-wedding present, if you make up a small album of your best shots. Everyone remembers weddings through pictures—the more the merrier.

People at weddings are usually paying attention to the proceedings. You get great opportunities to capture friends and relatives being themselves. If you have a loaded camera, ready for action, you should get a wonderful collection of memories.

71

PLACES

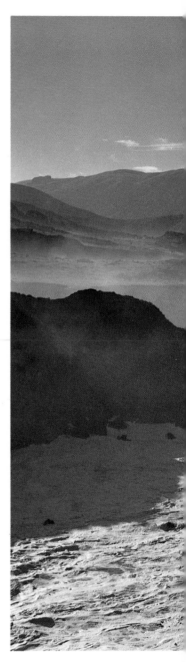

Landscapes closely follow people in popularity with most photographers. The reasons are as varied as the pictures, but several stand out—landscapes are beautiful and interesting; they provoke the imagination, and they provide a photographic challenge. Transferring the appearance and emotion of the scene from the mind to the film has been a lifetime quest for some photographers.

How often do photographers revel in the panorama stretched before them only to sigh with disappointment when they view their pictures? Although there are a number of hints that we'll discuss for better scenic shots, the most important advice we can give is: analyze *why* you're struck by a particular view and try to transfer your feelings to camera techniques. Ask these questions:

1. What elements of the scene interest you most? Trees, mountains, water, etc?
2. Do you want mostly sky, land, or water?
3. Is the scene more interesting as a horizontal or as a vertical?
4. Are colors or shapes more important?

Only you can answer these questions, of course, because you are the one who will be looking at the scene. The next few pages will offer some tools to help you get the answers into your pictures.

Pictures are reminders. As time passes, the memories get dimmer and dimmer. Moods and feelings are particularly difficult to recapture. Pictures help keep those memories bright—memories of the places you've seen and the wonders that leave you breathless. It's important to consider some of the ways to capture the sensations you feel in a particular place. Lighting and camera position are especially important. Notice in the picture at right how the slanting shadows of early morning help to define the shapes and bulk of the seaside cliffs? See also the subtle impression of distance offered by the haze in the scene. These ideas and others will be discussed in this chapter.

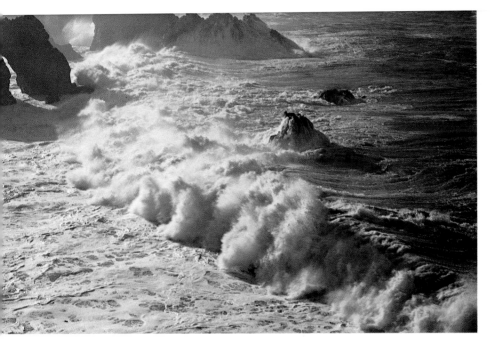

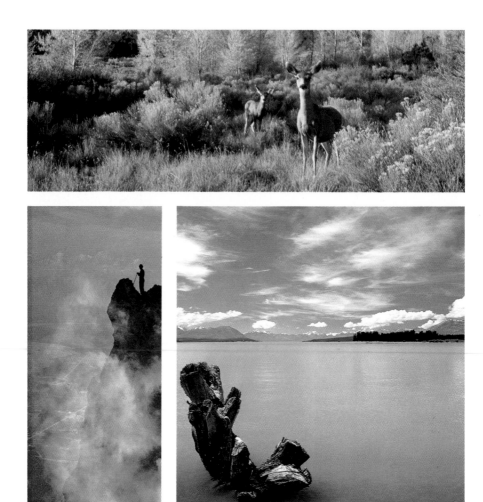

Question 1. Whatever part of the scene interests you the most, concentrate on it. No matter how vast the sight, you need one important center of interest. Otherwise the picture will lack impact. Making your camera respond generally means moving closer (making the subject bigger) and possibly shifting angles to eliminate anything extra and unwanted.

74

Question 2. If the sky is an important element in the picture, aim the camera to capture more sky, less land. If the sky only provides a horizon, aim the camera down for less sky.

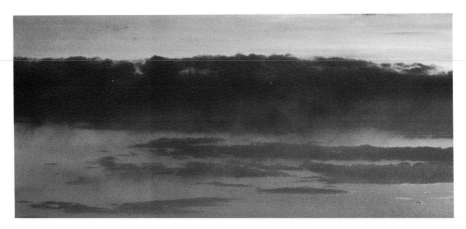

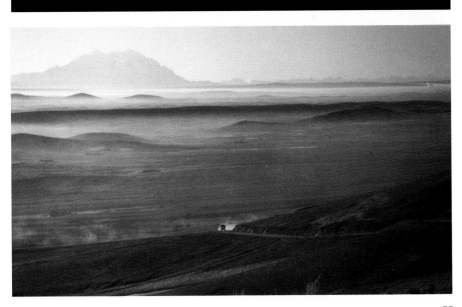

Question 3. If the scene is broad and magnificent, such as a mountain-range horizon, hold the camera horizontally. If the scene seems to stretch from your toes into the distance—a river or a highway—for instance—then hold the camera vertically.

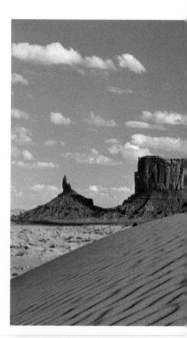

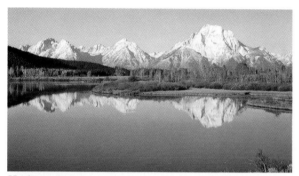

Horizontal

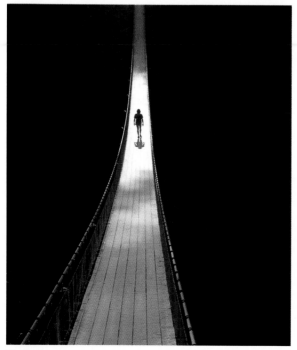

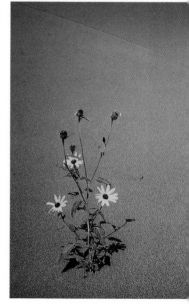

Vertical

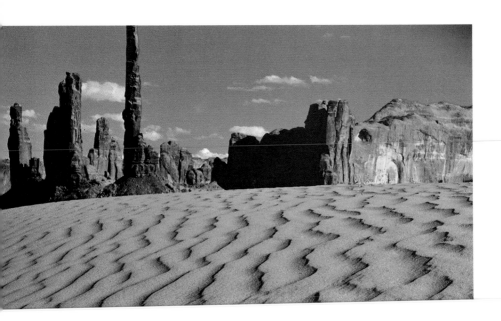

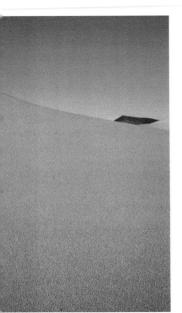

Question 4. Sometimes dark shapes and light shapes interact in a way that catches your eye. Find a position and aim your camera so that you concentrate on those shapes only. Anything else in the picture only serves to dilute the image. At other times you'll see colors interplay in a provocative way. Again, choose a location and aim your camera so that the areas of color dominate the picture.

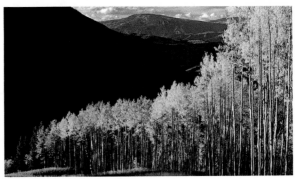

Dark and light shapes.

Composition

Good composition means placing the elements of a picture in a harmonious, interesting, and even unusual way to capture attention. In setting up a composition, consider the following:

Balance Do you want a symmetrical arrangement or a casual collection? A symmetrical design has obvious balance. But even an informal composition is balanced so that it feels complete and stable. Colors, shadows, and light areas tend to balance each other, and are affected by big shapes, little shapes, distance, and lines.

Rule of Thirds A traditional way that artists have grouped elements in pictures is called the rule of thirds. Place the center of interest and important subordinate elements near intersections of vertical and horizontal lines at 1/3 points of the picture.

Rule of thirds

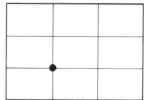

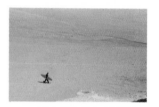

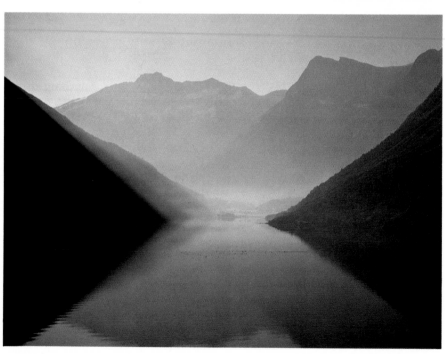

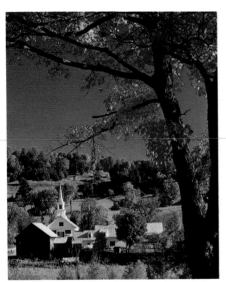

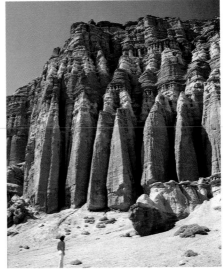

Framing   *Scale*

Perspective How do you make a two-dimensional picture express the depth and vastness of a three-dimensional scene? Carefully. Here are ideas.

Framing means almost surrounding your distant subject with some nearby foreground material, such as overhanging branches. The contrast between the near objects and the distant subject can help to establish distance. Framing is also helpful for disguising a dull, boring sky or hiding unwanted scene elements.

Similar to framing is the general use of objects in the foreground as subjects for scale to measure the background. Almost anything can be effective: a car, cactus, boulder, relative, motorcycle, boat (on water, of course), cabin, and more. The size of your scale subject will help give an impression of distance. If too close, viewers will forget the scene. At a medium distance the comparison may be most striking; at a greater distance the reference presents a more subtle view, but the viewer who stops for a second glance may be awed by how the landscape swallows up the extra subject.

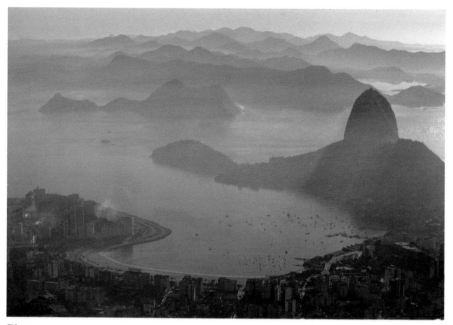

Planes

Planes Some stunning views, particularly from high up in the mountains and desert, show subjects at different distances. Parallel mountain ranges (running across your field of vision) become hazy as they become more distant. This phenomenon is called aerial perspective. It is particularly obvious in the photo above, taken in Brazil at an early-morning hour when mist still shrouded the cone-like peaks. In the desert, beige sand turns foggy blue near the horizon. Use these separate planes of different color to help establish distance and scale.

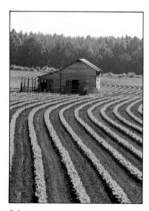

Lines Lines that lead far into the scene can also help establish distance. A fence, a row of telephone poles, a road, or a river, all shrink as they recede from the camera, and this will be captured on film. Lines can also help to draw near and distant areas together into a harmonious picture. The cultivated rows in the picture at left provide continuous threads that link foreground and background into a single, tranquil scene.

Lines

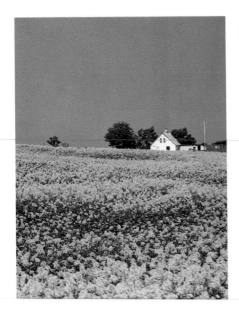

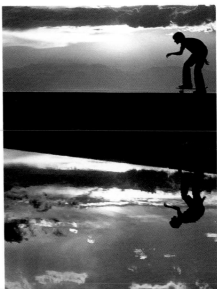

Frontlighting　　　　　　　　*Backlighting*

LIGHTING

Lighting Angles If you recall the discussion of lighting angles in the "People" section (page 51), you'll remember frontlighting, sidelighting, and backlighting. Although generalizing is always dangerous, sidelighting may be the most effective landscape lighting. Perhaps it's wise to broaden sidelighting to include any angle that does not produce direct front- or backlighting.

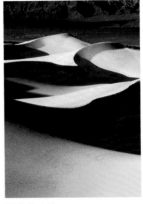

You need shadows to help show distance. Frontlighting gives no shadows. Backlighting can give dramatic shadows, but your subject may become a silhouette. Sidelighting from a wide series of angles casts shadows that help you gain an illusion of perspective. Waiting for the right times of day or carefully choosing your position may be the best answers.

Sidelighting

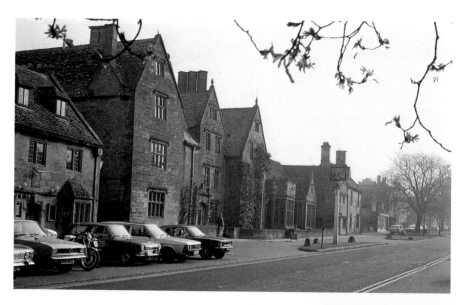

Time and Light As you've noticed, the landscape changes appearance dramatically from dawn to dusk and throughout the seasons. Obviously, seasonal changes mean green leaves, red leaves, or no leaves, as well as snow or soft grass. But the subtle changes come with changes in the light. Winter light is harsh but weak; summer light is rich but often oppressive. Sunlight in fall and spring is bright and cheerful. At noon the sun's rays beat straight down, flattening form and perspective. Early in the morning and late afternoon the light is a rich, warm color and long shadows streak across the scene.

Although you can't always choose the season, especially when traveling, you can often select the best time of day to make your landscape photographs. Early morning may be misty with light of a delicate rose color. Shadows are soft and violet, and the distance may be smoky. At noon the smaller shadows are hard and dense. Distance may be difficult to show. In the late afternoon, the light becomes more orange and the large shadows are warm and rich. The distance may be clear but will contrast in blue against the warmer foreground.

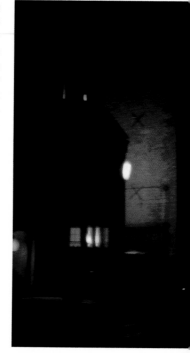

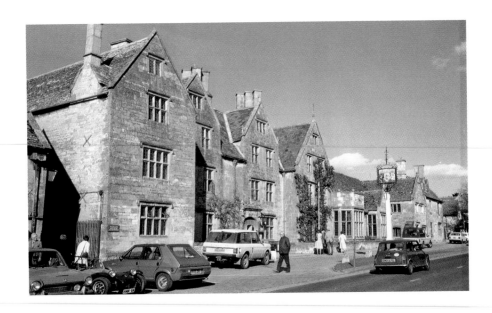

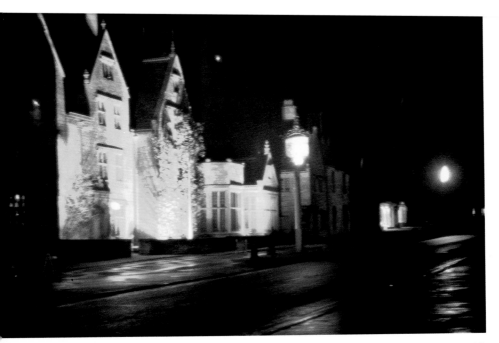

TRAVEL

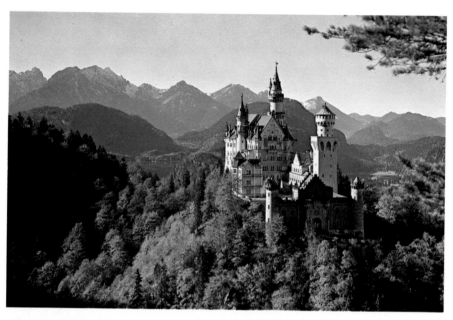

Many people take most of their year's pictures during vacation or travel times. They see new sights and enjoy exciting experiences—experiences they want to deposit in their memory banks and share with others.

Travel photography combines all the elements discussed in this book—people, landscapes, interesting objects, flowers, night scenes, and sports. The challenge is being ready for all at the same time. Here are some general ideas, followed by specific tips that should make your travel photography easier.

Research As you plan the details of your trip, list important sights that you'll want to photograph. Then you'll have a ready reference to assist your memory. Of course, you'll find special places of interest not listed in any guide book. Many of these will give your pictures a more authentic local flavor than the customary landmarks—the early-morning marketplace, people involved in unique craft work, unusual methods of transportation, and, of course, the preparation of those special meals.

Early-morning shadows and foreground branches create perspective in this gorgeous view of Neuschwanstein Castle near Füssen, Germany.

Right
Pictures of people add character to your travel memories. Ask permission and get a winning expression from a classical dancer in Cochin, India.

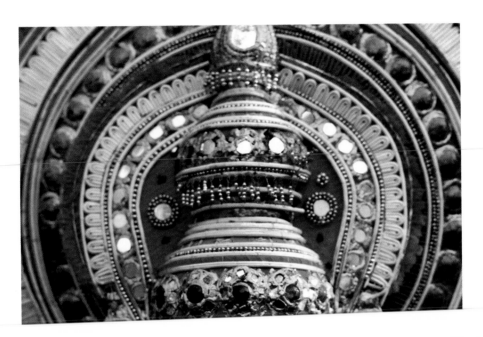

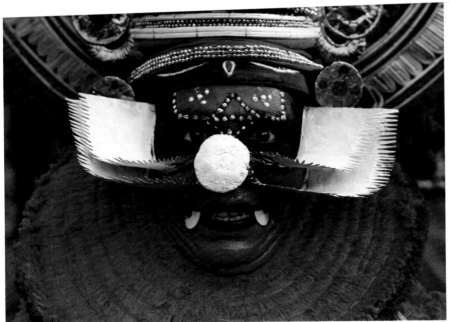

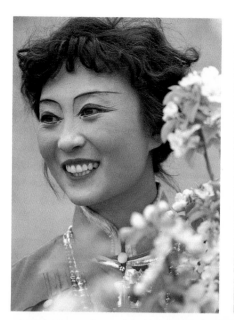

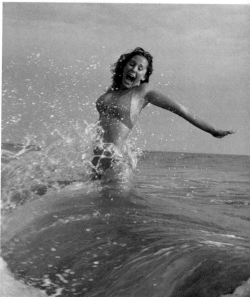

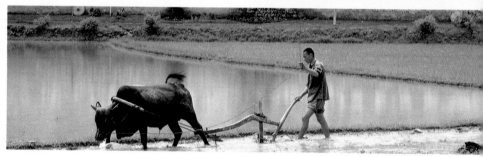

Take Plenty of Pictures Once back home, the typical sentiment is, "Why didn't we take more?" Film is a small part of your travel budget, but the pictures will be a large part of later enjoyment.

Look for the best angles and positions from which to photograph your subjects. Sometimes you'll find that you can improve the composition of your first picture by shifting your position.

When photographing colorful, fast-moving events, keep looking through the viewfinder. Take pictures as often as you see something you like.

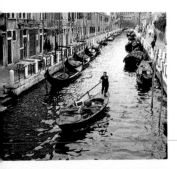
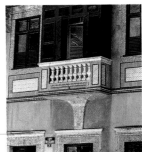
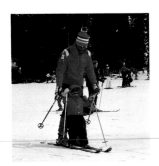
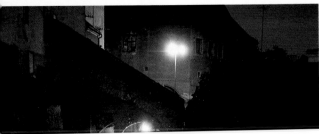
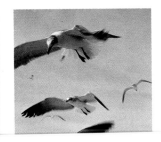
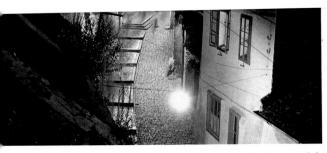
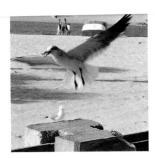

Many Subjects Be prepared to move in close, with permission of course, to people in native or ethnic dress. Photograph camel caravans, shop windows full of curios, floral displays, festivals, parades, local sports, children, building interiors, and illuminated sights at night. Remember that many of your best-treasured pictures will be of the subjects you found unique—the ones that you reacted to most strongly. Also, don't worry about bad weather. Fine photos can come from inclement conditions— umbrellas in the rain, fishing boats at anchor in the fog, and children playing in the snow.

Be Prepared Keep your camera with you at all times, ready and loaded, and be alert for good picture situations.

Tell a Story Your travel pictures should describe the vacation as completely as possible. Don't forget to capture events that will help you remember. Airplane flights, train trips, taxi rides, customs officials, hotels, tourguides—all these contribute to the later enjoyment of your vacation. Many travelers photograph signs as memory joggers. Signs are even better when familiar faces surround them.

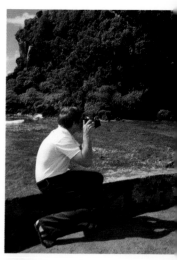

Personalize Your Pictures Have family or tour group members pose in pictures of monuments, scenic views, restaurants, and with the helpful local people you'll meet. You'll delight in the warmer significance of these scenes later.

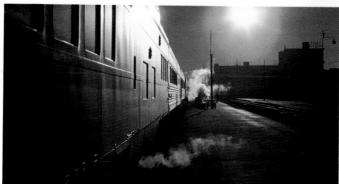

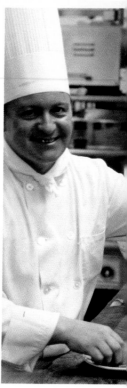

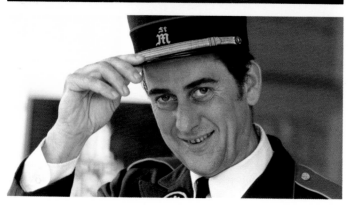

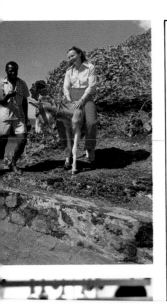

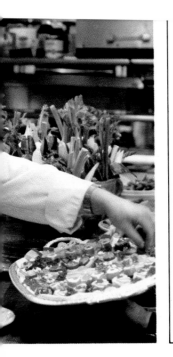

Tips Here are some specifics that might help.

1. Before you leave home, look at your list of possible pictures, and pack about twice as much film as you think you'll need.

2. Allow enough time to take a roll of film with your camera and have it processed before you leave. It's a good way to make sure that your camera is operating correctly.

3. During travel preparation, register all foreign-made photo equipment with U.S. customs, so that misunderstandings about duty won't arise on your return. Most Federal office buildings include a Custom House office where an official will inventory your equipment and give you the proper document to surrender to customs officials when you return. Sales receipts may be enough documentation.

4. Don't forget flash pictures. Take whatever bat-

5. When passing through airport security, ask for hand-inspection of your camera and all film, exposed and unexposed. It's not always possible. Security x-rays can be harmful to your film—the more x-rays the worse the harm. Anytime you avoid the x-ray scanners will help the final results.

6. For extra convenience in the U.S., take film processing mailers with you. Send the exposed film back in the mail to minimize exposure to x-rays. Your processed pictures should be waiting for you when you return.

7. It is a sensible practice to examine your camera at night after touring is finished for the day. Clean the lens if necessary, and check the battery if your camera uses one. Make sure that the carrying strap is secure.

8. Keep your camera with you—to avoid theft and to keep ready for picture opportunities. An unattended camera can be an inviting prize.

PETS

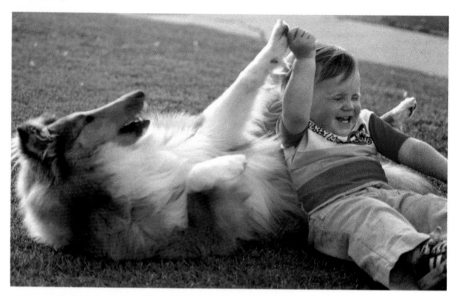

Pets have as much personality as people, and pictures should communicate those traits. You'll need some ingenuity, lots of patience, and a good location. Small animals, of course, can be photographed nearly anywhere. Larger pets will give you less choice. Above all, find a setting that appears natural.

Animals, like children, have limited patience and a short attention span. Set up your camera and

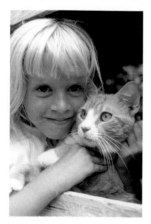

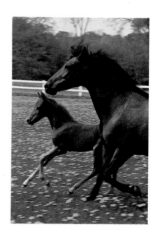

Horses might be best in a field.

A working dog might be best in a field, a house cat on a window sill or in front of the fire. Try to keep the background simple.

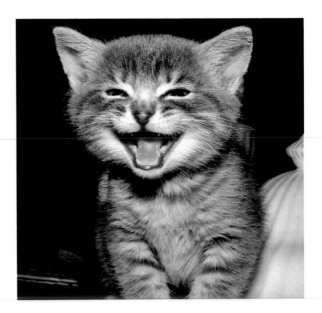

Flash is an effective way to separate a small animal from confusing surroundings indoors. Flash can also stop quick movement. Move in close enough to eliminate other elements in the picture.

Make sure that you stay in the minimum focus range of the camera. Also, see that you are still within the flash range of your camera. If you are still in focus, but too close for the flash, put one or two layers of white tissue over the flash to cut down the light. When you're all set to take a flash picture, try to spark an interesting

get completely ready to take pictures before you bring your subject on stage.

Ingenuity means keeping your pet in the same place and evoking appealing, enthusiastic expressions. Find or devise a noisemaker that will prick up your pet's ears for an alert look. Getting a pet to stay may call for a morsel of favorite food.

Be patient. When you see what you want, take plenty of pictures. Pets soon grow restless.

Get fairly close—enough so that your subject fills the viewfinder. Place the camera down at the pet's eye level, just as you would for a small child. The perspective gives a less distorted view, and animals appreciate the eye-level approach.

Some animals have special photogenic habits. Famous animal photographer Walter Chandoha made one of his first commercially successful pet photos of his cat Minguina, who made a long stretch in front of a mirror after every nap. Chandoha got ready and snapped her in the middle of the stretch—just what an eager art director wanted for an advertisement.

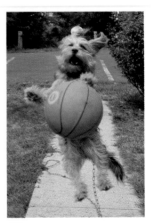

Most pets can move pretty fast when inspired. Practice the stunt you want to capture with an unloaded camera. When everything looks right, start taking pictures.

91

ZOOS

Everybody likes the zoo, and your zoo photos should show it. You can take pictures of the animals and pictures of people enjoying the animals. For best results in photographing the animals themselves, get as close as safely possible. Dangerous inhabitants are usually behind bars, wire, or glass. From behind the barriers in a safe position, aim your camera through the wire or between the bars or put it right next to the glass. Make sure to stay behind zoo-imposed barriers. Wild animals are always unpredictable. There's no sense offering yourself as a free meal if the city has already provided one.

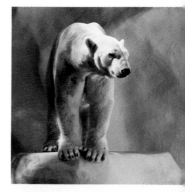

Where there are fewer restrictions, it's easier to get unobstructed photos. As always, see if you can find a position with superior lighting and background. Move around until you find the best.

The petting zoo is often one of the most fertile areas for great spontaneous pictures—especially with your kids. Most youngsters are thrilled and awed by all the furry, friendly creatures, and their faces show it. Move in close enough to capture those rapturous expressions.

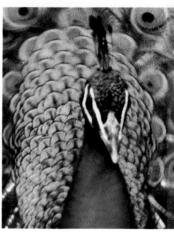

Some zoos have indoor displays where you can take flash pictures (pages 152-161) or existing-light pictures (see page 165) of the exhibits. Put camera and flash next to the glass where possible. Where you're separated from the glass, take your pictures at an angle so that flash reflections won't bounce back at your camera.

You can get fantastic results at the attractions where spectators are caged in autos and the inhabitants roam free. The wild animals are familiar with autos and will venture quite close. Use extreme caution, however, and carefully obey the rules. A charging carnivore has more primitive things in mind than portrait photography. If you're in a car with the windows down, just stay inside the window. If the windows are closed and the car is moving, hold the camera next to but not touching the glass. You'll avoid reflections and get sharper pictures. Use as fast a shutter speed as possible to overcome car or animal movement.

Surprisingly, time of day may be important for zoo pictures. At peak visitation periods during the weekend, the animals may retire to their hideaways just to avoid the crowds. Midday is usually a time for napping in the animal kingdom. Try to schedule a special trip with friends or family to see the creatures when they're likely to be most active—during the week, preferably in the morning before feeding time.

92

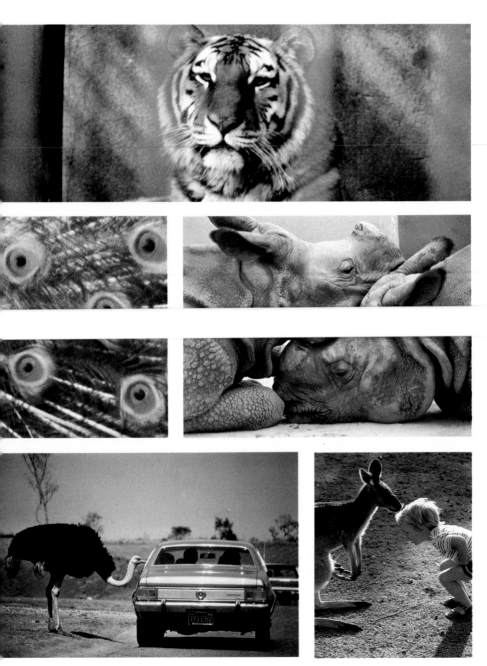

FLOWERS AND PLANTS

Any flower garden is a cornucopia of nature's greatest treasures—dazzling colors and soft fragrances combined in a master patchwork of cosmic design. Some "gardens" are wild, growing free, while others are carefully planned and cultivated. In either case, there are some simple techniques that should give you exciting pictures.

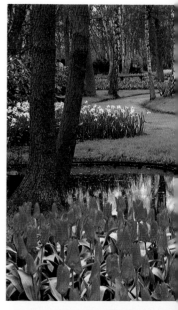

Concentrate on the garden—move in close enough to picture only the blooms. Better yet, take pictures at different distances to show the overall view and then smaller segments of floral glory. Get very close with close-up lenses. (See page 182.) Move around so that you have the best background and picture design. Take pictures when the light makes nature's work most attractive. The best times are early in the morning with soft shadows and sparkling dew or the rich warm light of late afternoon.

Take pictures throughout the growing season so that you have a complete record to share with distant friends or relatives.

Look for exciting pictures of nature subjects in all the seasons. Fall leaves, snow-covered pine needles, and the first crocuses give extra dimension to the year's picture-taking.

Close-Up Tips A piece of colored construction paper will provide a simple background that concentrates attention on your subject. Flash or a piece of white cardboard will reflect light into shadow areas. Since you'll be very close, cover a flash with two or more layers of tissue for correct exposure. If the breeze is batting your subject around, make a quick windbreak of tomato stakes and sheet plastic. For that extra-fresh look, create some artificial dew with an atomizer.

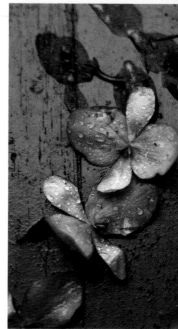

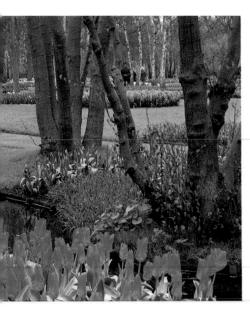

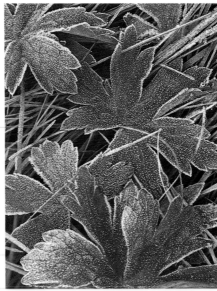

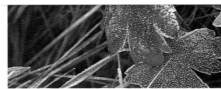

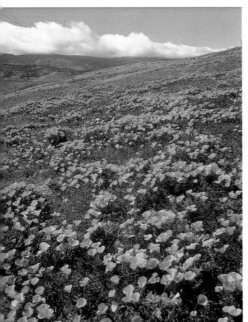

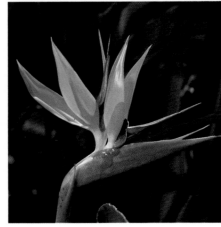

BUILDINGS

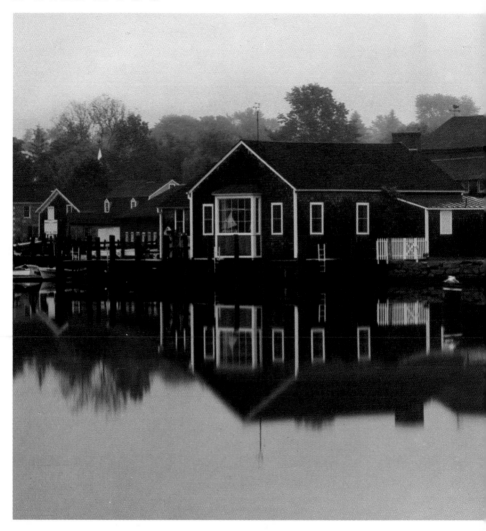

What's important about a particular building? Or, rather, why do you like a special building? What are the features that attract you? Once you've isolated these aspects, concentrate on them.

In the illustration above, the photographer sensed peace and stability in the weatherbeaten harbor structures. This feeling is augmented by the nearly perfect reflection. Although cropped for best

96

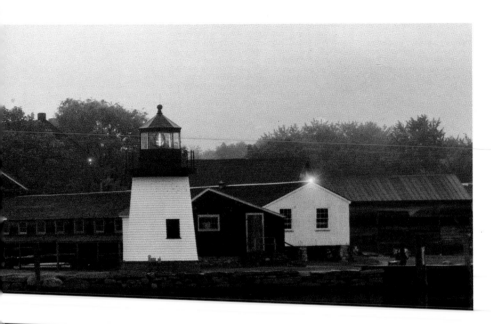

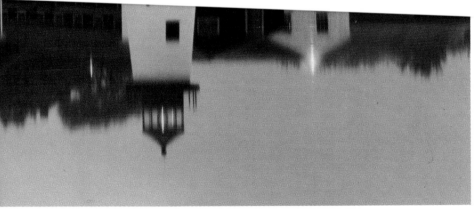

page design, the breadth of the long low buildings is captured by horizontal framing. The misty surroundings create a mood of New England nostalgia which seems to await the arrival of a transatlantic square-rigger. Another case might show a martial line of brilliantly gingerbreaded row houses. Naturally, you'll want to capture the pattern of the group, as well as individual details.

Details might be ornate or stately entrances, wrought-iron work, or designs in the brick or stonework of the facade. Again, wait for a time of day when the light shows off your subject, and move in close to isolate what you want to capture.

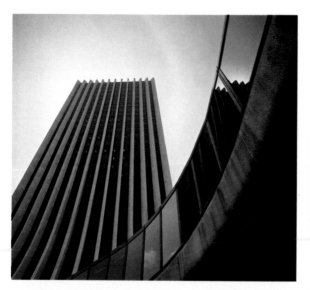

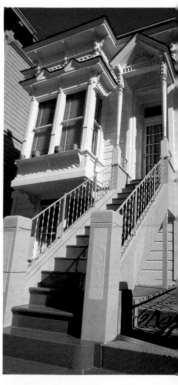

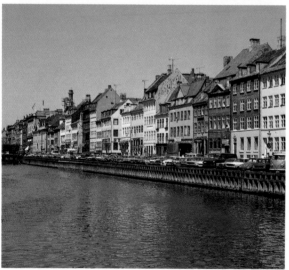

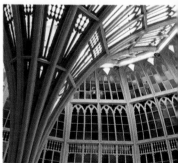

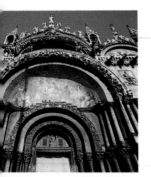

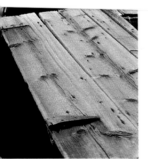

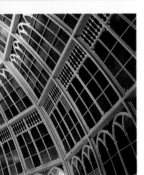

COLLECTIBLES AND OBJETS D'ART

Many hobbyists make or collect things that they want to show other like-minded people. They also see things on display that they want to record. Same important rules—move in close (with a close-up lens, if necessary. See page 182). Find a camera position that sees a simple background, and use lighting that shows off the object's best features. If necessary, use reflectors to fill in shadows. One good way to control your results is to cover a table with plain cloth or paper, preferably not white, that contrasts with your subject. Raise the cloth or paper up out of sight in the background to provide an undistracting backdrop. Outdoors in sunlight you can control the lighting by turning the table. Indoors with photolamps (see page 58), you can move the lights.

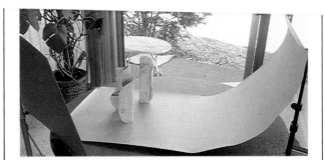

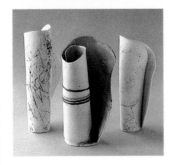

The free-form ceramic statuettes pictured at left were photographed in the set-up shown above. Indirect window light provided the main illumination, while a white reflector card filled the dark-side shadows.

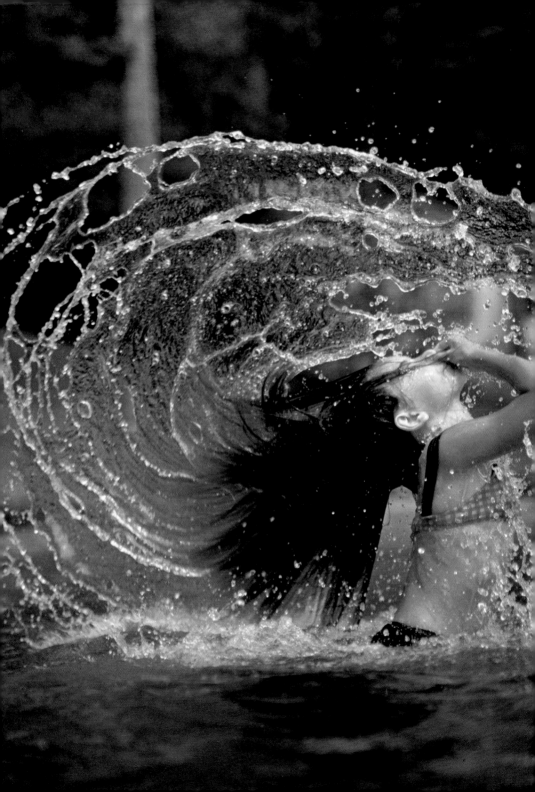

ACTION

There are some familiar ideas for capturing action successfully as well as several specific techniques. Following a few general tips are ideas about portraying movement.

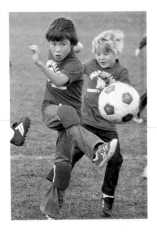

Get as close as you safely can. Choose a position that will dramatize the incident. Look for an uncluttered background and good lighting. Preset your camera controls and focus on the spot where you plan to capture your subject. When the moving body arrives at the spot, snap the picture. When composing the picture, leave a little room in front of your subject—it looks more natural.

STOPPING THE ACTION

You can usually freeze movement sharply in one of four ways. You can set a fast shutter speed on your camera (see pages 138-141). The faster the shutter speed, the more likely your chances of a sharp

can pan your camera with the subject.

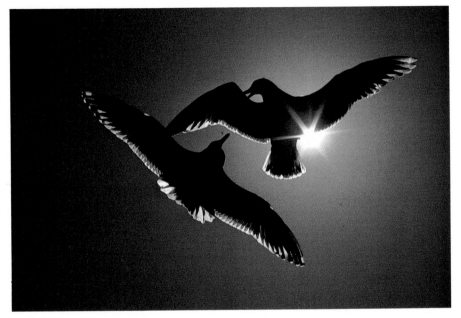

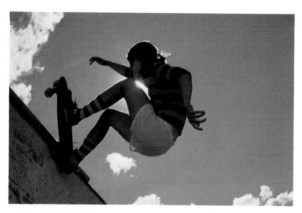

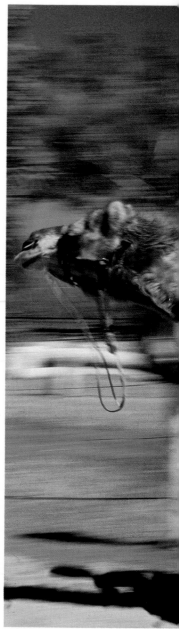

Peak of Action Some motions have a midpoint where everything stops momentarily. A diver at the top of an upward spring or a basketball player up for a dunk both stop before descending. A baseball pitcher or hitter, a tennis player, a golfer all pause before moving and stop after follow-through. Practice for a while without film. Follow a diver to the mid-air pause and pretend you're snapping that fraction of a second. Get a golfing friend to practice swings. See if you can capture the stationary highpoint of both backswing and follow-through.

Panning Panning works with running kids, dogs, horses, bicycles, race cars, speed boats, or airplanes during take off. You may have to pan for two reasons. First, the subject may be moving so fast that even a fast shutter speed cannot stop the action. Second, good composition is difficult because the subject is in your viewfinder for such a short time. Swing both your camera and body so that the moving subject stays in the same place in your viewfinder. This, too, takes practice. Rotate your body smoothly and concentrate on pressing the shutter release at the best point for picture design. Follow through after you snap the shutter. Unless you can choose a very fast shutter speed, chances are good that the subject will be sharp and the background will be blurred into attractive streaks of color.

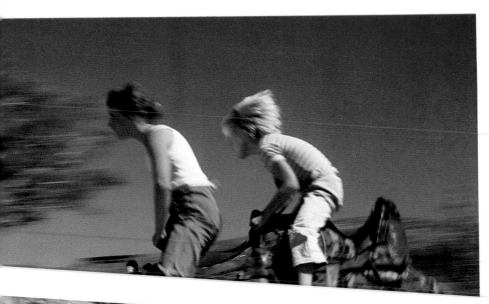

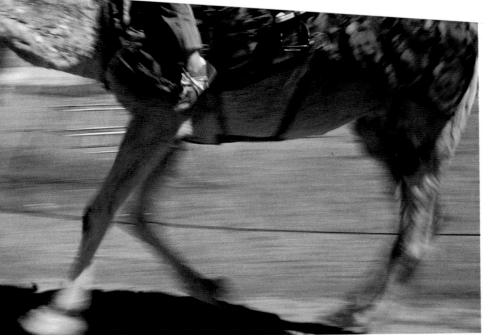

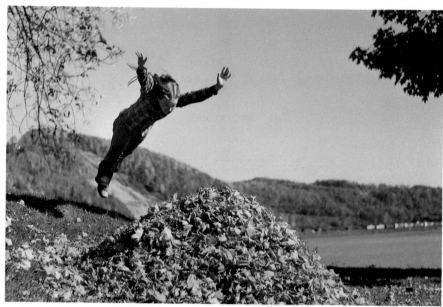

Toward the camera

Direction The direction of movement may affect your choice of technique. A subject coming toward or retreating from you is easier to capture sharp than one crossing your field of vision. You can use a slower shutter speed for action toward or away from you, and you'll find that you have more time to make a good composition. Subjects moving at a 90° angle to you and your camera invite panning and your fastest shutter speeds.

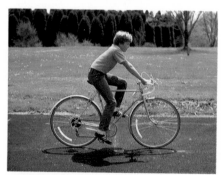

1/500 second at 90°

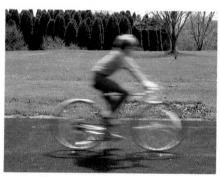

1/30 second at 90°

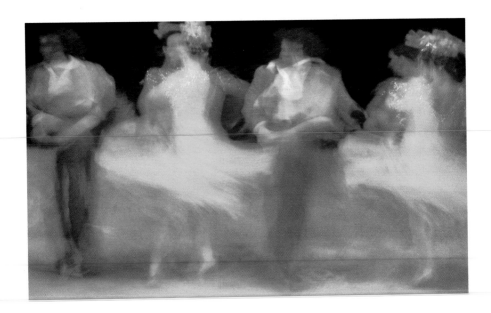

BLURRED ACTION

Blurred motion can convey the idea of speed and movement. Set a very slow shutter speed (1/30 to 1/8 second) on your camera. You can pan or hold the camera steady while the subject's blurred movements cover a little bigger slice of time on your film. When the camera is mounted on a tripod or other solid support, only the subject will be blurred. Add your own movement by handholding the camera.

SPORTS TIPS

Get close to the players. Ask permission for a side-line spot at amateur and school competition. At professional events choose an unobstructed position as near the action as possible.

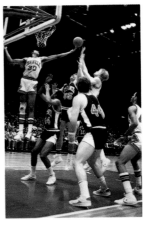

Prefocus on the spot where you'll get the best picture. Have your camera loaded and the exposure controls set. It's very helpful to know the game, because you can anticipate key plays and key players. Photograph night games and indoor events by the existing light. See pages 162-165.

NIGHT

The world spends half its time in light and half in darkness. Picture-taking at night can be just as exciting as daytime photography.

You'll find subjects everywhere—bright lights, fireworks, holiday displays, and outdoor activities. Snapshot camera owners can use flash outdoors at night. A high-speed film will extend the flash range. Owners of automatic or adjustable cameras can take pictures with flash or with the existing light. High-speed films, slow shutter speeds, and a large maximum aperture will help capture almost anything that can be seen. See pages 162-165 for more existing-light recommendations.

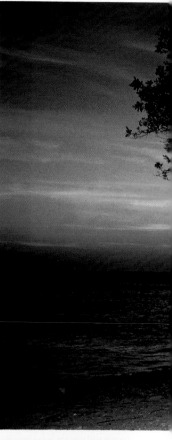

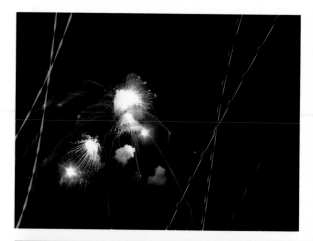

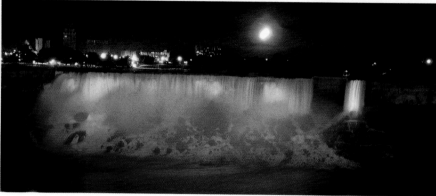

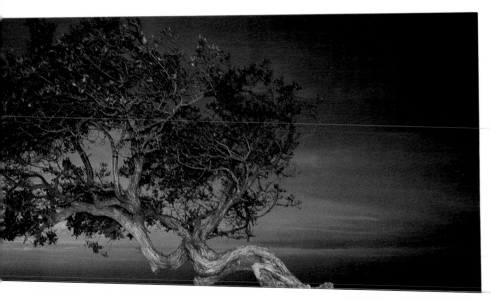

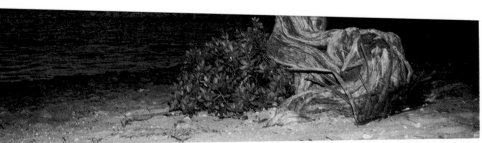

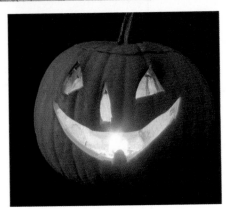

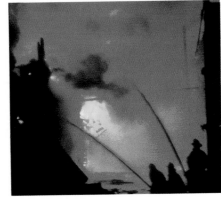

BAD WEATHER

Everybody takes pictures when the sun is out. But on some days, it rains, snows, mists, or is just plain overcast. The truth is that some of your best pictures can happen on days with poor weather. Think of the benefits.

People look their best out of the sun. Their faces open up with bright, natural, unshadowed expressions. Light overcast days are perfect for outstanding portraits. Just make sure that your background doesn't include much dull sky and move in close to your subject. You may even find that rain and snow give people, kids especially, an opportunity to wear colorful clothing and engage in activities you'll want to capture. In rain or snow, take care to protect your camera. Keep it warm and dry under a slicker or parka.

Scenery takes on a very different appearance on a dull day. Although the sky appears gloomy and grim, the colors of grass and trees, red barns, and white fences can appear brighter. Fog will lend an ethereal quality to many scenes—subjects may appear partly shrouded in mist. Subjects may appear bluish in pictures made while the sun is hiding. Attach an 81A filter* to your camera lens to warm up the colors a bit. You won't need to change your exposure.

Snow and cold give a soft, blurry appearance in pastel shades. With your camera protected from flakes and the cold, you'll find a world full of children, sleds, snowmen, skiers, and colorful outerwear. At night, you can take unusual flash pictures of nearby subjects with snowflakes hovering all around.

Rain brings some charming surprises. Bright umbrellas and colorful rain gear, for instance. Reflections in puddles or on rain-drenched streets give another dimension to your pictures. Keep your camera out of the water, but don't hesitate to shoot activity in a rainshower. Find a good position to snap the action from under an overhang, or inside a car with the window open.

*See pages 170-171 for more on filters.

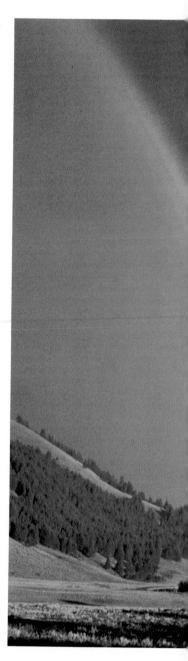

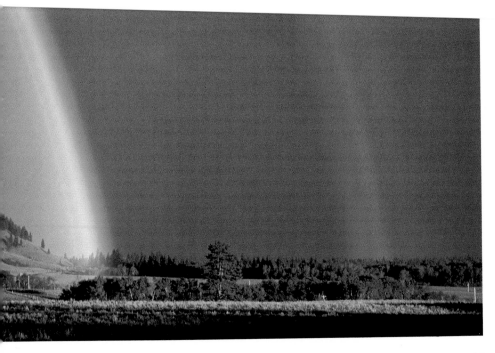

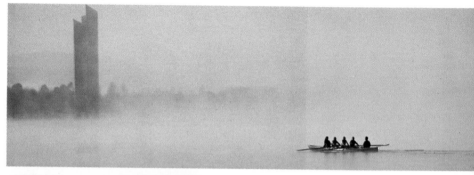

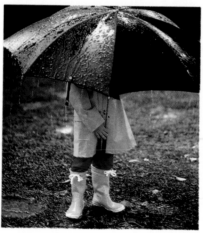

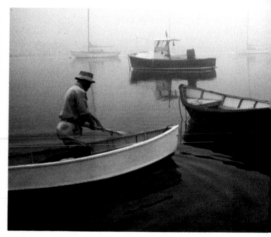

Overcast skies give delightful casual portraits, because your subjects won't be squinting into the sun. Try not to include much of the dull sky, and you'll find bright, colorful subjects all around. Again, high-speed film will help you get well-exposed pictures with a snapshot camera. Remember that your family and other people don't suspend activity when the sun goes under. Sometimes a gloomy day will inspire children to try something new. If they don't think of anything, suggest an interesting activity that will get them occupied and yield good pictures.

Mist or fog can lend a ghostly, ethereal appearance to familiar scenes. Nearby subjects will be distinct, but more distant subjects will seem to be

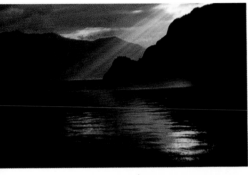

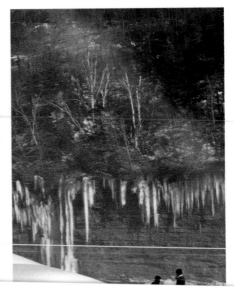

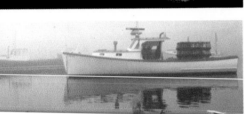

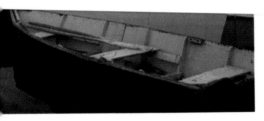

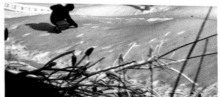

fading into another dimension. Often, there's bright light coming through the mist, spotlighting bright objects or making trails through the heavy air. Early morning is a perfect time to search out misty scenes. If the sky is dark overhead, use a high-speed film in a snapshot camera.

EXPOSURE

Bad weather is darker, and you'll need more exposure than in sunlight. See pages 132-141 for film choice and exposure setting information. Automatic cameras, of course, will adjust to scene lighting with very little help from you. Use high-speed film in a snapshot camera.

SHOWING YOUR PICTURES

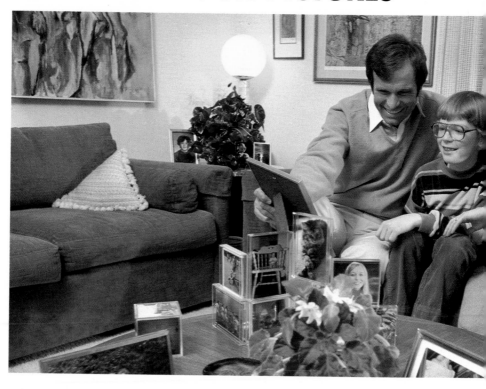

Good pictures are meant to be seen. Here are some ideas for getting more mileage from your best efforts. (Make sure you read page 115 for information about storing and protecting your photos.)

PHOTO ALBUMS
Albums abound in shapes and sizes from a purse-size book to coffee-table volumes. You can also make your own with a loose-leaf binder, thin cardboard pages, and photo cement or white glue. Many people assemble their albums chronologically—it seems sensible. They also label the pictures *and* the negative-envelopes so that they can get reprints at a much later date.

Some people get more in albums by cutting up the prints and inserting the best parts. There's wasted space in almost every print.

A photo album can be the chronicle of years or an up-to-date newsbrief filled with your latest snapshots.

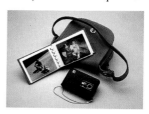

112

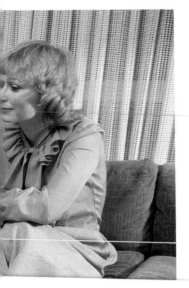

ENLARGEMENTS AND HOME DÉCOR

Another way to get your best images out of the box and into view is to display enlargements. Available from your photofinisher in different sizes (5x7, 8x10, 11x14, and 16x20 inches) and shapes to fit your film format, enlargements are ideal for framing or for gifts. Hung on a wall, displayed on a desk, or even commanding an important place in your albums, enlargements have a powerful ability to cross the barriers of time and say, "You were there." For more ideas on decorating with photographs, see the KODAK Photo Book *Photo Décor,* available from your photo dealer.

Traditional and unusual ways of displaying prints are available from your local photo, stationery, department, or discount

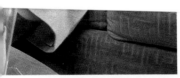

such different ideas as photo cubes, wall clocks, mobiles, and collage boards.

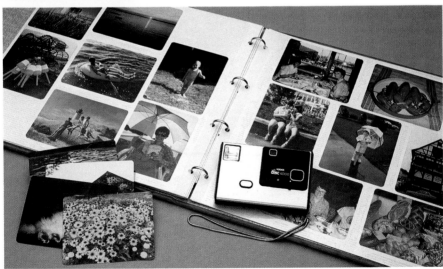

GREETING CARDS

A card with a picture of you or you and your family is truly a personal communication. Children grow, houses change, and so do the seasons. You can commission special greetings from your photofinisher with pictures and words all printed together, or you can attach a print to the inside of other cards. You can send 3 1/2 x 5-inch prints as postcards. Make sure you use a pen that will write on the slick, plastic back of the print. Some people plan ahead and have favorite shots reprinted to enclose in letters to distant friends and relatives. A photo Christmas card each year keeps the people on your mailing list in closer touch with a growing family.

PROCESSING SERVICES

In addition to reprints, enlargements, and photo-greeting cards, your photofinisher can make slides from negatives, prints and enlargements from slides, and copyprints from other prints. Some photofinishers can help you crop the negatives you want enlarged to improve the picture design.

Greeting cards for many occasions are available from your photofinisher. Can you guess which holiday cards receive the most attention?

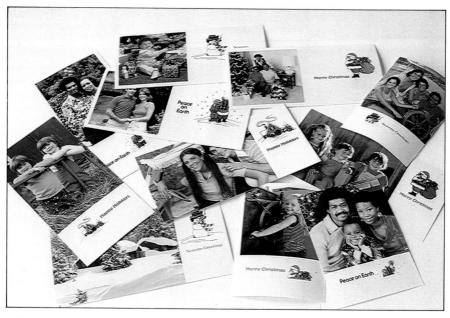

STORING PICTURES

With a little care and forethought, your pictures will provide you with many years of pleasure. Here are some general ideas for prolonging the lives of prints, slides, and negatives.

Storage Locations You want a place with moderate temperature (under 70° F [21°C]) and fairly low humidity (under 50% relative humidity) which probably eliminates most basements and attics. Heat can become excessive in an attic, and humidity in either place may be harmful. A spot near a chimney, heat run, or in direct ~~light can cause problems~~

Containers An album is the best way to display and protect your prints. Since the prints will be in intimate contact with the pages, make sure that the materials used in the construction of the album will not harm the prints. Check with your photo dealer about the cover, pages, plastic sleeves, mounting corners or hinges, and the ink used for identification. This becomes especially important if you have prints without the negatives. If you have the negatives, you can have them reprinted.

Album prints should not be subjected to pressure, nor should the image sides of the prints be in direct contact with each other. Protect the faces of the prints in an album with a suitable plastic sheeting.

If you're making your own album, be sure that the adhesive you use for adhering the prints is photographically safe. Starch paste, animal glue, and rubber cement are not advised. One of the safest methods is mounting prints on album pages with special dry-mounting tissue. Ask your photo dealer for specific recommendations.

You'll want to find a safe home for negatives and extra prints. The envelopes provided by most photofinishers are suitable for storing prints and negatives because they contain no contaminants that would ruin the images.

dients that will quickly photos. The same applies to furniture drawers, attics, and basements where fumes from mothballs, cosmetics, chemicals, glues, or wood-finishing products can cause damaging chemical reactions.

Don't store prints and negatives under pressure—they may stick together. In fact, if you have real favorites, they should be separated into plastic photo sleeves for safekeeping.

SLIDE SHOWS

Most people who take slides like to see that big bright image up on the screen. Because it's so big, it can be shared with many people at the same time, and modern projection equipment can show many slides in a comparatively short time. On the other hand, everyone nods in sympathy when a friend mentions that three of last evening's hours were devoted to someone's slide show or home movies. With a little planning and restraint, you can have your audiences clamoring for more.

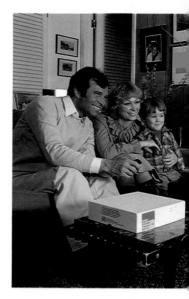

First, arrange your slides so that they tell a story, even if it's a simple chronological story of vacation travel. You'll find that narration is easier when you can proceed logically from one topic to the next. Second, use only your best slides. Pass over pictures that are fuzzy or incorrectly exposed. Resist the temptation to show everything. Third, don't leave any one slide on the screen too long—10 seconds is a

Selecting pictures

Choose only your best pictures— ones that are sharp and correctly exposed. Poor-quality pictures are tiring to view and lower the impact of your show. One easy way to look at slides is with the help of an inexpensive illuminator, available from most photo dealers. Project your final choices to check their sharpness.

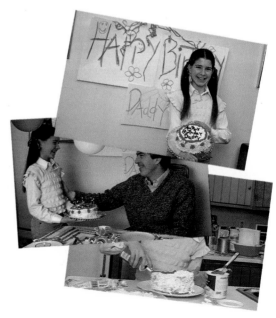

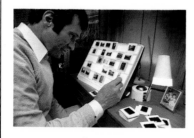

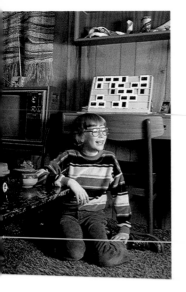

useful average time. If you have to spend a long time explaining a picture, chances are that it's not a very good illustration. Your audience is used to TV and movies where things generally happen pretty fast. Fourth, consider one hour the maximum time that people can sit still comfortably. Fifth, rehearse your presentation a few times, so that you're familiar with the order of the slides and so that your narration will flow easily. Sixth, get everything—screen, projector, and chairs—set up in advance. And make sure that you have a spare projector bulb and know how to change it.

These are easy preplanning steps, but you may be surprised at the enthusiasm of your audience. If you think you want to delve deeper into slide presentations, consult Keith Boas' article in *The Ninth Here's How*—a KODAK Photo Book available from most photo dealers.

Telling a Story

The easiest way to tell a story with pictures is to put them in chronological order. Since every story has certain key elements or events, use the pictures that best portray the highpoints. You don't have to explain or show every step. Just include the necessary pictures. Too many will dilute the message.

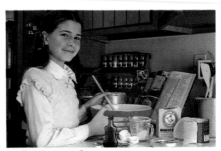

1. Getting ready.

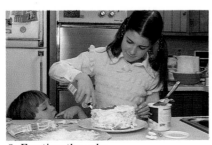

2. Frosting the cake.

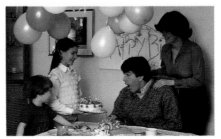

3. Making the presentation.

PHOTO REPORTS

There are times when photos are more striking than words alone. Reports for business, school, and even your community are more effective when amplified by pictures. You can create a slide show or illustrate a written report with captioned prints, or consider enlargement displays in public places. Here's what's important. The pictures should clearly show exactly what you want them to show. Use no more than you need—too many dilute impact. Make sure that the technical quality is good—sharp and well-exposed pictures. Captions or narration should be short and to the point.

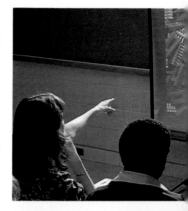

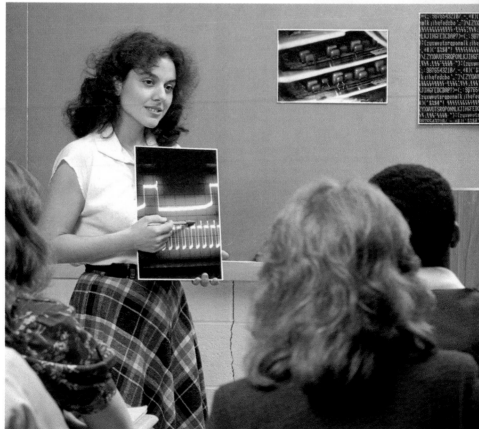

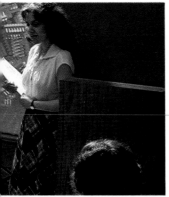

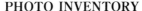

PHOTO INVENTORY

Nobody likes to face the idea of calamity, but that's why insurance companies exist. In case of a loss, it's helpful to provide as much evidence as possible. Pictures can be a valuable resource.

Take a moment to make a mental inventory of your possessions and how much it would cost to replace them. With this incentive, you might want to load and use your camera. A series of photographs can effectively document your goods, particularly when combined with the sales receipts.

Start with your home—the outside and the inside. Take pictures outside when the scene is bright and when important features aren't hidden in shadow. Shoot from all important viewpoints, and maybe a few more for extra precaution. When inside, take pictures of the four walls in each room with flash or existing light. (Don't forget to include some of the floor with costly rugs or carpet.)

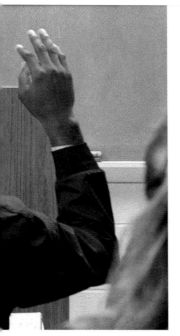

a closer distance the smaller items such as silver flatware, fine china, paintings, objets d'art, clothes, tools, small appliances, sports equipment, antique furniture, and jewelry. The same applies to lawn and garden equipment, outside furniture, and so on.

Keep the prints and negatives or slides in your safe deposit box in case you ever need them to prove a loss.

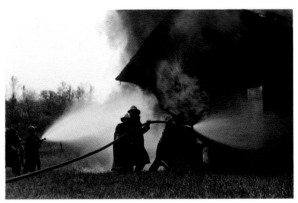

HAS IT HAPPENED TO YOU?

Sometimes things go wrong, and you get results you didn't plan *or* want. Here are some of the most common problems, the reasons, and some suggested solutions.

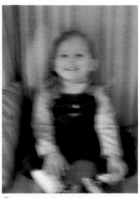

Camera movement

Problem	Reason	Solution
Fuzzy, unsharp pictures	Shutter speed too slow.	For pictures of still subjects, use a shutter speed no slower than 1/30 second if handholding the camera. For fast-moving subjects, use the fastest shutter speed possible—usually no slower than 1/250 second. (See page 141.)
	Incorrect handling.	Make sure you hold the camera very steady and gently press the shutter release. (See page 44.)
	Incorrect focus.	Make sure you focus correctly on your subject. Refer to your camera manual. (See page 45.)
	Dirty lens.	Keep your lens clean of dust and smears. (See page 186.)

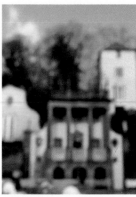

Out of focus

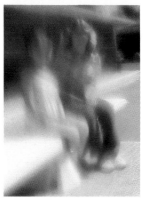

Dirty lens

Problem	Reason	Solution
Pictures too light, too dark	Incorrect film speed setting on camera or on handheld meter.	Set or check the film speed every time you load a new roll of film. (See page 36.)
	Dead or weak meter battery.	Check battery periodically according to camera instruction manual. Replace at least once a year.
	No adjustment for side- and back-lighting.	See page 142 for information about adjusting for different lighting angles.

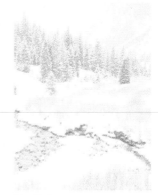

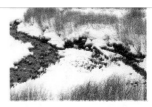

Too light

light		person.
Blank negatives (no prints) or black slides	Shutter does not open.	See camera repair person.
	Film does not advance through camera.	Check loading procedures in instruction manual or have repair person check film-advance mechanism.
	Lens cap not removed.	Make sure you remove lens cap.
Pictures consistently too light or dark	Exposure meter may need adjustment.	See repair person.

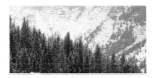

Correct exposure

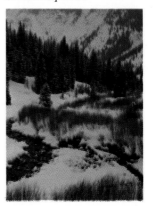

Too dark

Problem	Reason	Solution
Flash pictures too light, dark	Light—too close to subject. Dark—too far from subject.	Check snapshot camera distance range or check focus setting with adjustable/automatic camera. (See page 153.)
	Film speed on camera/flash unit wrong.	Check to see that correct film speed is set on flash unit or camera. (See page 154.)
	Aperture setting wrong.	Make sure that aperture setting on camera agrees with information on flash calculator dial. (See pages 155-156.)
Flash too dark	Dark—electronic flash may not have fully recycled.	Allow flash to recycle fully until ready light shows or maybe a bit longer.
	Weak batteries.	(See page 157.) Change batteries.
People or animals with glowing eyes	Flash positioned too close to lens for subject with open retina.	Turn on all room lights. If possible, remove flash from camera to increase distance between lens and flash. Increase flash-to-subject distance. Have person avert eyes.

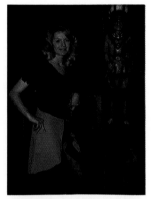

Too dark

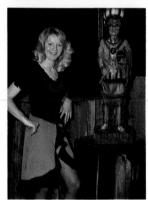

Correctly exposed

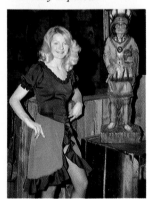

Too light

Problem	Reason	Solution
Flash pictures: black slides, blank negatives, and no prints	Flash didn't fire.	Battery dead, poor connection between flash and camera. (See page 154.)
Glare spots in flash pictures	Flash fired into reflective background.	Adjust your position so that any reflective material (mirrors, paneled walls, eyeglasses) is at an angle.
Flash pictures unevenly exposed	Foreground object closer than main subject—gets overexposed.	Use a position where the main subject is closest to the flash.
partly exposed	shutter speed.	camera manual for correct shutter speed with flash. (See page 154.)

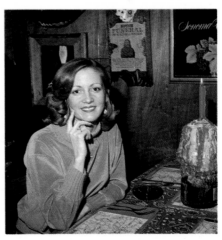

Foreground object

Object removed

Wrong shutter speed

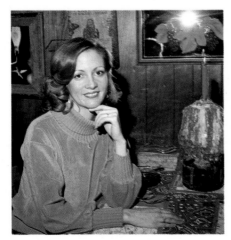

Reflection from shiny surface

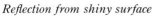

Position changed to avoid reflection

123

Problem	Reason	Solution
Pictures with dark obstructions	Finger in front of lens. Material inside camera.	Check camera-holding position to make sure hand or fingers don't obstruct lens. Carefully check inside camera for foreign matter obstruction.
	Camera strap or case in front of lens.	Check that lens is clear of strap and case before taking picture.
Pictures with unusual color	Bluish—tungsten film used in daylight.	Make sure that the film matches the lighting conditions. If not, add a filter. (See page 168.)
	Yellowish-red—daylight film used in tungsten light.	If using daylight film in tungsten light, consider a filter. (See page 168.)
	Mottled, streaked, maybe greenish or muddy—film outdated.	Make sure you use fresh film and get it processed promptly. Check packing material for expiration date. Do not leave film in extremely hot places.

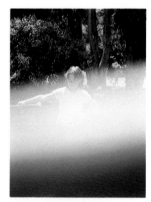

Finger blocking lens

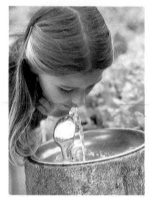

Tungsten film in daylight

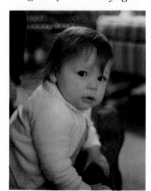

Daylight film in tungsten light

124

Problem	Reason	Solution
Pictures overlapped	Too many pictures on roll.	Don't try to squeeze one more shot at the end of the roll.
	Film winding mechanism needs adjustment.	See a competent repair person.
Light streaks and spots on pictures	Direct rays of light strike lens.	Don't shoot directly into the sun or other bright light source.
Consistent streaks and spots	Fogging: light leak in camera.	Have camera checked by competent repair
	Camera back opened accidentally.	Never trip camera without checking to see if it has film inside.
	Film handled in direct sunlight.	Load and unload your camera in the shade or other subdued light.
	Sticking shutter.	Have camera checked by competent repair person.
	X-ray exposure.	Ask for hand inspection of camera and film at airport security. (See page 89.)

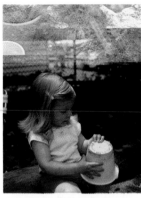

Overlapped pictures

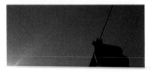

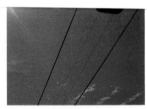

Direct rays of light

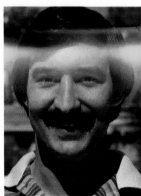

Camera back opened

SIMPLIFYING THE TECHNICALITIES

The more you know about any skill or activity, the better the results. This section of *How to Take Good Pictures* is devoted to how photography works and how to extend your knowledge for even better pictures under a greater variety of conditions.

We'll approach our goal—good pictures—in two ways. First we'll take a tour of a typical 35 mm camera to see what functions all the controls perform. We'll look at film to see what makes it work for you. We'll tie film and camera together into a discussion of exposure that will help you get better results in many tricky situations.

Then, after discussing the sketchy fundamentals of how you can control camera and film, we'll talk about some individual techniques that you'll want to sample. Flash, filters, existing light, and more will show you the delight of creation, where *you* control *your* photography.

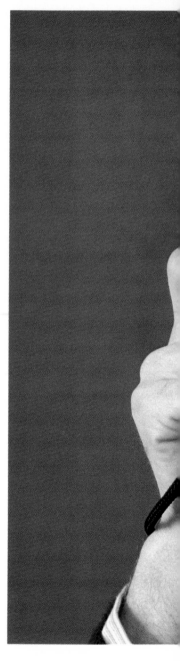

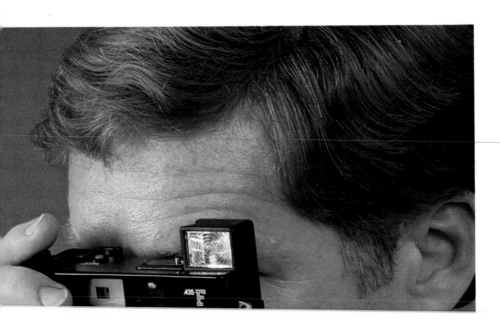

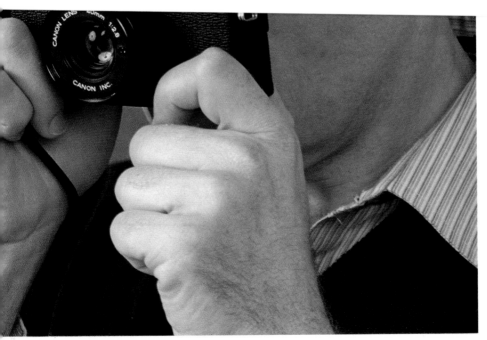

CAMERA CONTROLS

All cameras have controls. The simplest camera might have only one control—the shutter release which you press to take a picture.

More complicated cameras may have several controls. Earlier in the book, we gave a short discussion of 35 mm camera operation—enough to help you start. Now we'll take an imaginary automatic 35 mm camera that is fairly complex and describe the function of all the moving parts you need to know about. Your camera may have some or all of the features we'll describe. And very likely some of the devices will be in different positions from those shown here. Compare these diagrams to those in your camera instruction manual.

For greater clarity, we've even repeated some functions. For example, if your camera has a pop-up flash, you probably won't have a flash hot shoe or a flash-cord socket.

Top Front View
1. *film-advance lever*
2. *film-frame counter*
3. *shutter release*
4. *shutter-speed dial*
5. *flash hot shoe*
6. *rewind knob*
7. *pop-up flash*
8. *pop-up flash button*
9. *viewfinder window*
10. *lens*
11. *aperture ring and mode selector (automatic, manual, possibly flash)*
12. *focusing ring*
13. *film-speed selector dial*
14. *self-timer*
15. *flash-cord socket*

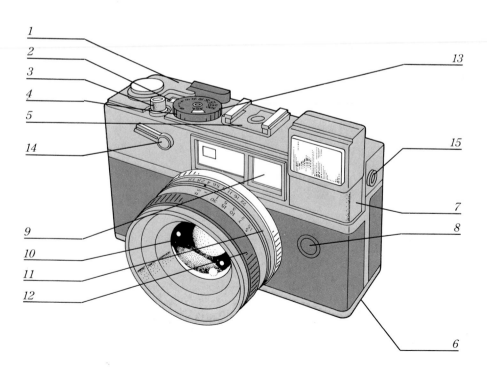

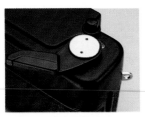 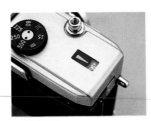 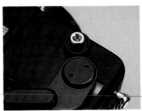

1. **Film-advance lever:** *By moving this lever one or more strokes after taking a picture, you advance the film to the next frame.*

2. **Film-frame counter:** *This shows you how many pictures you have taken: from loading steps to 12, 20, 24, or 36.*

3. **Shutter release:** *You press this button to take a picture.*

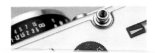 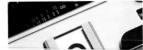 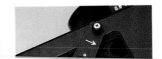

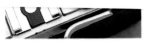 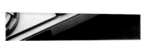 

4. **Shutter-speed dial:** *This selects the shutter speed. It may include the film-speed selector or the automatic operation switch.*

5. **Flash hot shoe:** *This accepts an electronic flash unit. When you attach the flash, the electrical connection is complete.*

6. **Rewind knob:** *This knob usually has a fold-out lever to help rewind exposed film back into the magazine.*

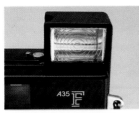 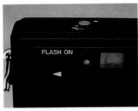 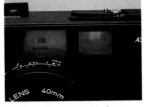

7. **Pop-up flash:** *Raise and activate built-in flash with the button shown in callout 8. Turn off the flash by pressing down.*

8. **Pop-up flash button:** *This button raises and activates the built-in flash unit.*

9. **Viewfinder window:** *This is the other side of the window you look through to compose your picture.*

129

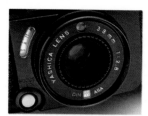 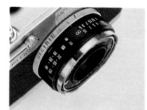 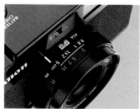

10. Lens: *The lens on your camera gathers and organizes light rays to make a sharp picture on your film.*

11. Aperture ring: *With this you select the lens aperture. The aperture ring may also control automatic, manual, or flash functions.*

12. Focusing ring: *You turn this to get sharp pictures of your subject. It may show distances as symbols or in feet and metres.*

Back View

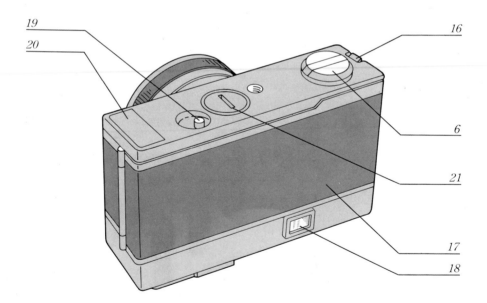

16. *release for film-compartment door*
17. *film-compartment door*
18. *viewfinder window*
19. *film-advance release button*
20. *pop-up flash battery compartment*
21. *meter-battery compartment*

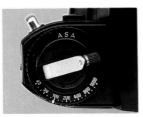
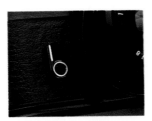
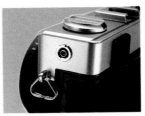

13. **Film-speed selector dial:** *Every time you load film into your camera, set the film speed on the selector dial.*

14. **Self-timer:** *This device automatically snaps the shutter after it is triggered, which allows you to include yourself in the picture.*

15. **Flash cord socket:** *Plug the flash cord (PC cord) into this socket to complete the electrical connection between the flash and the camera.*

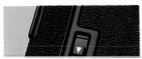
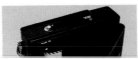
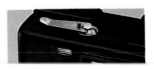

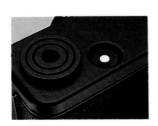
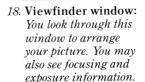

16. **Release for film-compartment door:** *After you rewind the exposed film, open the compartment door with this latch.*

17. **Film-compartment door:** *By operating the latch in callout 16, this door can be opened to load or unload film.*

18. **Viewfinder window:** *You look through this window to arrange your picture. You may also see focusing and exposure information.*

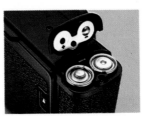
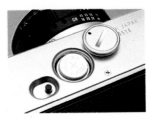

19. **Film-advance release button:** *This button releases the film-advance mechanism so that you can rewind the film.*

20. **Pop-up flash battery compartment:** *This compartment holds the batteries that supply the power to your built-in electronic flash.*

21. **Meter-battery:** *The battery for automatic or manual cameras with exposure meters should be changed at least once a year.*

FILM

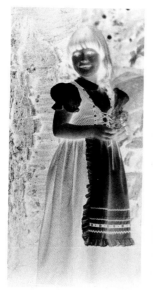
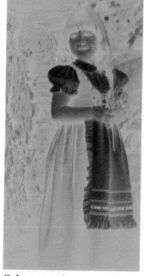
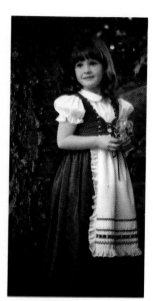

Black-and-white negative   *Color negative*   *Color slide*

In addition to the film information on page 48 here is more information that will help you understand the next section on exposure.

SIZE

Film comes in different sizes and lengths: disc and 110 for pocket-sized cameras, 126 for larger snapshot cameras, and 135 for 35 mm cameras. Films in 110- and 126-sizes generally give a choice of 12 or 24 exposures for color prints, 20 exposures for color slides. Film in 135-size magazines offers several possibilities—12, 24, and 36 exposures for color prints and 20 and 36 exposures for color slides.

SLIDES OR PRINTS

Do you want slides to project or prints from negatives to pass around and put in albums? Slides projected on a screen are brilliant and beautiful, but slide film requires near-perfect exposure for good results. Prints are lovely, too, convenient to share, and negative film is somewhat tolerant of exposure error. You can have enlargements made from either.

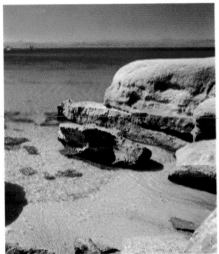

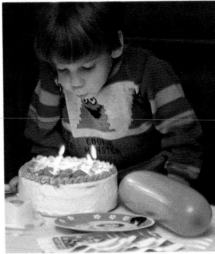

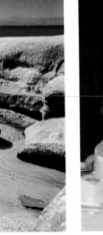

Bright—low or medium-speed film   *Dim—high or very high-speed film*

SPEED

indicated by an assigned ISO, ASA, or DIN number. Low- and medium-speed films—ISO (ASA) 25, 32, 64, 100, 125, 200—are intended for general picture-taking in daylight, while high- and very high-speed films—ISO (ASA) 320, 400, and 1000—are intended for low light. If you take pictures on dark days, indoors, or at night without flash, you'll want a high- or very high-speed film.

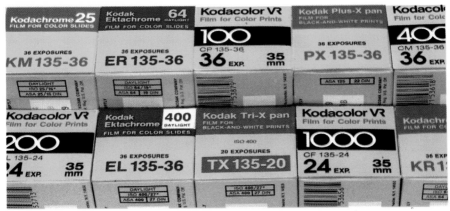

There are other considerations, too. Sharp pictures of action require fast shutter speeds (see the "Exposure" section, pages 138-141).

On the other hand, there's a good reason for choosing a low-speed film. With careful examination, prints or slides from high-speed films don't appear quite as sharp as those from the other films. For scenic pictures you may decide that it's important to have as sharp an image as possible—from an ISO (ASA) 25 film, perhaps.

Choosing a film speed is often a function of what's most important—extreme speed or extreme sharpness. If you don't need the extremes, stick to one of the medium-speed films, ISO (ASA) 64 to 200, which will be very sharp and still allow you enough speed for moderately fast action or a fairly wide range of lighting conditions.

COLOR BALANCE

Most films give natural-appearing colors in daylight or with flash. Some negative films respond almost as well to tungsten or fluorescent light. If you want correct color rendition in lighting other than daylight, choose a film balanced for a particular light source, or use color-correction filters. (See page 168 in the "Filters" section.)

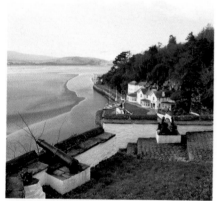

Daylight—daylight film

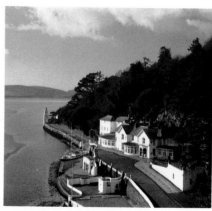

Daylight—tungsten film

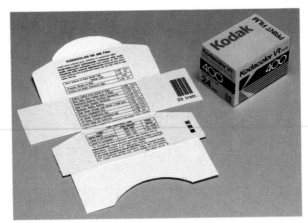

"When all else fails, read the instructions." Actually, the film data inside the box or on a sheet can be very helpful if your meter quits. Some of the information may even prove to be valuable casual reading.

FILM INSTRUCTIONS

Some of the handiest information around is in the instructions packaged with some films for automatic and adjustable cameras. You'll find data on

filtration, see the inside of the box.

CARE

All film has a useful life. Usually there's an expiration date printed on the film box. Take pictures and have the film processed before that date.

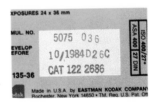

Extremes in humidity and temperature are film's worst enemies. In heat and high humidity, protect your film and camera as well as you can. For instance, don't store them in the attic or basement. Don't leave them in direct sunlight, the glove compartment of your car, or a similar high-temperature environment. When taking pictures in cold dry air, keep your camera and film close to your body so that cold film won't get brittle and snap when it is advanced or rewound. Keeping your camera warm will also help prevent static electricity marks on your film.

Try to change film in the shade, even if it's the shade of your own body to help eliminate fog marks on your film from direct, bright sunlight.

EXPOSURE

Although automatic cameras successfully choose exposure settings without human help, understanding the rudiments of exposure can improve your picture-taking. There are four factors—scene brightness, film sensitivity, shutter speed, and aperture—which affect exposure.

Extremely dim light. High- or very high-speed film—ISO (ASA) 250-1250— would be a must in this case.

SCENE BRIGHTNESS

Scene brightness can vary widely, from a sunny day at a beach with white sand to a somber plaza lighted only by a shaded street light. To record these extremes and all the variations in between, your photographic apparatus must be flexible.

FILM SENSITIVITY

As discussed on pages 133-134, film comes in a wide range of sensitivities, or speeds, for a wide range of lighting conditions and applications. Film speed helps determine camera exposure settings. Once you match the film to the situation, an ISO (ASA) 100 film for fair weather for instance, then you or the camera must adjust the shutter speed and aperture.

Bright light. A low- or medium-speed film— ISO (ASA) 25-200— would work well here.

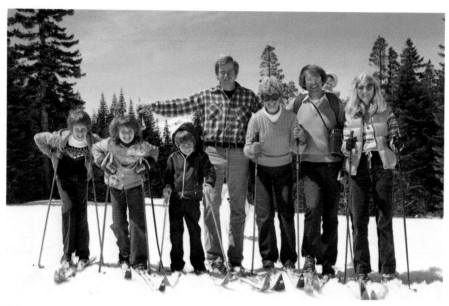

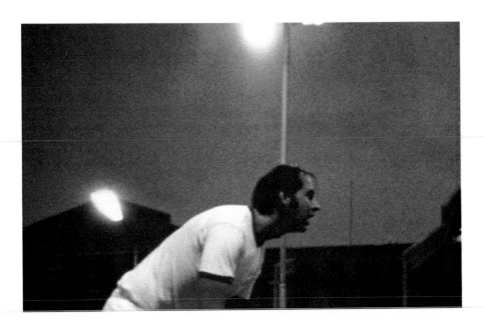

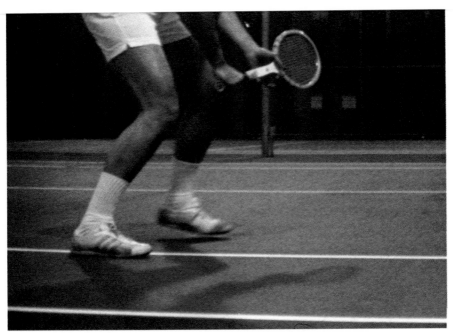

SHUTTER SPEED

The shutter speed controls the *length of time* that the shutter stays open. The longer the shutter is open, the more light it lets in. When open, it's usually for a very brief time, anywhere from 1/1000 second to 1/30 second. You can see the different speeds on your camera's shutter speed control: 1000 (1/1000), 500, 250, 125, 60, 30, and sometimes 15, 8, 4, 2 (1/2), and 1 second. The B setting is used to make time exposures. Each shutter speed is roughly half or double its immediate neighbor. The shutter will let in half as much light at 1/125 as it will at 1/60 second, but twice as much as if set at 1/250. (Older cameras may have slightly different shutter speeds, such as 500, 200, 100, 50, 25, 15, 10, 5, 2, 1. There's no cause for concern. Operation is exactly the same as with newer values. It might be helpful, however, to have the shutter speeds on an older camera checked for accuracy.)

Changing the aperture or the shutter speed will change the amount of light that reaches the film. Automatic cameras will compensate for the gain or loss in light. The picture series at right shows the effect of one-stop changes in the aperture setting. Changing the shutter speed would have produced the same results. Most people would consider the image at lower left to be correctly exposed.

APERTURE

The aperture controls the *amount* of light you let into the camera. The aperture on most automatic cameras is adjustable from a large opening, *f*/2.8, to a small opening, *f*/22. Contrary to what you'd expect, the *smaller the number, the bigger the aperture.* The *f*-number represents a ratio between the size of the aperture and the focal length of the lens. *f*/11 would mean that the aperture diameter is 1/11 the focal length of the lens. Customary aperture numbers are *f*/22, *f*/16, *f*/11, *f*/8, *f*/5.6, *f*/4, *f*/2.8, *f*/2 and occasionally *f*/1.8, *f*/1.7, or *f*/1.4.

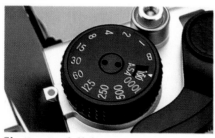

Shutter speed dial

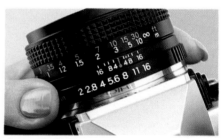

Aperture ring

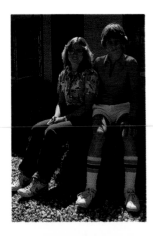
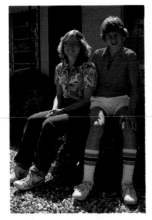
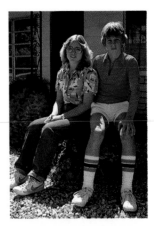

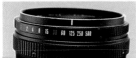
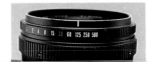
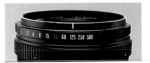

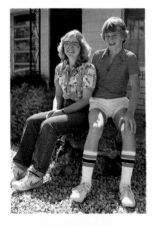
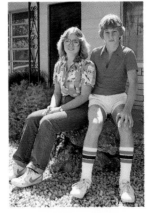
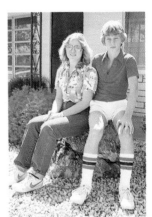

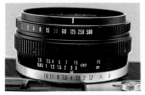
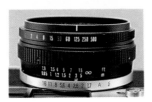
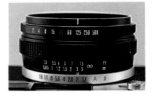

SHUTTER SPEED PLUS APERTURE

The *f*-numbers work in one sense the same way as shutter speeds. An aperture set at *f*/2.8 lets in twice as much light as its neighbor on the scale, *f*/4, but only half as much as its neighbor on the other side, *f*/2. The big surprise is that the unit spacing for shutter speeds and *f*-numbers is comparable. A change from one shutter speed to the next gives the same exposure result as changing from one *f*-number to the next. This means that several different combinations of *f*-number and shutter speed will give good exposure under the same lighting conditions with the same film. For instance, if you set aperture and shutter speed at *f*/8 and 1/125, respectively, you can get the same exposure as if you had set *f*/5.6 and 1/250, *f*/4 and 1/500, *f*/2.8 and 1/1000, *f*/11 and 1/60, *f*/16 and 1/30, or *f*/22 and 1/15-second.

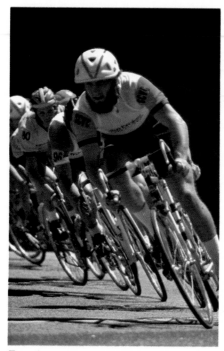

Fast shutter speed

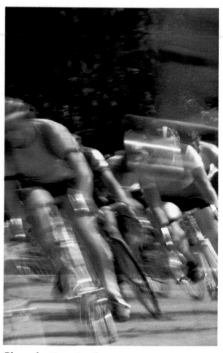

Slow shutter speed

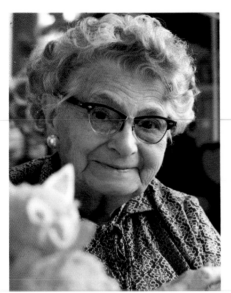
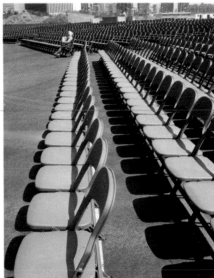

What's the reason for all the numbers? If you think back a second, you'll realize that you need the extensive adjustments to cope with all the possibilities in lighting that you're likely to come across. There are other reasons as well. Fast shutter speeds such as 1/250, 1/500, and 1/1000 will stop rapid action. Slow shutter speeds such as 1/30, 1/15, and 1/8 second are often used intentionally to blur certain action subjects into a swirl of color and motion. Moderate shutter speeds are used for general photography—fast enough to negate hand movement, but slow enough to permit middle-size apertures and medium-speed film.

On the other hand, changing the aperture changes the depth of field (explained in detail on pages 144-145). Large apertures such as $f/2.8$ and $f/2$ give a shallow depth of field where only your subject, or part of your subject, is in sharp focus. Small apertures such as $f/16$ and $f/22$ give great depth of field. Experienced photographers use all these controls—film speed, shutter speed, and aperture size—to keep as much control over the resulting picture as possible.

141

EXPOSURE METERS

Getting the right exposure for a given situation is often a matter of opinion. Some photographers prefer their slides a little darker than others. Generally, though, acceptable exposure will still show some detail in the brightest areas and some in the darkest.

Most people use manually adjustable cameras with built-in exposure meters or automatic cameras in which a built-in meter sets the shutter speed, the aperture, or both. In any case, the meter will gather the exposure information for you. Always take a reading very close to the subject before stepping back and composing the picture. Check your camera or exposure meter instruction manual for information on its operation.

There are times when a camera exposure meter will not make the right exposure decision. What you must do is recognize the situation and compensate. Here are typical situations and compensations:

Sidelighted subject	increase exposure 1/2 stop
Backlighted subject	increase exposure 1 stop
Small bright subject against dark background	decrease exposure 1 stop
Small dark subject against bright background	increase exposure 1 stop
Average subject in extremely bright scene, such as snow or sand	increase exposure 1 stop

Although camera exposure meters take much of the work out of determining and setting exposure, they often miss in the situations described at left. With an adjustable camera that has a built-in meter, make your meter reading, and then adjust as recommended at left.

On some automatic cameras, there is a way to override manually the automatic exposure feature. It may be a dial that offers up to a two-stop increase or decrease in exposure. It may also be a way to switch the camera to completely manual operation.

Other cameras are entirely automatic with no apparent way to alter the camera-selected settings. To increase the exposure by one stop, set the film-speed indicator to a value half of the speed of the film you're using. To increase exposure by two stops, cut the film speed to one quarter of the real value of the film in the camera. The reverse is true for decreasing exposure. Double the film speed setting for a one-stop decrease in exposure and quadruple it for a two-stop decrease. *DO NOT FORGET TO RETURN THE FILM-SPEED SETTING TO THE CORRECT VALUE AFTER YOU'VE MADE YOUR SPECIAL-SITUATION PICTURE.*

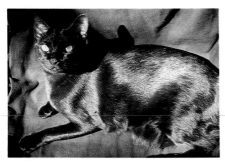

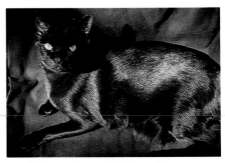

Meter recommendation   *Decrease exposure one stop*

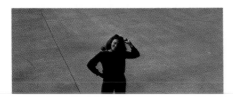

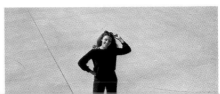

Meter recommendation   *Increase exposure one stop*

EXPOSURE SUMMARY

1. Use medium-speed film in normal outdoor situations, high- or very high-speed film in dim scenes, and low-speed film for the sharpest pictures possible.
2. Use a shutter speed at least as fast as 1/125 second for most situations to prevent camera movement from blurring your picture.
3. Fast shutter speeds capture action; slow shutter speeds blur action.
4. Large apertures give shallow depth of field; small apertures give great depth of field.
5. Usually several combinations of shutter speed and aperture will give correct exposure. Review the reasons for choosing shutter speeds and apertures.
6. Check the manual for your exposure meter or automatic camera to compensate for very bright and very dark subjects.
7. Sidelighting and backlighting often require more exposure than frontlighting—one half and one stop, respectively.

Note: If the film speed selector on your camera cannot register a very high-speed film such as ISO (ASA) 1000, compensate by setting it to 500 for this instance and using the next faster shutter speed or the next smaller aperture.

DEPTH OF FIELD

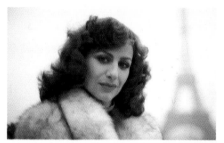
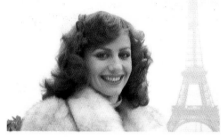

Shallow depth of field—f/2　　　　　*Great depth of field—f/22*

When you focus your camera lens on a subject, you are unknowingly including a greater area in focus. Each aperture setting gives a different depth of field—that is, the distance range that is in acceptably sharp focus. Small apertures such as *f*/11, *f*/16, and *f*/22 give the greatest depth of field, while large apertures such as *f*/2.8, *f*/2, and *f*/1.4 give very little depth of field.

Many single-lens-reflex cameras incorporate a previewer that shows how much of the scene is sharp at different apertures. Other cameras usually include a depth-of-field scale that surrounds the distance scale on the lens barrel. By looking at the indicators for the *f*/number you are using, you can see how much of the scene will be sharp in front of and behind the subject.

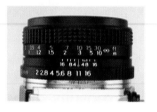

Depth of field also depends on the camera-to-subject distance. With the same aperture, depth of field will be shallower if you focus on a nearby object than if you focus on a distant one.

You can include more foreground than background by focusing closer than your main subject but still keeping the subject within the depth of field. The reverse is also true.

You can use your understanding of depth of field to preset your camera in a fast-action situation so that you won't have to refocus as the activity gets close and then recedes. Set the smallest aperture your action shutter speed will allow and then focus on the spot where most of the action will take place. Even if things drift back and forth a little, your pictures will still be in focus.

By aligning the indicators for the aperture setting (f-number) on the depth-of-field scale with the distances on the focusing ring, you can see the range that will be in sharp focus. The aperture above is f/11. The indicators—between 16 and 8 on the depth-of-field scale—show that anything at a distance between 7 and 15 feet from the camera will be in acceptably sharp focus.

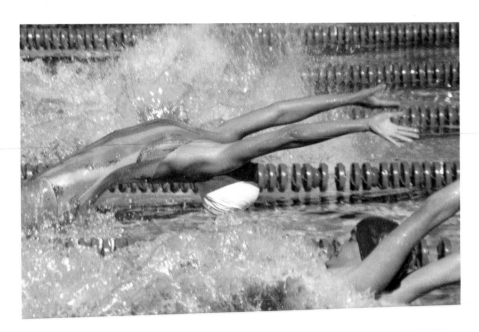

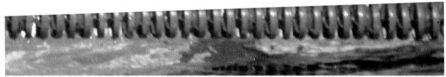

With a small aperture and preset focus, you can concentrate on the action.

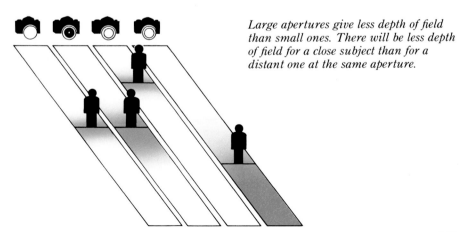

Large apertures give less depth of field than small ones. There will be less depth of field for a close subject than for a distant one at the same aperture.

LIGHTING

Light is the basis for all picture-taking. Light in the morning is a striking change from light at noon. Bright days are vastly different from cloudy days. Shady spots, open fields, and home interiors, summer, fall, winter, and spring all have their unique light properties—all somehow adaptable for good pictures. Let's first discuss the angles of light that apply for almost any situation.

ANGLES OF LIGHT

There are three basic lighting angles—frontlighting, sidelighting, and backlighting. Frontlighting means that light is coming from behind the photographer, brightening the side of the subject facing the photographer. A sidelighted subject has light striking one side, and backlighting illuminates the side of the subject away from the photographer. Frontlighting is common for most picture-taking, but it may not give the most effec-

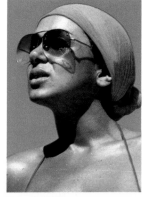

Frontlighting

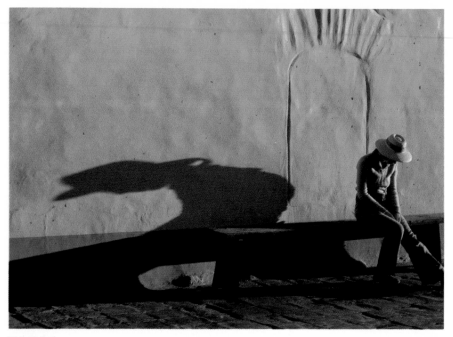

Sidelighting

146

tive photos. People tend to squint when looking into the sun and dark shadows surround their eyes. Frontlighting is also flat, giving few shadows that help create a feeling of perspective.

Sidelighting is more dramatic, with shadows streaking across the picture, helping to establish shape and three-dimensionality. Sidelighting can also give portraits increased impact. Many photographers prefer backlighting for close-up pictures of people, because their subjects never have to look near the sun. Expressions are relaxed and natural and there are no contrasting shadow and lighted areas. Backlighting may also give striking scenic pictures, especially early or late in the day, with long shadows racing back toward the camera from rich, black silhouettes. Sidelighting and backlighting require exposure adjustments for properly exposed subjects (not silhouettes). See page 142-143 in "Exposure" for more information.

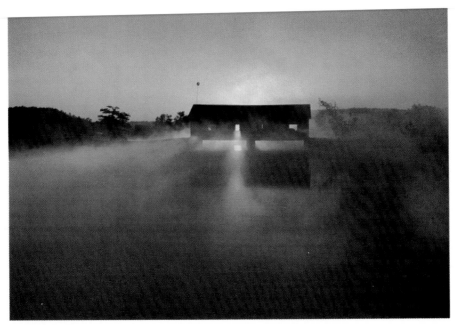

Backlighting

IN THE SUN OR OUT

You also have a choice between photographing a subject in bright sunlight or in shade. It depends on the subject. If you want hard, black shadows, photograph in sunlight. If you want a softer quality of light (although a little cooler-colored) take your subject into a shady spot that's clear overhead. There will be plenty of light, but no harshness.

Light overcast days are excellent for some picture-taking. If you have diffused sunlight that creates soft shadows, you have perfect lighting for a portrait.

COPING WITH SUNLIGHT

Sunlight gives shadows. You can reduce the intensity of these shadows by using a crinkled foil or white reflector to bounce light back at the subject. Experiment by angling a white or foil-covered piece of cardboard in different directions to see how much reflection you want.

You can also use light from a flash device to fill in shadows. (See page 160 in "Flash" for more information.)

DIFFERENT TIMES OF DAY

The color and intensity of sunlight changes throughout the day. Early morning photographers (dawn to 9 a.m.) are rewarded with a soft, pale, sometimes rosy light, painting long shadows that

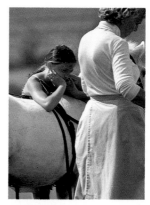
Bright sun

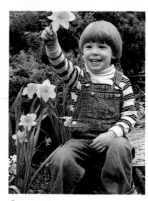
Overcast

Dawn

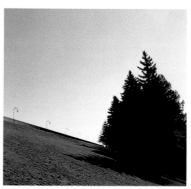
9 AM

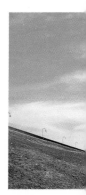
Noon

148

are freshened by dew. It's beautiful light for landscapes, especially if you find a few patches of low-lying ground fog. People benefit from this light, too. From 10 a.m. to 4 p.m., sunlight is brilliant and harsh, dropping small, dense shadows. Ordinarily it's not very attractive unless that's the mood you want. From 4 p.m. to sunset, the light deepens in warm tones and lavishly smooths rich shadows across the land. It's dramatic lighting for side-lighted landscapes and sometimes even people. Between sunset and complete darkness comes perfect lighting and color for existing-light cityscapes. (See pages 162-165.)

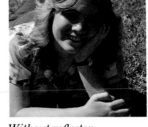

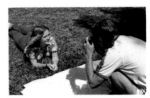

Without reflector

INTENSITY

Although our eyes don't see it, there's a vast difference in the intensity of light as it changes. A shaded spot is much darker than a sunlighted area, as is any scene on a cloudy day. Indoors, it's *much* darker than outdoors. ...

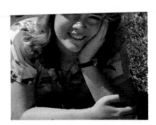

Bedsheet reflector

... your camera make the adjustments necessary for changing lighting conditions. (See pages 136-143, "Exposure," and page 133, "Film," for more information about scene brightness.)

Light gives our pictures a chance to appear. It is endlessly variable, and if you study its effects, you'll be able to apply your knowledge to making better pictures in any situation.

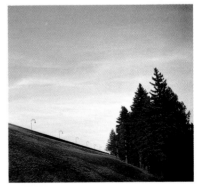

With reflector

4 PM

Sunset

SEASONS

As the seasons change, so does the nature of light. Have you ever noticed how much stronger midsummer light is than spring or winter light? Remember those crisp autumn days when the edges of every leaf seem to snap out toward you? Indeed, the lighting is different. Winter with snow finds the sun at a low angle casting weak shadows, reflecting off snow and ice everywhere. Your meter may be fooled by all the whiteness into recommending underexposure. For snow scenes, increase your exposure one stop (see page 142 in "Exposure") over the meter reading. Springtime also brings weakened sunlight, not reinforced by snow reflections. It's beautiful light for people and other subjects not flattered by strong contrast between shadow and light areas. The sun in summer seems to beat down with a vengeance, almost too strong for most picture-taking. By carefully watching the angles and time of day, you can take endless, excellent pictures in summertime, when all the world comes out to play. Clear, strong (but not overpowering) sunlight characterizes autumn. Brilliant for landscapes, it can also give lovely shade-lighted portraits.

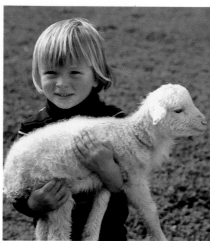

Spring

Summer

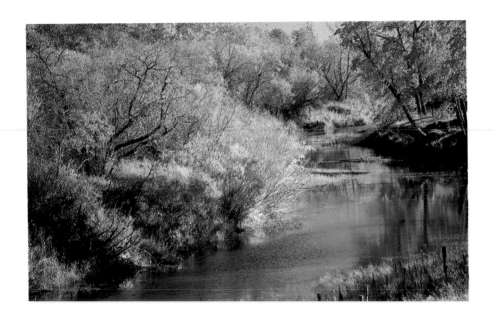

Fall

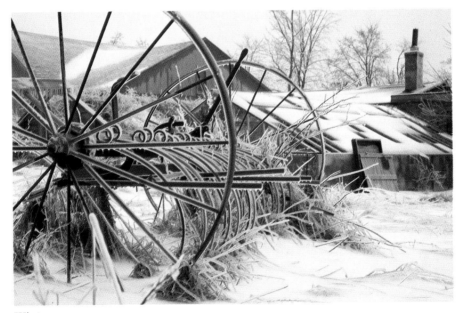

Winter

FLASH

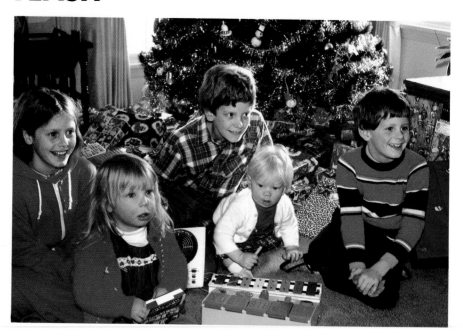

When it's too dark to take pictures, the logical decision is to use flash. Some cameras even tell you when it's necessary. There is nothing tricky about flash photography, provided you know the basics and understand your equipment.

GENERAL TIPS

Reflections Watch out for reflective backgrounds or eyeglasses in the scene. If you take a flash picture directly at either, you'll get an unattractive glare spot in your picture. Stand at an angle to mirrors, windows, or shiny paneling. Ask subjects wearing glasses to turn their heads slightly or remove their glasses.

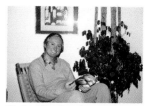

Reflection in glass

Red Reflections Some people's eyes (and some pets') can reflect flash with an eerie, often red glow. To prevent this internal reflection of the flash, turn on all the room lights—the extra brightness will help reduce the size of the iris. Then, if possible, increase the distance between flash and camera

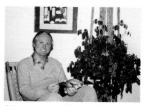

Change position.

152

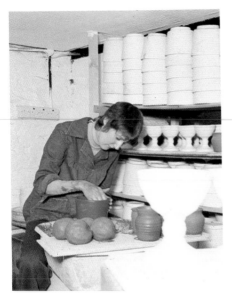 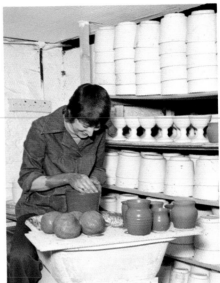

lens. Some cameras will accept a flash extender. Finally, back off to a point within the flash range where the reflections will be less noticeable.

Flash Range With snapshot cameras, photograph subjects within the flash range recommended for your camera, flash type, and film. With other cameras, the range for good flash exposure is determined by the film speed, the aperture setting, and possibly the flash mode.

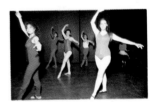

Subjects scattered at different distances.

Overexposed Foreground Any person or object closer than the minimum limit of the flash range will be overexposed and too bright in your flash picture. Compose the scene so that the main subject is closer than anything else, but still within the flash range.

Several Subjects Subjects at different distances from the camera will receive different amounts of flash light—some will be too bright or too dark. Make sure that all your subjects are roughly the same distance from the flash.

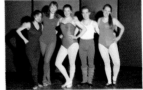

Subjects grouped at same distance.

153

SNAPSHOT CAMERAS

To get well-exposed pictures with your snapshot camera, keep your subject in the correct flash distance range—usually 4 to 9 feet with flashcubes, use fresh batteries, and keep the camera-battery contacts clean. With flashcubes, magicubes, or flipflash, check to see that an unused bulb is in position before making an exposure. If you have an add-on or built-in electronic flash unit, see the general information below.

ELECTRONIC FLASH

The most popular flash accessory for 35 mm cameras is the electronic flash unit. Different systems are detailed in the following pages. Before searching for your flash and camera combination, read the general tips below.

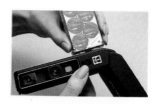
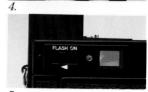

1. On a camera with built-in flash, make sure that the film-speed setting is correct for good exposure. Set your film speed on a separate flash unit.

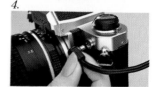

2. If necessary, set the shutter speed recommended by your camera manual for electronic flash. Because the flash duration is typically 1/1000 or less, shutter speed does not affect exposure. If set too fast, however, you'll get partly exposed pictures with a focal-plane shutter or underexposed pictures with a leaf shutter.

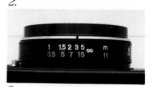

3. Focus carefully. Camera-to-subject distance determines exposure with built-in flash.

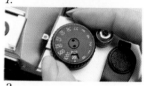

4. Cameras that don't have built-in flash have an accessory shoe that may be electrically sensitive—a hot shoe. Slide a flash unit with a matching hot foot into the shoe to make the necessary connection. Older cameras or flash units may not be hot. Plug the cord (PC cord) that usually comes with the flash unit into flash and camera. If there is a choice of camera sockets, choose the one marked X—the other is for flashbulbs.

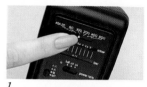

5. Flash units take a few seconds to get ready (recycle) for the next picture. The ready light will glow when the flash is ready. When the ready light takes a long time to glow, change the batteries or recharge the flash unit.

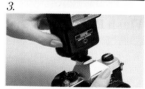

BUILT-IN AND
DEDICATED AUTOMATIC

Some 35 mm cameras have a built-in flash unit or can be matched with a special flash unit—a "dedicated" system. Turn on the flash, focus, and take a picture. The camera and flash combination makes exposure settings automatically. Cameras with built-in flash rely on the film speed set on the camera. Separate flash units may need to have the film speed set on a dial.

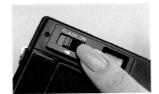

Press a button to raise and activate the flash.

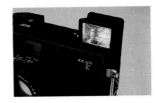

Other cameras work automatically with any flash, provided that you follow instructions and preset any necessary adjustments, such as flash mode switch or the guide number. (See page 157.) It's necessary to set the focus carefully for sharp pictures *and* for correct exposure. (Focusing also controls the aperture.)

SENSOR-CONTROLLED AUTOMATIC

set the film speed on the flash, and select an aperture and a corresponding flash mode, the sensor will govern how much light the flash emits by measuring the intensity of light reflected by the subject. For each aperture and mode combination, the sensor will be able to control flash output over a certain distance range. Read the instruction manual carefully for correct operation of sensor-controlled automatic flash units.

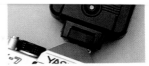

The sensor inside the circle governs flash output.

With a sensor-automatic flash unit, you decide what distance range you'll need, choose the appropriate flash mode, and set the aperture. The flash will do the rest to give good exposure. Make sure to set the film speed on the flash unit. The unit pictured is set at its yellow mode which gives a range of 1.6 to 8.5 feet with an ISO (ASA) 100 film at f/8.

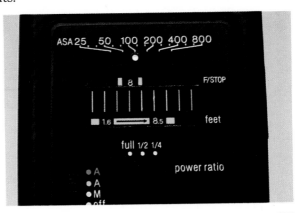

MANUAL FLASH UNITS,
MANUAL OR AUTOMATIC CAMERAS

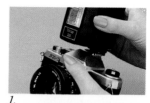

1.

Older or inexpensive flash units operate at full power for every picture. You have to adjust the camera for correctly exposed flash pictures. Since the shutter speed will always be the same (as recommended by the camera instruction manual— usually 1/30, 1/60, or 1/125 second) you have to set the aperture. Here's a typical operation given in a step-by-step sequence.

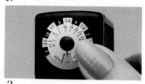

2.

1. Attach the flash unit to the camera. If the camera does not have a hot shoe, connect camera and flash with a PC connecting cord*.
2. Set the film speed on the calculator of the flash unit.
3. Set the correct flash shutter speed on the camera.
4. Turn on the flash unit.
5. Focus on your subject.

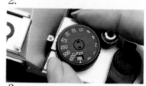

3.

6. Check the lens distance scale for the distance between flash and subject, assuming that the flash is attached to the camera. (Exposure is always based on the distance between *flash* and *subject*—not camera and subject.)
7. Apply the distance to the flash unit calculator to find the correct aperture.
8. Set the aperture on the camera.
9. Take the picture.

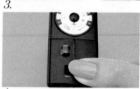

4.

The process usually takes only a few seconds. Many people preset their cameras at 10 feet, particularly at parties and take pictures from that distance only.

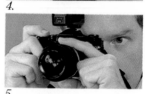

5.

*Older cameras may require you to choose a socket for the PC cord or select a synchronization setting. If faced with a choice of sockets, plug the cord into the socket marked X for electronic flash. The other socket is for a flash-bulb unit. Set a synchronizing switch at X as well. Check your camera manual for additional flash synchronization instructions.

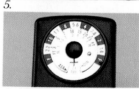

6. *and* 7.

Note: If the film-speed dial won't register the 1000-speed film you're using, set it to 500 and select a lens opening one stop smaller than indicated.

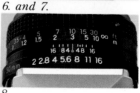

8.

GUIDE NUMBERS

The proliferation of automatic flash systems has nearly erased the memory of a formula used to calculate aperture settings for flash pictures. It may be handy in a pinch.

It works like this. If you know the guide number for your flash unit/film combination, you can easily set the aperture when you know the flash-subject distance. Merely divide the guide number by the distance—the resulting number is the aperture, or very close to it. See the example below.

Guide Number Formula The guide number of the flash unit is 65 with ISO (ASA) 100 film. Flash-to-subject distance is 8 feet.

$$65 \div 8 = f/8 \text{ (round when necessary)}$$

Often the guide number for a particular unit is given for only one film speed. Do the same calculations but add or subtract f-stops as indicated by the

using. (If you're using ISO (ASA) 100 switch to ISO (ASA) 200 film, perform your usual guide number calculation and then select the next smaller f-stop.)

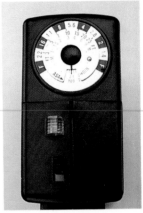

If you need the guide number for a flash unit that has an exposure calculator, set the film speed, and read the guide

The guide number changes for different film speeds.

CARE AND HANDLING

An electronic flash unit's worst enemies are weak batteries and infrequency of use. Particularly with rechargeable models that use nickel-cadmium cells, try to take a few flash pictures every month. Better yet, remove and store batteries in the freezer to preserve their life and protect the flash unit's contacts. Remove the batteries with the power on and the capacitor fully charged to protect the flash unit during storage. Before taking pictures after storage, allow frozen batteries several hours of thawing time to reach room temperature. Then, put them in the unit and form the capacitor by firing the flash manually several times. Remember that weak batteries can shorten the life of your flash unit, and it should enjoy a long life.

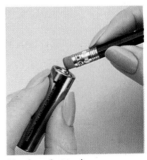

Replace batteries as recommended. Extend their useful life by occasionally cleaning the contacts with a pencil eraser.

157

FLASH OFF CAMERA

Moving the flash off the camera flatters many subjects. The lighting gives enough shadow for a three-dimensional appearance.

Removing the flash from the camera may defeat the automatic function of a dedicated flash system. If so, determine exposure by using the manual method described on page 156. Most sensor-

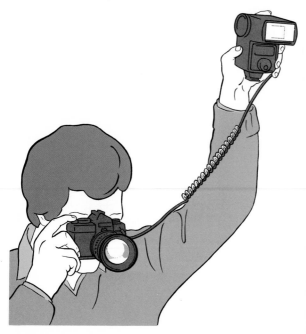

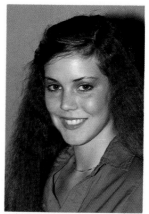

Flash on camera

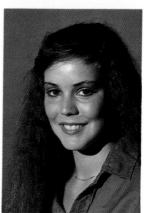

Flash off camera

operated automatic units will perform if the sensor is aimed at the subject, and certainly most manual units will work. All you need is an extension PC cord to connect camera and flash. Remember that *flash-to-subject distance* determines aperture setting. It won't be very different if you hold the unit at arm's length. But if a friend or family member holds the flash unit at a distance different from the camera-subject distance, make your exposure adjustments based on *flash-to-subject* distance.

BOUNCE FLASH

Bouncing the flash off the ceiling or a nearby wall is another way to improve your subject's appearance. The indirect light is softer, less harsh, and often the soft shadows can help you create a feeling of three-dimensional form.

Again, the idea and execution are fairly simple. Some sensor-governed automatic units will work correctly, provided that the sensor is aimed at your subject. If this is impossible, operate the unit manually, as you will have to do with some

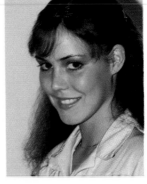

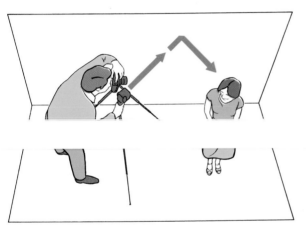

dedicated automatic flash units or a manual unit. Here's how.

Choose a location near a white or light-neutral colored wall or ceiling. The wall may be preferable because it won't cast shadows under a person's eyes. Calculate the distance that the light must travel from flash-to-wall-to-subject. Estimate the aperture necessary for that distance and then open up the aperture an additional two f-stops. For instance, let's say that the distance is 15 feet (7 feet from flash to wall and 8 feet back to the subject) and your flash calculator recommends an aperture of f/5.6. Instead of f/5.6, set f/2.8 on the aperture ring.

Your wall and ceiling situations are unique. It's a wise idea to experiment a little with slide film and keep records to fine tune your exposure.

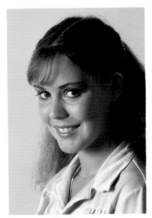

Bounce flash

FILL-IN FLASH

One way to reduce the contrast of shadow and lighted areas in bright sunlight is to fill those shadows with light from an electronic flash unit. (The results may also be satisfactory with a snapshot camera. Try it and see.)

Manual and Sensor-Governed Units The idea is to add a hint of light to a subject in frontlighting, sidelighting, backlighting, or even in the shade. Too much flash light may make your picture appear artificial. Follow these simple guidelines for most manual and sensor-governed automatic flash units.

1. Set the shutter speed recommended for flash photography. Set the aperture for the prevailing lighting conditions with that shutter speed.
2. Set the calculator on your manual or sensor-governed automatic flash unit to a number two or three times as great as the speed of the film you're using. This way the flash will not overpower existing-lighting conditions.
3. Locate yourself and your subject at the distance recommended on the flash calculator for the aperture already set on the camera.
4. Take a flash picture.

Dedicated Automatic Flash Fill On cameras with built-in flash units, just extend the flash and take a picture. There isn't much you can control. Try taping a layer of white tissue over the flash to soften the light. Because cameras that have matched, separate flash units vary in their approach to fill-in flash, read the instructions for your outfit carefully. Make sure you don't cover the sensor with tissue.

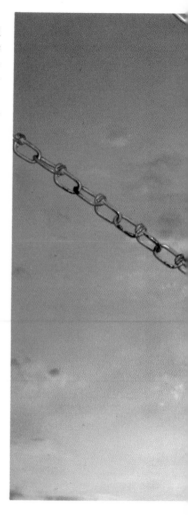

ACTION

The duration of an electronic flash is usually much shorter than your fastest shutter speed. This high-speed capability can stop even very fast action in dark places—children playing, pets jumping, Ping-Pong players smashing, and so on. Exposure is based on flash-to-subject distance. Remember that bounce flash provides more natural light.

160

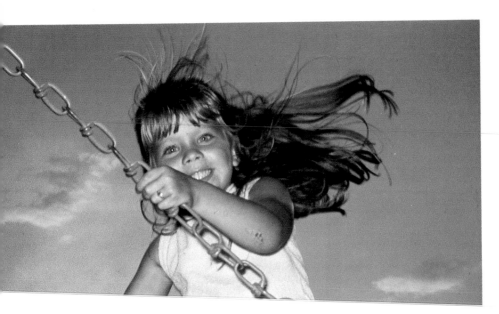

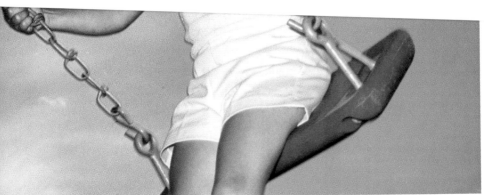

Flash is a useful tool that will serve you in many more ways than merely brightening dark interiors. Fill-in flash will brighten the shaded side of a subject outdoors which allows people to look away from the sun. They can relax their faces and eyes from squinting and offer more cheerful, natural expressions. Flash can also stop fast action for a picture, as in the case of the swinging child above.

EXISTING LIGHT

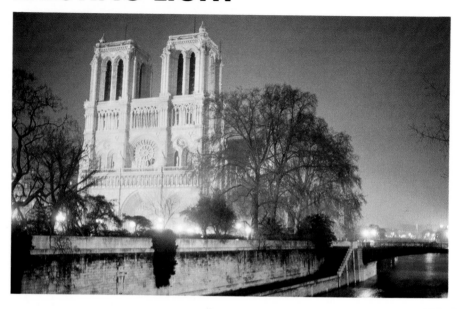

Taking pictures by existing light means picture-taking in dim lighting without flash. You need high- or very high-speed film [ISO (ASA) 250–1250] and a lens with an *f*/2.8 maximum aperture or larger. Read the following pointers and have a look at the exposure suggestions on page 165.

Take exposure meter readings as close to your subject as possible. Avoid reading parts of the scene that include a bright light source, such as this candle. The small spot of bright light may confuse your exposure meter into recommending underexposure.

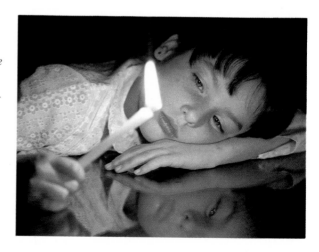

SOME POINTERS

1. Don't include a bright light source when making a meter reading. The light will fool your meter into recommending underexposure.
2. Make meter readings close to your subject.
3. With an automatic camera, get as close as possible to your subject to take the picture.
4. The side of your subject facing the light should probably be the one you photograph.
5. Since your shutter speeds may be fairly slow—often at 1/30 second—hold your camera steady.
6. If you use a shutter speed slower than 1/30 second, brace your camera against something solid or mount it on a tripod.

duces the light available.

8. KODAK EKTACHROME Films and equivalents can be push-processed one additional stop by your photofinisher. If you're using an ISO (ASA) 400 film, set the film speed dial at ISO (ASA) 800 when you ask for special (push) processing. Expose the whole roll at the same film speed.

9. A wide range of exposures may be acceptable in many existing-light situations. Experiment with different exposures to see what you prefer.

10. At the very large apertures you'll be using (f/2.8 or f/2), depth of field is very shallow. (See pages 144-145 for more on depth of field.) Make sure to focus carefully

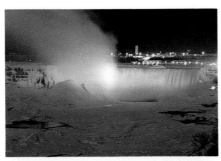
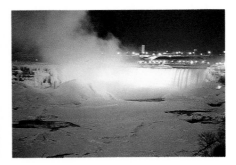

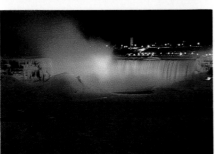

Many existing-light scenes can be captured with a wide range of exposures, as you see in these views of Niagara Falls. It's wise, in fact, to take several pictures at different exposure settings, so that you'll have several to choose from. Left: 2 seconds at f/4, ISO (ASA) 800. Top left: 4 seconds at f/4, ISO (ASA) 800. Top right: 8 seconds at f/4, ISO (ASA) 800.

Suggested Exposures Consider the exposure settings shown in the table at right as guidelines. It's wise to bracket your exposures, especially with slide film, because many existing-light scenes can fool an automatic camera or built-in exposure meter. Typical existing-light subjects may be acceptable in a wide range of exposures, especially outdoors at night.

☐ *For color slides, use tungsten film. You can use daylight film, but your slides will look yellow-red.*

☐ *For color slides, use daylight film or tungsten film with No. 85B filter and 1 stop more exposure.*

☐ *For color slides, use either daylight or tungsten film.*

For color prints you can use KODACOLOR films for all the scenes listed.

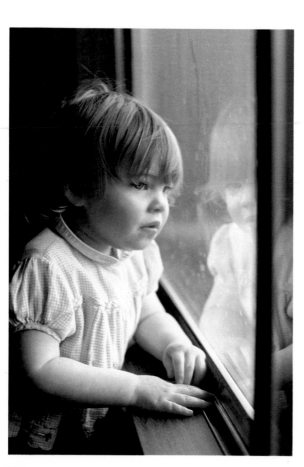

In a window-light portrait like this, you'll probably get best results when you take your exposure reading from the bright side of your subject's face. Emphasize that side when you compose the picture.

164

Suggested Exposures for Existing-Light Pictures

Picture Subject	ISO (ASA) 64-100*	ISO (ASA) 125-200	ISO (ASA) 400††	ISO (ASA) 1000
AT HOME				
Home interiors at night				
Areas with bright light	1/15 sec f/2	1/30 sec f/2	1/30 sec f/2.8	1/60 sec f/4
Areas with average light	1/4 sec f/2.8	1/15 sec f/2	1/30 sec f/2	1/30 sec f/4
Candlelighted close-ups	1/4 sec f/2	1/8 sec f/2	1/15 sec f/2	1/30 sec f/2.8
Indoor and outdoor holiday lighting at night, Christmas trees	1 sec f/4	1 sec f/5.6	1/15 sec f/2	1/30 sec f/2.8
OUTDOORS AT NIGHT				
Brightly lighted downtown street scenes (Wet streets add interesting reflections.)	1/30 sec f/2	1/30 sec f/2.8	1/60 sec f/2.8	1/125 sec f/4
Brightly lighted nightclub or theatre districts—Las Vegas or Times Square	1/30 sec f/2.8	1/30 sec f/4	1/60 sec f/4	1/125 sec f/5.6
Neon signs and other lighted signs	1/30 sec f/4	1/60 sec f/4	1/125 sec f/4	1/125 sec f/8
Floodlighted buildings, fountains, monuments	1 sec f/4	1/2 sec f/4	1/15 sec f/2	1/30 sec f/2.8
Skyline—distant view of lighted buildings at night	4 sec f/2.8	1 sec f/2	1 sec f/2.8	1 sec f/5.6
Skyline—10 minutes after sunset	1/30 sec f/4	1/60 sec f/4	1/60 sec f/5.6	1/125 sec f/8
Fairs, amusement parks	1/15 sec f/2	1/30 sec f/2	1/30 sec f/2.8	1/60 sec f/4
bursts.)				
Burning buildings, campfires, bonfires	1/30 sec f/2.8	1/30 sec f/4	1/60 sec f/4	1/125 sec f/5.6
Night football, baseball, racetracks†	1/30 sec f/2.8	1/60 sec f/2.8	1/125 sec f/2.8	1/250 sec f/4
Niagara Falls				
White lights	15 sec f/5.6	8 sec f/5.6	4 sec f/5.6	4 sec f/11
Light-colored lights	30 sec f/5.6	15 sec f/5.6	8 sec f/5.6	4 sec f/8
Dark-colored lights	30 sec f/4	30 sec f/5.6	15 sec f/5.6	4 sec f/5.6
INDOORS IN PUBLIC PLACES				
Basketball, hockey, bowling	1/30 sec f/2	1/60 sec f/2	1/125 sec f/2	1/250 sec f/2.8
Stage shows				
Average	1/30 sec f/2	1/30 sec f/2.8	1/60 sec f/2.8	1/125 sec f/4
Bright	1/60 sec f/2.8	1/60 sec f/4	1/125 sec f/4	1/250 sec f/5.6
Circuses				
Floodlighted acts	1/30 sec f/2	1/30 sec f/2.8	1/60 sec f/2.8	1/250 sec f/2.8
Spotlighted acts (carbon-arc)	1/60 sec f/2.8	1/125 sec f/2.8	1/250 sec f/2.8	1/250 sec f/5.6
Ice shows				
Floodlighted acts	1/30 sec f/2.8	1/60 sec f/2.8	1/125 sec f/2.8	1/250 sec f/4
Spotlighted acts (carbon-arc)	1/60 sec f/2.8	1/125 sec f/2.8	1/250 sec f/2.8	1/250 sec f/5.6
Interiors with bright fluorescent light	1/30 sec f/2.8	1/30 sec f/4	1/60 sec f/4	1/125 sec f/5.6
School—stage and auditorium	—	1/15 sec f/2	1/30 sec f/2	1/30 sec f/4
Church interiors—tungsten light	1 sec f/5.6	1/15 sec f/2	1/30 sec f/2	1/30 sec f/4
Stained-glass windows, daytime— photographed from inside	Use 3 stops more exposure than for the outdoor lighting conditions.			

*With ISO (ASA) 25-32 film, increase exposure by 2 stops.

†When lighting is provided by tungsten lamps and you want color slides, use Tungsten films.

**If your camera doesn't have this lens opening, use the next larger opening.

††KODAK EKTACHROME 400 Film (Daylight) may be rated at ISO (ASA) 800 when push processed. Merely decrease suggested exposure in this column by one stop.

FILTERS

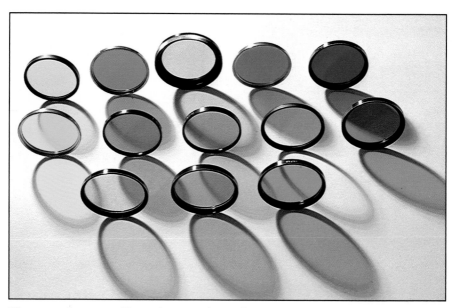

Photographers use filters for a variety of reasons. With color film, filters can enhance or diminish effects of lighting color. They can also correct the color of light for film of a particular balance. (See "Film," page 134.) Haze and reflections can be diminished and saturation of colors can be increased with a polarizing filter. Deep color filters primarily used for black-and-white film can be used for special effects with color film. With black-and-white film, filters can increase contrast, correct tonal relationships, reduce haze, and control reflections.

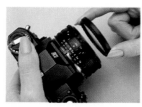

Many glass-mounted filters are available that will screw directly into the front of your lens.

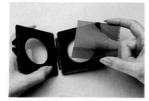

Other filters are available as acetate squares. The squares fit into special frames.

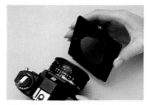

The frames screw into the front of your lens, and can be adapted for a number of lens sizes.

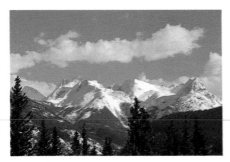

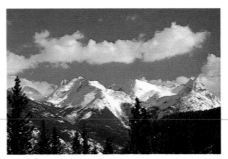

Without polarizer

With polarizer

COLOR FILM

Polarizer The polarizing filter reduces reflections from airborn moisture in the sky (haze) and from non-metallic sources. This means that sky, grass, and other subjects will show more accurate, richer

Polarizers will reduce reflections from non-

effect. You may also adjust the effect on most polarizing filters by turning the outer filter ring. A polarizing filter always requires a 1⅓-stop exposure increase. Adjust an automatic camera manually because the meter may not give correct exposure.

reflection you eliminate by operating the adjusting ring on the filter. You may want to retain some sparkle in water scenes.

Without polarizer

With polarizer

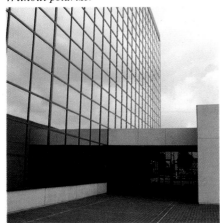

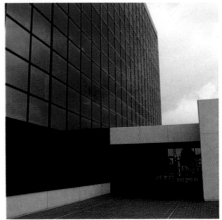

Color Correction Filters In the section on "Film," page 134, we discussed films with different color balance. It's convenient if the film in your camera always matches the light where you're photographing. When it doesn't, you can attach the appropriate filter. See the table at right for possible film, light, and filter combinations. Notice also that the table gives exposure adjustment information. Since all filters block some of the light entering the camera, you must always give extra exposure. Operate your camera manually if possible. Meter the scene without a filter attached, make the necessary adjustment, and then add the filter for your picture. (This may not be necessary with through-the-lens metering.) One note here—typical household lighting is tungsten 2900 K. There are also special lights for photography called photolamps 3200 K and 3400 K which require a different film and slightly different filters.

Table Instructions

Conversion filters change the color quality of a light source to match the quality of the light for which a color film is balanced. The table at right shows which filter to use with various film and light combinations. The table also shows how much additional exposure to give for the filters listed.

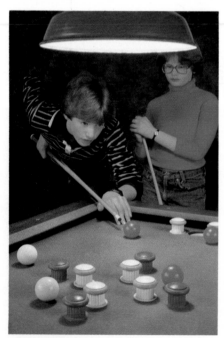

Tungsten light, daylight film, no filter.

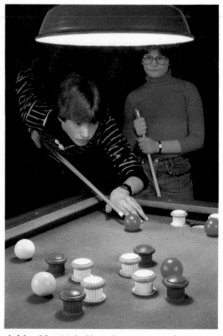

Add a No. 80A filter for correct color.

Conversion Filters for KODAK Color Films

KODAK Color Films	Balanced for	Filter and *f*-Stop Change		
		Daylight	Photolamp (3400 K)	Tungsten (3200 K)
All KODACOLOR Films	Daylight, Blue Flash, or Electronic Flash	No filter	*No. 80B + 1⅔ stops	*No. 80A + 2 stops
KODACHROME 25 (Daylight)		No filter	No. 80B + 1⅔ stops	No. 80A + 2 stops
KODACHROME 40–5070 (Type A)	Photolamps (3400 K)	No. 85 + ⅔ stop	No filter	No. 82A + ⅓ stop
KODACHROME 64 (Daylight) and EKTACHROME 64 (Daylight)	Daylight, Blue Flash, or Electronic Flash	No filter	No. 80B + 1⅔ stops	No. 80A + 2 stops
EKTACHROME 200 (Daylight)		No filter	No. 80B + 1⅔ stops	No. 80A + 2 stops
EKTACHROME 400 (Daylight)		No filter	No. 80B + 1⅔ stops	No. 80A + 2 stops
EKTACHROME 160 (Tungsten)	Tungsten (3200 K)	No. 85B + ⅔ stop	No. 81A* + ⅓ stop	No filter

Note: Increase exposure by the amount shown in the table.   *For critical use.
If your camera has a built-in exposure meter that can
make a reading through a filter used over the lens,
see your camera manual for instructions on exposure with filters.

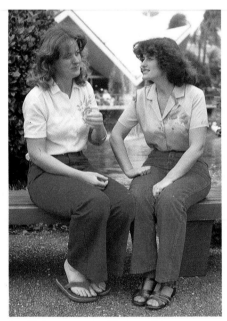

Daylight, tungsten film, no filter.

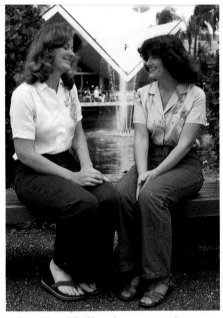

Add a No. 85B filter for correct color.

169

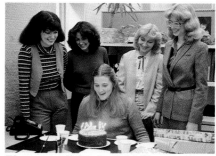

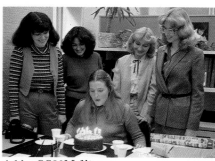

Fluorescent light, daylight film, no filter.   *Add a CC30M filter.*

The table at right gives filter recommendations for fluorescent light. You'll get best results on color negative film for prints. If you're unsure about lamp type, use the average filter combination. These filters are supplied as 3-inch acetate squares. Glass averaging filters in screw-in mounts are also available. FLD denotes an averaging filter for fluorescent light with daylight film and FLB works with tungsten film and fluorescent light.

Table Instructions
You can correct color rendition with fluorescent light by using CC (Color Compensating) filters over the camera lens. The table at right tells you which filters to use and how much you have to increase the exposure to compensate for the light absorbed by the filters.

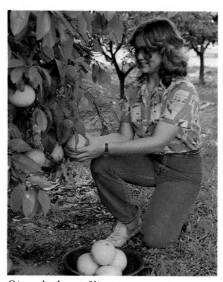

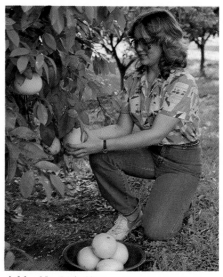

Open shade, no filter.   *Add a No. 81A filter.*

KODAK Color Compensating Filter (CC) for Fluorescent Light

Type of Fluorescent Lamp	KODAK Color Film		
	Daylight		Tungsten
	KODACHROME 25 EKTACHROME 200 All KODACOLOR Films*	KODACHROME 64 EKTACHROME 64 EKTACHROME 400	EKTACHROME 160
Daylight	40M + 40Y + 1 stop	50M + 50Y + 1½ stops	No. 85B + 40M + 30Y + 1⅔ stops
White	20C + 30M + 1 stop	40M + ⅔ stop	60M + 50Y + 1⅓ stops
Warm White	40C + 40M + 1½ stops	20C + 40M + 1 stop	50M + 40Y + 1 stop
Warm White Deluxe	60C + 30M + 2 stops	60C + 30M + 2 stops	10M + 10Y + ⅔ stop
Cool White	30M + ⅔ stop	40M + 10Y + 1 stop	60R 1⅔ stops
Cool White Deluxe	20C + 10M + ⅔ stop	20C + 10M + ⅔ stop	20M + 40Y + ⅔ stop
Average Fluorescent†	10C + 20M + ⅔ stop	30M + ⅔ stop	50M + 50Y + 1 stop

Note: Increase exposure by the amount shown in the table.
See your camera manual for exposure instruction if the built-in meter can make readings through a filter.
*For critical use with KODACOLOR 400, VR 400, and VR 1000 Films.
†These filters yield less than optimum results. Use them only when you can't determine fluorescent lamp type.

color picture slightly. Intended for advanced or professional use to get precise matches of film and lighting, they can be very handy for a subject in the blue light of open shade or the fiery light of sunset.

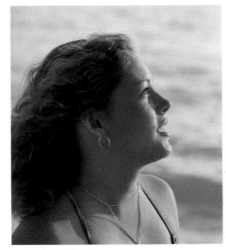

Sunset, no filter.

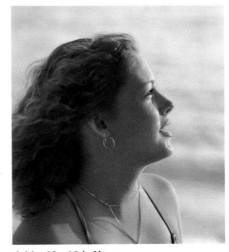

Add a No. 82A filter.

Creative Colors The filters used for black-and-white photography come in a wealth of rich hues. Sometimes one of these can make a brilliant addition to your color pictures. Naturally, blue filters make your pictures blue, and red filters make them red. Exposure is a matter of personal prefer-

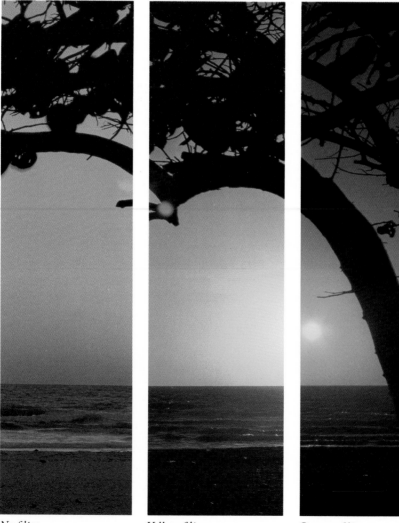

No filter   *Yellow filter*   *Orange filter*

ence. Normally it's wise to increase the exposure slightly, but not as much as recommended for correct exposure with that filter and black-and-white film. Experiment a little to see how you like the effects best.

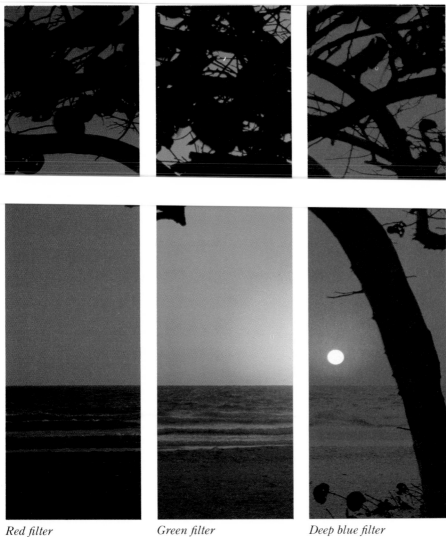

Red filter   *Green filter*   *Deep blue filter*

BLACK-AND-WHITE FILM

Black-and-white film records all colors in many tones of gray—from black through countless grays to white. Subjects that appear nearly white in prints have received a great deal of exposure; dark subjects not nearly as much. Filters transmit their own color of light and subtract others, depending on their color and density. A red flower photographed through a red filter will be nearly white, and the green leaves very dark gray.

Exposure Filters for black-and-white film require exposure compensation. See the table at right for filter and exposure recommendations.

Table Instructions
The table at right shows typical uses for filters with black-and-white film. To apply the exposure information, meter the scene without a filter, make the necessary exposure change, attach the filter, and take the picture.

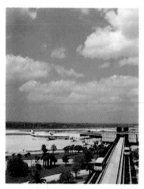

Color film

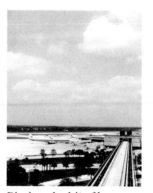

Black-and-white film, no filter

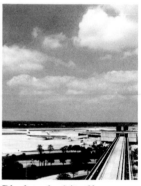

Black-and-white film, No. 8 yellow filter

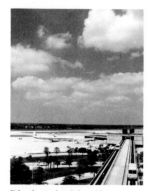

Black-and-white film, No. 25 red filter

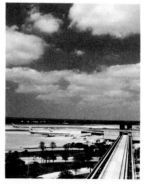

Black-and-white film, No. 25 red filter and polarizer

Filters can help bring out striking contrasts in black-and-white landscape photos. A No. 8 yellow filter gives the scene a tonal rendition similar to the color version. A red or polarizing filter will heighten the contrast. Adding the red filter to the polarizer makes the scene even more dramatic.

174

Filter Recommendations for Black-and-White Films

Subject	Effect Desired	Suggested Filter	Increase Exposure by:
Blue Sky	Natural	No. 8 Yellow	1 stop
	Darkened	No. 15 Deep Yellow	1⅓ stops
	Spectacular	No. 25 Red	3 stops
	Almost black	No. 29 Deep Red	4 stops
	Night effect	No. 25 Red, plus polarizing screen	4⅓ stops
Marine Scenes When Sky Is Blue	Natural	No. 8 Yellow	1 stop
	Water dark	No. 15 Deep Yellow	1⅓ stops
Sunsets	Natural	None or No. 8 Yellow	1 stop
	Increased brilliance	No. 15 Deep Yellow or No. 25 Red	1⅓ or 3 stops
Distant Landscapes	Addition of haze for atmospheric effects	No. 47 Blue	2⅔ stops
	Very slight addition of haze	None	None
	Natural	No. 8 Yellow	1 stop
	Haze penetration	No. 15 Deep Yellow	1⅓ stops
		No. 29 Deep Red	
Nearby Foliage	Natural	No. 8 Yellow or No. 11 Yellowish-Green	1 or 2 stops
	Light	No. 58 Green	2⅔ stops
Outdoor Portraits Against Sky	Natural	No. 11 Yellowish-Green No. 8 Yellow, or polarizing screen	2, 1, or 1⅓ stops
Flowers—Blossoms and Foliage	Natural	No. 8 Yellow or No. 11 Yellowish-Green	1 or 2 stops
Red, "Bronze," Orange, and Similar Colors	Lighter to show detail	No. 25 Red	3 stops
Dark Blue, Purple, and Similar Colors	Lighter to show detail	None or No. 47 Blue	None or 2⅔ stops
Foliage Plants	Lighter to show detail	No. 58 Green	2⅔ stops
Architectural Stone, Wood, Fabrics, Sand, Snow, etc. When Sunlit and Under Blue Sky	Natural	No. 8 Yellow	1 stop
	Enhanced texture rendering	No. 15 Deep Yellow or No. 25 Red	1⅓ or 3 stops
Interiors in Tungsten Light	Natural	No. 11 Yellowish-Green	2 stops

Contrast and Separation One of the main uses for filters in black-and-white photography is to separate subjects of different colors into strikingly different tones. Black-and-white film may see the red tones and the blue tones as nearly equal. A red filter will make the red tones white and the blue tones dark. A blue filter, however, will make the blue tones lighter and the reds dark. See the examples at right.

Use color filters to separate tones in black-and-white pictures. In the comparison at right, note the different values given to the red and blue areas by the red and blue filters.

Color correction Black-and-white film is affected by different qualities of light. Tungsten light is much redder than sunlight. A yellow-green filter can help the film render the correct tonal relationships in a scene lighted by tungsten light.

Polarizer A polarizing filter will also help reduce haze and reflection in black-and-white pictures while increasing contrast. The guidelines for handling and exposure adjustment are the same as for color film. (See page 167.)

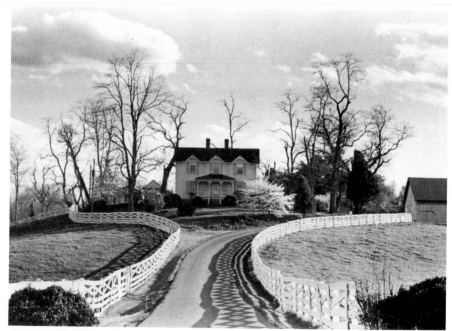

Filters can increase contrast between sky and clouds.

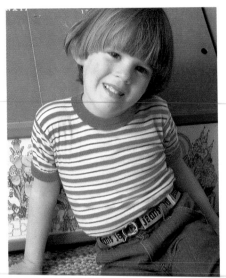

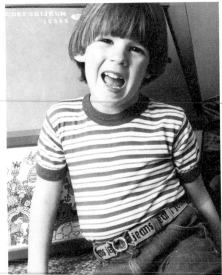

Color film

Black-and-white film, no filter

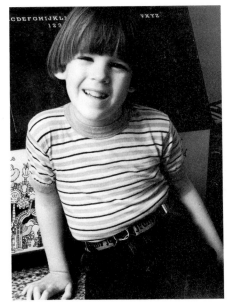

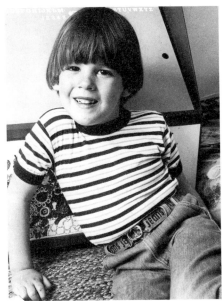

Black-and-white film, red filter

Black-and-white film, blue filter

LENSES

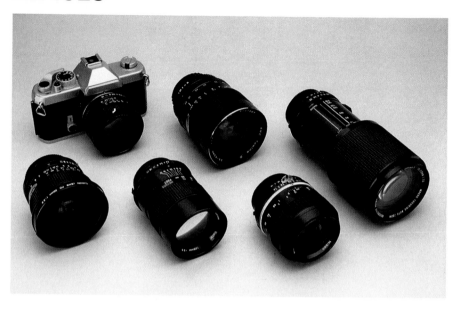

Single-lens-reflex cameras typically are sold with a normal lens which sees perspective and image size about the same as your naked eye. It is probably a fast lens with an $f/2.8$ or larger maximum aperture. The normal lens is designed for the kind of general picture-taking people do at home, on vacation, and at special events. What about other lenses?

TELEPHOTO LENSES

Telephoto lenses make subjects look bigger and they show less of the scene than a normal lens would. The magnification alters perspective by compressing distance relationships and consequently decreases depth of field. The strength of a telephoto lens is determined by its focal length—an optical measurement. The normal lens on a 35 mm camera is roughly 50 mm long. A 100 mm lens will give 2X magnification and a 200 mm lens 4X magnification.

Portrait photographers prefer a moderate telephoto lens (75 to 135 mm with a 35 mm camera) for a large image at a comfortable distance from the subject. The altered perspective gives a pleasing

Telephoto lens

178

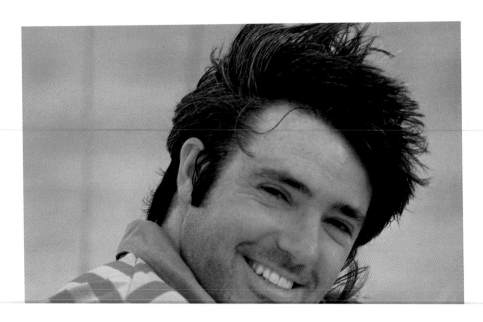

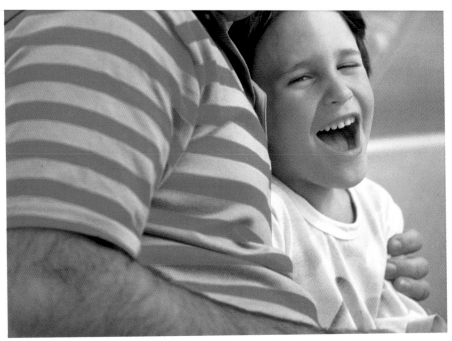

view of the subject's features and the shallow depth of field makes it easy to blur the background at large apertures. Strong telephoto lenses—200 mm and more—can help you get closer to sports, wildlife, and other distant subjects.

Camera movement is also magnified by telephoto lenses. Use a fast shutter speed (at least the reciprocal of the focal length, i.e., 1/250 second for a 200 mm lens) or give the camera solid support with a tripod to get sharp pictures.

WIDE-ANGLE LENSES

Wide-angle lenses see more of a scene than normal or telephoto lenses and subjects will be correspondingly smaller. Compared with a normal focal length lens, the distance between near and far objects and the depth of field are extended with a wide-angle lens when the subject distance remains the same.

Situations such as narrow streets and building

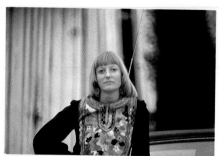

100 mm telephoto lens

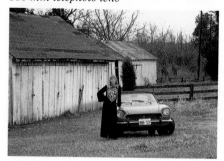

500 mm telephoto lens

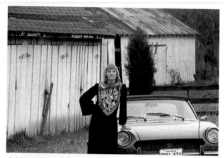

50 mm normal lens

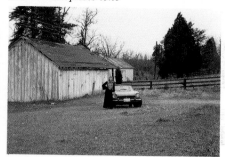

200 mm telephoto lens

interiors demand wide-angle lenses. But be careful with people. The perspective can be grotesque with close subjects.

Moderate wide-angles—28 to 35 mm—are so useful that many photographers consider them normal lenses. Very wide-angle lenses—18 to 25 mm—are more extreme and are generally used for special applications or to amplify distortion.

ZOOM LENSES
Zoom lenses offer an economical and convenient alternative to a large assortment of single-focal-length lenses. They come in a wide variety of focal-length ranges and give excellent results. For traveling a typical zoom lens choice would be a 28 to 85 mm zoom and an 80 to 200 mm zoom. These two lenses plus your fast normal lens for dim light could capture nearly any subject, yet occupy little space in your luggage.

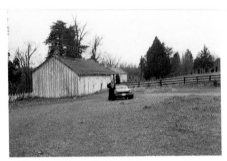

35 mm wide-angle lens

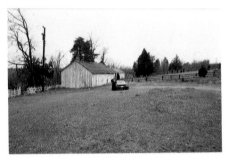

28 mm wide-angle lens

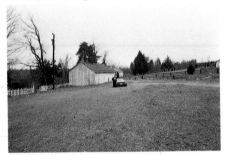

24 mm wide-angle lens

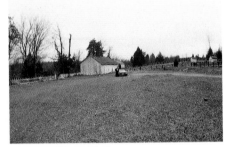

16 mm wide-angle lens

CLOSE-UPS

With many cameras, you can usually find a way to isolate small subjects such as a single big flower or a tidy group of lesser blossoms. The easiest way is with an accessory called a close-up lens, which allows you to get closer than the minimum focusing distance for your camera. More advanced cameras have a threaded connector at the end of the lens where you can screw in close-up lenses or filters. Less advanced cameras might require you to tape a close-up lens over the camera lens.

Close-up lenses come graded in diopters—typically +1, +2, and +3. The higher the number, the closer you can get, and the bigger your image will be. If you have a camera that has a viewfinder separate from the lens, it might be best to use only one close-up lens, a +2 for instance, so that you get completely familiar with how it works. (As you'll see later, close-up lenses require a little measuring and calculation for accurate results.) A single-lens-reflex camera, however, shows you in the viewfinder almost exactly what will be on the film, so you can use any close-up lens, or even a combination of close-up lenses for the best treatment of your subject.

The viewfinder for any rangefinder camera is adjusted to give you accurate framing (you get what you see) from the minimum focusing distance to infinity. At the closer distances you'll use with a close-up lens, the viewfinder will not show exactly what the film will record. And, since depth of field is so shallow at close focusing distances, you'll want the camera lens to be at the precise distance recommended by the close-up lens instruction sheet or in the table on page 185. To aim your camera from the correct distance, attach a string to the camera with a knot tied at the recommended distance. Extend the string until the knot just touches the subject. Then you're at the right distance. When you hold the string out, make sure the camera lens is pointed directly at the subject. Then drop the string and snap the picture. With practice, this becomes a simple and effective way to make close-ups.

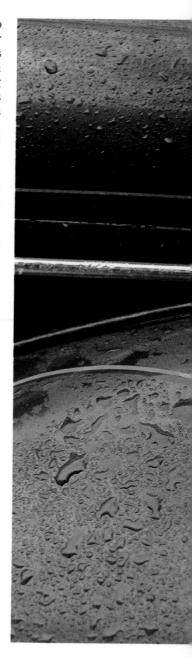

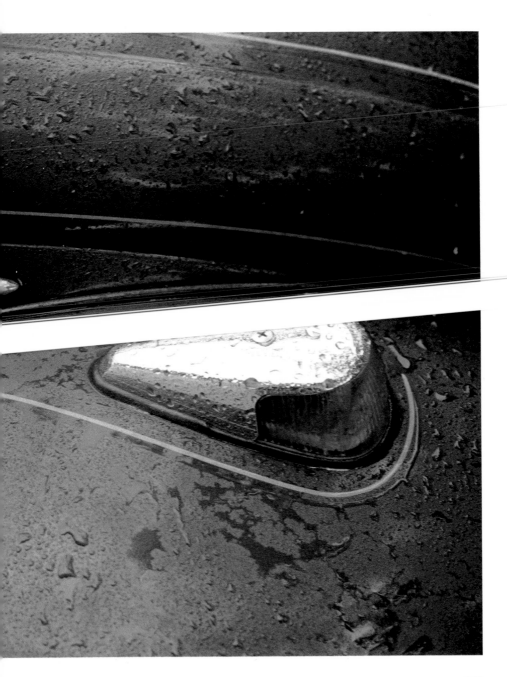

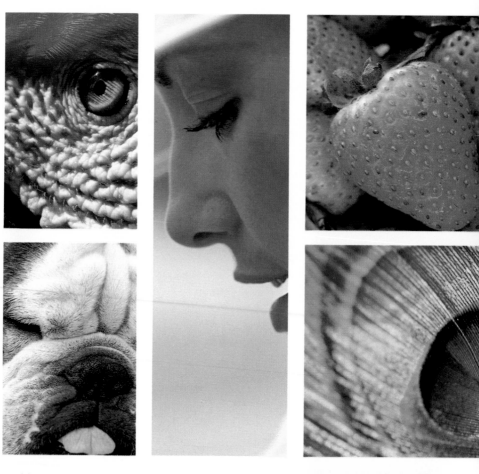

Almost as easy, and much more accurate is a lightweight cardboard measuring device. Cut to the recommended distance, the board should have a lengthwise line at center that you line up from camera lens to subject. The board should be only as wide as the long dimension of the field of view for that close-up lens. That way, you'll know how much of the subject will be included in the picture. Make sure the camera isn't tilted up or down, remove the cardboard, and take your picture.

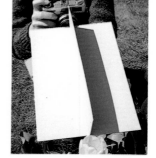

Cardboard measuring device

184

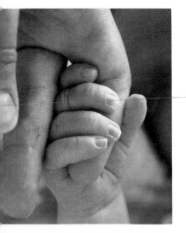

Shown below is information you'll want to use for taking close-up pictures with a rangefinder camera. The left column shows different close-up lenses and lens combinations at various camera lens focus settings. The next column gives lens-to-subject distances for you to measure. The columns on the right give the field size (subject area) for the combinations shown at left. Just remember to measure the distance carefully from the front rim of your close-up lens to the subject. Aim the camera lens directly at the subject. Incidentally, close-up lenses require no exposure compensation.

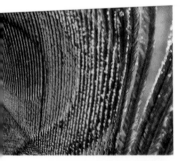

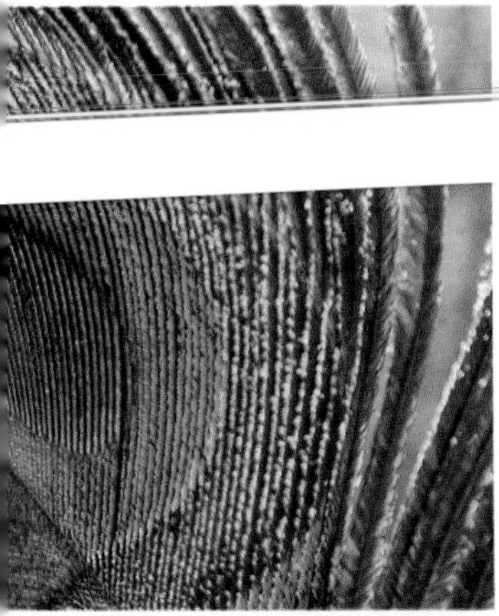

Close-Up Lens Data

Close-up Lens and Focus Setting	Lens-to-Subject Distance	Approximate Field Size (in inches)	
		38–40 mm Lens on a	50 mm
+1 Inf	39	23⅛ x 34½	18 x 27
+1 15	32¼	18⅞ x 28⅛	14⅝ x 21⅞
+1 6	25½	14⅝ x 21¾	11⅜ x 16⅞
+1 3½	20⅜	11½ x 17⅛	8⅞ x 13¼
+2 Inf	19½	11⅝ x 17¼	9 x 13½
+2 15	17¾	10⅜ x 15½	8 x 12
+2 6	15½	8⅞ x 13¼	6⅞ x 10¼
+2 3½	13⅜	7⅝ x 11⅜	5⅞ x 8¾
+3 Inf	13⅛	7¾ x 11½	6 x 9
+3 15	12¼	7⅛ x 10⅝	5½ x 8¼
+3 6	11⅛	6⅜ x 9½	5 x 7⅜
+3 3½	10	5⅝ x 8½	4⅜ x 6½
+3 plus +1 Inf	9⅞	5¾ x 8⅝	4½ x 6¾
+3 plus +1 15	9⅜	5½ x 8⅛	4¼ x 6⅜
+3 plus +1 6	8⅝	5 x 7⅜	3⅞ x 5¾
+3 plus +1 3½	8	4½ x 6¾	3½ x 5¼
+3 plus +2 Inf	7⅞	4⅝ x 6⅞	3⅝ x 5⅝
+3 plus +2 15	7½	4⅜ x 6½	3⅜ x 5⅛
+3 plus +2 6	7⅛	4⅛ x 6⅛	3⅛ x 4¾
+3 plus +2 3½	6⅝	3¾ x 5⅝	2⅞ x 4⅜
+3 plus +3 Inf	6⅝	3⅞ x 5¾	3 x 4½
+3 plus +3 15	6⅜	3¾ x 5½	2⅞ x 4¼
+3 plus +3 6	6	3½ x 5⅛	2⅝ x 4
+3 plus +3 3½	5⅝	3¼ x 4¾	2½ x 3¾

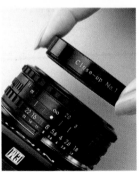

Attaching +1 close-up lens

185

CAMERA CARE

Although a precision instrument, your camera is designed for hard use. It does deserve whatever care you can provide. Here are some guidelines:

1. Protect your camera from dirt and bumps with a ready case.
2. Keep the inside clean by using a soft brush or air syringe at film-change time. You can also use canned compressed air, but follow instructions on the can or in your camera instruction manual carefully. Misuse could damage your camera. Also, aim the air stream precisely—it's possible to blow debris *into* the camera.
3. Keep the lens protected from dirt and finger-prints with a lens cap.
4. Clean the lens by first brushing or blowing off surface debris. Then use photographic lens tissue (not the kind for eyeglasses) and a drop or two of lens cleaning fluid to wipe off smudges.
5. Protect your camera from water—particularly

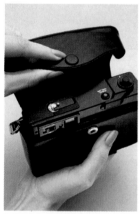

1. Use a camera case.

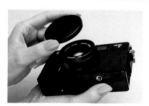

3. Protect the lens.

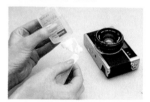

4. Clean the lens.

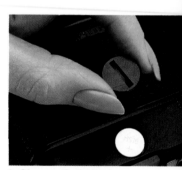

6. Change the batteries.

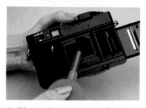

2. Keep the camera clean.

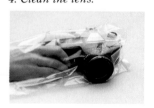

5. Shield your camera.

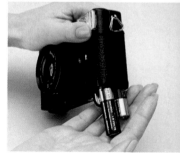

7. Remove for storing.

salt spray—in a plastic bag or zippered camera case. Attach a UV filter to the lens to protect the vulnerable glass surface from water, dust, sand, and other airborne particles.

6. Change the batteries for meter, flash, and motorized film-advance according to the camera instruction manual.

7. Remove the batteries when storing your camera. If left for long periods, they could corrode the camera electrical contacts.

8. Allow a camera used in cold air to warm up gradually when brought indoors to help prevent condensation. Keep the lens cap attached.

9. Do not leave your camera in a very warm place, such as the glove compartment of your car. Avoid damp basements, too.

10. At the first sign of malfunction, have your camera checked over by a competent repair

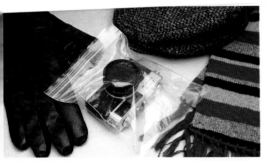

8. Allow slow warm-up.

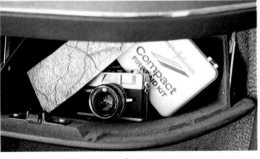

9. Avoid extreme heat.

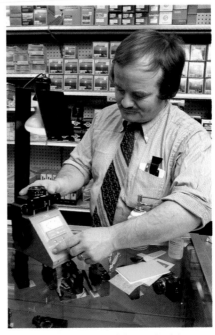

10. Check problems with a technician.

PHOTO CREDITS

The following list of photographer credits does not include the dozens of comparison, equipment, and technique photos made by Kodak staff photographers and employees Donald Buck, Neil Montanus, Marty Czamanske, and Marty Taylor. Free-lance photographers Mark Hobsen, Tom Beelmann, and Jerry Antos made significant contributions as did art director William Paris and designer Roger Pring.

Much appreciation is due Kodak Limited who contributed comparison and technique photos taken in Great Britain and in Europe under the supervision of Mr. Jack Oakley.

Many of the illustrations came from the files of the Kodak International Newspaper Snapshot Contest and the Scholastic Photo Contest. Although a proportion of the entrants are accomplished amateur photographers, a larger number are snapshooters in homes just like yours. The joy and spontaneity of these images should be inspiring and encouraging to picture-takers everywhere.

BIBLIOGRAPHY

KODAK Guide to 35 mm Photography
(AC-95S)

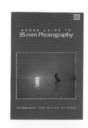

This book is for the new 35 mm camera owner or for the more advanced photohobbyist who wants to brush up on the basics. *KODAK Guide to 35 mm Photography* discusses in detail camera handling, Kodak films, exposure, daylight photography, flash, interchangeable lenses, composition, action pictures, existing light, filters, and close-up photography.

Photographing with Automatic Cameras
(KW-11), a KODAK Workshop Series book

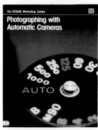

Here's a book aimed at providing photographers with an understanding and working knowledge of their automatic cameras and related equipment. It teaches the basics through clear language and pictures.

Electronic Flash (KW-12),
a KODAK Workshop Series book

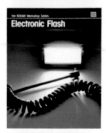

Electronic Flash starts with basics and gives thorough coverage—great advice for the novice and a handy review for someone with experience. Complete technical information plus well-illustrated ideas should give a confident head start in flash photography.

Using Filters (KW-13),
a KODAK Workshop Series book

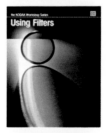

This book shows the reader how filters work and how they can be used for color and black-and-white photography. It covers how filters help to reproduce realistic colors and black-and-white tones. Also, there's advice about the creative aspects of filters, complete filter systems, homemade filters, diffusers, accelerators, and far more.

Adventures in Existing-Light Photography
(AC-44)

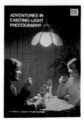

High-speed film, a camera with a fast lens, and this colorful 80-page guide are all you need to take exciting, uncontrived pictures anywhere, anytime, without a flash or additional photolamps. It's packed with hundreds of ideas you can use to take pictures at home or traveling, indoors or outdoors. Includes easy-to-use exposure tables and advice on films and processing.

INDEX

191

lives out in the cytoplasm (or main body) of the cell. The mitochondrion has its own membrane and DNA. (4)

Your results will reveal your deep ancestry along a single line of descent (paternal or maternal) and show the migration paths ancestors followed over time. Your results also place you on a particular branch of the human family tree.
I took the Y-chromosome test for men.
The analysis of my DNA showed that I belonged to Y-chromosome Haplogroup R1b, M343 (subclade R1b1b2, M269). (5)
This haplogroup, R1b, M343 (subclade R1b1b2, M269), is very common in parts of Spain and Ireland, where more than 90% of men belong to it. Therefore, whether you are a Redmond, or Hennessey, Walsh, McGuire, Corbett, O'Leary, Kinsley, Murphy, O'Grady, Currie, Collins or Ross or any other Irish family, this history applies to you, with rare exceptions.

Initial Thoughts on Analysis

The results of the DNA analysis were intriguing.
They showed clearly the dispersion of modern humans from the Near East throughout the entire world. In addition, the DNA suggested that humans had their origin in the Near East, even though the interpretation provided claimed human origins were in Eastern Africa. Also, given the patterns of dispersion of modern man, the popular thesis on the evolution of man from earlier species, leading back to a common ancestor with the monkey, seemed dubious at best.
These initial conclusions on the value of DNA analysis were reinforced by statements from others who have written about DNA analysis and its impact. For example, I.L. Cohen, researcher and mathematician, member of the New York Academy of Science and officer of the Archaeological Institute of America wrote:

"At that moment, when the DNA/RNA system became understood, the debate between Evolutionists and Creationists should have come to a screeching halt." (6)

Francis S. Collins, who led the Human Genome project, said that creation has become intelligible to us through science. He says with joyful astonishment: "The language of God was revealed" (7)

The more one studied the data, the more did DNA analysis suggest a suddenly emerging and rapidly spreading modern man, not a man slowly evolving from a distant and little known past.

To confirm this, a variety of other sources were checked, including genealogical studies, historical manuscripts, a variety of written works and, finally, various religious sources. This information provided a fascinating and credible story of my ancestry that matched the DNA analysis much better than the brief summary provided to me to explain the analysis of my DNA.

The results are shown in the following pages which, it is hoped, will offer a good explanation of the origins of modern man through one of his ancestral lines, that of our haplogroup.

marker M60, are found only in Africa, everyone originates in Africa. (15)

Wells gives additional reasons why he makes these two African markers the oldest. One is the fossil evidence. Another is the practice of ancient cultural traditions by people with markers M60 and M91, such as being hunter-food gatherers. A third is greater genetic diversity with age. A fourth is having an ancient language, specifically one with clicks. (16)

These reasons are not convincing.

Genetic diversity may not increase with age, as we shall discuss below, when commenting on the mtDNA data.

The practice of cultural traditions, such as being hunter-food gatherers can be a result of population pressures on small groups, forcing them to inhospitable fringes and limiting their ability to develop their economies, rather than prove the antiquity of the group.

Also, while click languages may be considered complex, they cannot, as a result, be identified as the oldest. Fred Field, of the California State University, in his excellent study of languages, writes that within linguistics, there are at least four commonly held principles concerning the nature of language: 1. every language is, in principle, infinite; 2. all human languages are equally complex or challenging; 3. there are no primitive languages; 4. wherever humans have been found to exist, there is language. He continues that language and the language facility reflect the cognitive abilities that every human being shares. Assuming his second principle, other languages such as Sanskrit can readily replace click languages as the most ancient language. (17) Indeed, as we shall see below, the earliest probable language has been identified as pre-Sanskrit.

Reinforcing doubts on the status of click languages as the most ancient is information on the the origin of writing which points to the Near East. As Woolley writes:

11

"All the archaeological evidence available seems to prove that true writing was first developed in southern Mesopotamia ... the Egyptians took over the principle of writing ready-made from the Sumerians...that India owed its art of writing to the Sumerians cannot be proved, but it is highly probable ... On the whole it is probable the Chinese derived from Sumer the principle of writing". (18)

Fossil claims for a human origin in Eastern Africa are very dubious.

Stephen Jay Gould, professor at Harvard, writes in the May 1977 issue of *Natural History*

"it is essentially an open confession that, although evolutionary trees are displayed in every textbook, it was a 'trade secret of paleontology' that these were based on inference and not on fossil evidence". (19)

Taylor writes that the actual fossils are so incomplete they are open to any interpretation:

"The overwhelming problem in the study of fossil man is that the actual fossil remains are extremely rare, and when they are found, the pieces are so broken, distorted, and incomplete that entirely different interpretations are possible. The field is thus wide open for speculation which, indeed, has been carried out with abandon, particularly in the case of flesh reconstructions, which become the interface between the knowledge of the scientist and the view offered to the lay public."(20)

Others have questioned the differences in these species. For example, William Hoesch writes:

"Fossils classified as *H. erectus* all share a set of "primitive" traits including a sloping forehead and large brow ridges, yet these all fall comfortably within the range of what are called normal humans today."

And

"Studiously avoided in most museum depictions is the fact that fossils with a *H. erectus* anatomy that are younger than 400,000 years number well over 100, including some as young as 6000 years. Even more amazing is this: fossil humans that are easily interpreted as "anatomically modern" (i.e., non-*H. erectus*) have been found in rocks that are much *older* than 1.5 million years. From a dozen different sites have come cranial fragments, including one good skull, teeth, several arm and leg bones, a fossil trackway, and stone structure that each screams out

12

"modern human." The trackways at Laetoli, Tanzania, dated at 3.6 million years, and tibia (leg bone) and humerus (arm bone) from Kanapoi, Kenya, dated at 3.5 million, are especially significant for these pre-date even "Lucy," the celebrated upright-walking ape". (21)

Erick Von Fange, a professor at Concordia University in Ann Arbour, writes:

"Hard work for the past 150 years has brought scientists no closer to finding the so-called 'missing link' between man and animal than when the search began. Every year or two another article appears in *National Geographic* with spectacular new discoveries about human evolution. Without exception they are without substance. The fossils are either fully human or fully apelike with nothing in between." (22)

Richard Leakey who, with his father, was one of the leading archaeologists in East Africa and who was well aware of some of the Ethiopian fossils, wrote:

"Echoing the criticism made of his father's *habilis* skulls, he added that Lucy's skull was so incomplete that most of it was 'imagination made of plaster of Paris', thus making it impossible to draw any firm conclusions about what species she belonged to."(23)

More recent finds have been made at other sites in Ethiopia such as Herto, Middle Awash. Many of these are intermediate hominid fossils, claimed to be "immediate ancestors of anatomically modern humans". (24) As we shall see below, such claims are rejected by many.

Other finds have been made in Israel, China and Spain of fossils that are claimed to be older than the African ones. The Israeli findings, for example, at Qesem Cave near Rosh Ha'ayin, are of fossils dated as older than the African ones from Ethiopia. This has led to claims of a Middle East origin for modern man.

"The findings of Professor Avi Gopher and Dr Ran Barkai of the Institute of Archeology at Tel Aviv University, published last week in the American Journal of Physical Anthropology, suggest that modern man did not originate in Africa as previously believed, but in the Middle East."(25)

13

In summary, doubts on the antiquity of the M91 and M60 Y-chromosome haplotypes, as well as on dating and other aspects of the archaeological and fossil evidence for Eastern Africa are convincing enough to allow one to reject the Eastern African origin of the first modern man, Adam.

So, if we can proceed with the assumption that, with M168, man started in the near East, can we say the same about woman?

Eve Started in the Near East as well

As noted above, Wells, and others who support evolution, state that Eve came from East Africa. (26) However, the evidence seems stronger for a Near East origin in the case of mtDNA than it is even for Adam and the Y-chromosome analysis.

The key evidence supporting an origin in Eastern Africa for Eve is the presence, in Africa only, of the L0, L1 and L2 haplogroups. The following chart shows this:

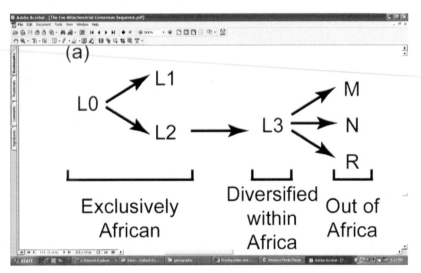

14

Some geneticists reject this interpretation and propose alternate ones. For example, Carter and others suggest the following, which they then explain: (27)

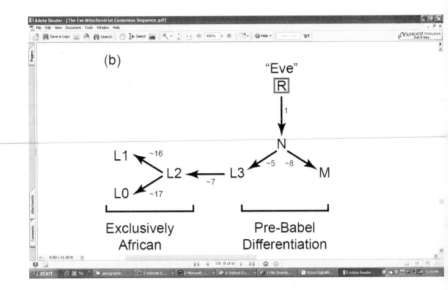

"Eve 1.0 is identical to the root node of macrohaplogroup R. From R, the closely related M, N and L3 lineages diverged (small numbers indicate the approximate number of mutations that separate the nodes for each lineage…) One of the L3 lineages entered Africa and gave rise to the African-specific lineages, L2, L1, and L0…. Most of the differences we see in these lineages (specific to sub-Saharan Africa) are due to rare, homoplasic, or private alleles."

In a comparable manner to those who use the fossil record, language and culture in interpreting the Y-chromosome results to claim an African origin, researchers in mtDNA use other facts to point to an African origin.

Carter and his team identify some of these facts. They state that option A, the origin in Africa, relies on certain assumptions, including

15

"the need for mutations to accumulate in all lineages at an equal rate (a molecular clock), that mtDNA undergoes no recombination, and that all new mutations are free from natural selection".

His team then shows how all three assumptions are wrong.

"If the molecular clock is violated, a reliable phylogenetic tree for worldwide mtDNA haplotypes cannot be built. Tests for a molecular clock have failed in African L2 clades of mtDNA. (Also) one of the newer studies (by Zsurka, 2007) seems to have found conclusive evidence for mitrochondrial recombination... (Thirdly) several studies indicate that selection may also operate on mtDNA". (28)

Further his team does not accept the emphasis on mtDNA clades from Africa made by the evolutionists to show an African origin:

"the African clades form... a cascading pattern with deep branches and the non-African lineages form a star-like pattern with short branches. The evolutionary explanation is that these groups have been in Africa for tens of thousands of years longer than the lineages that left Africa. However, there are a number of alternative explanations, all of which support the biblical model. For instance, if the groups that eventually made up the African populations were restricted to smaller tribal sizes until recently, drift would have occurred more quickly and they would have diverged from the rest of the world, and from each other, at a higher rate. Likewise, if the African groups have a different DNA repair system than the others (either defective or differential), this would also explain their more rapid divergence...Generation time is another consideration... (as is) lifespan differences ... many private mutations characterize the African sequence. Private mutations are best explained as very recent mutations that have not yet spread into the population. This is also further evidence of a young mitochondrial genome."(29)

They also reject the use of chimpanzee mtDNA sequences because human and chimp sequences are substantially different and because the ancestral chimp sequence is not known, among reasons. (30)

In conclusion, one can accept a theory that states that the Near East was the starting point for Eve.

Assuming that Adam and Eve are most likely to have started in the Near East, we can now examine how, where and when they started.

How did We Start?

So, how did Adam and Eve start?

Those who support evolution claim modern man evolved from earlier species.

The National Geographic, in its atlas showing the timeline of the genographic program, notes: Dawn of Humans – shows a number of major hominid sites. Australopithecus hominids

"disappeared about 1 million years ago though for a while they co-existed with Homo erectus. HOMO HABILIS: In sub-Saharan Africa some two million years ago, it is likely that one Australopithecus species began the direct line of human evolution by giving rise to the first species of the Homo genus, Homo habilis." (31)

DNA analysis does not support this.

IBM and the National Geographic Society analyzed the DNA of the hominid or animal who lived concurrently with early Homo sapiens, and was often credited as being his precursor, Homo neanderthal.

Mitochondrial DNA analysis on a set of Neanderthal bones has identified Neanderthals as a distinct species from Homo sapiens. They were an evolutionary dead end. They lacked the cognitive abilities of humans. (32)

As a result of this find, many who support evolution have been removing Homo neanderthal from the progression of hominid types leading up to Homo sapiens. (33)

No tests have been possible to date with earlier hominids identified in the line of evolution, these including Homo erectus, Homo habilis and various species of Australopithecus, as scientists have not yet extracted any DNA for analysis from these early fossils. It is most unlikely that any of these have any links to Homo sapiens.

17

However, other scientific work has been done on earlier hominids that support a conclusion that Homo sapiens is unique. For example, Dr. Charles Oxnard of the University of Western Australia, completed the most sophisticated computer analysis of australopithecine fossils ever undertaken, and concluded that the australopithecines have nothing to do with the ancestry of man whatsoever, and are simply an extinct form of ape. (34)

Therefore, we can safely doubt the evolution of Homo sapiens from earlier species.

Now let us see where the first modern man started.

The first Modern Human site

We saw above how the Qesem Cave findings in Israel have been claimed to be the oldest Homo sapiens site found. Until then the first site known of Homo sapiens has been the Qafzeh Caves in Israel. The Skuhl cave is another early site, a few meters from Qafzeh. These are in lower Galilee, near Nazareth. Skuhl Cave is a rock shelter located on the slopes of Mount Carmel in Israel. The following graph shows this first site, noted as the black dot. If you visit the website quoted, you will see a larger graph and the black dot has a line connecting it to Israel. All the other dots represent Neanderthal and earlier hominid sites.These surround it. (35)

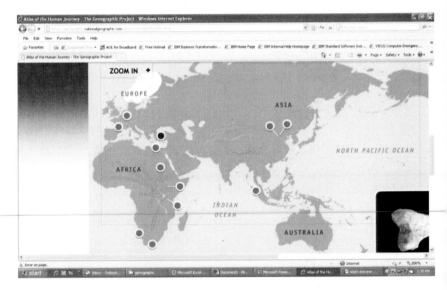

So it is reasonable to conclude that the earliest known site for Homo sapiens is in the Near East.

This has led some to comment on the weak nature of the claims for an East Africa origin for modern man. For example, Ofer Bar-Yosef, a professor at Harvard, writes:

"The sites in East Africa are poorly dated by comparison to Western Eurasia where debates continue due to wealth of evidence. In poorly known regions, 'the less you know – the clearer is the picture'." (36)

Now we can ask – when did they start?

According to the National Geographic, there were two distinct periods of settlement at the Qesem Cave: a first one, then a break, then a second one.

Few details are provided in the archaeological record to explain the break.

Dating Adam and Eve

Those who support the evolution of man from primitive species state we have been around for a long time.

19

The National Geographic atlas states:

"Adam is the common male ancestor of every living man. He lived in Africa some 60,000 years ago, which means that all humans lived in Africa until at least that time". (37)

Regarding the Y-chromosome male side, the interpretation of the analysis of my DNA states the time of the first man, or 'Adam', was between 31,000 to 79,000 years ago. The interpreters of the DNA added two columns to the markers, one with dates and the other associating those dates with archaeological and other data.

M343	30,000 yo (years ago)	Associated with Cro-Magnon
M173	30,000 yo	Associated with Aurignacian culture
M207	30,000 yo	Glaciers expanding
M45	35,000 yo	Hunter, food gatherers
M9	40,000 yo	Eurasian clan spreads far and wide
M89	45,000 yo	Moving through Middle East
M168	50,000 yo	Earliest lineage outside Africa

The dates are unrealistic. For example, three markers – M343, M173 and M207 – are given dates of around 30,000 years ago, and an additional three are given a ten thousand year period before that, showing that no new markers have formed for the past 30,000 years. This does not follow patterns of marker creation, as in my case. Indeed, we shall see below, that marker M343 is linked to events that occurred around 1000 years ago. Also that marker M173 is linked to events of some 3000 years ago. The dates provided to me are unacceptable guesswork.

Furthermore, some associations given with the dates in fact have a much wider timeframe than noted in the chart. For example, Cro-Magnon man has been dated from 40,000 years ago to 10,000 years ago. Furthermore, the association

20

of marker M343 with Cro-Magnon seems to be a dubious link, as we shall discuss below. Also, Aurignacian culture has been dated from 40,000 to as recent as 3500 years ago. (38)

Furthermore, we shall discuss below how marker M173 is more likely to be associated with Urnfield and Halstatt culture than with Aurignacian Culture. Finally, the dates noted for M45, M9 and M89 have few facts supporting them. Others who have studied the same Y-chromosome lineages as mine suggest a much shorter time period. Basically, they state that the Irish, like other Europeans, immigrated into Europe from the Near East as part of the Neolithic expansion, which was associated with the spread of agriculture. Therefore, all seven markers appeared recently, with estimates of the total time span ranging from 4577 to 10,500 years. (39)

Balaresque, Patricia et al	Neolithic expansion	4,577 to 9,063 years ago with spread of agriculture from Anatolia in the Middle East
Pinhasi, Ron, et al	Neolithic expansion	9,000 to 10,500 years ago spread from Middle East
Chikhi, Leones et al	Neolithic expansion	Below 10,000 years ago

Those who claim more ancient dates for the populating of Europe acknowledge that there was a Neolithic expansion into Europe. However, they emphasize that there was a Paleolithic people in Europe into which these Neolithic farmers from the Near East immigrated. Many of these studies note the Basques as being among these Paleolithic people.

However, some question that the Basques are part of an earlier Paleolithic group.

Lounes Chikhi writes:

"It is worth stressing again that the analyses presented here rest on the use of Basques (or Sardinians) as descendants of Palaeolithic people. Because the Basques are likely to contain an unknown proportion of Neolithic genes, there is reason to believe that the Palaeolithic contribution has actually been overestimated, even though we cannot say by how much." They conclude "the genetic contribution of Neolithic farmers had to be between 65 and 100% "(40)

Elsewhere he writes:

"All estimates of times since separation of populations other than Saami, but including Sardinians and Basques, were below 10,000 years. These dates are rather recent, and so hereafter we only give upper bounds of their estimates. We do not believe any of these figures should be taken at its face value; clearly, it is the trend of the data that contains useful information, and not the exact numerical estimates. However, the overall pattern emerging is one in which, even using a long generation time (25 years) and the lowest mutation rate, there is no evidence of European population splits predating the diffusion of Neolithic technologies, as inferred from archaeological evidence. Using the mutation rates recently estimated from pedigrees for Y-chromosome tetranucleotide microsatellites would further reduce the time elapsed since population separations." (41)

Another summary of Y-chromosome analyses of the Basque people concludes that the Basques were not part of the supposed Paleolithic peoples into whom Neolithic groups immigrated, but rather were part of the Neolithic expansion.

"Studies of the Y-chromosome found that on their direct male lineages modern Basques have a common ancestry with other Western Europeans. The similarity includes the predominance in their male populations of Y-chromosome Haplogroup R1b, now considered to have been spread through Europe from southwest Asia in the Neolithic period or later, between 4,000 to 8,000 years ago."(42)

To summarize, the DNA evidence shows that our ancestors arrived in Europe with the Neolithic immigrants and were part of the modern populating of Europe by Homo sapiens from the Near East, which could have happened anytime from 4000 to 7,000 years ago.

This is very different from the evolutionist interpretation, which suggests settlement in Europe some 45,000 years ago by Paleolithic peoples who were later joined by Neolithic immigrants from the Near East.

Does this mean there were no modern humans in Europe before the immigration of our ancestors in the Neolithic period? Not necessarily, as we shall see below when discussing the flood.

The significant difference in time suggested by the evolutionists versus those who have focused on DNA analysis and not archaeological and other data is also reflected in the mtDNA interpretation.

Evolutionists, when first considering mtDNA, suggested that the first Homo sapiens female was very ancient.

Doran Behar and others state:

"Both the tree phylogeny and coalescence calculations suggest that Khoisan matrilineal ancestry diverged from the rest of the human mtDNA pool 90,000–150,000 years before present" (43)

Wells states:

"Mitochondrial Eve represents the earliest female root of the human family tree. Her descendants, moving around within Africa, eventually split into two distinct groups…The older group is referred to as L0…Haplogroup L0 likely originated in East Africa around 100,000 years ago."(44)

However, considerable recent analysis, particularly of the molecular clock, casts serious doubts on such claims and suggests strongly that Eve lived in the recent past.

Michael Hammer, of the University of Arizona, writes

"We are finding that humans have very, very shallow genetic roots which go back very recently to one ancestor."(45)

Ann Gibbons writes:

"regardless of the cause, evolutionists are most concerned about the effect of a faster mutation rate. For example, researchers have calculated that "mitochondrial Eve", the woman whose mtDNA was ancestral to

23

that in all living people...lived 100,000 to 200,000 years ago in Africa. Using the new clock, she would be a mere 6000 years old." (46)

Pitman notes a 1987 mtDNA study of 136 women in which, after thousands of computer runs

"the 'African origin' for modern humans does not hold a statistical significance over other possibilities" (47)

He quotes Mark Stoneking, a Berkeley biochemist who was one of the original researchers on mtDNA who once thought offspring received all copies of mother's mitochondria and it mutated only every 300 to 600 generations, but now acknowledges that the theory of an African Eve has been invalidated.

Pitman continues:

"Scientists who study historical families and their genetic histories started questioning the mutation rates that were based on evolutionary phylogenetic assumptions. These scientists were "stunned" to find that the mutation rate was in fact much higher than previously thought. In fact it was about 20 times higher at around one mutation every 25 to 40 generations (about 500 to 800 years for humans). It seems that in this section of the control region, which has about 610 base pairs, humans typically differ from one another by about 18 mutations. By simple mathematics, it follows that modern humans share a common ancestor some 300 generations back in time. If one assumes a typical generation time of about 20 years, this places the date of the common ancestor at around 6000 years before present."

Finally, Pitman references a study by Evelyn Heyer et al, published in the *American Journal of Human Genetics* in 2001, which presented their findings of the mtDNA mutation rate in deep-rooted French-Canadian pedigrees. Their findings

"Confirmed earlier findings of much greater mutation rates in families than those based on phylogenetic comparisons...For the HVI sequences, we obtained 220 generations or 6,600 years, and for the HVII sequences 275 generations or 8,250 years."

To summarize, analysis of mtDNA mutation rates suggest Eve lived some 6000 years ago, rather than the 90,000 to 150,000 years ago proposed by evolutionists.

Also, we are looking at perhaps 300 generations between us and Adam and Eve.

Moreover, the time for these 300 generations could be 6000 years, if we accept the analysis provided above by Pitman. (48)

Scientific Dating Supports Recent Origin

Given that much of the proof for long periods is based on scientific dating of fossils, we must now examine how accurate this dating is.

Taylor, writing on carbon 14 and potassium argon dating, quotes Whitelaw who subjected 15,000 published carbon 14 dates to statistical analysis by ranking, and then applied the correction factors using the acknowledged 30 percent difference in rates, and the entire data reduce to a remarkably sharp beginning point, about 5,000 years ago. This is a good reason to question openly all the long ages given by the other radiometric methods, reckonings we have been assured are based on sound scientific principles. (49)

Taylor then comments on the carbon 14 data, writing:

"We may reasonably conclude that within the dating range of calibration standards, perhaps the past five thousand years, the carbon 14 method is probably a good indicator of true age, especially when carried out by the new high-energy technique. For material believed to be older than this, however, the results obtained are all subject to interpretation, according to the presuppositions of the investigator, and the exercise then passes from the area of true science into that of pseudoscience."(50)

He continues

"When it comes to the other radiometric methods, such as the potassium/argon, there are no independent test methods; thus there can be no primary calibration standards. The use of fossils to calibrate the radiometric method, meanwhile, is simply adding to an already circular situation. Any consistency found with various radiometric methods is simply consistency within test methods based on the radio-decay phenomenon and, as we have seen, these are all subject to the same assumptions. The acceptance of the extreme ages given by these radiometric methods is, therefore, not based on good science but rather on philosophical grounds, because they appear to give support to Lyell's geology (51)

Robert E. Lee writes:

"the radiocarbon method is still not capable of yielding accurate and reliable results. There are gross discrepancies, the chronology is uneven and relative, and the accepted dates are actually selected dates. This whole bless(ed) thing is nothing but 13th-century alchemy, and it all depends on which funny paper you read."(52)

Reinforcing the doubts on the validity of much of the ancient dates offered for fossils and other artifacts is evidence provided by magnetic field observations that suggest ancient dates are improbable.
Von Fange writes:

"For the past century and a half careful measurements of the earth's magnetic field have been conducted. The rapid decay of the magnetic field is startling. Assuming that this rate is constant, scientists are able to show mathematically how strong the magnetic field was in the distant past. Instead of an age in the millions or billions of years, however, the magnetic field can be projected back in time less than 20,000 years. The world could not exist with the powerful magnetic field projected beyond 20,000 years. This finding is strong evidence for a young earth." (53)

As a final reinforcement of the likelihood of a recent history for modern man, we can quote Taylor who comments on population growth:

"the world's population today would be almost exactly what would be expected from the four couples surviving the Genesis Flood some five thousand years ago and would take into account all the natural disasters."(54)

In conclusion, the evidence we have considered suggests that Adam and Eve started some 6000 years ago in the Near East and spread from there.

26

Historical data supports Recent Origins

Historical and other sources reinforce a recent history of modern man, as suggested by DNA evidence. Among these, we can note the following. (55)

Young's concordance	7000 BC creation earliest date
Douay Rheims bible	Flood 1656 year of the world (AM anno mundi); Joseph born 3934 AM
Ussher	4004 BC creation
Orthodox Jews	3760 BC creation
Masons	4000 BC creation
Scaliger	4713 BC creation
Mayans	3113 BC time since flood

Discussing Robert Young's concordance, Taylor writes:

"Robert Young's concordance, and in the popular twenty-second edition, under "creation", will be found a list of thirty-seven computations of the date of creation from a possible list of more than one hundred and twenty. Of these thirty-seven, thirty are based on the Bible and seven are derived from other sources -- Abyssinian, Arab, Babylonian, Chinese, Egyptian, Indian, and Persian. Not one of these ancient records puts the date of creation earlier than 7000 B.C. In all the hundreds of thousands of years over which hominid man is alleged to have evolved, it is surely more than coincidental that ancient civilizations, which were by no means ignorant of timekeeping by astronomical methods, should all begin their historical record at this arbitrary date. In addition, all the myths and legends, however bizarre, speak of instant creation just a few thousand years earlier."(56)

Discussing Scaliger, Cooper writes that Scaliger analyzed the three basic cycles upon which all workable calendars are built. These are the Solar Cycle, completed every 28 years, the Metonic cycle, completed every 19 years and the Roman indiction, started every 15 years. Scaliger realized that there must obviously be points when all three cycles begin and end together, so, noting carefully the age of each cycle at the moment when he began his calculations, he counted the years backwards until he came to that year when all three cycles began together. And that was the year 4713 BC. (57)

Major European historical documents also support a recent history.

Bill Cooper has done an excellent study of ancient European documents, in his book entitled *After the Flood*. Bill spent twenty-five years reading old chronicles and documents in the British Museum and other libraries and museums and has assembled an excellent collection of early manuscripts on the origin of European peoples.

These manuscripts include Nennius, *'Historia Brittonum'* (History of the Britons (Welsh)); Geoffrey of Monmouth, *Tysilio Chronicle'*; Anglo-Saxon Chronicle; Welsh Annals; *Ehelwerdi Chronicorum*; *Prosa Edda*; *Saltair of Cashel*; *Cin of Drom Snechta* (The Book of Invasions); *Beowulf*; and Traux, E, *Genesis According to the Miao People*.

They provide genealogies of the Irish, Anglo-Saxons, Danish, Norwegian and British peoples. In one genealogical comparison, he included known Roman authors. He shows a Chinese genealogy. (58)

All have fairly complete renderings of history. All go back to Noah, some even to Adam.

Their timelines are all recent. For example, one of the major works, Nennius, *History of the Britons*, notes that from Adam until the passion of Christ was 5228 years. (59)

Another, the Chronicum Scotorum notes:

"The first age of the world contains 1656 years according to the Hebrews, but 2242 according to the Seventy Interpreters; all which perished in the deluge…ten generations" (60)

Lest we too quickly reject the relevance and value of these historical documents, it is worth noting that some geneticists have commented favourably on these historical texts. For example, Laoise T Moore, and others, in their study of the

28

Y-chromosome signature of hegemony in Gaelic Ireland, write:

"our results do seem to confirm the existence of a single early-medieval progenitor to the most powerful and enduring Irish dynasty. They also lend support to the veracity and remarkable knowledge preservation of the genealogical and oral traditions of Gaelic Ireland."(61)

In conclusion, the evidence provided by DNA analysis, especially mtDNA analysis, does not contradict claims by many historical and other sources that modern Homo sapiens started around 4000 BC.

Chapter 2

From Adam to the Flood

While DNA analysis and archaeology can tell us a fair amount about our earliest ancestors, where and when they may have lived, more complete details must come from other sources, such as historical and religious materials. Therefore, to enhance the picture we have so far, let us now turn to some of these sources for additional details on the origin and early spread of modern human society.

The Bible Narrative on the Creation of Adam and Eve

Genesis provides us with our most familiar description of Adam and Eve. Let us quote it:

"Let us make man to our image and likeness: and let him have dominion over the fishes of the sea, and the fowls of the air, and the beasts, and the whole earth, and every creeping creature that moveth upon the earth.
And God created man to his own image: to the image of God he created him: male and female he created them.
And God blessed them, saying: Increase and multiply, and fill the earth, and subdue it, and rule over the fishes of the sea, and the fowls of the air, and all living creatures that move upon the earth...
And the Lord God formed man of the slime of the earth: and breathed into his face the breath of life, and man became a living soul...
Then the Lord God cast a deep sleep upon Adam: and when he was fast asleep, he took one of his ribs, and filled up flesh for it.
And the Lord God built the rib which he took from Adam into a woman: and brought her to Adam.
And Adam said: this now is bone of my bones, and flesh of my flesh she shall be called woman, because she was taken out of man."(62)

Others Comment on the Creation and Fall of Adam

Throughout the ages, various religious people have been given further details on the narrative provided by the Bible.

One of these was St. Anne Catherine Emmerich (1774-1824). A sickly nun, who was bedridden for years, she was visited almost daily by Jesus who asked her to write down accounts of the past as He described and showed them. She noted that Adam was created from dirt in the region in which Jerusalem was subsequently situated. (63)

Interestingly, the oral traditions of the Miautso people of China, refers to Adam as Dirt. (64)

What was Adam like in heaven? A priest, St.Louis Marie de Montfort (1673-1716), recounts the description he was given by Jesus:

"Eternal Wisdom made copies, that is, shining likenesses of his own intelligence, memory, and will, and infused them into the soul of man so that he might become the living image of the Godhead. In man's heart he kindled the fire of the pure love of God. He gave him a radiant body and virtually enshrined within him a compendium of all the various perfections of angels, animals and other created things.

Man's entire being was bright without shadow, beautiful without blemish, pure without stain, perfectly proportioned without deformity, flaw or imperfection. His mind, gifted with the light of wisdom, understood perfectly both Creator and creature. The grace of God was in his soul making him innocent and pleasing to the most high God. His body was endowed with immortality. He had the pure love of God in his heart without any fear of death, for he loved God ceaselessly, without wavering and purely for God himself. In short, man was so godlike, so absorbed and wrapped in God that he had no unruly passions to subdue and no enemies to overcome."(65)

Blessed Louise Piccarreta (1865-1947) also has some marvellous words on Adam and Eve in heaven.

"In God's relationship with mankind, there are three prime decrees, which the Most Holy Trinity has issued and which absolutely must take

31

effect. The "First Fiat of God" is the Decree of Creation, of all that exists outside of God Himself. Here, two humans are the principal objects of this decree: Adam and Eve who were created in a most perfect manner. They were created immaculate, without sin. In their original state of justice, they were full of grace because they possessed the fountain of all grace – the Divine Will – which was the crowning glory of their creation, super-added to their perfect human nature. They lived and acted by the vital principle of God Himself, namely the Divine Will, which eternally animates the Three Divine Persons.

Had our first parents maintained the Gift of the Divine Will at the time they were tested (a test that was to confirm this Kingdom within them) the other two decrees would not have been necessary." (66)

The other two decrees are the decree of redemption and the decree of sanctification. These are not discussed here.

Was he created as a child? Apparently not. According to the ancient manuscript, *The Fifteen Tokens of Doomsday*, Adam was created at thirty years of age. (67)

Genesis then relates that Adam and Eve succumbed to the temptations of the devil, and ate from the tree of life, which gave them knowledge of good and evil, where before they had known only good.

When they acknowledged before God that they had disobeyed Him, they were expelled from Paradise. It appears that Adam and Eve then moved to the area near Jerusalem. This matches the archaeological evidence presented above.

The Saltair na Raan, a collection of early Middle Irish poems, credited to a 9th century author, writes of the expulsion:

"For a week after the expulsion Adam was without fire, house, drink, food or clothing.
He laments to Eve their lost blessings and admits his fault…
Adam goes to seek for food and finds naught but herbs…
He proposes to Eve to do penance, to adore the Lord in silence, Eve in the Tigris for thirty days, Adam in the Jordan for forty and seven…
Forgiveness is granted to Adam and to all his seed save the unrighteous…

Adam and Eve then live alone for a year on grass, without proper food, fire, house, music or raiment; drinking water from their palms, and eating the green herbs in the shadow of trees and caverns...
God at last pities Adam and sends Michael to him with various seeds, And Michael teaches him husbandry and the use of animals." (68)

Genesis tells us that Adam's son, Cain, killed his younger brother Abel. After doing this, Cain was driven from the region of Jerusalem.
Genesis describes what happened to Cain's family, then later, others.

"The sons of God seeing the daughters of men, that they were fair, took to themselves wives of all which they chose....
Now giants were upon the earth in those days. For after the sons of God went in to the daughters of men, and they brought forth children, these are the mighty men of old, men of renown.
And God seeing that the wickedness of men was great on the earth, and that all the thought of their heart was bent upon evil at all times.
It repented Him that He had made man on the earth." (69)

Some religious writers have provided more detail on this passage. One is Francine Beriault. She writes of the meeting between the clan of Cain and the 'sons of God', whom she refers to as the fallen angels:

"When Cain left far away, he met beings unfaithful to God but who had to obey what they were seeing: the mark. God marked Cain so that the unfaithful ones would not touch Cain...
Cain left with his family, with his descendants, his lineage; he left and all those who left with Cain had that mark; therefore, the unfaithful ones couldn't kill them but they could frequent them, they could seduce, they could deceive and they could be with them, live with them. ..
Beings approached them slowly so as not to upset them: they learned to recognize their customs, they learned to recognize their words as words that nourished their interior, they learned to observe their manner of behaviour amongst themselves, they learned to listen to their requests to God, they learned how to be friends with them using what they had just learned. Slowly, they approached; slowly, they came closer but they themselves were incapable of being faithful, for they wanted nothing to

do with that faithfulness to God: they were learning in order to deceive, they were learning in order to manipulate, they were learning in order to dominate, they were learning in order to seduce, for they were beings of darkness: they were fallen angels.

They had assumed the shape of beings that had already been created on earth; they had, my children, committed vile acts with animals, and those animals allowed themselves to be possessed; what they were giving birth to were deformed beings – not of their own species – and this was happening over and over again, for the demons wanted to…create a race in the likeness of what they had known…

the beings of darkness were watching them, the beings of darkness were close to them, and they wanted to seduce them, they wanted to seduce the woman. Remember, my children that they had seen Eve's beauty, and Eve's beauty was upon these children – not that they were seduced by Eve's beauty, but they recognized, they recognized God's splendor, and they wanted to possess God's splendor to dominate it in order to control it and to enslave it: such was their hatred.

And so, they seduced the women: … they showed them that they could be even more beautiful; they showed them that they could be more feminine; they showed them that they could turn themselves into beings superior to man: to no longer be submitted to man; they showed them how to seduce, how to present themselves with controlling words: they showed them how to be vain. The women let themselves be seduced: they began to place movements upon their eyes, they turned them into women who seduce with make-up; women began to place adornments on their ears, on their nose, on their hands, fingers, feet, around their waist to attract men; they learned through these beings of darkness how to perfume themselves; they learned to consult the stars in order to learn who could be an object of seduction for them; they learned to know their own power: they were becoming so proud of themselves that they wanted to be goddesses.

And those beings of darkness were talking about divinity: they learned to use power: the power that attracts, that controls, that dominates, that places the being at their mercy; they learned to use formulas, formulas that cast spells with herbs; they learned to be sexual beings so inferior to animals that their acts were of tremendous impurity, for they slept with them, the demons. And they gave birth to vile beings; this became widespread my children: under their power, man became hideous, violent, wreaking havoc, destructive in every way, for those men had evil in their veins: evil flowed in the blood of those men. For they would eat what was being given to the idols, there was no longer grace within them; this was so deplorable…

34

And they went forward, they populated, they walked on earth...
they no longer wanted anything to do with God, they rejected all that was from God, for they wanted to offend God. (70)

We have covered the separation of Cain and his lineage and of the changes that occurred in this group because this lineage had a great influence on modern humans who lived before the flood. Almost all humans born after Seth admired the powers and capabilities of Cain and his lineage and followed them.
Genesis notes the disillusionment God had with what would become of these early modern humans.

"And God seeing that the wickedness of men was great upon the earth, and that all the thought of their heart was bent upon evil at all times,
It repented him that he had made man upon the earth. And being touched inwardly with sorrow of heart,
He said: 'I will destroy man whom I have created, from the face of the earth...
But Noe (Noah) found grace before the Lord."(71)

Until the disillusionment of God led to the flood, man lived on earth for some time. According to the Bible, man lived for 1656 years before the flood. Other sources, as we have seen above, vary this date somewhat, but not significantly. (72)
This was a time during which there developed a high degree of civilization. Cusack writes of this period in man's history:

"There can be no doubt that a high degree of cultivation, and considerable advancement in science, had been attained by the more immediate descendants of our first parents. Navigation and commerce existed, and Ireland may have been colonized. The sons of Noah must have remembered and preserved the traditions of their ancestors, and transmitted them to their descendants. Hence, it depended on the relative anxiety of these descendants to preserve the history of the world before the Flood, how much posterity should know of it...
men had " multiplied exceedingly upon the earth ;" and that the age of stone had already given place to that of brass and iron, which, no doubt, facilitated commerce and colonization, even at this early period of the

world's history. The discovery of works of art, of however primitive a character, in the drifts of France and England, indicates an early colonization. The rudely fashioned harpoon of deer's horn found beside the gigantic whale, in the alluvium of the carse near the base of Dummyat, twenty feet above the highest tide of the nearest estuary, and the tusk of the mastodon lying alongside fragments of pottery in a deposit of the peat and sands of the post-pliocene beds in South Carolina, are by no means solitary examples."(73)

Adam's Life

Adam lived for many years, dying when 930 years old.
According to the *Saltair na Raan*, "he had seventy sons and seventy daughters born to him after the transgression (of Cain)" (74)
When Adam eventually died, he was buried, according to Emmerich, in a cave under Mount Calvary. (75)
The *Saltair na Raan* notes:

"Adam's body is anointed with the Oil of Mercy and buried in Hebron, where it remained till the Deluge. His head was then swept to Jerusalem, and remained in the gateway till Christ's cross was planted therein." (76)

During and after Adam's life, humans, who started in the region of modern day Israel and Palestine and environs, started spreading out throughout the world.
We can look briefly at the spread of man from the Near East to other regions of the world and discuss who they encountered, what they built and how advanced society was becoming.

Humans Replace Neanderthals

As the first humans moved through Europe, they encountered a hominid species in many parts of the continent. These were the Neanderthals.
At one time it was thought that these creatures were a precursor to modern humans. However, as noted above,

IBM analyzed the DNA of samples and proved beyond any doubt that they had no link to humans. They were a distinct ape family. (77)

Many of their sites have been excavated in Europe and elsewhere. One of the more famous sites is Neander, Germany, from which their name comes.

The archaeological evidence indicates that humans and Neanderthals lived concurrently for a while in Europe before 2600 BC, a rough dating for the flood.

There appears to be no historical or other evidence that modern man, after the flood, encountered Neanderthals, so it seems likely they were wiped out in the flood.

Modern Human Settlements in Europe

The National Geographic explanation of the DNA analysis, in linking together the DNA tracking with archaeology and wider analysis, concludes that the move into Europe happened 30,000 years ago and was connected with the spread of Cro-Magnon man. It writes about this:

"The Cro-Magnon are responsible for the famous cave paintings found in southern France. These spectacular paintings provide archaeological evidence that there was a sudden blossoming of artistic skills as your ancestors moved into Europe. Prior to this, artistic endeavours were mostly comprised of jewelry made of shell, bone and ivory; primitive musical instruments; and stone carvings.

The cave paintings of the Cro-Magnon depict animals like bison, deer, rhinoceroses, and horses, and natural events important to Paleolithic life such as spring molting, hunting and pregnancy. The paintings are far more intricate, details and colorful than anything seen prior to this period. Your ancestors knew how to make woven clothing using the natural fibers of plants, and had relatively advanced tools of stone, bone and ivory. Their jewelry, carvings and intricate, colorful cave paintings bar witness to the Cro-Magnon's advanced culture during the last glacial age." (78)

Were these people connected with the first expansion into Europe by the descendants of Adam and not by our ancestors, who expanded in the Neolithic expansion?

Some facts support this. The characteristics of Cro-Magnon culture do not match the culture we will follow as we track the descendants of those who survived the flood as they moved through Central Asia to Europe, and which are also described by the National Geographic.

But they could match the culture of a society that expanded from the time of Adam to the time of the flood.

One indication of this is the fact that mastodons were among the animals they painted and these are not known to have existed in the post flood world.

Taylor offers us a good description of the Cro-Magnon culture, which notes the suddenness of their emergence, sophistication of their paintings and other aspects of their culture.

"The Cro-Magnon were truly human, possibly of rather noble bearing, some being well over six feet tall and all having a cranial volume slightly larger than men of today; the heavy eyebrow ridges and curved limb bones were absent from these specimens. Remarkably, Cro-Magnon man appears in the fossil record abruptly, and in perfection. That is, he is truly human in the anatomical sense and evidently accomplished in at least several arts, among which are the now famous cave paintings discovered at Altamira, Spain, and at Lascaux in France. The discovery of these paintings indicates the degree to which men's view of their ancestors had turned from the idea of the "fall" of man to that of ascent. In 1879 Marcelino de Sautuolo discovered the cave at Altamira, but none of the authorities would at that time believe they were genuinely ancient, and he died in 1888 an object of ridicule (Schiller 1971). The Lascaux cave was discovered in 1940 and by then cave paintings were acknowledged to be genuine and the public allowed to view them. However, it took several decades of careful juggling with time estimates before the mind-set of science could accommodate the fact that intelligent and skillful man was evidently contemporaneous with prehistoric animals such as the woolly mammoth that appear beautifully painted on the cave walls. The photographs usually shown in the opening chapters of art history books cannot do justice to these incredible paintings because they are in fact three-dimensional. The artist has cleverly made use of the natural contours of the cave walls and ceilings to form the rounding of the belly or the depression for the eye of each one of the colored figures. In 1972 Marshack disclosed a mass of evidence showing that these Cro-Magnon people were not only proficient artists but had a very good grasp of the movements of the heavenly bodies and kept daily records of the position of the moon. This raises the question now seriously being posed: Were these Cro-Magnon people the originators if not the actual builders of the dozens of stone megaliths dotted across Europe of which Stonehenge in England and Carnac in France are probably the best-known examples?

The fact that most of the Cro-Magnon artifacts have been found in caves does not necessarily mean that they all lived in caves, but rather that this is simply where their record has been preserved. There are indications that they did not necessarily dress in animal skins crudely draped about their bodies as usually depicted but had nicely cut clothes and even hairstyles. Surprisingly, a picture appeared in a Time-Life publication showing what appeared to be a mother and daughter wearing dresses and with their hair tied up

This is an exciting period for archaeohistory as many of the old preconceived notions of cavemen are giving way to a totally new picture in which it is recognized that these early ancestors were intelligent beings living in communities and in buildings, who quite possibly only used the caves for ritualistic purposes. (79)

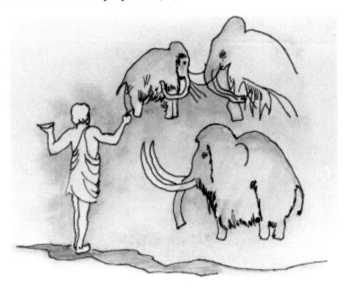

Cave paintings of mammoths, similar to those shown, have been discovered at Les Cambarelles, France. It is evident that intelligent man was contemporaneous with the mammoth. These paintings are one of the principal reasons the mammoth is assigned to a relatively recent era in the evolutionary time scale." (80)

The Wikipedia entry on the Cro-Magnons notes:

"They brought with them sculpture, engraving, painting, body ornamentation, music and the painstaking decoration of utilitarian objects. "

Given the differences between these peoples and those we know later as the Celts and their ancestors, we can consider these folk as the pre-flood ancestors, not as the early Celts who moved into Spain and France that we will discuss later.

Pre-Flood Settlement of Ireland

In a manner comparable to the Bible's recording of life before the flood, some ancient European manuscripts records stories of those who settled in Ireland before the flood.

One, the Irish text called *The Annals of the Kingdom of Ireland by the Four Masters*, also known as *The Annals of the Four Masters*, notes that some people had reached Ireland before the great flood. It records that in the year of creation 2242:

"Forty days before the Deluge, Ceasair came to Ireland with fifty girls and three men; Bith, Ladhra, and Fintain, their names. Ladhra died at Ard Ladhrann, and from him it is named. He was the first that died in Ireland. Bith died at Sliabh Beatha, and was interred in the carn of Sliabh Beatha, and from him the mountain is named. Ceasair died at Cuil Ceasra, in Connaught, and was interred in Carn Ceasra. From Fintan is *named* Feart Fintain, over Loch Deirgdheirc. "(81)

A variation on this story appears in another ancient manuscript the *Chronicum Scotorum*, which records:

"In this year the daughter of one of the Greeks came to Hibernia, whose name was h-Erui, or Berba, or Cesar, and fifty maidens and three men

40

with her. Ladhra was their conductor, who was the first that was buried in Hibernia."(82)

The *Cin of Drom Snechta* is quoted in the *Book of Ballymote* as authority for the same tradition. (83) Other sources, while not mentioning a flood, write about ancient settlement of Ireland. *Times Online*, The Times, January 9, 2009 in an article by Norman Hammond, Archaeology Correspondent, notes:

"Ireland's first farmers settled the island later than some sites from Ulster have long suggested, but did so in a short period which may also have seen parallel migration into western England and Scotland. Radiocarbon dates indicate that sites from Co Kerry in the South West to Co Derry in Northern Ireland were all settled within the century after 3700 BC.

The immigrants built rectangular timber houses up to a hundred square meters in area, cultivated cereals such as wheat and barley, used flint tools and made plain pottery bowls, Cormac McSparron notes in Archaeology Ireland.

They were not the first people in Ireland: Mesolithic fishers and gatherers lived in Kerry and Waterford, keeping cattle, and many years ago the site of Ballynagilly in Ulster yielded dates around 4000 BC associated with what seems to have been a cattle-keeping settlement. (84)

Glenn Allen Nolan, who has done genealogical research on his family, writes:

"Many of the radiocarbon dates obtained using older technology are not of 'gold standard', Mcsparron claims; only those run using AMS (accelerator mass spectronomy), from short-lived plant species such as nuts rather than long-lived timbers, and from securely understood archaeological contexts are reliable. Only 18 out of 66 Irish early Neolithic dates meet these criteria, but their pattern suggests 95 per cent likelihood that all the sites were settled and then abandoned within 90 years, between 3715 and 3625 BC. This matches data from peat bogs which suggest that land clearance did not begin until after 3850 BC.
Sites of almost exactly the same age as the Irish ones are known in Llandegai in northwest Wales and from Lismore Fields in the West Midlands, and coeval structures are known from Claish and Balbridie in northern Scotland.

41

It seems possible that settlers from the European mainland sailed up the Irish Sea and around the Atlantic coast, settling in a number of separate locations," Mcsparron says. A "significant element of colonization must have been involved" in the beginnings of settled agriculture in Ireland. Why these houses ceased to be built after around 3600 BC is a mystery, but possibly population growth led to the rise of larger settlements, and even to defended ones as competition for the best land developed." (85)

One conclusion that can be drawn from Nolan's comments is that they could validate a settlement not long before the flood that was wiped out by the flood.

Humans, Dinosaurs and Other Monsters

As modern humans moved through Europe, it appears they met dinosaurs, animals that we have long associated with pre-human life on earth in a distant past.

This is suggested by the content matter in collections of ancient stone carvings that have been uncovered in many areas of the world.

One famous collector of ancient artifacts is Klaus Dona, the Art Exhibition Curator for the Habsburg Haus of Austria. Klaus Dona has been able to gather more than 1700 pieces, all of which have no logical explanation. He has displayed these in exhibitions in Vienna, Berlin, Seoul, and Switzerland, and shown them on the internet in connection with radio and other interviews. Being physical pieces, they are irrefutable evidence and difficult to reject.

Klaus shows stone and ceramic carvings. They seem to belong to cultures distinct from cultures that developed after the flood.

He notes also that stones with the same writing have been found throughout the world, from Ecuador, to Bolivia, Columbia, USA, Australia, France, Malta, and Turkmenistan. A German professor, Kurt Schildmann, President of the German Linguistic Association, has deciphered this text, which he calls pre-Sanskrit. (86)

42

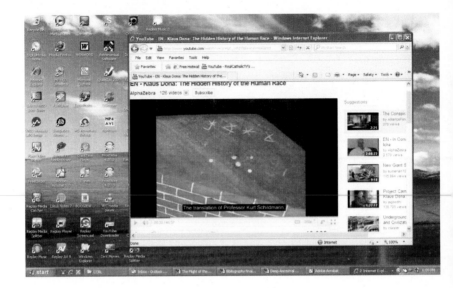

This shows the pre-Sanskrit script above the Orion constellation. This appears on the base of a pyramid. Translated, it says "the son of the creator comes".

A number of these artifacts are described by Klaus Dona in the following video http://www.youtube.com/watch?v=XmMwo1Xzgus&feature =related. Two of these pieces follow:

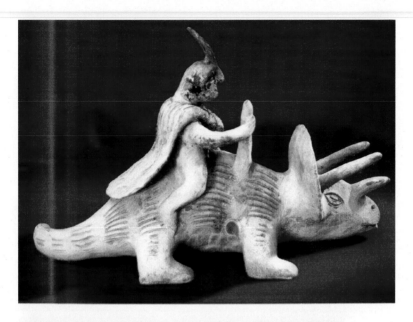

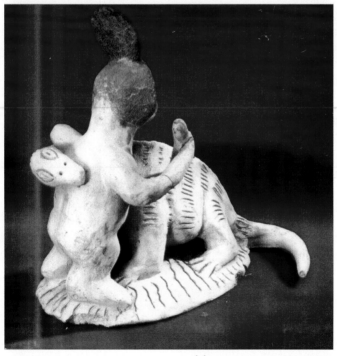

44

It has also been found in the interesting research of Paul Abramson, who has evidence of carbon 14 dating of dinasaurs, which place them as existing in the recent past. (87)

Monsters of sorts lived on after the flood.

The Bible talks of monsters. Job describes a behemoth that was a giant vegetarian and leviathian, an armour-plated amphibian. (88)

Also they are described in the historical records of many cultures, as noted by Cooper:

"Babylonian and Sumerian literature has preserved details of similar creatures, as has the written and unwritten folklore of peoples around the world. But perhaps the most remarkable descriptions of living dinosaurs are those that the Saxon and Celtic peoples have passed down to us". (89)

Cooper also notes that there are more than 200 sightings of reptilian monsters in the British Isles, from the one who ate King Morvidus ca 336 BC, to the water monster who almost ate a friend of St Columba, until the saint rebuked him.

Perhaps the most famous of the monsters was decribed in the poem Beowulf in which Beowulf, on a journey from Sweden to Denmark in 515 AD, slew the monster Grendel. Grendel stalked the marshes from which he would emerge in the dark of night to catch his prey. One night he killed 30 Danish warriors. Beowulf eventually died, fighting a giant reptile, 50 feet in length and 300 years of age. (90)

Did these exist on earth only prior to the flood? Some certainly, for we know, as discussed below, that many were destroyed in the flood.

However, it is clear that some who lived in the water, particularly the oceans, were spared. Indeed the Japanese captured one a few years ago. Reports noted:

"Japanese fishermen caught a dead monster, weighing two tons and 30 feet in length, off the coast of New Zealand in April (1977)...Paleontologists from the Natural Science Museum near Tokyo have concluded that the beast belonged to the plesiosaurus family – huge, small-headed reptiles with a long neck and four fins."(91)

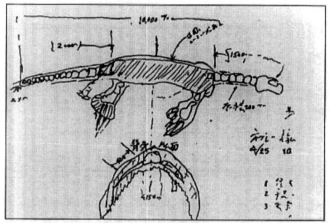

Figure 10.1 The drawing and measurements made by Michihiko Yano of the creature's skeleton that was dredged up off the New Zealand coast in 1977, and which the BBC and British Museum of Natural History would assure us was the body of a dead shark.

Emergence of Towns and Cities such as Atlantis

Evidence of the advances in the cultures that emerged can be seen in the towns and cities known prior to the flood.

Of all the cities that emerged in the centuries prior to the flood, Atlantis was undoubtedly the best known. Among the stories about this ancient city, probably the most famous are those of Plato, who wrote about it in 360 BC, in two dialogues - Timaeus and Critias.

In Critias, he describes the beginnings of Atlantis as a union between a god and a woman – an interesting similarity to Beriault and others who have written on Cain's lineage and specifically the women in it who intermarried with the fallen angels, as noted above.

"I have before remarked in speaking of the allotments of the gods, that they distributed the whole earth into portions differing in extent, and made for themselves temples and instituted sacrifices. And Poseidon,

46

receiving for his lot the island of Atlantis, begat children by a mortal woman, and settled them in a part of the island, which I will describe. Looking towards the sea, but in the centre of the whole island, there was a plain which is said to have been the fairest of all plains and very fertile. Near the plain again, and also in the centre of the island at a distance of about fifty stadia, there was a mountain not very high on any side. In this mountain there dwelt one of the earth born primeval men of that country, whose name was Evenor, and he had a wife named Leucippe, and they had an only daughter who was called Cleito.

The maiden had already reached womanhood, when her father and mother died; Poseidon fell in love with her and had intercourse with her, and breaking the ground, inclosed the hill in which she dwelt all round, making alternate zones of sea and land larger and smaller, encircling one another; there were two of land and three of water, which he turned as with a lathe, each having its circumference equidistant every way from the centre, so that no man could get to the island, for ships and voyages were not as yet...

And he named them all; the eldest, who was the first king, he named Atlas, and after him the whole island and the ocean were called Atlantic. To his twin brother, who was born after him, and obtained as his lot the extremity of the island towards the Pillars of Heracles, facing the country which is now called the region of Gades in that part of the world, he gave the name which in the Hellenic language is Eumelus, in the language of the country which is named after him, Gadeirus...

With such blessings the earth freely furnished them; meanwhile they went on constructing their temples and palaces and harbours and docks. And they arranged the whole country in the following manner:

First of all they bridged over the zones of sea which surrounded the ancient metropolis, making a road to and from the royal palace. And at the very beginning they built the palace in the habitation of the god and of their ancestors, which they continued to ornament in successive generations, every king surpassing the one who went before him to the utmost of his power, until they made the building a marvel to behold for size and for beauty."(92)

In Timaeus he wrote:

"Many great and wonderful deeds are recorded of your state in our histories. But one of them exceeds all the rest in greatness and valour. For these histories tell of a mighty power which unprovoked made an expedition against the whole of Europe and Asia, and to which your city put an end. This power came forth out of the Atlantic Ocean, for in those days the Atlantic was navigable; and there was an island situated in front of the straits which are by you called the Pillars of Heracles; the island was larger than Libya and Asia put together, and was the way to other islands, and from these you might pass to the whole of the opposite continent which surrounded the true ocean; for this sea which is within the Straits of Heracles is only a harbour, having a narrow entrance, but that other is a real sea, and the surrounding land may be most truly called a boundless continent.

Now in this island of Atlantis there was a great and wonderful empire which had rule over the whole island and several others, and over parts of the continent, and, furthermore, the men of Atlantis had subjected the parts of Libya within the columns of Heracles as far as Egypt, and of Europe as far as Tyrrhenia. This vast power, gathered into one, endeavoured to subdue at a blow our country and yours and the whole of the region within the straits; and then, Solon, your country shone forth, in the excellence of her virtue and strength, among all mankind. She was pre-eminent in courage and military skill, and was the leader of the Hellenes. And when the rest fell off from her, being compelled to stand alone, after having undergone the very extremity of danger, she defeated and triumphed over the invaders, and preserved from slavery those who were not yet subjugated, and generously liberated all the rest of us who dwell within the pillars."

Then, he noted, it all disappeared in a flood.

"But afterwards there occurred violent earthquakes and floods; and in a single day and night of misfortune all your warlike men in a body sank into the earth, and the island of Atlantis in like manner disappeared in the depths of the sea. For which reason the sea in those parts is impassable and impenetrable, because there is a shoal of mud in the way; and this was caused by the subsidence of the island." (93)

Was Atlantis the only city known during these times? Apparently not.

Many reports exist of other cities. A search on Google will find many references to underwater cities and structures on land found over the years.

For example, here is a reference to a city uncovered in the Pacific:

"In 1966, an oceanographic research expedition led by Dr. Robert J. Menzies of Duke University aboard the vessel Anton Brunn photographed what appeared to be carved rock columns under 6000 feet of ocean in the Milne-Edward Deep, a depression that reaches a depth of 19,000 feet. A cautious Dr. Menzies admitted that the discovery of what might be the ruins of an ancient city could be 'one of the most exciting discoveries of this century, insofar as ruins go. Some of the columns are half buried in mud while others stand upright. Many of them appear to have a kind of writing on them.'" (94)

The Transmission of Knowledge

If society was virtually wiped out in the flood, how do we have knowledge about it?

For one thing, those who lived before the flood had written documents.

Enoch, who lived before the flood, is credited with having written a history of man, as noted in one commentary on the Bible:

"Noah was a pivotal figure for the intellectual history of mankind just as he was for man's physical survival, and he carried the ancient knowledge of nature that had descended from Adam through his third son Seth to Enoch. Five generations separated Enoch from Seth, but such was the longevity of the patriarchs (Seth died aged 920) that traditions of learning could be constructed between them on the basis of personal knowledge. Adam lived for 930 years, so Enoch knew him. Enoch was generally credited with being the first author and making the earliest written records of the ancient wisdom. Enoch was alive on earth for only 365 years - not because he died, but because 'God took him' - so although Noah was separated from Enoch by only three generations, the chronology in Genesis makes it impossible for him to have known Enoch personally. But he would have known Enoch's son Methuselah, who lived for 967 years (for 243 years of which Adam himself was alive) and there was confidence among Biblical commentators that Noah would have inherited the learning of Enoch, especially since it had been written down.

Adam in his innocence and natural wisdom understood the voice of God, as God communicated with him in the Garden. After the Fall, only two men had that combination of wisdom and righteousness that allowed the record of Genesis to say that they 'walked with God': these two were Enoch and Noah. Little wonder, then, that it was important to extract as

49

much natural knowledge as possible from the building and management of the Ark.

After the Flood, Noah lived to the time of Abraham, so it was not difficult to imagine the authoritative descent extending a few more generations to Moses, the author of Genesis. In connection with both Noah's expertise in astronomy and the writings of Enoch, Walter Ralegh explained things as follows:

"it is very probable that Noah had seene and might preserve this booke. For it is not likely, that so exquisite knowledge therein (as these men had) was suddenly invented and found out, but left by Seth to Enoch, and by Enoch to Noah, as hath been said before. And therefore if letters and arts were knowne from the time of Seth to Enoch, and that Noah lived with Methuselah, who lived with Adam, and Abraham lived with Noah, it is not strange (I say) to conceive how Moses came to the knowledge of the first Age, be it by letters, or by Cabala and Tradition, had the undoubted word of God neede of any other proofe then self-authoritie.

It is interesting that Ralegh, as historian, argues to substantiate the authority of his primary author, Moses, but then points out that in any case, as scripture, the source has the authority of divine inspiration." (95)

An early version of the flood, by Berosus, a priest of Bel, the great god of Babylon, also noted that Noah had been asked to write a history of the world before the flood. He notes:

"The Deity, Cronus, appeared to him in a vision, and warned him that upon the 15th day of the month Daesius there would be a flood, by which mankind would be destroyed. He therefore enjoined him to write a history of the beginning, procedure and conclusion of all things; and to bury it in the city of the Sun at Sippara."

Berosus continues on to describe the flood. Then, after the survivors landed, they were told to return to Babylonia; and, it was ordained, search for the writings at Sippara, which they were to make known to mankind: moreover that the place, wherein they then were, was the land of Armenia. (96) Finally, the survivors of the flood knew the world they had left behind and described it to their descendants.

Chapter 3

From The Flood to the Dispersion

Our Ancestors and the Flood

According to the Bible, all modern humans that live today are descendants of Noah and his immediate family. All other humans were drowned in a great flood.

Noah's family line from Adam was as follows: Adam begot Seth, Seth begot Enos, who begot Cainan, who begot Malaleel, who begot Jared, who begot Henoch, who begot Methusala, who begot Lamech, who begot Noah. (97) Each of these lived hundreds of years and begot many children. Virtually all of these children joined Cain's descendants and became unfaithful to God.

When God saw how evil had spread throughout the world he decided to destroy it. Yet He relented with Noah, who had found grace with Him. (98) He decided to spare Noah and his family, and directed him to build an ark.

When the rains began, Noah went into the ark, taking his family and many animals with him. His family comprised three sons, Japheth, Sem and Cham, (99) and their wives.

Science and the Flood

Has science told us much about the flood? Those who promote evolution generally reject or ignore it. Those who view science within a faith framework will discuss it.

One scientist, Dr. Walter Brown, former Chief of Science and Technology Studies at the US Air War College, who accepts the biblical account, has written a book on the flood entitled *In the Beginning: Compelling Evidence for Creation and the Flood.* He has also provided the following

explanation of the flood in a video, available at http://www.youtube.com/watch?v=X16SE-N-8ys. In the video he discusses the hydroplate theory and shows how this explains the worldwide geography found today. Basically the earth had one super continent covered with lush vegetation. Mountains were smaller than today. Ten miles beneath the surface were vast quantities of water. A fracture occurred in the crust above the water and encircled the globe in two hours. The overlying rock crust opened and water pressured by ten miles of rock over it exploded twenty miles into the atmosphere. The spray from this produced torrential rains. In cold regions, such as Siberia, the water became ice crystals and produced massive ice dumps which buried animals such as the mammoths. In warmer climes, the water mixed with debris and produced massive sediments which buried mammals and much else. The split created the Atlantic ridge which circles the globe. It caused plates to separate and split the single continent that hitherto existed. As continental plates pushed they buckled. Some created sub ocean trenches. On land, they created ridges and mountains. These mountains follow the Atlantic ridge. Large basins opened and created inland lakes. Brown concludes that the event he describes supports the biblical version of the deluge in every detail. (100)
Others have explained how dramatically the flood affected life on the planet. Chris Parker writes:

"In the Karoo Bone yards or Karoo Supergroup in South Africa, there are an estimated 800 billion mostly vertebrate fossils—largely swamp dwelling reptiles. Composed mainly of sandstones and shales deposited in shallow water, the Karoo can be 20,000 feet thick. The fossil-rich beds stretch out for hundreds of miles…
….Massive fossil graveyards of dinosaurs still exist in other locations the world over. The Morrison beds in North America, the dinosaur beds in Montana, in the Rocky Mountains, in Alberta, the Dakotas, China, Colorado, Utah, Africa, etc., etc., contain literally millions of dinosaur fossils piled together in tremendous heaps.

Ten thousand Hadrosaurs were found on Egg Mountain, Montana alone, jumbled together in what appears to have been a mass death. The Flood produced the Sicilian hippopotamus beds, the fossils of which are so extensive that they are mined as a source of charcoal; the great mammal beds of the Rockies; the dinosaur beds of the Black Hills and the Rockies, as well as in the Gobi Desert; the fish beds of the Scottish Devonian stratum, the Baltic amber beds, Agate Spring Quarry in Nebraska, and hundreds more....

Many fossil graveyards are high up in mountainous areas. In Sicily, for example, four thousand feet above sea level on Mount Etna, there are two caves crammed with the bones of thousands of hippopotamus in each grave. On the island of Malta there are lions, tigers, mammoths, birds, beavers, hippopotamus and foxes all mixed together.

It has been estimated that some ten million animals lay buried along the rivers of northern Siberia. Thousands of tusks formed a massive ivory trade for the master carvers of China, all from the remains of the frozen mammoths and mastodons of Siberia."(101)

Ancient Documents and the Flood

There are many ancient documents that record a flood.

One very famous document is the Chaldean Account of the Deluge. George Smith translated this document, which is in Assyrian cuneiform tablets in the British museum. He speculated that its author lived in the epoch immediately following the flood. He stated that it was at least 1700 BC, and possibly much older. The Assyrians brought it to their archives. These tablets are now known as the eleventh tablet of the Gilgamesh epic. The flood took place during the reign of Xisuthras, the tenth king of the Chaldeans.

Here are the extracts recounting the flood:

"20. Surippakite son of Ubaratutu
21. make a great ship for thee . . . .
22. I will destroy the sinners and life . . . . .
23. cause to go in the seed of life all of it, to preserve them
24. the ship which thou shalt make
25. . . cubits shall be the measure of its length, and
26. .. cubits the amount of its breadth and its height.
27. Into the deep launch it."

28. I perceived and said to Hea my lord,
29. "Hea my lord this that thou commandest me
30. I will perform, it shall be done...
79. all I possessed I collected of the seed of life, the whole
80. I caused to go up into the ship, all my male and female servants,
81. the beasts of the field, the animals of the field, and the sons of the army all of them, I caused to go up.
82. A flood Shamas made, and
83. he spake saying in the night, 'I will cause it to rain from heaven heavily;
84. enter to the midst of the ship, and shut thy door,'
85. A flood he raised, and
86. he spake saying in the night, 'I will cause it to rain from heaven heavily.'...
99. the spirits carried destruction;
100. in their glory they swept the earth;
101. of Vul the flood, reached to heaven;
102. the bright earth to a waste was turned;
103. the surface of the earth, like .... it swept;
104. it destroyed all life, from the face of the earth . . . . .
105. the strong tempest over the people, reached to heaven.
106. Brother saw not his brother, it did not spare the people. In heaven
107. the gods feared the tempest, and
108. Sought refuge; they ascended to the heaven of Anu.
109. The gods, like dogs with tails hidden, couched down...
115. to evil were devoted all my people, and I prophesied
116. thus, 'I have begotten man and let him not
117. like the sons of the fishes fill the sea.'...
123. on the seventh day in its course, was calmed the storm, and all the tempest
124. which had destroyed like an earthquake,
125. quieted. The sea he caused to dry, and the wind and tempest ended.
126. I was carried through the sea. The doer of evil,
127. and the whole of mankind who turned to sin,
128. like reeds their corpses floated.
129. I opened the window and the light broke in, over my refuge
130. it passed, I sat still and
131. over my refuge came peace.
132. I was carried over the shore, at the boundary of the sea.
133. For twelve measures it ascended over the land.
134. To the country of Nizir, went the ship;...
178. When his judgment was accomplished, Bel went up to the midst of

54

the ship,
179. he took my hand and brought me out, me
180. he brought out, he caused to bring my wife to my side,
181. he purified the country, he established in a covenant and took the people." (102)

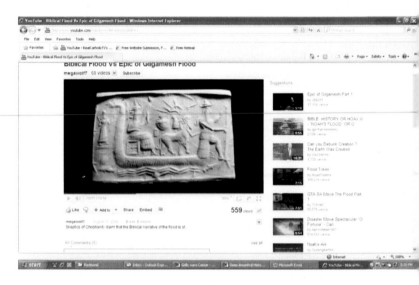

A depiction of the flood on a tablet relating the Epic of Gilgamesh. (103)

There are many legends of the flood from civilizations such as China, Babylon, Mexico, India, Rumania, Egypt, Sudan, Persia, Norway, Syria, Persia and Wales. The similarity of their content is remarkable. Perloff describes these similarities:

"In 95% of the more than 200 flood legends, the flood was worldwide; in 88 percent, a certain family was favoured; in 70 percent, survival was by means of a boat; in 67 percent animals were also saved; in 66 percent the flood was due to the wickedness of man; in 66 percent the survivors had been forewarned; in 57 percent they ended up on a mountain; in 35 percent birds were sent out from the boat; and in 9 percent exactly eight people were spared." (104)

Diodorus Siculus, in his book *The Library of History*, written in the 1st century BC, refers to the flood when he discusses the origins of Egypt:

"In general, he says that if in the flood which occurred in the time of Deucalion most living things were destroyed, it is probable that the inhabitants of southern Egypt survived rather than any others, since their country is rainless for the most part; or if, as some maintain, the destruction of living things was complete and the earth then brought forth again new forms of animals, nevertheless, even on such a supposition the first genesis of living things fittingly attaches to this country." (105)

Many of these stories have different names for the participants. For example, Diodorus refers to Deucalion, where we think of Noah. Deucalion, according to Micha F. Lindemans, was the son of Prometheus and Clymene. When Zeus punished humankind for their lack of respect by sending the deluge, Deucalion and his wife Pyrrha were the sole survivors. They were saved because of their piety. Prometheus advised his son to build an ark and they survived by staying on the boat.

The Start of new Human Expansion after the Flood

After the flood, notes Genesis:
"And the sons of Noah who came out of the ark, were Sem, Cham, and Japheth: and Cham is the father of Chanaan.
These three are the sons of Noah: and from these was all mankind spread over the whole earth". (106)

We are descendants of Noah's son Japheth.
Japheth was very well known in the ancient world, as Cooper notes:

"Japheth was regarded as the father of many peoples, particularly the Indo-European nations. The pagan Greeks perpetuated his name as Iapetos, the son of heaven and earth and again the father of many nations. We find his name in the vedas of India where it appears in Sanskrit as Pra-Japati, Father Japheth, who was deemed to be the sun and lord of creation, the source of life in other words for those descended from him.

Later, the Romans were to perpetuate his name as that of Ju-Pater, Father Jove, later standardized to Jupiter ... We shall see also that the early Irish Celts, the early Britons and other pagan European races traced the descent of their royal houses from Japheth, including the Saxons who knew him as Sceaf (pr. sheaf or shaif). And all these peoples, we must remember, were pagans whose knowledge or even awareness of the book of Genesis was non-existent. (107)

Japheth had seven sons, according to Genesis. They were Gomer, Magog, Madai, Javan, Tubal, Moshech and Tiras. (108)
We are the descendants of Magog.
Other European peoples are descendants of other sons. Javan, for example, is the father of most European people. These include the Franks, Romans, Britons, Albans, Vandals, Saxons, Bavarians, Thuringians, Goths, Valagoths, Burgundians and Lombards.
Tubal was the ancestor of the Iberians, Spanish and Italians. Two charts showing this can seen in Cooper's book in Appendix 3. (109) One is included in Appendix 1.

The Tower of Babel and the Dispersion of People

When did the separation of families start in earnest?
As the DNA analysis does not elaborate on the separation of peoples and their dispersal from the Near East, we can turn to historical and other documents for some information.
According to Genesis:

"And the earth was of one tongue and the same speech.
And when they removed from the east, they found a plain in the land of Sennaar, and dwelt in it...
And the Lord came down to see the city and the tower, which the children of Adam were building.
And he said: Behold, it is one people, and all have one tongue: and they have begun to do this, neither will they leave off from their designs, till they accomplish them in deed.

Come ye, therefore, let us go down, and there confound their tongue, that they may not understand one another's speech.
And so the Lord scattered them from that place into all lands, and they ceased to build the city."(110)

Clark's commentary on the Bible states:

"Noah and his family, landing after the flood on one of the mountains of Armenia, would doubtless descend and cultivate the valleys: as they increased, they appear to have passed along the banks of the Euphrates, till, at the time specified here, they came to the plains of Shinar, allowed to be the most fertile country in the east. That Babel was built in the land of Shinar we have the authority of the sacred text to prove; and that Babylon was built in the same country we have the testimony of Eusebius, Praep. Evang., lib. ix., c. 15; and Josephus, Antiq., lib. i., c. 5." (111)

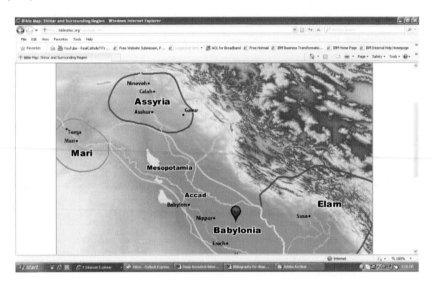

This map shows the Sinar, or Sennaar, region. (112)

Though Genesis does not note any individuals being responsible for building the Tower of Babel and angering God, commentaries on the Bible do.

For example, the Historical and Chronological Index to the Old Testament in the Douay-Rheims Bible, the one used by the Roman Catholic church since around 400 AD, notes

"Nimrod about threescore years after the flood, by force and subtlety drawing many followers, began a new sect of infidels. And afterwards was the principal author of building the Tower of Babel."(113)

Clark, commenting on Nimrod in Genesis 10:8-9 writes:

"Nimrod - Of this person little is known, as he is not mentioned except here and in 1 Chronicles 1:10, which is evidently a copy of the text in Genesis. He is called a mighty hunter before the Lord; and from Genesis 10:10, we learn that he founded a kingdom which included the cities Babel, Erech, Accad, and Calneh, in the land of Shinar. Though the words are not definite, it is very likely he was a very bad man. His name Nimrod comes from 1 no ,mugraT eht dna ;delleber eh ,daram, מרד Chronicles 1:10, says: Nimrod began to be a mighty man in sin, a murderer of innocent men, and a rebel before the Lord. The Jerusalem Targum says: "He was mighty in hunting (or in prey) and in sin before God, for he was a hunter of the children of men in their languages; and he said unto them, Depart from the religion of Shem, and cleave to the institutes of Nimrod." The Targum of Jonathan ben Uzziel says: "From the foundation of the world none was ever found like Nimrod, powerful in hunting, and in rebellions against the Lord." The Syriac calls him a warlike giant. The word דיצ tsayid, which we render hunter, signifies prey; and is applied in the Scriptures to the hunting of men by persecution, oppression, and tyranny. Hence it is likely that Nimrod, having acquired power, used it in tyranny and oppression; and by rapine and violence founded that domination which was the first distinguished by the name of a kingdom on the face of the earth. How many kingdoms have been founded in the same way, in various ages and nations from that time to the present! From the Nimrods of the earth, God deliver the world! (114)

Other writers comment unfavorably on Nimrod as well.

George Smith, who translated the Chaldean Account of Genesis in 1876, writes of Nimrod:

"Nearly thirteen hundred years before the Christian era, one of the Egyptian poems likens a hero to the Assyrian chief Kazartu, 'a great hunter... and it has already been suggested that the reference here is to the fame of Nimrod. A little later, in the BC 1100 to 800, we have in Egypt many persons named Nimrod, showing a knowledge of the mighty hunter there."(115)

Cooper writes:

"Nimrod was undoubtedly the most notorious man in the ancient world who is credited with instigating the Great Rebellion at Babel, and of founding astrology and even human sacrifice. Moreover, there is much evidence to suggest that he himself was worshipped from the very earliest times. His name, for example, was perpetuated in those of Nimurda, the Assyrian god of war; Marduk, the Babylonian king of the gods; and the Sumerian deity Amar-utu. ..

Nimrod was also worshipped by the Romans under the name of Bacchus, this name being derived from the Semitic bar-Cush, meaning the son of Cush. A mountain not far from Ararat, has been called Nimrud Dagh (Mount Nimrod) from the earliest times since the Flood, and the ruins of Birs Nimrud bear the remains of what is commonly reputed to be the original Tower of Babel. The Caspian Sea was once called the Mar de Bachu, or Sea of Bacchus, as is witnessed by the map appearing in Sir Walter Raleigh's History of the World, published in 1634. One of the chief cities of Assyria was named Nimrud, and the Plain of Shinar, known to the Assyrians as Sen'ar and the site of the Great Rebellion, was itself known as the Land of Nimrod. Iraqi and Iranian Arabs still speak his name with awe, and such was the notoriety of the man that his historical reality is beyond dispute" (116)

Flavius Josephus, in his *Antiquities of the Jews*, (94 AD) said that it was Nimrod who had the tower built and that Nimrod was a tyrant who tried to turn the people away from God.

"Now it was Nimrod who excited them to such an affront and contempt of God. He was the grandson of Ham, the son of Noah, a bold man, and of great strength of hand. He persuaded them not to ascribe it to God, as if it were through his means they were happy, but to believe that it was their own courage which procured that happiness. He also gradually changed the government into tyranny, seeing no other way of turning men from the fear of God, but to bring them into a constant dependence on his power... Now the multitude were very ready to follow the determination of Nimrod and to esteem it a piece of cowardice to submit to God; and they built a tower, neither sparing any pains, nor being in any degree negligent about the work: and, by reason of the multitude of hands employed in it, it grew very high, sooner than anyone could

60

expect; but the thickness of it was so great, and it was so strongly built, that thereby its great height seemed, upon the view, to be less than it really was. It was built of burnt brick, cemented together with mortar, made of bitumen, that it might not be liable to admit water. When God saw that they acted so madly, he did not resolve to destroy them utterly, since they were not grown wiser by the destruction of the former sinners [in the Flood]; but he caused a tumult among them, by producing in them diverse languages, and causing that, through the multitude of those languages, they should not be able to understand one another. The place wherein they built the tower is now called Babylon, because of the confusion of that language which they readily understood before; for the Hebrews mean by the word Babel, confusion."(117)

Some have described the layout of the Tower. For example, Gregory of Tours, writing ca. 594 AD, quotes the earlier historian Orosius, ca. 417AD, as saying the tower was

"laid out foursquare on a very level plain. Its wall, made of baked brick cemented with pitch, is fifty cubits wide, two hundred high, and four hundred and seventy stades in circumference. A stade contains five agripennes. Twenty-five gates are situated on each side, which make in all one hundred. The doors of these gates, which are of wonderful size, are cast in bronze. The same historian Orosius tells many other tales of this city, and says: 'Although such was the glory of its building still it was conquered and destroyed.'" (118)

The Chaldean Account of the Deluge notes:

"They say that the first inhabitants of the earth, glorying in their own strength and size and despising the gods, undertook to raise a tower whose top should reach the sky, in the place in which Babylon now stands; but when it approached the heaven the winds assisted the gods and overthrew the work upon its contrivers, and its ruins are said to be still at Babylon; and the gods introduced a diversity of tongues among men, who till that time had all spoken the same language." (119)

When did the Dispersion Happen

The dispersion of peoples appears to have happened in the fifth generation after Japheth. The Irish chronicles have Magog, then Iobaath, Baath, Izrau and Ezra. Other chronicles note the same. Cooper comments that different histories had the same five generations because there was a mixing of the patriarchal lines before Babel. He adds that all people had royal families and these may be descended from this line. Cooper adds that the concept of royalty and divinely ordered nations "would, of course, have been an act of open defiance towards God, and an attempt to repair or perhaps exploit the damage that was inflicted against a unifying of mankind at Babel". (120)

So the dispersal would have been some 100 to 150 years after the flood, depending on whether one uses 20 years or 30 years per generation.

The Historical and Chronological Index of the Douay Rheims Bible states that the separation of peoples happened 140 years after the flood. It notes that Heber, great grandson of Shem, did not consent to the building of the Tower, so his family were allowed to keep their language, which "for distinction's sake" was called Hebrew. (121)

After the dispersion, languages seem to have developed quickly. The manuscript *Chronicum Scotorum* notes:

"Fenius composed the language of the Gaeidhel from seventy-two languages, and subsequently committed it to Gaeidhel, son of Agnoman, viz, in the tenth year after the destruction of Nimrod's Tower." (122)

Commenting on dates, if we suppose that creation happened around 4000 BC, then the flood some 1600 years later, around 2400 BC, then the dispersion would have started around 2260 BC.

As people moved from the Sennaar region, some people headed west to the lands south of the Black Sea. Others headed northeast. Finally, some headed south towards Africa.

The DNA analysis notes that our ancestors were part of the group that headed north-east.

Some stayed in the Senaar Region. Nimrod and his followers built the tower in the centre that became the city and civilization of Babylon. They stayed there. Others of his line founded the cities and later, empires, of Assyria, Sumeria and Chaldea.

Changes in the DNA

The DNA analysis notes that our ancestors who had as the earliest marker, M168, now added another marker, M89. This man's descendants comprise 90 to 95% of all non-Africans.

After this change a group split and started moving towards Australia. According to the map provided by the National Geographic, they followed a coastal route. A second group split later, moving towards Anatolia and the Balkans. The main group to which our ancestors belonged moved north to the vast steepes of Central Asia.

We, and others who separated, and eventually moved into Europe, have been known in history as the Neolithic people. A discussion of the Neolithic and its link to the DNA analysis has been provided above.

Chapter 4

Emergence of Scythians and Others in Asia

Magog's Group Moves Northeast

After the separation of peoples that followed the building of the Tower of Babel, the descendants of Japheth spread out over the lands of the Near East.

Cooper has a map showing the split of Japheth's descendants. Magog's group is at the top left, to the northeast of the Black Sea. A second group of Magog's descendants, the Ashkenaz, moved below the Black Sea.

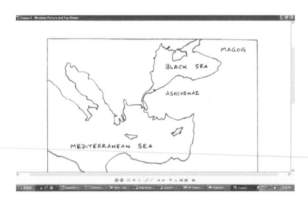

The Jewish historian Josephus wrote, around 50 AD, as quoted by Cusack, "Magog led out a colony, which from him were named Magoges, but by the Greeks called Scythians." (123)

Cooper, who provides the above map, notes that the Magogites and Ashkenaz were both known as Scythians:

"(Magog's) immediate descendants were known as the Magogites, being later known to the Greeks as the Scythians, according to the testimony of Josephus. However, given the subsequent history of the peoples of Ashkenaz, who are far more certainly identified as the later Scythians

(Gk. Skythai, and Assyr. Askuza), it is more likely that the early Magogites were assimilated into the peoples of Ashkenaz, thus making up merely a part of the Scythian hordes. The early Irish Celts traced their own lineage from Japheth through the line of Magog."(124)

The descendants of Magog can be seen north east of the Black Sea, which would be Georgia and southern Russia.
From there we moved again, into the vast steppes that cover this region of Asia from China to Eastern Europe.

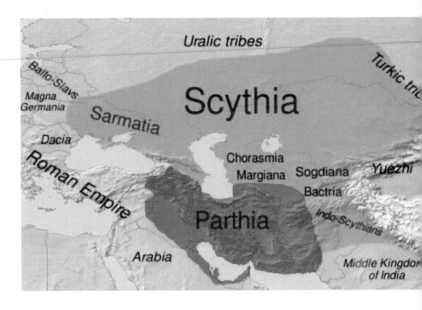

The map shown gives an idea of where we lived. This was the eastern end of the Great Plains that stretched from China to the Baltic States.
Writing on these plains, Tamara Talbot Rice states:

"The vast Eurasian steppes stretch some 4,350 miles from the base of the Carpathian Mountains in Europe to Mongolia in eastern Asia. They formed a single geographic unit of natural grassland that every spring was transformed into spectacular seas of wildflowers stretching as far as the eye could see.

This vast plain was perfectly suited to ranching and grain-raising. Archaeologists have discovered ample evidence to prove that, in antiquity, nomadic tribes regularly traversed it while following grazing herds and flocks in great cyclical routes during the spring, summer and fall.

However, climatic changes about 2,000 years ago turned large sections of the central-Asian steppes into a desert waste. It became so dry that it could no longer support the pastoral way of life practiced from 2,700 to 2,100 years ago." (125)

Let us look now at the Scythian culture that emerged.

Scythian Memories of Origin

Marcus Junianus Justinus, 2nd century AD, wrote that the Scythians claimed that they were more ancient than Egypt, of the power they developed in Asia, and of their relations with neighbours and their challenge to the power of Egypt.

"The nation of the Scythians was always regarded as very ancient; though there was long a dispute between them and the Egyptians concerning the antiquity of their respective races."(126)

He noted that the Egyptians said they were first because their climate was better. The Scythians would reply that after the floods, their lands, being higher, dried first and animals spread there, and indeed, their water flowed down to Egypt, which, therefore, dried later and thus grew later. (127)

Below we discuss recent DNA analysis of Tutankhamun, which links the Egyptian New kingdom to the Scythians and adds credence to these ancient written claims.

Herodotus, in Book 4 of his classic *The Histories*, relates the history of the Scythians that they provided him, along with another version he preferred. (128)

Herodotus states the Scythian rulers told him they had been there for a thousand years before Darius, the Persian king, attacked them. Darius ruled from 509 BC to 486 BC.

This means they knew they were in this region since 1500 BC anyway.

Following the dating we have been using so far, if they started separating from Babel in 2260 BC, it is reasonable to assume they were there at that time, and probably for a few centuries earlier.

Scythian Relations with Neighbours

Some of the earliest contacts with neighbours seem to have come with known distant relatives. They fought the Cimmerians, identified by Cooper as descendants of Gomer, the brother of Magog. They also fought the Medes, who, according to Cooper, descended from Madai, another brother of Magog. (129)

Regarding their relations with neighbours, Marcus Junianus Justinus wrote:

"They thrice aspired to the supreme command in Asia; while they themselves remained always either unmolested or unconquered by any foreign power. Darius, king of the Persians, they forced to quit Scythia in disgraceful flight. They slew Cyrus with his whole army. They cut off in like manner Zopyrion, a general of Alexander the Great, with all his forces. Of the arms of the Romans they have heard, but never felt them. They founded the Parthian and Bactrian powers. They are a nation hardy in toils and warfare; their strength of body is extraordinary; they take possession of nothing which they fear to lose, and covet, when they are conquerors, nothing but glory."(130)

One of their early great wars was against Egypt. Justinus wrote that Sesostris, King of Egypt proclaimed war against the Scythians and send messengers to announce conditions on which they might become his subjects. The Scythians replied that Egypt had far more wealth and they were going to take it. They advanced quickly against the Egyptians, who retreated. However "the morasses prevented the Scythians from invading Egypt" (131)

The Scythians then extended their power throughout much of Asia.

Diodorus writes:

"Now among the descendants of this king there were two brothers who were distinguished for their valour, the one named Palus and the other Napes. And since these two performed renowned deeds and divided the kingship between them, some of the people were called Pali after one of them and some Napae after the other. But some time later the descendants of these kings, because of their unusual valour and skill as generals, subdued much of the territory beyond the Tanaïs river as far as Thrace, and advancing with their armies to the other side they extended their power as far as the Nile in Egypt."(132)

Diodorus writes of their expansion after the Egyptian war.

"And after enslaving many great peoples which lay between the Thracians and the Egyptians they advanced the empire of the Scythians on the one side as far as the ocean to the east, and on the other side to the Caspian Sea and Lake Maeotis; for this people increased to great strength and had notable kings, one of whom gave his name to the Sacae, another to the Massagetae, another to the Arimaspi, and several other tribes received their names in like manner. It was by these kings that many of the conquered peoples were removed to other homes, and two of these became very great colonies: the one was composed of Assyrians and was removed to the land between Paphlagonia and Pontus, and the other was drawn from Media and planted along the Tanaïs, its people receiving the name Sauromatae. Many years later this people became powerful and ravaged a large part of Scythia, and destroying utterly all whom they subdued they turned most of the land into a desert."

In this incursion, which occurred between 630 and 625 B.C., the Scythians overran Palestine, but according to Herodotus, were turned back from Egypt by Psammetichus. A vivid picture of these foes from the north is preserved in Jeremias, chapters 4-5. (133) We can quote two passages:

"At the voice of the horsemen, and the archers, all the city is fled away: they have entered into thickets and have climbed up the rocks: all the cities are forsaken, and there dwelleth not a man in them:" and

"Their quiver is as an open sepulchre, they are all valiant.

And they shall eat up thy corn, and thy bread: they shall devour thy sons, and thy daughters: they shall eat up thy flocks, and thy herds: they shall eat thy vineyards, and thy figs: and with the sword they shall destroy thy strong cities, wherein thou trusted."

Justinus wrote that from the time of the invasion of Egypt, they subdued Asia and made it tributary. Agricultural populations provided food, others, such as the Medes, paid tribute, while others were plundered. Asia was tributary to them for fifteen hundred years, until Ninus, King of Assyria, ended the payment of the tribute. (134)

During the 90-year life of King Ateua, in the 4th century BC, the Scythians continued their westward expansion, settling in Thrace and becoming an important player in the Balkans. (135)

Economic and Cultural Life among the Scythians

The Scythians gradually developed royal rule. Herodotus and others mention a line that ruled from the 7th century BC. (136)

The Scythians were herdsmen for the most part, though some of the people were farmers.

As herdsmen, they wandered through the vast lands of the steepes. Herodotus, writing in the 4th century BC, said this gave them a great advantage in wars with neighbours.

"The Scythians indeed have in one respect, and that the very most important of all those that fall under man's control, shown themselves wiser than any nation upon the face of the earth. Their customs otherwise are not such as I admire. The one thing of which I speak is the contrivance whereby they make it impossible for the enemy who invades them to escape destruction, while they themselves are entirely out of his reach, unless it pleases them to engage with him. Having neither cities nor forts, and carrying their dwellings with them wherever they go; accustomed, moreover, one and all of them, to shoot from horseback, and living not by husbandry but on their cattle, their wagons the only houses that they possess, how can they fail of being unconquerable, and unassailable even?"(137)

Those in agriculture were poor and exploited. By the 4th century BC, the farmers were "socially deprived, dependent and exploited, who did not participate in the wars, but were engaged in servile agriculture and cattle husbandry."(138) The Scythians had developed expertise in metallurgy.

"Materials from the site near Kamianka-Dniprovska, purportedly the capital of the Ateas' state, show that metallurgists were free members of the society, even if burdened with imposed obligations. The metallurgy was the most advanced and the only distinct craft specialty among the Scythians." (139)

Trade became an important economic activity over time. By the 5th century BC, the Scythians were trading with the Greeks. This fostered a more defined stratification among the population. This reached a peak in the 4th century BC under King Ateas. In addition, the enhanced trading led to greater sedenterization.

Trade goods changed over time, with slaves becoming more important. The Scythians captured people and traded them to the Greeks. (140)

In religion, they had followed the practices of virtually all the emerging societies of these times in losing their knowledge of the God that Noah had followed and that the Hebrews still worshipped. In His place, they worshipped a variety of gods. Herodotus wrote of these gods:

"They worship only the following gods, namely, Vesta, whom they reverence beyond all the rest, Jupiter and Tellus, whom they consider to be the wife of Jupiter; and after these Apollo, Celestial Venus, Hercules, and Mars. These gods are worshipped by the whole nation: the Royal Scythians offer sacrifice likewise to Neptune…They use no images, alters, or temples, except in the worship of Mars; but in his worship they do use them."(141)

They sacrificed animals, and sometimes humans, to these gods.

A religious class emerged. Herodotus wrote that they had soothsayers, who foretold the future by means of willow wands. When the king is ill, soothsayers are called to identify who issued a false oath that caused the illness. They identify someone. If he claims innocence, more soothsayers are consulted. If they find him innocent, the first soothsayers are burned to death. If the man is found guilty, he and his male offspring are killed. He wrote that when a king dies, he is buried with a concubine, many servants and animals and a vast mound is placed above the grave. A year later, fifty more servants and horses are slain.

The burial sites, known as kurgan burials, are found in the steepe zone of North Pontic and other areas. Some date from the 5th century BC. (142)

They scalped and skinned their enemies and made drinking cups of their skulls.

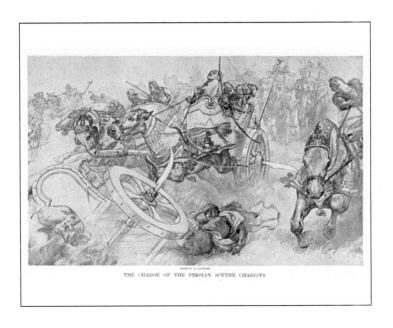

THE CHARGE OF THE PERSIAN SCYTHE CHARIOTS

Scythian war chariots (143)

71

Major Dispersions of Peoples Take Place

The DNA analysis provided by IBM and the National Geographic Society notes significant dispersion of peoples from the Near East into which the Scythians had moved. The chart below shows these splits that ultimately populated much of the world. The black lines are the Y-chromosome, while the grey are the mtDNA.

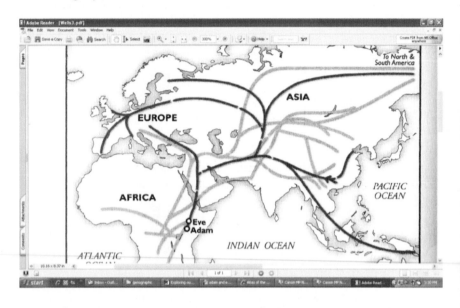

Archaeological research and historical documents identify many of these separations. We can now comment on some of the groups that separated as shown in the chart as well as on some groups that represented minor splits, but which are of importance and interest to our haplotype.

The Amazons

Perhaps one of the most unique splits was that which created a female warrior society known to the ancient world as the Amazons.

Justinus, the ancient Roman author, explained how they emerged:

"Among the Scythians, in the meantime, two youths of royal extraction, Ylinos and Scolopitus, being driven from their country by a faction of the nobility, took with them a numerous band of young men, and found a settlement on the coast of Cappadocia, near the river Thermodon, occupying the Themiscyrian plains that border on it. (The men fought neighbours and were killed.)

Their wives, when they found that to exile was added the loss of their husbands, took arms themselves, and maintained their position, repelling the attacks of their enemies at first, and afterwards assailing them in return. They relinquished all thoughts of marrying with their neighbours, saying that it would be slavery, not matrimony. Venturing to set an example not imitated through all generations, they established their government without the aid of men, and soon maintained their power in defiance of them. ..

Having thus secured peace by means of their arms, they proceeded, in order that their race might not fail, to form connexions with the men of the adjacent nations. If any male children were born, they put them to death. The girls they bred up to the same mode of life with themselves, not consigning them to idleness, or working in wool, but training them to arms, the management of horses, and hunting; burning their right breasts in infancy, that their use of the bow might not be obstructed by them; and hence they were called Amazons. They had two queens, Marpesia and Lampedo, who, dividing their forces into two bodies (after they were grown famous for their power), conducted their wars, and defended their borders separately and by turns. And that a reason for their success might not be wanting, they spread a report that they were the daughters of Mars. After subduing the greater part of Europe, they possessed themselves also of some cities in Asia. Having then founded Ephesus and several other towns there, they sent a detachment of their army home, laden with a vast quantity of spoil. (They fought Hercules, with the help of Scythians – they lost.)" (144)

Diodorus Siculus, writing in the 1st century BC described the decline of the Amazons:

"Heracles, the son of Alcmenê and Zeus, was assigned by Eurystheus the labour of securing the girdle of Hippolytê the Amazon. Consequently he embarked on this campaign, and coming off victorious in a great battle he not only cut to pieces the army of the Amazons but also, after taking captive Hippolytê together with her girdle, completely crushed this nation. Consequently the neighbouring barbarians, despising the weakness of this people and remembering against them their past injuries, waged continuous wars against the nation to such a degree that they left in existence not even the name of the race of the Amazons. For a few years after the campaign of Heracles against them, they say, during the time of the Trojan War, Penthesileia, the queen of the surviving Amazons, who was a daughter of Ares and had slain one of her kindred, fled from her native land because of the sacrilege. And fighting as an ally of the Trojans after the death of Hector she slew many of the Greeks, and after gaining distinction in the struggle she ended her life heroically at the hands of Achilles. Now they say that Penthesileia was the last of the Amazons to win distinction for bravery and that for the future the race diminished more and more and then lost all its strength; consequently in later times, whenever any writers recount their prowess, men consider the ancient stories about the Amazons to be fictitious tales. (145)

When did this happen? The Trojan War has been dated at 1194 to 1184 BC. (146)

A few of the Amazons, who had remained at home in their own country, established a power that continued, to the time of Alexander the Great. Their queen Minithya, or Thalestris, after obtaining from Alexander the enjoyment of his society for thirteen days, in order to have issue by him, returned into her kingdom, and soon after died, together with the whole name of the Amazons.

The Phoenicians

Writing on the origins of the Phoenicians, Cusack notes how a Scythian noble, who had been banished from his kingdom, had settled in Egypt, at the town of Chiroth, with his followers. This was at the time Moses was in Egypt. Herodotus confirmed that the Phoenicians anciently dwelt, as they allege, on the borders of the Red Sea. (147) When Moses led the Israelites out of Egypt, this Scythian noble gave provisions to the fleeing Israelites. This assistance was confirmed by Rabbi Simon, who wrote two hundred years before the birth of Christ, that Canaanites near the Red Sea helped the Israelites "and because these Canaan ships gave Israel of their provisions, God would not destroy their ships, but with an east wind carried them down the Red Sea".

When would this have been? As no exact date is known, a range of dates have been offered by different authors. It seems probable that Moses led the Israelites over the Red Sea anywhere from 1421 BC to 1313 BC. (148) Yet other documents note that, within a few generations, these Scythians moved, ending up in Spain, according to some around 764 BC.

They came to be known as the Phoenicians. As Cusack notes:

"It is not known at what time this ancient nation obtained the specific appellation of Phoenician. The word is not found in Hebrew copies of the Scriptures, but is used in the Maccabees, the original of which is in Greek, and in the New Testament. According to Grecian historians, it was derived from Phoenix, one of their kings, and brother of Cadmus, the inventor of letters. It is remarkable that our annals mention a king named Phenius, who devoted himself especially to the study of languages, and composed an alphabet and the elements of grammar. Our historians describe the wanderings of the Phoenicians, whom they still designate Scythians, much as they are described by other writers." (149)

She refers to Greeks using the script developed by the Phoenicians. Herodotus had also discussed the Greeks importing the Phoenician script.(150) Nennius, who wrote in the seventh century, from the oral testimony of trustworthy Irish Celts, gives corroborative testimony, on this origin.

The colony was eventually forced to leave Chiroth, being expelled by the grandson of the Pharaoh who drowned in the Red Sea, probably because of their help to the Israelites, but also because they may have posed a threat to the Egyptian state. Cusack notes their subsequent journey:

"(They) wandered through Africa for forty-two years, and passed by the lake of Salinas to the altars of the Philistines, and between Rusicada and

75

the mountains Azure, and he came by the river Mulon, and by sea to the Pillars of Hercules, and through the Tuscan Sea, and he made for Spain."

Spanish historians mention this settlement and claim the Phoenicians as their principal colonizers. The *Hispania Illustrata*, a rare and valuable work, on which no less than sixty writers were engaged, fixes the date of the colonization of Spain by the Phoenicians at 764 BC. Cusack notes:

"De Bellegarde says: "The first of whom mention is made in history is Hercules, the Phoenician, by some called Melchant." It is alleged that he lived in the time of Moses, and that he retired into Spain when the Israelites entered the land of promise. This will be consistent with old accounts, if faith can be placed in the inscription of two columns, which were found in the province of Tingitane, at the time of the historian Procopius. A Portuguese historian, Emanuel de Faria y Sousa, mentions the sailing of Gatelus from Egypt, with his whole family, and names his two sons, Iberus and Himerus, the first of whom, he says, "some will have to have sailed into Ireland, and given the name Hibernia to it."(151)

Rankin notes that "the luxurious contents of the burial at Vix in the Cote d'Or proves the existence in the sixth century BC of a flourishing community engaged in trade with the Greek world, no doubt through Massalia. (152)The Phoenicians were known as great navigators. Cusack discusses the information Herodotus provided on their circumnavigation of Africa seven centuries before the Christian era.

"Herodotus gives an account of the circumnavigation of Africa by the Phoenicians, which may have some coincidence with this narrative. His only reason for rejecting the tradition, which he relates at length, is that he could not conceive how these navigators could have seen the sun in a position contrary to that in which it is seen in Europe. The expression of his doubt is a strong confirmation of the truth of his narrative, which, however, is generally believed by modern writers.

This navigation was performed about seven centuries before the Christian era, and is, at least, a proof that the maritime power of the Phoenicians was established at an early period, and that it was not impossible for them to have extended their enterprises to Ireland. The traditions of our people may also be confirmed from other sources. Solinus writes thus: "In the gulf of Boatica there is an island, distant some hundred paces from the mainland, which the Tyrians, who came from the Red Sea, called Erythroea, and the Carthaginians, in their language, denominate Gadir, *i.e.*, the enclosure."(153)

Rankin quotes a poem, entitled Ora Maritima, written by Rufus Festus Avienus, proconsul of Africa in 366 AD, which described the shores of the known world and which noted these Phoenicians, whom he called Celts.

"A vigorous tribe lives here, proud-spirited, energetic, and skillful
On all the ridges trade is carried on:
The sea froths far and wide with their famous ships, and they cut through
the swell of the beast-haunted ocean.
These people do not build their boats with pine wood
(they make their ships out of skins joined together)
They run the vast salt sea on leather hide...
If anybody has the courage to urge his boat
Into the waves away from the Oestrymnides
Under the pole of Lycaon (in the Northern sky)
Where the air is freezing, he comes to the Ligurian land, deserted
By its people: for it has been emptied by the power of the Celts
A long time since in many battles." (154)

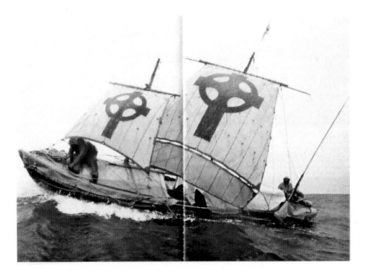

The boats mentioned by Rufus Festus Avienus were curraghs, boats still used in this century by the people of the Aran Islands. He notes that Pliny mentioned the British used them, and Strabo said the Lusitani of Spain had them. The place mentioned by Avenieus may have been the Bay of Biscay. The picture above shows a reconstruction of one used by St Brendan. (155)

The following map, noted by Hecataeus, gives an understanding of how the Phoenicians saw the world in which they roamed.

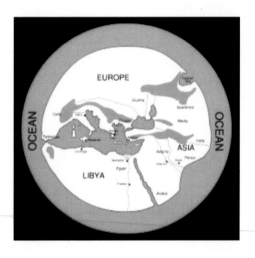

A map by Hecataeus ; he wrote travels around the world. (156)

According to some writers, they ventured very far. Cahill writes, "traces of the buildings of these Iberian Celts may have been found as far afield as New Hampshire – which would make the Celts the first Europeans to reach the New World". (157)

Parthians

One group of the Scythians that remained in Asia but evolved into a distinct group was the Parthians. Justinus writes that they were originally exiles from Scythia, which was apparent from their very name, for exiles in the Scythian language were called Parthi. (158) He goes on to write of the wars, their methods of fighting and their culture.

"The Parthians, in whose hands the empire of the east now is, having divided the world, as it were, with the Romans, were originally exiles from Scythia. This is apparent from their very name; for in the Scythian language exiles are called *Parthi*. During the time of the Assyrians and Medes, they were the most obscure of all the people of the east. Subsequently, too, when the empire of the east was transferred from the Medes to the Persians, they were but as a herd without a name, and fell under the power of the stronger. At last they became subject to the Macedonians, when they conquered the east; so that it must seem wonderful to everyone, that they should have reached such a height of good fortune as to rule over those nations under whose sway they had been merely slaves. Being assailed by the Romans, also, in three wars, under the conduct of the greatest generals, and at the most flourishing period of the republic, they alone, of all nations, were not only a match for them, but came off victorious; though it may have been a greater glory to them, indeed, to have been able to rise amidst the Assyrian, Median, and Persian empires, so celebrated of old, and the most powerful dominion of Bactria, peopled with a thousand cities, than to have been victorious in war against a people that came from a distance; especially when they were continually harassed by severe wars with the Scythians and other neighbouring nations, and pressed with various other formidable contests.

The Parthians, being forced to quit Scythia by discord at home, gradually settled in the deserts betwixt Hyrcania, the Dahae, the Arei, the Sparni and Margiani. They then advanced their borders, though their neighbours, who at first made no opposition, at length endeavoured to prevent them, to such an extent, that they not only got possession of the vast level plains, but also of steep hills, and heights of the mountains; and hence it is that an excess of heat or cold prevails in most parts of the Parthian territories; since the snow is troublesome on the higher grounds, and the heat in the plains.

The government of the nation, after their revolt from the Macedonian power, was in the hands of kings. Next to the royal authority is the order of the people, from which they take generals in war and magistrates in peace. Their language is something between those of the Scythians and Medes, being a compound of both. Their dress was formerly of a fashion peculiar to themselves; afterwards, when their power had increased, it was like that of the Medes, light and full flowing. The fashion of their arms is that of their own country and of Scythia. They have an army, not like other nations, of free men, but chiefly consisting of slaves, the numbers of whom daily increase, the power of manumission being allowed to none, and all their offspring, in consequence, being born slaves. These bondmen they bring up as carefully as their own children, and teach them, with great pains, the arts of riding and shooting with the bow. As any one is eminent in wealth, so he furnishes the king with a proportionate number of horsemen for war. Indeed when fifty thousand cavalry encountered Antonius, as he was making war upon Parthia, only four hundred of them were free men.

Of engaging with the enemy in close fight, and of taking cities by siege, they know nothing. They fight on horseback, either galloping forward or turning their backs. Often, too, they counterfeit flight, that they may throw their pursuers off their guard against being wounded by their arrows. The signal for battle among them is given, not by trumpet, but by drum. Nor are they able to fight long: but they would be irresistible, if their vigour and perseverance were equal to the fury of their onset. In general they retire before the enemy in the very heat of the engagement, and, soon after their retreat, return to the battle afresh; so that, when you feel most certain that you have conquered them, you have still to meet the greatest danger from them. Their armour, and that of their horses, is formed of plates, lapping over one another like the feathers of a bird, and covers both man and horse entirely. Of gold and silver, except for adorning their arms, they make no use.

Each man has several wives, for the sake of gratifying desire with different objects. They punish no crime more severely than adultery, and accordingly they not only exclude their women from entertainments, but forbid them the very sight of men. They eat no flesh but that which they take in hunting. They ride on horseback on all occasions; on horses they go to war, and to feasts; on horses they discharge public and private duties; on horses they go abroad, meet together, traffic, and converse. Indeed the difference between slaves and freemen is that slaves go on foot, but freemen only on horseback. They dispose of bodies by leaving them to be torn apart by birds or dogs; the bare bones they at last bury in the ground. (159)

The Great Move East of Major Segments

With the emergence of marker M9 in our haplogroup's DNA, major dispersions of people started taking place.

Indeed, the descendants of the man with this marker, in which our ancestors are included, populated much of the planet.

The National Geographic in their analysis calls this large clan the Eurasian Clan.

Many among their numbers were seasoned hunters who followed the herds along the great steepes of Asia.

When they came to the massive mountain ranges of south-central Asia – the Hindu Kush, the Tian Shan and the Himalayas, new splits occurred.

Some, including our ancestors, moved north into Central Asia.

Others moved south into what are now Pakistan and the Indian subcontinent.

Others moved into the Northern Hemisphere and eventually into North and South America. Acording to the DNA analysis, most people native to the Northern Hemisphere trace their roots to the Eurasian Clan. Nearly all North Americans and East Asians are descended from the man who started marker M9, as are most Europeans and many Indians.

After a time, an ancestor gave rise to another genetic marker M45.

We were still living in Central Asia at this time. Many had moved north of the mountainous Hindu Kush and onto the game-rich steepes of present day Kazakhstan, Uzbekistan and southern Siberia.

During this period climate was changing and desert like conditions were appearing on the southern steepes. These conditions pushed our ancestors northwards.

A creationwiki article on China notes:

"Today. China, although inhabited in the main by descendants of Magog, also includes some descendants of Gomer, Javan, and Esau." (160)

In time, another ancestor's marker changed and M207 started. The descendants of his man split into two groups.
One moved towards India.
The other, our ancestors, continued towards Europe.
Let us look briefly at groups that moved east.

Scythian Similarities with Indian Migrants

Rankin offers some interesting comparisons between the groups that went to India and those that later moved into Europe.

"Most had a royal or aristocratic social structure, and were divided into distinct, but not always rigid classes. Aggressive leadership in war probably evolved from the need for firm guidance of communities on the move, either seasonally, or in more distant migrations. The possession of wheeled transport and a relatively developed metal technology enhanced their social organization and enabled these restless and adaptable tribes to become dominant in most of the places where they settled." (161)

Not only general vocabulary and certain morphological features are involved, but more specialized lexical items concerning personal qualities and relationships, functions within the respective societies, names of commonly used tools and instruments. (162)
There are many similarities between Italic and Celtic and Indo-Iranic languages.
The words for person with magical power, freeman and many others are similar.
There were parallels in custom.

"Ancient Celts and Indians both seem to have attributed to kings a truth peculiar to their sacral and kingly function and continuous with the truth that supports the whole cosmos...There are also evidences of truth-ordeals and ceremonies concerning oaths in both societies...both societies had several grades of marriage." (163)

Family structure embraced three past and three forward generations. Ritual obligations went back to the great grandfather and forward to the great grandchildren. (164)

Scythian Moves into Kazakhstan, Mongolia and Siberia

Some of the moves to the east, such as that of the Kurgan people, appear to have taken place around 1000 BC. (165) Genetic research on fossils found at sites in the Altai Republic, Kazakhstan, Mongolia and Siberia has identified individuals belonging to the Scythians.

Keyser and others have worked on the mtDNA of skeletons from the Siberian Kurgan people. (166) They write:

"To help unravel some of the early Eurasian steppe migration movements, we determined the Y-chromosomal and mitochondrial haplotypes and haplogroups of 26 ancient human specimens from the Krasnoyarsk area dated from between the middle of the second millennium BC. to the fourth century AD. In order to go further in the search of the geographic origin and physical traits of these south Siberian specimens, we also typed phenotype-informative single nucleotide polymorphisms. Our autosomal, Y-chromosomal and mitochondrial DNA analyses reveal that whereas few specimens seem to be related matrilineally or patrilineally, nearly all subjects belong to haplogroup R1a1-M17 which is thought to mark the eastward migration of the early Indo-Europeans. Our results also confirm that at the Bronze and Iron Ages, south Siberia was a region of overwhelmingly predominant European settlement, suggesting an eastward migration of Kurgan people across the Russo-Kazakh steppe. Finally, our data indicate that at the Bronze and Iron Age timeframe, south Siberians were blue (or green)-eyed, fair-skinned and light-haired people and that they might have played a role in the early development of the Tarim Basin civilization."

A further quote from the same source notes:

"Y-Chromosome DNA testing performed on ancient Scythian skeletons dating to the Bronze and Iron Ages in the Krasnoyarsk region found that all but one of 11 subjects carried Y-DNA R1a1, with blue or green eye color and light hair common, suggesting mostly European origin of that particular population. Additional testing on the Xiongnu specimens revealed that the Scytho-Siberian skeleton (dated to the 5th century BCE) from the Sebÿstei site also exhibited R1a1 haplogroup. A search in the YHRD database as well as the authors' own database revealed no perfect haplotype matches for the Southern Siberian skeletons tested. However close matches were found for all but two. A haplotype found in samples 10 and 16 closely matched a haplotype found at high frequency in Altaians and considered a founder haplotype among them, as well as appearing among eastern Europeans and Central Anatolia. The haplotype of samples 24 and 34 closely matched types in Poland, Germany, Anatolia, Armenia, Nepal and India. The haplotype of specimen 26 has close matches in Western, Central, and Southern Asia as well as Europe and Siberia. It is the most frequent type in Ukraine. Haplotype S28 finds the most frequent matches in modern populations, being carried by northern and eastern Europeans and Southern Siberians." (167)

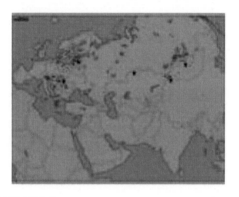

This chart shows the current distribution pattern of the mtDNA haplotypes found in the ancient Siberians studied by Keyser. The squares show present day individuals having the same haplotype. (168) As can be seen, the haplotype is concentrated in Europe.

Maternal genetic analysis of Saka period male and female skeletal remains from a double inhumation kurgan located at the Beral site in Kazakhstan determined that the two were most likely not closely related and were possibly husband and wife. The HV1 mitochondrial sequence of the male was similar to the Anderson sequence which is most frequent in European populations. Contrary, the HV1 sequence of the female suggested a greater likelihood of Asian origins. The

84

study's findings were in line with the hypothesis that mixings between Scythians and other populations occurred. This was buttressed by the discovery of several objects with a Chinese inspiration in the grave. No conclusive associations with haplogroups were made though it was suggested that the female may have derived from either mtDNA X or D. (169) DNA research has been done on the content of the mounds in the Altai Republic. Mitochondrial DNA extracted from skeletal remains obtained from excavated Scythian kurgans has produced a myriad of results and conclusions. Analysis of the HV1 sequence obtained from a male Scytho-Siberian's remains at the Kizil site in the Altai Republic revealed the individual possessed the N1a maternal lineage. The study also noted that haplogroup mtDNA N1a was found at a relatively high frequency in the southern fringes of the Eurasian steppe in Iran (8.3%). From this, a possible link to ancient populations presumed to have come from Europe that lived in the neighboring northwestern parts of the Subcontinent and Iran was suggested.

Additionally, mitochondrial DNA has been extracted from two Scytho-Siberian skeletons found in the Altai Republic (Russia) dating back 2,500 years. Both remains were determined to be of males from a population who had characteristics "of mixed Euro-Mongoloid origin". ("European" in this context means Western Eurasian).One of the individuals was found to carry the F2a maternal lineage, and the other the D lineage, both of which are characteristic of East Eurasian populations. Also found in the Altai Republic was the mummy of a Scythian warrior, which is believed to be about 2,500 years old, was a 30 to 40 year old man with blond hair and was found in the Altai, Mongolia."(170)

Scythian Similarities with Emerging Celts

The Scythians developed distinct cultural and religious habits during these years of migration, then settlement. Rankin notes how the early Irish repeatedly connected their ancestry with the Scythians, and quotes Wagner who described the most notable cultural resemblances between western insular Celts and Thracians, Phrygian, and Scythic tribes as follows:

1. Rider-god: Eochaidh (Dagde), Rhesus, and the Thracian Rider-god.
2. Hermes the oath-god of the Thracians and Scythians; Lugh in the Irish tradition.
3. Ceremonial use of drink in religious and guasi-religious group bonding.
4. Raiding habits: Homeric boelasiai, Tain Bo Cualgne.
5. Wakes, funeral games: rejoicing at death as the inception of a better afterlife.
6. River and well worship amongst Thracians, Irish, and Brythonic Celts.
7. The three-headed rider-god (specimen found at Philip-popolis); Celtic tricephalic statues.
8. Pastoral emphasis: small respect for agriculture. (171)

broadcast by the Discovery Channel on February 17, 2010. In that broadcast, the camera panned over a printout of the DNA test results of King Tutankhamun. (177) These results showed STR (Short Tandem Repeats) values for 17 markers. Whit Atley, a doctor of physics and biochemistry and a specialist in genetic genealogy, who runs a valuable website called the Haplogroup Predictor, inputted the STR data and generated the haplogroup which marked those STR data. (178)

The data showed that King Tutankhamun had a 99.6% fit with the R1b haplogroup. The R1b haplogroup, as we noted above, is found in 89% of the Welsh, 88% of the Basque, 70% of the Dutch, 82% of the Irish and 77% of the Scotch. (179) Tutankhamun's paternity was confirmed through further DNA testing linking him to his father Akhenaten and grandfather Amenhotep III. (180) His mother was Nefertiti. (181) Indications were that this group originated in the Black Sea area of Anatolia or the Caucasus Mountains. (182)

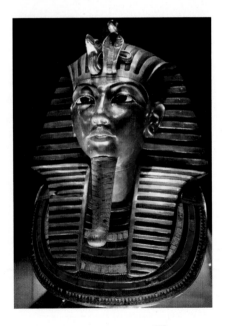

89

This is the mask of Tutankhamun's mummy in the Egyptian museum. (183)

Below is the mummified head that was analyzed. (184)

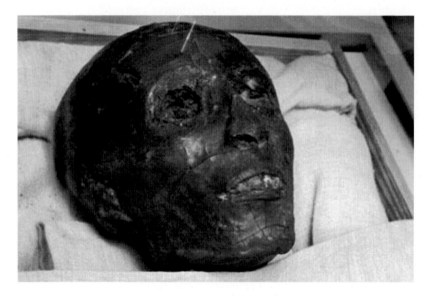

The *EU Times*, which released information on the announcement, provided the following map which showed where most of King Tutankhamun's haplotype group eventually settled.

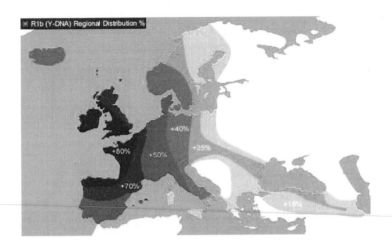

Commemoration of the victories of this group as they moved towards and into Egypt is found in objects buried with him. For example the following cartouches of his birth and throne names are displayed between rampant Sekhmet lioness warrior images (perhaps with his head) crushing enemies of several ethnicities, while Nekhbet flies protectively above. (185)

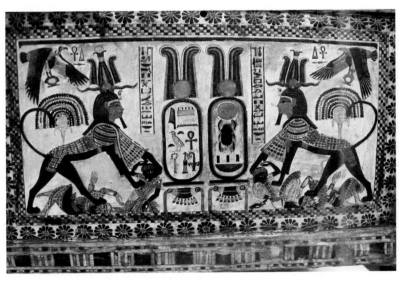

The New Kingdom of Egypt, also referred to as the Egyptian Empire is the period in ancient Egyptian history between the 16th century BC and the 11th century BC, covering the Eighteenth, Nineteenth, and Twentieth Dynasties of Egypt. The New Kingdom followed the Second Intermediate Period and was succeeded by the Third Intermediate Period. It was Egypt's most prosperous time and marked the peak of its power. Radiocarbon dating suggests that the New Kingdom range for its beginning is 1570-1544 BC. The later part of this period, under the Nineteenth and Twentieth Dynasties (1292-1069 BC) is also known as the Ramesside period, after the eleven pharaohs that took the name of Ramesses. (186)

Tutankhamun ruled from c.1333 BC to 1323 BC. His original name, Tutankhaten, means "Living Image of Aten", while Tutankhamun means "Living Image of Amun". In hieroglyphs, the name Tutankhamun was typically written Amen-tut-ankh, because of a scribal custom that placed a divine name at the beginning of a phrase to show appropriate reverence. (187)

He was a great builder. He initiated building projects, in particular at Thebes and Karnak, where he dedicated a temple to Amun. Many monuments were erected, and an inscription on his tomb door declares the king had "spent his life in fashioning the images of the gods". He restored traditional festivals, including those related to the Apis Bull, Horemakhet, and Opet. His restoration stela says:

"The temples of the gods and goddesses ... were in ruins. Their shrines were deserted and overgrown. Their sanctuaries were as non-existent and their courts were used as roads ... the gods turned their backs upon this land ... If anyone made a prayer to a god for advice he would never respond."

Tutankhamun was one of the few kings worshiped as a god and honored with a cult-like following in his own lifetime. A stela discovered at Karnak and dedicated to Amun-Re and

Tutankhamun indicates that the king could be appealed to in his deified state for forgiveness and to free the petitioner from an ailment caused by wrongdoing. Temples of his cult were built as far away as in Kawa and Faras in Nubia.

Chapter 5

Expansion throughout Europe

DNA Analysis and the Move into Europe

Descendants of the man with marker 173 who moved into Europe become the "first modern humans to move into Europe and eventually colonize the continent", according to the information provided in my DNA analysis. (188)
The DNA analysis I received further states that this move is marked by the emergence of the Aurignacian culture. Perhaps, in a general sense this was so. However, historical and archaeological evidence specifically link our ancestors to the Urnfield and Halstatt cultures. So let us now look at these cultures.

Urnfield and Hallstatt Cultures in Austria 1300-800 BC

The Urnfield culture was a Bronze Age culture that lasted from the thirteenth to the eight centuries BC. Rankin writes that the members of this culture were speakers of a kind of Celtic. This is often called proto-Celtic. He notes that there are many place names of almost certain Celtic derivation in these areas of habitation. (189)
Rankin notes that one of the early centres of this culture was Noreia in Austria. The geographer Hecataeus, in his book Europe, refers to Nyrax, a Celtic city. (190)
This culture became pre-eminent in Central Europe. It was characterized by a dramatic increase in population in the region, probably due to innovations in technology and agricultural practices. (191)
This culture led on to the Hallstatt culture, a bronze and iron culture, which dominated from the eight century BC

onwards. It derived its name from the rich grave finds at Hallstatt, Austria. Rankin writes of this:

"Settlement along the Danube is marked by the "remains of destroyed Hallstatt sites. Fortified townships (oopida) along the south bank of the Danube have distinctly Celtic names in antiquity: Vindobona, Carnuntum, Brigetio and Arrabona are clear examples. These oppida may be taken to be a line of defense against northern tribes here and elsewhere in Europe where they occur." (192)

The Hallstatt culture was succeeded by the La Tene culture, which developed out of it under the impetus of Mediterranean influence from Greek and later Etruscan societies. This culture flourished during the late Iron Age, from 450 BC to the Roman conquests in the 1st century BC. (193)

During this period cultures emerged that later became states in Eastern Europe.

In what is now Czechoslovakia, are traces of LaTene culture, which Rankin notes as likely Celtic. He notes many characteristics of this culture, which were Celtic.

"In the offida of Slovakia, the craft of the smith was well developed, and this might suggest that it was closely connected with the needs of a warrior class of the kind we find evidenced in Celtic societies elsewhere. Torques are found imprinted on Celtic coinage: there are coins imitating those of Philip II which may have been the currency of the Boii. Distinctly Celtic motives, such as the boar, appear on coinage of the second century BC. Names, Celtic beyond reasonable doubt, occur on coins of this region – for example the names of leaders such as Nonnos and Biatec constitute the earliest written inscriptions of the area." (194)

A similar culture was defining itself in what is now Hungary. Celts seem first to have appeared in Hungary in the La Tene period. They probably arrived in Pannonia about the same time as their kinsmen invaded Italy in the first decade of the fourth century BC.

"We know that in the eastern part of Hungary there were speakers of an Iranic dialect who were of Cimmerian decent and had become assimilated to the Scythians who had defeated them and settled in their territory. These were the Sigynnae. (Herodotus 5.9) Their name may have the meaning 'merchant' in an IE dialect spoken in Pannonia before the arrival of the Celts. "(195)

The land that is now Poland also developed Celtic cultures.

"The region which in modern times became Poland also was touched by Celtic migration. These Celts came from Bohemia (which bears the name of the Bopii) through the Ktodzko valley and impinged upon an already established Lusatian/Hallstatt culture. They seem to have come as a full community, with farmers and craftsmen as well as warriors."(196)

Rankin quotes Herodotus, in his second book, where he compares the Nile with the Danube which

"rises among the Celts and the city of Pyrene and flows through Europe, splitting it in the middle. The Celts, he says live outside the pillars of Heracles, and have common boundaries with the Cynesioi who live to the west of all the other inhabitants of Europe."

Analyzing this quote Rankin says Herodotus knew the Celts lived in Spain and Central Europe. (197)

Rankin notes that "it is reasonable to accept that in the fourth and third centuries BC the Celtic peoples dominated northern and central Europe from the Black Sea to Spain. This is the message of the Greek and Roman authors, who, together with the archaeologists of the present time, are convincing on this point. (198).

Thus, we see that by 500 BC, Celtic influence was very strong throughout Europe.

Nolan gives a good idea of this in his discussion of the move of his branch of the Celtic family into France:

"The Belgae made their way into Gaul, which consists in the modern world of Britain, France, Belgium, Luxembourg, Monaco, the Netherlands; Iberia (Spain and Portugal). Historians describe these Britannic Celts, Érainn, spreading their La Tène culture in the British Isles before moving into Ireland circa 500 B. C. E. Trinity College geneticists from Dublin, Ireland estimate the migration may have occurred much earlier 4,000-1,000 B. C. E. claiming that the Celtic people of Ireland and Scotland have a commonality with the people of

Portugal and Spain. This 2004 Trinity College genetic study revealed kinships between the Celts of Ireland and Scotland, the people of Galicia, an ancient association of Celtic tribes residing above the banks of the Douro River in the Iberian Peninsula, and the non-Celtic Basque region. The Gaul's conquered parts of Asia Minor and the term Gaul refers to an ancient name given the territory south and west of the Rhine, west of the Alps, and north of the Pyrenees. These ancient Celtic associations, though, could be representative of Ken Nordtvedt's calculation of a time to most recent common ancestor for U152 (R1b1b2a2g) (R1b1b2h*) (R1b1c10) that falls within the range for the volcanic destruction of the city and territory of Nola in ancient Italy circa 1800 and 1750 B. C. with a 3,780 year most recent common ancestor estimate for R-U152 and R-U106 stating that the MRCA for R-U152 is within range of that estimate and the MRCA for R-U106 occurs at the 3,270 year marker making the MRCA for it 500 years younger than R-U152." (199)

Celtic Extent in Europe 500 BC

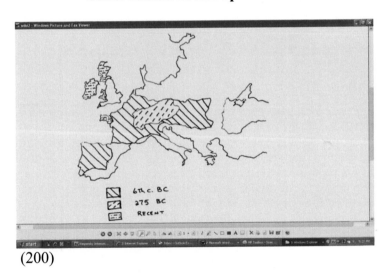

(200)

A comprehensive list of the Celtic tribes or groups throughout Europe is provided in http://en.wikipedia.org/wiki/List_of_Celtic_tribes

Celtic Trade in Europe

The Celts had developed a large trading network in Europe by 500 BC. One description of it notes:

"An Iron Age culture spanning from 450 BC to the fall of Gaul in 51 BC. Trade now included wines, fine Etruscan pottery, bronze and iron goods, iron weapons, jewellery and even some gold: Chieftains were even buried with their war chariots. At their greatest extent, around 200 BC, the culture of the Iron Age people formerly known as 'Celts' lay from the Pyrenees east skirting northern Italy and northern Greece to present day Bulgaria. Trade routes made use of the 7 major rivers of Central Europe, namely Garonne, Rhône, Seine, Saône, Rhine, Po and the upper Danube. The use of iron weapons against less advanced tribes, ensured their supremacy. Trade routes between Egypt and Britain have been proved with the discovery of blue glass beads in Wiltshire identical to those found at Deir el-Bahari and have been subsequently dated at about 1400 BC." (201)

Celtic Social Life within Europe

Rankin (202) describes the social strata of Celtic society at this time:

"Kings, warrior-aristocrats and at least two grades of client hood, one more respectable than the other. Insular literature of later centuries gives us a picture of a relatively complex social system composed not only of noble warriors and druids, but of various groups devoted to particular skills and professions, or agricultural and service functions. The learned classes consisted of druids and various grades of poets. There is archaeological evidence for the emergence in the Halstatt culture of a social pattern which differed from that of the Urnfield in constructing, undoubtedly for a minority, elaborate and richly furnished tombs. The Halstatt grave at Vix (6th century BC), the burial of a young woman, illustrates this by its store of magnificent Greek bronze and ceramic ware, its interred four-wheeled chariot, and other valuable articles."

Writing on rulers, Rankin notes:

"Like the Greeks and Romans, the Continental Celts of historical times had substantially moved away from kingly rule, though they preserved the name of king in designating their great overlords in war, such as Dumnorix ('world-king') and Veringetorix ('great king of those who march to attack') ... Kings survived in Ireland well into the medieval period."

Writing on the culture, Rankin identifies seven characteristics of the Celts that had emerged: the druidic priesthood, head-hunting, the cult of the severed head, human sacrifice, distinctive laws of hospitality, a heroic warrior class, and orders of bards and poets.

DNA Changes as Celts move into France

When we moved into France and Spain, one man's chromosomes changed and the marker M343 was started.
With this change, we now have the final of the Y-chromosome changes to date in our ancestral line.
Today, roughly 70% of the men in southern England belong to this haplogroup, while in parts of Spain and Ireland, that number exceeds 90%.

The Celtic Name in Europe

The earliest recorded mention of the Celtic name in France was by Hecataeus of Miletus, the Greek geographer who, in 517 BC, wrote about a people living near "Massilia" (Marseille). The Latin name "Celtus" (pl. "Celti" or "Celtae") seems to have been borrowed from Greek (Κέλτης pl. Κέλται or Κελτός pl. Κελτοί), according to testimony of Caesar itself taken from a native Celtic tribal name. Pliny the Elder referred it as being used in Lusitania as a tribal surname which epigraphic findings confirm. Strabo referred to them as Keltai, sometimes compounding the names into Kelti-Iberian or Kelto-Scythian. (203)
Until this time, they had been referred to by other names. The Romans often called them Galli. The Greeks referred to them as Galatai. (204)

99

We have noted above how the Celts living in Marseilles are mentioned by Rufus Festus Avienus as Celts.

The Celtic Groups in Marseilles Fence

Aristotle is said to have written a Constitution of Massalia in which he told the story of its foundation as follow:

"The Phoenicians of Ionia in the course of their trading founded Massalia. Euxenus of Phocaea was the guest-friend of Nanos, for this was the name of their king. Nanos was arranging his daughter's marriage, and by chance Euxenus arrived and was invited to the feast. Now the marriage (selection of bridegroom) was conducted in the following fashion: the girl had to come in after the dinner and to give a bowl of wine mixed with water to the one amongst the suitors she wanted. The one she gave it to, this would be her bridegroom. The girl came in, and through chance, or for some other cause, she gave it to Euxenus. The girl's name was Petta. When this happened, and with the father asking him to accept her on the grounds that the choice was inspired by the god, Euxenus took her as his wife, changing her name to Aristoxene. And there is a family in Massalia to this day descended from this girl, called the Protiadai: Protos was the name of the son of Euxenus and Aristoxene." (205)

In the years preceding the attack on Rome, Massalia reached a level of power and wealth that provoked fear and jealousy in the other peoples of southern Gaul. He quotes Trogus, a Celt of the tribe of Vocontii, whose grandfather had received Roman citizenship from Pompey the Great for his services in the war against Sertorius; his maternal uncle had led squadrons of cavalry against Mithridates; his father was in the army of Julius Caesar; he was in charge of negotiations with the Gauls.

"There were great conflicts with the Ligurians and equally great wars with the Gauls, which increased the city's glory by the addition of victory to victory, and made her famous among the neighbouring peoples. Also she defeated the armies of Carthage when war broke out over the seizure of fishing vessels, and created security for those who had been oppressed. The city also formed alliances with the tribes of Spain, and almost from the beginnings of her history she remained scrupulously faithful to a treaty concluded with Rome, and energetically aided her ally in all her wars by means of auxiliary forces." (206)

Diodorus distinguished between the Celts and the Gauls, stating that the peoples who dwell in the interior above Massalia, those on the slopes of the Alps, and those on this side the Pyrenees mountains are called Celts, whereas the peoples who are established above this land of Celtica in the parts which stretch to the north, both along the ocean and along the Hercynian Mountain, and all the peoples who come after these, as far as Scythia, are known as Gauls.

The Romans, however, included all these nations together under a single name, calling them one and all Gauls.(207)

Life of the Gauls in France

Nolan notes this map (208), one of Gaul around 58 BC:

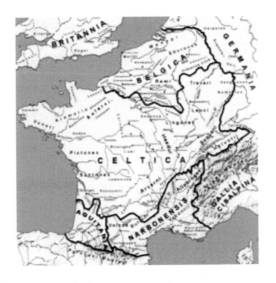

Diodorus, who wrote between 60 BC and 30 BC, described life among the Gauls. The following paragraphs are based on his description. (209)

101

Gaul is inhabited by many tribes of different size; for the largest number some two hundred thousand men, and the smallest fifty thousand, one of the latter standing on terms of kinship and friendship with the Romans, a relationship which has endured from ancient times down to our own day. There is much gold in their land and both men and women wear it. For around their wrists and arms they wear bracelets, around their necks heavy necklaces of solid gold, and huge rings they wear as well, and even corselets of gold. He described their customs:

"The Gauls are tall of body, with rippling muscles, and white of skin, and their hair is blond, and not only naturally so, but they also make it their practice by artificial means to increase the distinguishing colour which nature has given it. For they are always washing their hair in lime-water, and they pull it back from the forehead to the top of the head and back to the nape of the neck, with the result that their appearance is like that of Satyrs and Pans, since the treatment of their hair makes it so heavy and coarse that it differs in no respect from the mane of horses. Some of them shave the beard, but others let it grow a little; and the nobles shave their cheeks, but they let the moustache grow until it covers the mouth. Consequently, when they are eating, their moustaches become entangled in the food, and when they are drinking, the beverage passes, as it were, through a kind of a strainer. When they dine they all sit, not upon chairs, but upon the ground, using for cushions the skins of wolves or of dogs. The service at the meals is performed by the youngest children, both male and female, who are of suitable age; and near at hand are their fireplaces heaped with coals, and on them are caldrons and spits holding whole pieces of meat. Brave warriors they reward with the choicest portions of the meat."

They had an awareness of eternity and a remarkable relaxed attitude towards death which arose from their belief that they would never die, as Diodorus notes:

"They invite strangers to their feasts, and do not inquire until after the meal who they are and of what things they stand in need. And it is their custom, even during the course of the meal, to seize upon any trivial matter as an occasion for keen disputation and then to challenge one another to single combat, without any regard for their lives; for the belief of Pythagoras prevails among them, that the souls of men are immortal and that after a prescribed number of years they commence upon a new life, the soul entering into another body."

In war, they used chariots and hand to hand fighting. They scalped their enemies and cut off their heads and kept them, as Diodorus notes:

"(When) they go into battle the Gauls use chariots drawn by two horses, which carry the charioteer and the warrior; and when they encounter cavalry in the fighting they first hurl their javelins at the enemy and then step down from their chariots and join battle with their swords.... When their enemies fall they cut off their heads and fasten them about the necks of their horses; and turning over to their attendants the arms of their opponents, all covered with blood, they carry them off as booty, singing a paean over them and striking up a song of victory, and these first-fruits of battle they fasten by nails upon their houses, just as men do, in certain kinds of hunting, with the heads of wild beasts they have mastered. The heads of their most distinguished enemies they embalm in cedar-oil and carefully preserve in a chest."

These habits of behaviour in war were clearly long lasting, having been practiced since early Scythian times. Diodorus describes the clothing:

"The clothing they wear is striking — shirts which have been dyed and embroidered in varied colours, and breeches, which they call in their tongue bracae; and they wear striped coats, fastened by a buckle on the shoulder, heavy for winter wear and light for summer, in which are set checks, close together and of varied hues ...For armour they use long shields, as high as a man, which are wrought in a manner peculiar to them, some of them even having the figures of animals embossed on them in bronze, and these are skillfully worked with an eye not only to beauty but also to protection. On their heads they put bronze helmets which have large embossed figures standing out from them and give an appearance of great size to those who wear them; for in some cases horns are attached to the helmet so as to form a single piece, in other cases images of the fore-parts of birds or four-footed animals."

They had bards and enjoyed boasting and telling stories.

"The Gauls are terrifying in aspect and their voices are deep and altogether harsh; when they meet together they converse with few words and in riddles, hinting darkly at things for the most part and using one word when they mean another; and they like to talk in superlatives, to the end that they may extol themselves and depreciate all other men. They are also boasters and threateners and are fond of pompous language, and yet they have sharp wits and are not without cleverness at learning. Among them are also to be found lyric poets whom they call Bards. These men sing to the accompaniment of instruments which are like lyres, and their songs may be either of praise or of obloquy."

The Druid Religion in Gaul

Their religious leaders were Druids. Diodorus wrote of the Druids:

"Philosophers, as we may call them, and men learned in religious affairs are unusually honoured among them and are called by them Druids. The Gauls likewise make use of diviners, accounting them worthy of high approbation, and these men foretell the future by means of the flight or cries of birds and of the slaughter of sacred animals, and they have all the multitude subservient to them." (210)

Cusack would later write in glowing terms of these religious leaders.

"Druidism was the religion of the Celts, and druidism was probably one of the least corrupt forms of paganism. The purity of the divinely-taught patriarchal worship, became more and more corrupted as it passed through defiled channels. Yet, in all pagan mythologies, we find traces of the eternal verity in an obvious prominence of cultus offered to one god above the rest; and obvious, though grossly misapplied, glimpses of divine attributes, in the many deified objects which seemed to symbolize his power and his omnipotence The Celtic druids probably taught the same doctrine as the Greek philosophers.

The metempsychosis, a prominent article of this creed, may have been derived from the Pythagoreans, but more probably it was one of the many relics of patriarchal belief which were engrafted on all pagan religions. They also taught that the universe would never be entirely destroyed, supposing that it would be purified by fire and water from time to time. This opinion may have been derived from the same source. The druids had a *pontifex maximus*, to whom they yielded entire obedience,—an obvious imitation of the Jewish custom. The nation was entirely governed by its priests, though after a time, when the kingly power developed itself, the priestly power gave place to the regal. Gaul was the head-quarters of druidism; and thither we find the Britons, and

104

even the Romans, sending their children for instruction. Eventually, Mona became a chief centre for Britain. The Gaedhilic druids, though probably quite as learned as their continental brethren, were more isolated; and hence we cannot learn so much of their customs from external sources. There is no doubt that the druids of Gaul and Britain offered human sacrifices; it appears almost certain the Irish druids did not.

Our principal and most reliable information about this religion, is derived from Caesar. His account of the learning of its druids, of their knowledge of astronomy, physical science, mechanics, arithmetic, and medicine, however highly coloured, is amply corroborated by the casual statements of other authors. He expressly states that they used the Greek character in their writings, and mentions tables found in the camp of the Helvetia written in these characters, containing an account of all the men capable of bearing arms. "(211)

Stone Monuments

It is worthwhile here to comment briefly on some of the stone monuments, particularly the large circular ones, such as Stonehenge, and what links, if any, there were to the Celtic peoples.

We have noted above that some authors credit the construction of these monuments to earlier Cro-Magnon groups.

However, other writers have linked the Celts to these famous stone monuments, such as Stonehenge.

For example, Hennig, in editing the writings of Diodorus notes the following comment by Diodorus, who is discussing the Hyperboreans, who lived beyond the Celts.

The editor writes:

"There seems good to see in this people who live "beyond the north wind," as their name signifies, an early acquaintance of the Greeks, through the medium of the Celts, with Britain and its inhabitants. In this chapter Apollo would be the Celtic sun-god Borvon, and the "sacred precinct" of Apollo would be the famous Stone Age remains of Stonehenge."(212)

The Wikipedia article on the settlement of France notes:

105

"It is most likely from the Neolithic that date the megalithic (large stone) monuments, such as the dolmens, menhirs, stone circles and chamber tombs, found throughout France, the largest selection of which are in the Brittany and Auvergne regions. The most famous of these are the Carnac stones ... and the stones at Saint-Sulpice-de-Faleyrens." (213)

Also, Philip Schaff in his multi volume History of the Christian Church notes:

"There are still remains of druidical temples – the most remarkable at Stonehenge on Salisbury plain, and at Stennis in the Orkney islands – that is, circles of huge stones standing in some places twenty feet above the earth, and near them large mounds supposed to be ancient burial-places; for men desired to be buried near a place of worship. (214)

Further research is probably needed before any conclusions can be made on the origin of these monuments.

The Molmutine Laws

The Celts had a legal system, called the Molmutine Laws. Cooper writes of these laws:

" the laws of Dunvallo, the father of Belinus and Brennius, which were known as the Molmutine Laws and which Geoffrey tells us were still held in high esteem by the Britons (Welsh) of Geoffrey's own day. However, not only were they held in high esteem in Geoffrey's day, they also have survived to the present, and they clearly reveal their pagan origins. The light that they shed upon the society in which the early Britons lived is set out in Appendix 6 of this book, where Flinders Petrie tells us in his own words about the laws and their application. But the history of the early Britons can be carried back further still, much further back, to the 12th century BC in fact, the time of the very foundation of the British nation." (215)

Relations and Links with Neighbours

As the Celts moved through Europe, they mixed with other populations. These included the Celtiberians, the Belgae and others. We can look at how a few of these relationships developed.

Tribal groups in Spain

The Celts in the Iberian Peninsula were traditionally thought of as living on the edge of the Celtic world of the La Tène culture that defined classical Iron Age Celts. Iberia experienced one of the highest levels of Celtic settlement in all of Europe. A comprehensive list of the many groups in Spain and Portugal is provided in Wikipedia. (216)

The Celtiberians

Diodorus writes of the Celtiberians:

"Now that we have spoken at sufficient length about the Celts we shall turn our history to the Celtiberians who are their neighbours. In ancient times these two peoples, namely, the Iberians and the Celts, kept warring among themselves over the land, but when later they arranged their differences and settled upon the land altogether, and when they went further and agreed to intermarriage with each other, because of such intermixture the two peoples received the appellation given above. And since it was two powerful nations that united and the land of theirs was fertile, it came to pass that the Celtiberians advanced far in fame and were subdued by the Romans with difficulty and only after they had faced them in battle over a long period. And this people, it would appear, provide for warfare not only excellent cavalry but also foot-soldiers who excel in prowess and endurance. They wear rough black cloaks, the wool of which resembles the hair of goats. As for their arms, certain of the Celtiberians, carry light shields like those of the Gauls, and certain carry circular wicker shields as large as an aspis,and about their shins and calves they wind greaves made of hair and on their heads they wear bronze helmets adorned with purple crests. The swords they wear are two-edged and wrought of excellent iron, and they also have dirks a span in length which they use in fighting at close quarters. And a peculiar practice is followed by them in the fashioning of their defensive weapons; for they bury plates of iron in the ground and leave them there until in the course of time the rust has eaten out what is weak in the iron and what is left is only the most unyielding, and of this they then fashion excellent swords and such other objects as pertain to war. The weapon which has been fashioned in the manner described cuts through anything which gets in its way, for no shield or helmet or bone can withstand a blow from it, because of the exceptional quality of the iron. Able as they are to fight in two styles, they first carry on the contest on horseback, and when they have defeated the cavalry they dismount, and assuming the rôle of foot-soldiers they put up marvellous battles." (217)

Celts and the Germanic Peoples

The Germanic tribes lived to the west of the Celts. The Celts held them at bay for centuries. Over time, border Celt communities integrated with Germanic tribes. Certain tribes of Gaul, such as the Aedui, boasted Germanic descent. The Belgae also were a mixture of German and Celt. (218)

Celtic Expansion into Italy

The growth and expansion of the Celts in what is now France led to pressures for a move into new lands. Thanks to the Roman historian Livy, we know a great deal about this expansion.

Livy wrote that when Tarquinius Priscus was king of Rome, 616 BC to 579 BC, the supreme power among the Celts, who formed a third part of the whole of Gaul, was in the hands of the Bituriges. He noted that they furnished the king for the whole Celtic race. Ambigatus was king at that time. Livy wrote of him:

"During his sway the harvests were so abundant and the population increased so rapidly in Gaul that the government of such vast numbers seemed almost impossible. He was now an old man, and anxious to relieve his realm from the burden of over-population."(219)

This ruler was known to the Celtic peoples who had settled in Britain. Cooper writes that in the Welsh chronicle, Bellovesus is known as Beli and Segnius as the prince of the Burgundians; in Geoffrey of Monmouth they are called Belinus and Segnius the King of the Allobroges or Burgundians. (220)

Cremin comments on the reasons for the expansion:

"Emigration was facilitated by the Celts' superior iron technology, by their skill in carpentry and wheelwrighting, which enabled entire groups to transport dependents and chattels, and also probably by the rising status of the individual." (221)

Ambigatus therefore asked his sister's sons, Bellovesus and Segovesus, both enterprising young men, to settle in whatever locality the gods would by augury assign to them. He told them to invite as many as wished to accompany them, sufficient to prevent any nation from repelling their approach.

When the auspices were taken, Segovesus was assigned the Hercynian Forest. This was a dense forest that stretched eastward from the Rhine River across southern Germany.

Bellovesus was assigned Italy. He invited the surplus population of six tribes-the Bituriges, the Averni, the Senones, the Aedui, the Ambarri, the Carnutes, and the Aulerci. Starting with an enormous force of horse and foot, he came to the Tricastini. (222)

Justinus, another Roman author, wrote that the people that went with the two sons numbered three hundred thousand men. (223)

As they moved towards the Alps, they came to the assistance of fellow Celts, the Massilians, who were being attacked by the Salyi. This led them to a route through the Alps, by the passes of the Ticinus and the valley of the Douro. After crossing the Alps, they fought and defeated the Tuscans, and then took land belonging to the Insubres, where they built a city called Mediolanum. Numerous other Celtic groups then followed Bellovesus into Italy, as Livy notes:

"Subsequently another body, consisting of the Cenomani, under the leadership of Elitovius, followed the track of the former and crossed the Alps by the same pass, with the goodwill of Bellovesus. They had their settlements where the cities of Brixia and Verona now stand. The Libui came next and the Saluvii; they settled near the ancient tribe of the

Ligurian Laevi, who lived about the Ticinus. Then the Boii and Lingones crossed the Pennine Alps, and as all the country between the Po and the Alps was occupied, they crossed the Po on rafts and expelled not only the Etruscans but the Umbrians as well. They remained, however, north of the Apennines. Then the Senones, the last to come, occupied the country from the Utis to the Aesis."(224)

Justinus wrote that they founded many cities, including Milan, Como, Brescia, Verona, Bergamo, Trent, and Vicenza. (225)

One of the last groups to be attached was the people of Clusium. These sent ambassadors to Rome seeking their help. Livy notes that this request had come some two hundred years after the Celts first moved into Italy.

This led to a war between the Celts and the Romans.

Celts Attack Rome in 390 BC

The Romans accepted the request from the people of Clusium and joined the attack on the Celts. They lost. The Celts then sent representatives to Rome to negotiate a tribute payment. Their demands were rejected so they decided to attack. Livy described the panic that ensued in Rome "The whole country in front and around was now swarming with the enemy, who, being as a nation given to wild outbreaks, had by their hideous howls and discordant clamour filled everything with dreadful noise. (226) Bennus led the Celtic forces. They attacked the city, forcing many to flee, killing others and burning much of the city. A truce was then arranged. Numerous Roman authors, including Livy, Justinus and Diodorus Siculus wrote about this. Livy notes:

"A conference took place between Q. Sulpicius, the consular tribune, and Brennus, the Gaulish chieftain, and an agreement was arrived at by which 1000 lbs. of gold was fixed as the ransom of a people destined ere long to rule the world. This humiliation was great enough as it was, but it was aggravated by the despicable meanness of the Gallic Celts, who produced unjust weights, and when the tribune protested, the insolent Gaul threw his sword into the scale, with an exclamation intolerable to Roman ears, "Woe to the vanquished!" (227)

They did not keep the tribute long. Diodorus Siculus notes that the Gauls on their way from Rome laid siege to the city of Veascium, which was an ally of the Romans. The citizens of Veascium, along with a newly formed Roman force, counterattacked and defeated the Celts regaining possession of all their baggage, included in which was the gold which had been paid by Rome and practically all the booty which had been gathered in the seizure of the city

Celts in Italy after the Attack on Rome

Rankin writes that the Celts, after attacking Rome, stayed in northern Italy, parts of which became so Celtic or Gallic in character that the region became known as Cisalpine Gaul. They only ceased to be an acute menace to Italy after their defeat in the battle of Telamon in 225 BC. In 192 BC, the tribes of Northern Italy finally submitted to Rome, but the Celtic challenge to Rome was never forgotten (228)

Celts Move towards Eastern Europe

Around the same time that some Celtic groups were moving into Italy, others were moving further east. Justinus described their move.

"Of these adventurers part settled in Italy, and took and burnt the city of Rome; and part penetrated into the remotest parts of Illyricum under the direction of a flight of birds (for the Gauls are skilled in augury beyond other nations) making their way amidst great slaughter of the barbarous tribes, and fixed their abode in Pannonia. They were a savage, bold, and warlike nation, and were the first after Hercules (to whom that undertaking procured great admiration for his valour, and a belief in his immortality), to pass the unconquered heights of the Alps, and places uninhabitable from excess of cold. After having subdued the

111

Pannonians, they carried on various wars with their neighbours for many years." (229)

Celtic groups pushed into the Carpathian region and the Danube basin. Splinter groups moved south via two major routes: one following the Danube river, another eastward from Italy. By the 3rd century BC, the native inhabitants of Pannonia were almost completely celticized. La Tene finds are found widely in Pannonia,. These finds are deemed to have been locally produced Norican-Pannonian variation of Celtic culture. Even in these distant eastern lands, the Celts maintained contacts with their kin in Iberia. (230)

The fertile lands around the Pannonian rivers enabled the Celts to establish themselves easily, developing their agriculture and pottery, and at the same time exploiting the rich mines of modern Slovenia. Thus it appears that the Celts had created a new homeland for themselves in Southeastern Europe- centred in a region stretching from Vienna to the river Tizsa.

The Boii controlled most of northern Pannonia during the second century BC, and are also mentioned to have occupied the territory of modern Slovakia. We learn of other tribes inhabiting Pannonia, belonging to the Boian confederation. There were the Taurisci in the upper Sava valley, west of Sisak, as well as the Anarti, Osi and Cotini in the Carpathian basin. In the lower Sava valley, the Scordisci wielded much power over their neighbours for over a century. (231)

Celts Attack Greece

In 281 BC the Celts turned their attention towards Greece. The collapse of Lysimachus' successor kingdom in Thrace started this initiative Authors have given different reasons for the move. Pausanias said it was greed for loot, Justin claimed it to be a result of overpopulation, and Memnon said it was the result of famine. According to Pausanias, an initial probing raid was led by a Cambaules which withdrew when they realized they were too few in numbers.

In 280 BC a great army, comprising about 85,000 warriors, coming from Pannonia and split into three divisions, marched South in a great expedition to Macedon and central Greece. 20,000 of those, headed by Cerethrius, moved against the Thracians and Triballi. Another division, led by Brennus and Acichorius moved against Paionians while a third division, headed by Bolgios, aimed for Macedonians and Illyrians. (232)

The Roman author Justinus has given us the following description of the attack on Greece. (233) The Celts, under the leadership of Belgius, sent an embassy to Ptolemaeus, the king of Macedonia, to have him accept submission and pay tribute. Justinus notes that Ptolemaeus rejected this writing:

"Ptolemaeus boasted to his courtiers that the Gauls sued for peace from fear of war. Nor was his manner less vaunting before the ambassadors than before his own adherents, saying that " he would grant peace only on condition that they would give their chiefs as hostages, and deliver up their arms; for he would put no trust in them until they were disarmed." The deputies bringing back this answer, the Gauls laughed, and exclaimed throughout their camp, that "he would soon see whether they had offered peace from regard for themselves or for him." Some days after a battle was fought, and the Macedonians were defeated and cut to pieces. Ptolemaeus, after receiving several wounds, was taken, and his head, cut off and stuck on a lance, was carried round the whole army to strike terror into the enemy. Flight saved a few of the Macedonians; the rest were either taken or slain."

The Macedonians reassembled and counterattacked under another chief, Sosthenes. They defeated Belgius. This victory was short lived. Another Celtic leader, Brennus, learning of the initial victories of Belgius, assembled an army of one hundred and fifty thousand foot and fifteen thousand horse soldiers and attacked Macedonia. He defeated the army under Sosthenes, and then proceeded to plunder the lands of Macedonia. Brennus then marched on to fight the people of Delphi. In the midst of their fighting, near the Temple of Apollo at Delphi on Mount Parnassus, an earthquake struck, then hail. Justinus described the scene:

"for a part of the mountain, broken off by an earthquake, overwhelmed a host of the Gauls and some of the densest bodies of the enemy were scattered abroad, not without wounds, and fell to the earth. A tempest then followed, which destroyed, with hail and cold, those that were suffering from bodily injuries. The general Brennus himself, unable to endure the pain of his wounds, ended his life with his dagger. The other general, after punishing the advisers of the war, made off from Greece with all expedition, accompanied with ten thousand wounded men. But neither was fortune more favourable to those who fled; for in their terror, they passed no night under shelter, and no day without hardship and danger; and continual rains, snow congealed by the frost, famine, fatigue, and, what was the greatest evil, the constant want of sleep, consumed the wretched remains of the unfortunate army. The nations and people too, through whom they marched, pursued their stragglers, if to spoil them."

The Celts were pursued and defeated. Some scholars say the Greek campaign was a disaster for the Celts. However, others claim that permanent occupation was not their aim; rather they were intent on plundering the riches of the Greeks - which they did. Moreover, although they were expelled from Greece, their power in southeastern Europe did not end.

After leaving Greece, the Celts went in two directions, some to Asia, and others back to the Danube. Justinus writes:

"The Gauls, after their disastrous attack upon Delphi, in which they had felt the power of the divinity more than that of the enemy, and had lost their leader Brennus, had fled, like exiles, partly into Asia, and partly into Thrace, and then returned, by the same way by which they had come, into their own country. Of these, a certain number settled at the conflux of the Danube and Save, and took the name of Scordisci. The Tectosagi, on returning to their old settlements about Toulouse, were seized with a pestilential distemper, and did not recover from it, until, being warned by the admonitions of their soothsayers, they threw the gold and silver, which they had got in war and sacrilege, into the lake of Toulouse; all which treasure, a hundred and ten thousand pounds of silver, and fifteen hundred thousand pounds of gold, Caepio, the Roman consul, a long time after carried away with him. But this sacrilegious act subsequently proved a cause of ruin to Caepio and his army. The rising of the Cimbrian war, too, seemed to pursue the Romans as if to avenge the removal of that devoted treasure. Of these Tectosagi, no small number, attracted by the charms of plunder, repaired to Illyricum, and, after spoiling the Istrians, settled in Pannonia."

A good listing of the different Celtic tribes in the east can be found in Wikipedia. (234)

The Druids and their Influence in Eastern Europe

An interesting insight into the power and influence of the druids comes from a recounting of the Great Battle of Thessaly, in central Greece, recounted in the work *The Civil war of the Romans*. Before that battle, Sextus Pompeius decided to go for advice, not to go to a temple of Jove or Apollo or any other god or goddess, but to the druid witches of Thessaly:

"for he thought he would obtain his certain knowledge from the druidesses of the land wherein he was, that is, from the witches of Thessaly. For their cities and hamlets were near to the great encampment. Wondrous and strange were the art and the science of the Thessalian druidesses. Every prodigy in the world their demons used to reveal to them, and their science was whatever was more wondrous and incredible than its fellow. For poisonous plants and magic-working herbs were more numerous in that land of Thessaly than in the rest of the lands of the world. For when the famous druidess Medea, daughter of Aeëtes king of the Colchians, came with Jason son of Aeson into Greece, she found in the land of Thessaly, although she was the chief witch of the world, much more than her witchcraft and druidic spells and poisonous herbs. The places on the globe wherein the Science of magic was most common, namely, the city of Memphis, and the land of Egypt, Babylon and the countries of the Chaldees, were all exceeded by the Thessalian witches. For they used to work their magic spells on the mundane elements, so that their own shapes were not left upon them. They used to lengthen the night and shorten the day as they wanted. They used not to leave the air or the firmament in its own power, for when they desired

115

they would stop the firmament from its mundane course. They would bring thunders and storms into the air, and rainy clouds and darkness over the sun at the time when his lightnings were manifest and his rays were clear...

Howsoever, every animal in all the world which is hurtful to man, both lion and bear and toad and tiger and viper and serpent and other poisonous snake, was in fear of those witches and the phantoms; and it availed none of them to pour its poison against them, for more savage and more devilish were the poisons of the Thessalians than the poisons of any of these animals.

Now although in the land of Thessaly there was many an evil witch reverenced in that art, one witch was there who surpassed them all and to whom all used to yield recognition and authority. A lath of a blue-haired hideous hag was she: Erictho her name, a sage of witchcraft she. Wizards' inventions and new spells were made by herself on every day. She used to visit hell and the fields of the river Styx and the abodes of Pluto king of hell whenever she desired. Her dwelling and her habitation and her couch were in clefts of rocks and in cavernous holes of the earth and in tombs of the dead.

She frequented no assembly nor city nor human dwellings out of them, unless the darkness of mist or rain or night should have come. She culled and gathered her poisonous herbs and her magical gear throughout the districts that were near her. And the ploughed corn-field or the meadow untilled. on which she used then to tread, its grass or its corn would not grow for a long time afterwards. She never used to demand prophecy save from the demons of hell. These would answer her forthwith at the first spell; and they durst not wait for the second spell from her."

She conjured spirits from hell to tell Sextus Pompeius that he would win. (235)

Changes in Celtic Control in the Baltic States

The latter half of the first century BC brought much change to the power relations in Pannonia. The defeat of the Boian confederation by the Geto-Dacian king Burebista significantly curtailed Celtic control of the Carpathian basin, and some of the Celticization was reversed. Yet, more Celtic tribes immigrated. The Hercuniates and Latobici migrated from Germania. New tribes are encountered, bearing Latin names, such as the Arabiates, possibly representing new creations carved out of the defeated Boian confederation. (236)

Then came the Romans, whose changes we shall discuss below.

Celts Move into Asia and Galatia

In 278 B.C., 20,000 Gauls, under Leonorius, Luterius, and fifteen other chieftains, crossed over to Asia Minor, in two divisions. They helped Nicomedes I, King of Bithynia, defeat his younger brother. As a reward for their services, he gave them a large tract of country, in the heart of Asia Minor, henceforward to be known as Galatia.

The Galatians developed as three groups:

- Tolistboboii, on the west, with Pessinus as their chief town;
- Tectosages, in the centre, with their capital Ancyra; and
- Trocmi, on the east, round their chief town Tavium. (237)

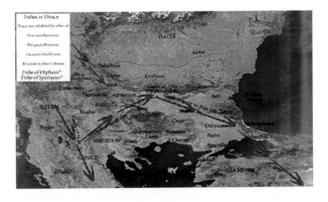

As soon as these Gauls, or Galatians, had gained a firm footing in the country assigned to them, they began to send out marauding expeditions in all directions. They became the terror of their neighbours, and levied contributions on the whole of Asia Minor west of the Taurus. Commenting on this, Justinus wrote.

"The kings of the east then carried on no wars without a mercenary army of Gauls; nor, if they were driven from their thrones, did they seek protection with any other people than the Gauls. Such indeed was the terror of the Gallic name, and the unvaried good fortune of their arms, that princes thought they could neither maintain their power in security, nor recover it if lost, without the assistance of Gallic valour."

Justinus wrote how these people, living in Asia, were the same as their confreres in Italy.

"these Gauls, who inhabited Asia, differed only in situation from the Gauls who had settled themselves in Italy; that they had the same extraction, courage, and mode of fighting; and that, as to sagacity, the Asiatic Gauls must have more than the others, inasmuch as they had pursued a longer and more difficult march through Illyricum and Thrace, having traversed those territories with almost more labour than it had cost them to acquire those in which they settled."(238)

They became overlords of the local peoples and acquired much wealth. Indeed, Josephus, the great Jewish writer, quotes Herod warning the Jews against revolt by comparing them negatively against others, stating: "Are you richer than the Gauls, stronger than the Germans, wiser than the Greeks". (239)

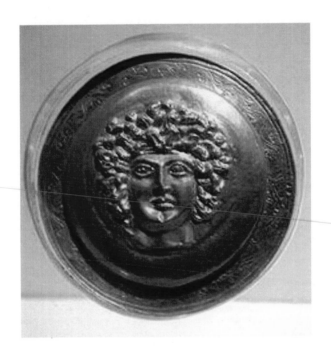

A Galatian head as depicted on a gold Thracian objet d'art 3rd c BC (240)

Their settlements are shown in the following map. (241)

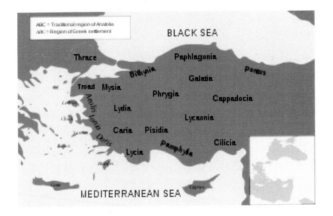

These Celts were warriors, respected by Greeks and Romans. They hired themselves out as mercenary soldiers, sometimes fighting on both sides in the great battles of the times. For years the chieftains and their war bands ravaged the western half of Asia Minor, as allies of one or other of the warring princes, without any serious check, until they sided with the Seleucid prince Antiochus Hierax, who reigned in Asia Minor. Hierax tried to defeat king Attalus I of Pergamum (241–197 BC), but instead, the Hellenized cities united under Attalus's banner, and his armies inflicted several severe defeats upon them in 232 BC, forcing them to settle permanently and to confine themselves to the region to which they had already given their name.

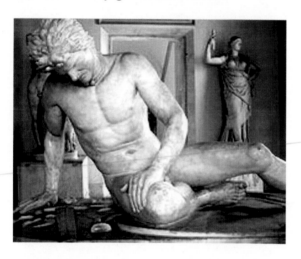

Attalus I of Pergamon commissioned a statue, called The Dying Gaul, between 230 BC and 220 BC, to celebrate his victory over the Celtic Galatians in Anatolia. Epigonus, the court sculptor of the Attalid dynasty of Pergamon, may have been its sculptor. The statue depicts a dying Celt with remarkable realism, particularly in the face, and may have been painted. He is represented as a Gallic warrior with a typically Gallic hairstyle and moustache. The figure is naked save for a neck torc. He lies on his fallen shield while his sword and other objects lie beside him. (242)

The military prowess of the Celts (Gauls) was noted by Herod Agrippa, when he warned the Jewish people against the disasters that lay ahead for them if they revolted:

" if great advantages might provoke any people to revolt, the Gauls might do it best of all, as being so thoroughly walled round by nature; on the east side of the Alps, on the north by the river Rhine, on the south by the Pyrenean mountains, and on the west by the ocean.—Now, although these Gauls have such obstacles before them to prevent any attack upon them, and have no fewer than three hundred and five nations among them, nay have, as one may say, the fountains of domestic happiness within themselves, and send out plentiful streams of happiness over almost the whole world, these bear to be tributary to the Romans, and derive their prosperous condition from them; and they undergo this, not because they are of effeminate minds, or because they are of an ignoble stock, as having borne a war of eighty years, in order to preserve their liberty; but by reason of the great regard they have to the power of the Romans, and their good fortune, which is of greater efficacy than their arms." (243)

Political Life in Galatia

The constitution of the Galatian state was described by Strabo: conformably to custom, each of the three groups, or tribes, was divided into four cantons, each governed by a chief ('tetrarch') of its own with a judge under him, whose powers were unlimited except in cases of murder, which were tried before a council of 300 drawn from the twelve cantons and meeting at a holy place, twenty miles southwest of Ancyra, written in Greek as Drynemeton (Gallic daru-nemeton holy place of oak). It is likely it was a sacred oak grove, since the name means "sanctuary of the oaks" (from drys, meaning "oak" and nemeton, meaning "sacred ground"). The local population of Cappadocians were left in control of the towns and most of the land, paying tithes to their new overlords, who formed a military aristocracy and kept aloof in fortified farmsteads, surrounded by their bands. (244) We shall discuss the Galatians more below.

Chapter 6

Settlement of Britain and Ireland

The Celts move into Britain

The people who occupied Britain before the Celtic immigration were the Britons. They were descendants of Javan, brother of Magog. Cooper describes their immigration into Britain under the leadership of Brutus:

"Brutus journeyed from Italy to Greece, and there he came into contact with certain slaves. These were the descendants of the soldiers who had fought against Greece in the Trojan Wars of the 13th century BC. They had been enslaved by Priam, son of Achilles, 'in vengeance for his father's death', and were subsequently to continue their slavery under Pandrasus, king of the Dorian Greeks. Learning that he was descended from their own ancient kings, the Trojans accepted Brutus into their fellowship and elected him as their leader, and under him they successfully rose against their captors. Defeating Pandrasus in battle, they set sail to look for a land in which to settle. Sailing their fleet out of the Mediterranean between the Pillars of Hercules (the Straits of Gibraltar), they came across another group of Trojans led by Corineus, who were likewise escaping abroad from their captors. They combined forces and landed in Gaul with Brutus being acclaimed as their overall king. There they fought and defeated the Picts under king Goffar... The Trojans again set sail, and came ashore at Totnes in Devon at some time in the 12th century BC. The land and its people were subsequently to derive their names from Brutus. Then Brutus founded the city of Trinovantum, or New Troy, which was later to become the city of London. Brutus, the first king of the Britons, reigned over his people in this island for twenty three years, i.e. from 1104-1081 BC. (245)

They replaced an earlier group who lived there, the Formorians, also described by Cooper:

"Now, although Brutus is said to have been the first colonizer of Britain, the chronicles do emphatically state that he had to displace an indigenous race of 'giants'. Whether physical gigantism is here intended cannot be certainly resolved, as the early British word 'gawr' (like the Hebrew *gibbor)* could mean simply a great warrior as well as a giant man. But we

123

do know from the biblical record that gigantism was a particular physical trait amongst certain of Ham's descendants, Goliath of Gath being the best known example, which lends both the British and Irish accounts a degree of hitherto unsuspected corroboration. The Formorians, it seems, were the displaced natives of Britain who were trying to seek a foothold on the Irish mainland only to be repelled by the Nemedians, thereafter having to live, like many other displaced peoples, by scavenging and piracy."

We know that many Celts had immigrated into Britain by 400 BC from the writings of Pytheas of Massilia, 4th century BC, who called the country Brettanike, a Celtic name, suggesting the Celts were long established there in his time. (246)

According to Nolan, who analyzed language differences in Celtic immigrants, immigration came in phases.

"There was a unifying language spoken by the Celts, called not surprisingly, old Celtic. Philogists have shown the descendence of Celtic from the original *Ur*-language and from the Indo-European language tradition. In fact, the form of old Celtic was the closest cousin to *Italic*, the precursor of Latin.

The original wave of Celtic immigrants to the British Isles are called the *q-Celts* and spoke *Goidelic*. It is not known exactly when this immigration occurred but it may be placed sometime in the window of 2000 to 1200 BC. The label *q-Celtic* stems from the differences between this early Celtic tongue and *Italic*. Some of the differences between *Italic* and *Celtic* included that lack of a **p** in *Celtic* and an **a** in place of an the *Italic* **o**.

At a later date, a second wave of immigrants took to the British Isles, a wave of Celts referred to as the *p-Celts* speaking *Brythonic*. *Goidelic* led to the formation of the three Gaelic languages spoken in Ireland, Man and later Scotland. *Brythonic* gave rise to two British Isles languages, Welsh and Cornish, as well as surviving on the Continent in the form of Breton, spoken in Brittany.

The label *q-Celtic* stems from the differences between this early Celtic tongue and the latter formed *p-Celtic*. The differences between the two Celtic branches are simple in theoretical form. Take for example the word *ekvos* in *Indo-European*, meaning **horse**. In *q-Celtic* this was rendered as *equos* while in *p-Celtic* it became *epos*, the **q** sound being replaced with a **p** sound. Another example is the Latin *qui* **who**. In *q-*

Celtic this rendered as *cia* while in *p-Celtic* it rendered as *pwy*. It should also be noted that there are still words common to the two Celtic subgroups.

As an aside, take note that when the Irish expansion into Pictish Britain occurred, several colonies were established in present day Wales. The local inhabitants called the Irish arrivals **gwyddel** *savages* from which comes **geídil** and **goidel** and thus the Goidelic tongue. (247)

A number of clans and groups developed in the years that followed, as shown in the following map (248)

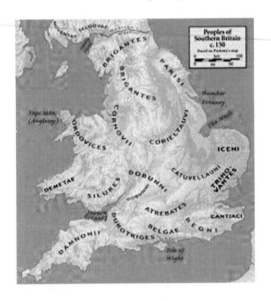

Comments can be offered on a few. (249)

The Atrebates tribe was a Belgic people descended from, and having close connection with, the tribes of north west Gaul (centered on the area around present-day Arras). They were based in eastern Hampshire and Berkshire as well as the western parts of Surrey and Sussex. Their capital was at Calleva Atrebatum - Silchester, Hampshire. The tribe was one of the few Celtic tribes to have issued coinage, just prior to the Roman invasion.

125

The Catuvellauni originally occupied Hertfordshire around Verulamium (St Albans). Under their strong leader Cunobelin, they attacked and eventually subjugated the Atrebates, becoming one of the major players in Southern Central Britain. They developed contacts with the Romans, as see shall discuss below.

The Parisi or Parisii occupied a small area centred on Humberside sandwiched between the Brigantes to the north and the more advanced Coritani to the south. Their capital was at Peturia and it is thought they descended from the tribes of north-central Gaul - and incidentally gave their name to the French capital.

Celtic Culture in Britain

The Celtic culture in Britain has been identified as La Tene. It was a transition between the bronze and iron ages and the Celts have been particularly associated with their skillful use of iron.

The artwork of the La Tène period is often quite complex and sophisticated, conflicting with the usual image of native barbarians existing in a wild and violent society. The Celtic preference was to decorate themselves, as evident by the high level of artistic sophistication present in personal belongings like swords, mirrors and jewellery, rather than decorate their buildings, which were primitive by comparison.

The usual living accommodation was a circular hut having a single room with walls made from mud and a thatched roof. The Celts would live in extended family groups, occupying a village often located in a defensive position such as a hill fort. These families would belong to large tribal groups that controlled certain areas of the country. At the time of the Roman invasion of Britain two of the most influential tribes were the Icenii in Norfolk and the Brigantes in northern England.

Celtic society was divided into three main classes: the warrior aristocracy, the Druids who were the religious leaders and all the rest. Women were also regarded highly amongst the Celts, which was unusual during ancient times, some like Boudicca and Cartimandua even becoming tribal leaders.

The Celts were a warlike people who tended to have battles that frequently devolved into individual combats; where the victor would cut off the head of the loser and display it on a pole outside his hut. Many of the Celts would fight naked, simply covered by artwork made from a blue dye extracted from a plant called woad. It is believed that this dye, as well as being used for tattoos to intimidate the enemy, also had a medicinal value, being able to constrict the skin; which was useful for treating wounds. In addition to using infantry and cavalry tactics, they also employed chariots in battle. (250)

Julius Caesar wrote extensively of Celtic culture in 54 BC when he was planning his attack on the Celts. The following paragraphs are taken from his books. (251)

"The interior portion of Britain is inhabited by those of whom they say that it is handed down by tradition that they were born in the island itself: the maritime portion by those who had passed over from the country of the Belgae for the purpose of plunder and making war; almost all of whom are called by the names of those states from which being sprung they went thither, and having waged war, continued there and began to cultivate the lands. The number of the people is countless, and their buildings exceedingly numerous, for the most part very like those of the Gauls: the number of cattle is great. They use either brass or iron rings, determined at a certain weight, as their money. Tin is produced in the midland regions; in the maritime, iron; but the quantity of it is small: they employ brass, which is imported. There, as in Gaul, is timber of every description, except beech and fir. They do not regard it lawful to eat the hare, and the cock, and the goose; they, however, breed them for amusement and pleasure. The climate is more temperate than in Gaul, the colds being less severe.

127

The most civilized of all these nations are they who inhabit Kent, which is entirely a maritime district, nor do they differ much from the Gallic customs. Most of the inland inhabitants do not sow corn, but live on milk and flesh, and are clad with skins. All the Britains, indeed, dye themselves with woad, which occasions a bluish color, and thereby have a more terrible appearance in fight. They wear their hair long, and have every part of their body shaved except their head and upper lip. Ten and even twelve have wives common to them, and particularly brothers among brothers, and parents among their children; but if there be any issue by these wives, they are reputed to be the children of those by whom respectively each was first espoused when a virgin."

Caesar noted that there were two main classes of people, a noble class and an oppressed class. The noble class included druids and knights.

"Throughout all Gaul there are two orders of those men who are of any rank and dignity: for the commonality is held almost in the condition of slaves, and dares to undertake nothing of itself, and is admitted to no deliberation. The greater part, when they are pressed either by debt, or the large amount of their tributes, or the oppression of the more powerful, give themselves up in vassalage to the nobles, who possess over them the same rights without exception as masters over their slaves. But of these two orders, one is that of the Druids, the other that of the knights. The former are engaged in things sacred, conduct the public and the private sacrifices, and interpret all matters of religion. To these a large number of the young men resort for the purpose of instruction, and they [the Druids] are in great honor among them. For they determine respecting almost all controversies, public and private; and if any crime has been perpetrated, if murder has been committed, if there be any dispute about an inheritance, if any about boundaries, these same persons decide it; they decree rewards and punishments; if any one, either in a private or public capacity, has not submitted to their decision, they interdict him from the sacrifices. This among them is the most heavy punishment. Those who have been thus interdicted are esteemed in the number of the impious and the criminal: all shun them, and avoid their society and conversation, lest they receive some evil from their contact; nor is justice administered to them when seeking it, nor is any dignity bestowed on them. Over all these Druids one presides, who possesses supreme authority among them. Upon his death, if any individual among the rest is pre-eminent in dignity, he succeeds; but, if there are many equal, the election is made by the suffrages of the Druids; sometimes they even contend for the

128

presidency with arms. These assemble at a fixed period of the year in a consecrated place in the territories of the Carnutes, which is reckoned the central region of the whole of Gaul. Hither all, who have disputes, assemble from every part, and submit to their decrees and determinations. This institution is supposed to have been devised in Britain, and to have been brought over from it into Gaul; and now those who desire to gain a more accurate knowledge of that system generally proceed thither for the purpose of studying it."

He continues to describe the Druids, their many years of study, their skill at memorizing verses and the like, and their use of the Greek language for writing. Also remarkable was their belief that their souls do not become extinct, but pass after death from one body to another. This eliminated fear in war and produced great valour among the Celtic peoples. Many of his observations were similar to those of observers of the Celtic culture in earlier times, as well as of the more ancient Scythian culture.

"The Druids do not go to war, nor pay tribute together with the rest; they have an exemption from military service and a dispensation in all matters. Induced by such great advantages, many embrace this profession of their own accord, and [many] are sent to it by their parents and relations. They are said there to learn by heart a great number of verses; accordingly some remain in the course of training twenty years. Nor do they regard it lawful to commit these to writing, though in almost all other matters, in their public and private transactions, they use Greek characters. That practice they seem to me to have adopted for two reasons; because they neither desire their doctrines to be divulged among the mass of the people, nor those who learn, to devote themselves the less to the efforts of memory, relying on writing; since it generally occurs to most men, that, in their dependence on writing, they relax their diligence in learning thoroughly, and their employment of the memory. They wish to inculcate this as one of their leading tenets, that souls do not become extinct, but pass after death from one body to another, and they think that men by this tenet are in a great degree excited to valor, the fear of death being disregarded. They likewise discuss and impart to the youth many things respecting the stars and their motion, respecting the extent of the world and of our earth, respecting the nature of things, respecting the power and the majesty of the immortal gods."

Caesar noted the following on the knights:

"The other order is that of the knights. These, when there is occasion and any war occurs (which before Caesar's arrival was for the most part wont to happen every year, as either they on their part were inflecting injuries or repelling those which others inflicted on them), are all engaged in war. And those of them most distinguished by birth and resources, have the greatest number of vassals and dependents about them. They acknowledge this sort of influence and power only."

They were good at war and enjoyed it. They arrayed themselves as fiercely as possible, sometimes charging into battle fully naked, dyed blue from head to toe, and screaming like banshees to terrify their enemies. They took tremendous pride in their appearance in battle, if we can judge by the elaborately embellished weapons and paraphernalia they used. Golden shields and breastplates shared pride of place with ornamented helmets and trumpets. The Celts were great users of light chariots in warfare. From this chariot, drawn by two horses, they would throw spears at an enemy before dismounting to have a go with heavy slashing swords. Celtic warriors would cut off the heads of their enemies in battle and display them as trophies. They mounted heads in doorposts and hung them from their belts. To the Celt the seat of spiritual power was the head, so by taking the head of a vanquished foe they were appropriating that power for themselves. It was a kind of bloody religious observance. They also had a habit of dragging families and baggage along to their battles. (252)

The characteristics of war just noted here are similar to what was practiced for a long time, going back to Scynthia. Life for the oppressed class was more monotonous.

Some Celts were farmers when they weren't fighting. One of the interesting innovations that they brought to Britain was the iron plough. Earlier ploughs had been awkward affairs, basically a stick with a pointed end harnessed behind two oxen. They were suitable only for ploughing the light upland soils. The heavier iron ploughs constituted an agricultural revolution all by themselves, for they made it possible for the first time to cultivate the rich valley and lowland soils. They came with a price, though. It generally required a team of eight oxen to pull the plough, so to avoid the difficulty of turning that large a team, Celtic fields tended to be long and narrow, a pattern that can still be seen in some parts of the country today. (253)

Caesar discussed the gods they followed:

"They worship as their divinity, Mercury in particular, and have many images of him, and regard him as the inventor of all arts, they consider him the guide of their journeys and marches, and believe him to have great influence over the acquisition of gain and mercantile transactions. Next to him they worship Apollo, and Mars, and Jupiter, and Minerva; respecting these deities they have for the most part the same belief as other nations: that Apollo averts diseases, that Minerva imparts the invention of manufactures, that Jupiter possesses the sovereignty of the heavenly powers; that Mars presides over wars. To him, when they have determined to engage in battle, they commonly vow those things which they shall take in war. When they have conquered, they sacrifice whatever captured animals may have survived the conflict, and collect the other things into one place. In many states you may see piles of these things heaped up in their consecrated spots; nor does it often happen that any one, disregarding the sanctity of the case, dares either to secrete in his house things captured, or take away those deposited; and the most severe punishment, with torture, has been established for such a deed. "

Other sources have identified different gods, including Dagda, father of the gods, Morrigan, queen of the gods, Bel, god of rebirth and the growth of crops, and Dis pater, the god of the afterlife. (254)

They had developed legends of their ancestry:

"All the Gauls assert that they are descended from the god Dis, and say that this tradition has been handed down by the Druids. For that reason they compute the divisions of every season, not by the number of days, but of nights; they keep birthdays and the beginnings of months and years in such an order that the day follows the night."

He found them very ingenious in their economy.

"They are a nation of consummate ingenuity, and most skillful in imitating and making those things which are imparted by any one; for they turned aside the hooks with nooses, and when they had caught hold of them firmly, drew them on by means of engines, and undermined the mound the more skillfully on this account, because there are in their territories extensive iron mines, and consequently every description of mining operations is known and practiced by them."

Other sources note that the use of iron had amazing repercussions. First, it changed trade and fostered local independence. Trade was essential during the Bronze Age, for not every area was naturally endowed with the necessary ores to make bronze. Iron, on the other hand, was relatively cheap and available almost everywhere.

The Celts lived in huts of arched timber with walls of wicker and roofs of thatch. The huts were generally gathered in loose hamlets. The time of the "Celtic conversion" of Britain saw a huge growth in the number of hill forts throughout the region. These were often small ditch and bank combinations encircling defensible hilltops. Some are small enough that they were of no practical use for more than an individual family, though over time many larger forts were built. The curious thing is that we don't know if the hill forts were built by the native Britons to defend themselves from the encroaching Celts, or by the Celts as they moved their way into hostile territory. Usually these forts contained no source of water, so their use as long term settlements is doubtful, though they may have been useful indeed for withstanding a short term siege. Many of the hill forts were built on top of earlier camps. (255) Caesar wrote that in death, the elite were honoured:

"When they died, if rich, much was buried with them. Their funerals, considering the state of civilization among the Gauls, are magnificent and costly; and they cast into the fire all things, including living creatures, which they supposed to have been dear to them when alive; and, a little before this period, slaves and dependents, who were ascertained to have been beloved by them, were, after the regular funeral rites were completed, burnt together with them. "

132

During these years, we start seeing cemeteries of ordinary people, buried in a hole in the ground.

Celtic lands were owned communally, and wealth seems to have been based largely on the size of cattle herd owned. The lot of women was a good deal better than in most societies of that time. They were technically equal to men, owned property, and could choose their own husbands. They could also be war leaders, as was Boudicca (Boadicea), whom we shall mention later. They would be there for some nine hundred years before they were pushed by the Angles and Saxons into Cornwall, where they would become Cornish, and into Wales, where they would become the Welsh.

One of the most famous of the British Celts was King Arthur and his Knights of the Round Table. (256)

Let us now look at the Celtic settlement of Ireland.

Formorians in Ireland

The Formorians may have been the earliest modern settlers in Ireland, being driven from Britain by Brutus when he took that land. Keating notes they arrived some two hundred years before Partholan, around 1680 BC. They lived on fish and fowl. (257) Those who write about later immigrants thought little of these people. The author of the *Chronicum Scotorum* notes that "they were demons, truly, in the guise of men, i.e. men with one hand and one leg each". (258) The *Annals of the four Masters* wrote of them:

"and to fight with the "Formorians in general," an unpleasant pugilistic race, who, according to the Annals of Clonmacnois, "were a sept descended from Cham, the sonne of Noeh, and lived by pyracie and spoile of other nations, and were in those days very troublesome to the whole world." (259)

133

Cooper writes that they were well known pirates. They were known as great warriors and giant men. Goliath of Gath was perhaps their best known. (260)

Waddell, who links them with people known as the Van or Fen, noted they were a matriarchal society. He stated they had a serpent cult and many early monuments can be found with this motif. He says they had been cave dwellers in East Asia from whence they came. (261)

Partholan

The next to enter Ireland was Partholan, who settled in the estuary of the river Kenmare.

Cooper, quoting the *Annals of the Four Masters*, gives his date of arrival as 1484 BC. The *Chronicum Scotorum* notes that this was in the sixtieth year of the age of Abraham. (262) Others think it may have been later. Cusack writes:

"a British prince, the son of Gulguntius, or Gurmund, having crossed over to Denmark, to enforce tribute from a Danish king, was returning victorious off the Orcades, when he encountered thirty ships, full of men and women. On his inquiring into the object of their voyage, their leader, *Partholyan*,made an appeal to his good nature, and entreated from the prince some small portion of land in Britain, as his crew were weary of sailing over the ocean. Being informed that he came from Spain, the British prince received him under his protection, and assigned faithful guides to attend him into Ireland, which was then wholly uninhabited; and he granted it to them, subject to an annual tribute, and confirmed the appointment of Partholyan as their chief.

This account was so firmly believed in England, that it is specially set forth in an Irish act (11th of Queen Elizabeth) among the "auncient and sundry strong authentique tytles for the kings of England to this land of Ireland." The tradition may have been obtained from Irish sources, and was probably "improved" and accommodated to fortify the Saxon claim, by the addition of the pretended grant; but it is certainly evidence of the early belief in the Milesian colonization of Ireland, and the name of their leader." (263)

Cusack adds that he arrived with wives, sons and a thousand followers. He added that they built burial mounds in the areas in which they lived.

Dennis Walsh has written of these court cairns and passage cairns:

"In all some 300 Passage cairns have been identified, with many found along a line from County Meath to County Sligo. This form of megalithic structure is distinguished as a round mound of earth and stone having, roughly in the center, a burial chamber which is reached by a passage leading in from the edge of the mound.

The astronomical alignment of some of these cairns, notably at Newgrange and Loughcrew, seem to place credence to the view they were used for ceremonial, and possibly astrological, purposes.

Wedge tombs (about 400) are considered to be built mainly between 2000 and 1500 BC, and Bell-Beaker pottery are often associated with them. Similar tombs also associated with Beaker finds are common in the French region of Brittany, and the origin of the Irish series seems connected to this region.

There were also stone circles. Of the more than 200 stone circles, almost 100 are concentrated in the southwestern counties of Cork and Kerry, many of them consisting of no more than five stones." (264)

Walsh continues on to describe the culture:

"Neolithic migrant men and women were Ireland's first farmers who raised animals and cultivated the soil. The earliest Neolithic pottery found in Ulster (Lyles Hill pottery) is similar to pottery found in northern Britain, suggesting that some of the earliest Neolithic colonists may have come to Ireland from northern Britain.

Domesticated cattle, sheep and goats were imported to Ireland at the beginning of the Neolithic period, together with cereals. The oldest known Neolithic house in Ireland (or Britain) was a wooden house, 6.5m by 6m, uncovered at an excavation at Ballynagilly, near Cookstown, County Tyrone."

After three hundred years, the population, some 9000, was decimated in a disease. (265)

The Arrival of Nemedius

In 1145 BC a group under Nemedius settled in Ireland.
The *Annals* described those who arrived. (266)

"Neimhidh came to Ireland. On the twelfth day after the arrival of
Neimhidh with his people, Macha, the wife of Neimhidh, died. These
were the four chieftains who were with him: Sdarn, Iarbhainel the
Prophet, Fearghus Leithdheirg, and Ainninn. These were the four sons of
Neimhidh. Medu, Macha, Yba, and Ceara, were the four wives of these
chieftains."

He erected forts and cleared plains, as his predecessors had
done. The Annals then note that for two hundred and sixteen
years Neimhidh and his race remained in Ireland. After this
Ireland was a wilderness for a period of two hundred years.
(267) A later outbreak of plague took its toll on the
population, the remainder of whom are recorded as having
fought off an invasion of Ireland by the Formorians.(268)
After the attack, the Nemedians split into three groups. The
Annals notes this dispersion:

"Three bands were said to have emigrated with their respective captains.
One party wandered into the north of Europe, and are believed to have
been the progenitors of the Tuatha De Dananns; others made their way to
Greece, where they were enslaved, and obtained the name of Firbolgs, or
bagmen, from the leathern bags which they were compelled to carry; and
the third section sought refuge in the north of England, which is said to
have obtained its name of Briton from their leader, Briotan Maol. "(269)

In 701 BC, the Firbolgs, who had gone to Greece, returned to
Ireland.
When the Firbolgs returned to Ireland, they continued to
foster their relations with kin they had in Spain. *The Annals
of the Four Masters* notes:

"It was in the reign of this Lugh that the fair of Tailltean was established,
in commemoration and remembrance of his foster mother, Taillte, the
daughter of Maghmor, King of Spain, and the wife of Eochaidh, son of
Erc, the last king of the Firbolgs."

Some years after the Firbolgs returned to Ireland they had to face the returning Tuatha de Danaun. This was around 504 BC.

The *Annals* described the Tuatha return and conquest:

"The tenth year of the reign of Eochaidh, son of Erc; and this was the last year of his reign, for the Tuatha De Dananns came to invade Ireland against the Firbolgs; and they gave battle to each other at Magh Tuireadh, in Conmaicne Cuile Toladh, in Connaught, so that the King Eochaidh, son of Erc, was killed, by the three sons of Neimhidh, son of Badhrai, of the Tuatha De Dananns; Ceasarb, Luamh, and Luachra, their names. The Firbolgs were vanquished and slaughtered in this battle. Moreover, the hand of Nuadhat, son of Eochaidh, son of Edarlamh (the king who was over the Tuatha De Dananns), was cut off in the same battle. The aforesaid Eochaidh was the last king of the Firbolgs. Nine of them had assumed kingship, and thirty seven years was the length of their sway over Ireland. "(270)

After establishing themselves, the Tuatha De Danaan brought with them their coronation stone. Cusack has described this stone, which appears to be the same one used today by the British monarchs.

"The Tuatha Dé Dananns are also said to have brought the famous Lia Fail, or Stone of Destiny, to Ireland. It is said by some authorities that this stone was carried to Scotland when an Irish colony invaded North Britain, and that it was eventually brought to England by Edward I., in the year 1300, and deposited in Westminster Abbey. It is supposed to be identical with the large block of stone which may be seen there under the coronation chair."(271)

After they were defeated by the next group to enter Ireland, the Milesians, they lived on in Irish myth and legend as the fairies of Irish history.

"It appears from a very curious and ancient tract, written in the shape of a dialogue between St. Patrick and Caoilte MacRonain, that there were many places in Ireland where the Tuatha Dé Dananns were then supposed to live as sprites and fairies, with corporeal and material forms, but endued with immortality. The inference naturally to be drawn from these stories is, that the Tuatha De Dananns lingered in the country for many centuries after their subjugation by the Gaedhils, and that they lived in retired situations, where they practiced abstruse arts, from which they obtained the reputation of being magicians." (272)

Milesians move into Ireland

The next group to move into Ireland was the Milesians. They invaded around 504 BC.

Nolan writes that they came from the Basque country in northern Spain, quoting research that concluded that the Iberian peninsula was the probable focal point of this migration to Ireland 4,000-1,000 BC, that genetically the Irish, Scots, Welsh, and the Cornish people have similar genetics with the Basque people of the western Pyrenees, and that they are of probable descent from an ancient culture residing on the Atlantic coast. (273)

Cooper writes that they came via the Spanish peninsula from the city of Miletus on the Turkish mainland. Miletus was an Ionian outpost whose population consisted of, among others, Scythians and Phoenicians at that time was being threatened by the expanding Persian Empire, which conquered them in 494 BC. Miletus was an Ionian outpost whose population consisted of, among others, Scythians and Phoenicians.

"The children of Milidh, known to us as the Milesians, had landed unobserved in the mouth of the river Slaney in what is today the county of Wexford, from where they marched to Tara, the central seat of government. The word Milesian is still used (though with increasing rarity) to denote the Irish people themselves, or things pertaining to Ireland. And of further interest to our enquiry is the fact that the Milesians were newly arrived (via the Spanish peninsula) from the city of Miletus, whose ruins still stand on the Turkish mainland, and which was finally destroyed by the Persian army in the year 494 BC. Given that the Irish records state ca 504 BC for the landing of the Milesian colony in Ireland, this is a spontaneous and unexpected chronological correlation that is close enough to give us serious pause for thought. For there's many an Egyptologist who wishes that he could get that close with Egyptian chronology!

138

The lives of the people of Miletus had been made precarious for decades prior to the fall of their city due to the increasingly threatening ambitions of the Persian army, and nothing would have been more natural than that a colony of Milesians should decide to flee in search of a safe haven. They would seek a land that was sufficiently far away to be safe, was fertile, and which was well known to the Phoenician mariners of the eastern Mediterranean, as was Ireland. And that the city of Miletus should also be known to us as an Ionian outpost whose population consisted of, amongst other races, Scythians and Phoenicians, tells us that we should take the claims of the early Irish chroniclers very seriously indeed.

So it is clear that at the very least, the early Irish chroniclers were passing on an account, albeit garbled in places, of authentic historical events and personages, and of the equally historic descent of their own race from Phoenician and Scythian stock. And on the subject of that descent, Cusack adds yet again to our store of knowledge:" (274)

The *Chronicum Scotorum* has its own interesting version of the arrival of the Milesians:

"Milidh proceeded from Spain to Scythia, and from Scythia to Egypt, after the slaying of Reflor...contending for the sovereignty of Scythia. His great fleet consisted of 100 ships...they came to Pharaoh, the king of Egypt. They learned the arts of that country. They remained eight years with Pharaoh in Egypt...Scota, Pharaoh's daughter, married Milidh...After that Milidh went with his host on the great sea...(then) the Caspian Sea...They stopped in Dacia...Caicher, the Druid, said to them,'we shall not stay until we reach Erinn'...They subsequently passed by Gothia, by Germany, by Bregann, until they occupied Spain. It was uninhabited until their arrival...Two sons were born here Eremon and hErennan...(Two others had been born earlier) in Scythia Donnwas born, and Ebhir in Egypt...(they then went on to Erinn)."(275)

The *Annals* described the battle with the Tuatha De Danaan:

"The fleet of the sons of Milidh came to Ireland at the end of this year, to take it from the Tuatha De Dananns; and they fought the battle of Sliabh Mis with them on the third day after landing. In this battle fell Scota, the daughter of Pharaoh, wife of Milidh; and the grave of Scota is to be seen between Sliabh Mis and the sea. Therein also fell Fas, the wife of Un, son of Uige, from whom is named Gleann Faisi. After this the sons of Milidh fought a battle at Tailtinn, against the three kings of the Tuatha

139

De Dananns, Mac Cuill, Mac Ceacht, and Mac Greine. The battle lasted for a long time, until Mac Ceacht fell by Eiremhon, Mac Cuill by Eimhear, and Mac Greine by Amhergin.

Their three queens were also slain; Eire by Suirghe, Fodhla by Edan, and Banba by Caicher. The battle was at length gained against the Tuatha De Dananns, and they were slaughtered wherever they were overtaken. There fell from the sons of Milidh, on the other hand, two illustrious chieftains, in following up the rout, namely Fuad at Sliabh Fuaid, and Cuailgne at Sliabh Cuailgne." (276)

Now began early modern Irish history. The great Irish families start from here, as Cusack notes:

"The genealogical tree begins, therefore, with the brothers Eber and Eremon, the two surviving leaders of the expedition, whose ancestors are traced back to Magog, the son of Japheth. The great southern chieftains, such as the MacCarthys and O'Briens, claim descent from Eber; the northern families of O'Connor, O'Donnell, and O'Neill, claim Eremon as their head. There are also other families claiming descent from Emer, the son of Ir, brother to Eber and Eremon; as also from their cousin Lugaidh, the son of Ith. From these four sources the principal Celtic families of Ireland have sprung;" (277)

As we see in the genealogy, Eber and Eremon were able to trace their own descent from Gadelas, the father of the Gaels and the Gaelic languages, but just how seriously did the early Irish take the question of pedigree? Were they serious enough to take the trouble to keep accurate records over long periods of time? Once more, Cusack answers the question for us:

"The Books of Genealogies and Pedigrees form a most important element in Irish pagan history. For social and political reasons, the Irish Celt preserved his genealogical tree with scrupulous precision. The rights of property and the governing power were transmitted with patriarchal exactitude on strict claims of primogeniture, which claims could only be refused under certain conditions defined by law ... and in obedience to an ancient law, established long before the introduction of Christianity, all the provincial records, as well as those of the various chieftains, were required to be furnished every third year to the convocation at Tara, where they were compared and corrected." (278)

140

Milesian Culture

The economic culture developed by the Milesians was a dynamic and vibrant one. They had a flourishing metal industry and bronze, copper and gold objects were exported widely to Britain and the continent. (279)

The Annals of the Four Masters praised this work, crediting the first smelting of gold to Tighearn and its smelting to Uchadan. The latter was credited with a lot

"It was by him that goblets and brooches were first covered with gold and silver in Ireland. It was by him that clothes were dyed purple, blue, and green." (280)

The quality of the craftsmanship is evidenced by the famous Gundestrup cauldron, perhaps the most famous artwork of this time.

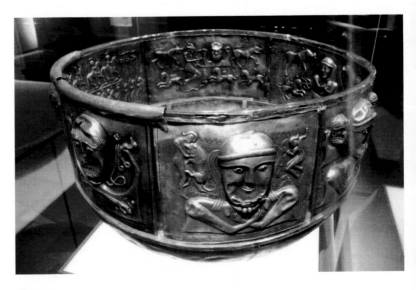

This cauldron, found in a Danish swamp, was thrown by an Irish devotee in the first century BC. (281)

The knowledge of Ireland was widespread in the Western world, as noted by Dennis Walsh:

"The earliest possible written reference to Ireland is in the *Peripolous* of Himilco, the Carthaginian who wrote in the 6th century BC. In it he references Celtic tribes on the North Sea, as well as in France and Spain. Writing in the late 4th century BC Pytheus refers to the British Isles as the *Pretanic islands*, from *Priteni*, terms which allude to a Celtic connection for the islands. A Greek name for the island as *Ierne*, as mentioned by Strabo in his work *Geography*. In *De Bello Gallico*, written about 52 BC, Caesar refers to name *Hibernia*. Ptolemy produced the first map (of Hibernia) with identifiable features about the middle of the 2nd century AD. In his *Ora Maritima* (4th century AD), based on a Greek original of the early 6th century BC, Festus Rufus Avienus refers to Ireland as *Insula sacra* (holy island) and to the inhabitants as *gens hiernorum*. The modern country's name of Éire (Gaeilge for Ireland) is thought to be derived, among others, from an early tribal group of Ireland referred   to   as   the   Érainn   (aka   Iverni). Some of the early descriptions of the [continental] Celts are from Poseidonios whose original works were written before 70 BC and survive in the works of later writers, e.g. Diodorus Siculus, Strabo, and Athenaus. Poseidonios describes a threefold division of Celtic society, the institutions of the druids, bardic praise poetry and clientship. Each of these are known in early Celtic Ireland as well as on the continent, where that which we call "Celtic" originated in central Europe. "(282)

The Celts in Ireland had extensive links with Celtic groups in Britain and the European mainland. Cooper discusses Livy's description of the Gauls and their move into Italy and comments on the relations between the British and the continental Celtic royal families.

"It is here, however, that Livy sheds some interesting light upon the Celtic royal families of the early 4th century BC. According to both Geoffrey and the Welsh chronicle, the father and mother of Belinus and Brennius were Dunvall Molmutius (Welsh Dyftial Moel Myd) and Tonuuenna (Welsh Tonwen). We know from the genealogy around which both Geoffrey's and the Welsh account are built, that Dunvallo was of British descent. Which means that Tonuuenna, whose genealogy is not given, could easily have been the sister of the Gaulish king, Ambitgatus, as is implied in Livy when he calls Bellovesus (the British Belinus and son of Tonuuenna) the nephew of Ambitgatus. There is

142

nothing at all unlikely or improbable in such a relationship. Indeed, marriage between the British and continental Celtic royal families would have been an entirely natural and expected event." (283)

The following may shows the different groups that had emerged around 100 AD. (284)

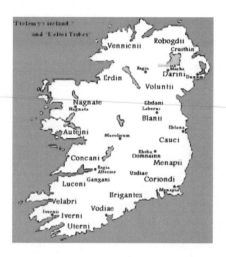

Practices exercised in war, as we noted above, continued among these Celts. We can comment here on the human sacrifice that occurred. Cahill writes:

"They sacrificed prisoners of war to the war gods and newborns to the harvest gods. Believing that the human head was the seat of the soul, they displayed proudly the heads of their enemies in their temples and on their palisades; they even hung them from their belts as ornaments, used them as footballs in victory celebrations, and were fond of employing skull tops as ceremonial drinking cups. They also sculpted heads – both shrunken, decapitated heads and overbearing, impassive godheads – and a favourite motif was the head of a tri-faced god, for three was their magical number, and gods and goddesses often manifested themselves as three."(285)

Let us now turn to the contacts between this Celtic empire in Europe and the emerging power of the Roman Empire.

143

Chapter 7

The Roman Empire and the Celtic World

By 500 BC, the Celtic peoples had established a firm presence in a wide area of Europe. The following map by Strabo, who lived from 64 BC to 24 AD, and wrote a 17-volume work called *Geographia*, shows this extent. (286)

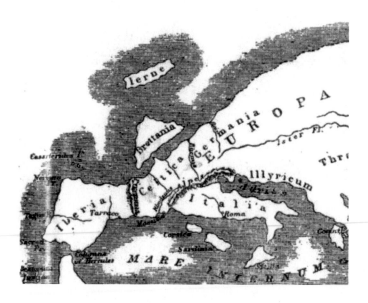

It was into these Celtic lands that the expanding Roman Empire moved. The first of the peoples to come under the Romans, were the Celts who had moved into the northern parts of Italy.

Romans defeat the Italian Celts

The Romans, in their expansion northwards, had fought the Samnites. In the third major war against these people, fought in 298-290 BC, the latter received help from the Celts. Among others who joined the league against Rome were the Etruscans, Sabines, Lucanians and Umbrians. Between 298 and 290 BC the Romans defeated each of the coalition members individually. Their conquest ensured their hold on central Italy.

From 285-282 BC the Romans fought with the Celts of northern Italy, conquering the Gallic Senones in 282 BC.

A century later, from 200 BC to 190 BC, the Romans moved against the Celtic tribes of the Po River valley, including the Boii and Insubres groups.

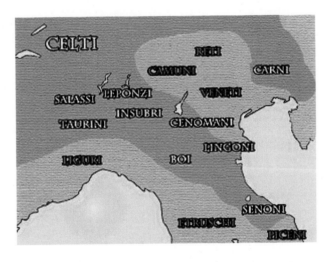

This conquest gave them control of Cisalpine Gaul. The rest of Cisalpine Gaul was conquered by Caesar in 59 BC. (287)

The Conquest of Transalpine Gaul

Transalpine Gaul is approximately modern Belgium, France and Switzerland. There were many Celtic tribes or groups throughout these lands. (288) Diodorus writes that Gaius Julius Caesar, who has been deified because of his deeds, subdued the most numerous and most warlike tribes of the Celts, and advanced the Roman Empire as far as the British Isles. The first events of this war occurred in the first year of the One Hundred and Eightieth Olympiad, when Herodes was archon at Athens. (289)

In The Gallic Wars, Julius Caesar notes that Gaul was divided into three parts:

"one of which the Belgae inhabit, the Aquitani another, those who in their own language are called Celts, in our Gauls (noted as Celtica), the third. All these differ from each other in language, customs and laws. The river Garonne separates the Gauls from the Aquitani; the Marne and the Seine separate them from the Belgae."(290)

The Gauls had been having difficulties with Germanic peoples. A powerful group under Ariovistus had moved into the lands of the Gauls, initially to assist some groups. They liked the lands and conquered them. Some of the Gauls went to Caesar for assistance.

Caesar had been fighting a group pillaging lands of Roman allies. Caesar defeated this Germanic group and drove them beyond the Rhine. The Gauls returned to their lands. (291)

While he was there, the Belgae entered into a confederacy with the Gauls to fight the Romans. Their numbers were large. Caesar writes that the Bellovaci Belgae had committed 100,000 men, Suessiones, whose king had been Divitiacus, king of Gaul and Britain, and his successor Galba, committed 50,000 and

" the Atrebates 15,000; the Ambiani, 10,000; the Morini, 25,000; the Menapii, 9,000; the Caleti, 10,000; the Velocasses and the Veromandui as many; the Aduatuci 19,000; that the Condrusi, the Eburones, the Caeraesi, the Paemani, who are called by the common name of Germans [had promised], they thought, to the number of 40,000."

Caesar described their manner of attack

"The Gauls' mode of besieging is the same as that of the Belgae: when after having drawn a large number of men around the whole of the fortifications, stones have begun to be cast against the wall on all sides,

146

and the wall has been stripped of its defenders, [then], forming a testudo, they advance to the gates and undermine the wall: which was easily effected on this occasion; for while so large a number were casting stones and darts, no one was able to maintain his position upon the wall."

Caesar fought them with eight legions, each having up to six thousand soldiers. It is well worth reading *The Gallic Wars* by Julius Caesar to better understand his fight against the experienced and talented opponents, the Celts. In the end, Caesar won. He writes:

"These things being achieved, [and] all Gaul being subdued, so high an opinion of this war was spread among the barbarians, that ambassadors were sent to Caesar by those nations who dwelt beyond the Rhine, to promise that they would give hostages and execute his commands. Which embassies Caesar, because he was hastening into Italy and Illyricum, ordered to return to him at the beginning of the following summer.

He himself, having led his legions into winter quarters among the Carnutes, the Andes, and the Turones, which states were close to those regions in which he had waged war, set out for Italy; and a thanksgiving of fifteen days was decreed for those achievements, upon receiving Caesar's letter; [an honor] which before that time had been conferred on none. "

However, he had not succeeded in suppressing the Celts. They continued to fight. Another confederation united for war. They included the Osismii, the Lexovii, the Nannetes, the Ambiliati, the Morini, the Diablintes, and the Menapii. They were defeated.

Next the Romans fought the Venetii, in 56 BC, in a sea battle. The Veniti were a powerful tribe who made most of their camps along the coasts in impressive cliff castles and were great sailors. It is thought that they may have also called for help from their close cousins in South-west Britain In 56 BC the Veneti assembled a great fleet of over 200 ships in Morbihan Bay and put all their efforts into this one battle. The smaller Roman vessels were more maneuverable and soon dealt with the larger Celtic force. (292)   Caesar commented on this battle:

"For their ships were built and equipped after this manner. The keels were somewhat flatter than those of our ships, whereby they could more easily encounter the shallows and the ebbing of the tide: the prows were raised very high, and, in like manner the sterns were adapted to the force of the waves and storms [which they were formed to sustain]. The ships were built wholly of oak, and designed to endure any force and violence whatever; the benches which were made of planks a foot in breadth, were fastened by iron spikes of the thickness of a man's thumb; the anchors were secured fast by iron chains instead of cables, and for sails they used skins and thin dressed leather. These [were used] either through their want of canvas and their ignorance of its application, or for this reason, which is more probable, that they thought that such storms of the ocean, and such violent gales of wind could not be resisted by sails, nor ships of such great burden be conveniently enough managed by them." (293)

Caesar won the battle, executed the leaders and sold into slavery the others he had captured.   The Celts who could, fled west to the Channel Islands and north to the southwest peninsula of Britain for safety
For the next two years, Caesar focused on the conquest of Britain.   However, the Gauls were not yet ready to settle under the onerous Roman rule.
A new rebellion arose in Transalpine Gaul, led by Vercingetorix. Vercingetorix adopted a burnt earth policy in this war, destroying food and other supplies to deny them to the Romans. His success led other Celtic groups to join him. Their forces ultimately amounted to eight thousand cavalry and two hundred and forty thousand infantry.   In the battles that ensued, the Romans won. The revolt was finally put down in 51 BC. Further battles followed, including one with the Bellovaci. In the end, Caesar left legions in all parts of Gaul to keep it under control.
Caesar writes that, in the end, he made peace with the Gauls by a policy of leniency, by treating the states with respect, making rich presents to the leading men, imposing no new

burdens, and making the terms of their subjection lighter. (294)

Romans Attack Britain

After his early successes against the Gauls, Caesar decided to attack the Celts in Britain because they had helped the Gauls. The first attack came in 55 BC. He brought with him two legions, totaling 10,000 men. (295) As he wrote:

"During the short part of summer which remained, Caesar, although in these countries, as all Gaul lies toward the north, the winters are early, nevertheless resolved to proceed into Britain, because he discovered that in almost all the wars with the Gauls succors had been furnished to our enemy from that country; and even if the time of year should be insufficient for carrying on the war, yet he thought it would be of great service to him if he only entered the island, and saw into the character of the people, and got knowledge of their localities, harbors, and landing-places, all which were for the most part unknown to the Gauls."

Caesar found them a formidable enemy. He wrote:

"But the barbarians, upon perceiving the design of the Romans, sent forward their cavalry and charioteers, a class of warriors of whom it is their practice to make great use in their battles, and following with the rest of their forces, endeavored to prevent our men landing."

Providing more detail later, he added:

"Their mode of fighting with their chariots is this: firstly, they drive about in all directions and throw their weapons and generally break the ranks of the enemy with the very dread of their horses and the noise of their wheels; and when they have worked themselves in between the troops of horse, leap from their chariots and engage on foot. The charioteers in the meantime withdraw some little distance from the battle, and so place themselves with the chariots that, if their masters are overpowered by the number of the enemy, they may have a ready retreat to their own troops. Thus they display in battle the speed of horse, [together with] the firmness of infantry; and by daily practice and exercise attain to such expertness that they are accustomed, even on a declining and steep place, to check their horses at full speed, and manage

149

and turn them in an instant and run along the pole, and stand on the yoke, and thence betake themselves with the greatest celerity to their chariots again."

Unable to win, Caesar returned to the mainland. A year later, in 54 BC, he returned to Britain. This time he brought 800 ships of troops. The Celts united under a war leader named Cassivellaunus. Caesar wrote that the Celts fought him at the Thames:

"When he had come thither, greater forces of the Britons had already assembled at that place, the chief command and management of the war having been entrusted to Cassivellaunus, whose territories a river, which is called the Thames, separates, from the maritime states at about eighty miles from the sea. At an earlier period perpetual wars had taken place between him and the other states; but, greatly alarmed by our arrival, the Britons had placed him over the whole war and the conduct of it."

Again, he had to quit Britain without having conquered it. This time it was to fight the Gauls who had rebelled again. He defeated them, and then went back to Rome. Plans may have been made for a full-scale invasion of Britain, but civil war in Rome (47-45 BC) and other turmoil led to Caesar's death at the hands of Brutus on the 15th March 44 BC. Plans for the conquest of Britain by the Romans were put on hold. One writer commented on the land and people they saw.

"During Rome's earlier armed reconnaissance of South East Britain, her armies had met and demanded tribute from the Celtic Trinovantes of Suffolk and Essex, who paid with large amounts of grain. The country was seen to be quite fertile with great forests and useful raw materials. They noted its predominantly agricultural economy with farms - arable in the south-east and livestock elsewhere. The Romans found Britain to be populated by many distinct Iron Age tribes, each tribe quite fearsome but with no overall military structure or 'mutual defense'. The Catuvellauni tribe originally occupied Hertfordshire around Verulamium (St Albans). Under their strong leader Cunobelin, they attacked and eventually subjugated their neighbours the Atrebates, becoming one of the major players in Southern Central Britain."(296)

In 43 AD, the Romans had another opportunity to invade Britain. The leader of the Atrebates, one Verica, son of

Commius, a former client king of the Romans, fled to the continent and asked the Roman Emperor Claudius for help to repel the Catuvellauni. This gave Claudius just the excuse he needed to invade Britain.

Southern Britain was invaded in 43AD, with a larger full-scale invasion some twelve years later. Provincial cities such as Londinium (London), *Corinium Dobunnorum* (Cirencester),*Lindum* (Lincoln), Eburacum (York) as well as major towns such as *Glevum* (Gloucester), *Virconium Cornoviorum* (Wroxeter), *Verulamium* (St. Albans) and *Aquae Sulis* (Bath) were founded. The *capital* of Britannia was built on the former Camulodunum (Colchester), until it was destroyed by the revolt of the Iceni under their warrior Queen Boudicca (Boadicea) some 18 years later in 60/61AD. The provincial city for the South West was founded at *Isca Dumnoniorum* - present day Exeter - and was built around the Roman garrison fort of the *Legio Secundus*. (297)

Romans decide not to Invade Ireland

Around 10 AD the Romans considered, and then abandoned, plans to invade Ireland. Cusack writes:

"The passage in Tacitus which refers to the proposed invasion of Ireland by the Roman forces, is too full of interest to be omitted: —" In the fifth year of these expeditions, Agricola, passing over in the first ship, subdued in frequent victories nations hitherto unknown. He stationed troops along that part of Britain which looks to Ireland, more on account of hope than fear, since Ireland, from its situation between Britain and Spain, and opening to the Gallic Sea, might well connect the most powerful parts of the empire with reciprocal advantage. Its extent, compared with Britain, is narrower, but exceeds that of any islands of our sea. The genius and habits of the people, and the soil and climate, do not differ much from those of Britain. Its channels and ports are better known to commerce and to merchants. Agricola gave his protection to one of its petty kings, who had been expelled by faction; and with a show of friendship, he retained him for his own purposes. I often heard him say, that Ireland could be conquered and taken with one legion and a small

151

reserve; and such a measure would have its advantages even as regards Britain, if Roman power were extended on every side, and liberty taken away as it were from the view of the latter island." (298)

The Romans Move against the Celts in Central Europe

In addition to conquering many of the Celtic societies in Western Europe, the Romans moved against those in the east. Rankin describes the conquest that took place from 88 BC to 35 BC

"In 88 BC...the Celtic Scordisci were defeated by a Roman army...and the Pannones were able to get back their lands. In turn, the Dacians, led by their king Bouribistes, defeated the Scordisci, Boii, and Taurisci in 60 BC. Vast tracts of land previously occupied by Boii were desolated and formed what Strabo called the Boian desert. Finally, in 35 BC, Octavian, seeking a defensible boundary for the Roman imperium, pushed into Illyricum and crushed the Pannones. He destroyed the inter-tribal organization but shrewdly left the residual Celtic area intact and in alliance with Rome as an insurance against further awkwardness on the part of the Pannones...On the other bank of the Danube, the vacuum created by Octavian's campaign was filled by Iranian-speaking peoples, the Jasygs, a splinter conglomerate of Scythians and Dacians, together with the dacians proper, who took over lands which the Celts and Pannones could no longer hold." (299)

To further weaken Celtic hegemony in Pannonia, the Romans moved the Pannonian-Illyrian Azali to northern Pannonia. The political dominance previously enjoyed by the Celts was overshadowed by newer confederations, such the Marcomanni and Iazyges. Their ethnic independence was gradually lost as they were absorbed by the surrounding Dacian, Illyrian and Germanic peoples, although Celtic names survive until the 3rd century AD. (300) After their defeat by the Greeks, the Celts settled in the Balkans, in places such as Singidunum, later known as Begrade.

Romans Conquer Celts in Galatia

In the great battle of Magnesia, 180 B.C., a body of Galatian troops fought against the Romans, on the side of Antiochus the Great, King of Syria. He was defeated by the Romans, under Scipio Asiaticus, and lost 50,000 of his men. Next year the Consul Manlius entered Galatia, and defeated the Galatians in two battles graphically described by Livy. Galatia was henceforth dominated by Rome through regional rulers. On account of ill-treatment received at the hands of Mithradates I King of Pontus, the Galatians took the side of Pompey in the Mitradatic wars, in 64 B.C. As a reward for their services, Deiotarus, their chief tetrarch, received the title of king, and his dominions were greatly extended. Henceword the Galatians were under the protection of the Romans, and were involved in all the troubles of the civil wars that followed.

In the settlement of 64 BC, Galatia became a client-state of the Roman Empire, the old constitution disappeared, and three chiefs were appointed, one for each tribe. But this arrangement soon gave way before the ambition of one of these chiefs, or tetrarchs, Deiotarus, the contemporary of Cicero and Julius Caesar, who made himself master of the other two tetrarchies and was finally recognized by the Romans as 'king' of Galatia. (301)

They supported Pompey against Julius Caesar at the battle of Pharsalia in 48 B.C. Amyntas, their last king was set up by Mark Antony, 39 B.C. His kingdom finally included not only Galatia Proper but also the great plains to the south, together with parts of Lyesonia, Pamphylia, Pisidia, and Phrygia, i.e. the country containing the towns Antioch, Iconium, Lystra and Derbe. Amyntas went to Actium, 31 BC, to support Mark Antony; but like many others he went over, at the critical moment, to the side of Octavianus, afterwards called

Augustus. Augustus confirmed him in his kingdom, which he retained until he was slain in ambush in 25 BC .

After the death of Amyntas in 25 BC, Galatia was incorporated by Octavian Augustus into the Roman Empire, becoming a Roman province. Near his capital Ancyra (modern Ankara), Pylamenes, the king's heir, rebuilt a temple of the Phrygian goddess Men to venerate Augustus (the Monumentum Ancyranum), as a sign of fidelity. Few of the provinces proved more enthusiastically loyal to Rome. The Galatians also practiced a form of Romano-Celtic polytheism, common in Celtic lands. (302)

For the next 400 years, large parts of the Celtic world remained under Roman rule. Some Celtic societies, such as Ireland, Scotland and Wales remained free. The next major change that came to Celtic culture involved the introduction of Christianity.

Chapter 8

The Celts Become Christians

As the Roman Empire declined after centuries of dominance in Europe and beyond, a new influence emerged on the scene, that of Christianity. As it became and has remained an important component of Irish life we will now consider it. The first to adopt Christianity were the Celts living in Asia, specifically, in Galatia.

Galatia

The Galatians first learned about Christ from St. Paul. In his second mission through East Asia, he was told by the Holy Spirit not to preach, so he only passed through. Then, on his third mission, between 53 and 57 AD, receiving no opposition from the Holy Spirit, he preached in Galatia. (303)
The Galatians were very responsive to the preaching of St. Paul and other early Jewish converts. Indeed, it was among the Galatians that early disputes arose over how the faith was to be interpreted, especially over the Judaistic nature of the emerging Christian church and whether converts had to be circumcised and follow the law of Moses or not. Paul said neither was necessary. He convinced the leaders of the church to agree. The decisions made at that time subsequently determined the Christian religion in the Roman Empire. Paul preached against sorcery and idolatry, practiced throughout the pagan world. He preached equality, stating:

"And putting on the new, him who is renewed unto knowledge, according to the image of him that created him. Where there is neither Gentile nor Jew, circumcision nor uncircumcision, Barbarian nor Scythian, bond nor free. But Christ is all, and in all". (304)

Ahern noted, when discussing Paul's Epistle to the Galatians:

"The Epistle implies that the Galatians were well acquainted with the doctrines of the Trinity, the Divinity of Christ, Incarnation, Redemption, Baptism, Grace, etc. As he had never to defend his teaching to these points against Judaizers, and as the Epistle is so early, it is clear that his teaching was identical with that of the Twelve, and did not, even in appearance, lend itself to attack." (305)

Ramsay comments quite favourably on those who converted as:

"those who desire education, who have shaken off the benumbing and degrading influence of the native magic and superstition, who judge for themselves as to the real value of the facts of life, who lay claim to insight" (306)

The Galatians became committed Christianity in the centuries that followed. Ramsay notes that the Bishops of Ancyra played a great part in many Church decisions from 312 AD onwards. Moreover, the metropolitan Bishop of Ancyra ranked second only to Caesareia in the Patriarchate of Constantinople. (307)

It is interesting to note that despite many centuries of separation, there were still numerous cultural similarities between the Galatians and their European relations   For example, St Jerome, who lived from 347 to 420 AD, wrote that the Galatians of Ancyra and the Treveri of Trier, in what is now the German Rhineland,   spoke the same language (308).

In an administrative reorganization about 386-95 AD two new provinces succeeded it, Galatia Prima and Galatia Secunda or Salutaris, which included part of Phrygia. The fate of the Galatian people is a subject of some uncertainty, but they seem ultimately to have been absorbed into the Greek-speaking populations of west-central Anatolia. (309)

Spread of Christianity in Europe

Christianity started spreading throughout Europe right from the time of the Apostles. For two hundred years, Christians alternated between being tolerated and being persecuted. Then, after Emperor Constantine issued the Edict of Milan in 313 AD that officially tolerated the existence of Christianity, the church was free to prosetelize. (310)

Conversion of Spain to Christianity

Legends credit the start of conversion in Spain to St. James. According to these, St. James, after returning to Palestine in 44 AD, was taken prisoner by Herodes Agrippa and tortured to death. In the night Jacob's disciples stole the body and brought him, in a sarcophagus of marble, on board of a small boat. The current of the sea drove the boat to the Spanish coast, into the port of the Roman province's capital, Iria Flavia. Here the Apostle was buried at a secret place in a wood. This site is now the city of Santiago de Compostela. Centuries later, in 831, the tomb was discovered. King Alphonse II declared Saint James the patron of his empire and built a chapel there. Many miracles happened afterwards, including help when he fought side to side with King Ramiro I in the decisive battle against the Moors. (311) Whether the above is true or not, we know that Spain was known to the early Christians, and mentioned by them. St. Paul identified Spain as a target for conversion in his Epistle to the Romans. He visited Spain in 62 AD. Christianity was spreading there in the 1st century AD and by the 2nd century AD had spread into most cities. Most of Spain's present languages and religion, and the basis of its laws, originate from this period.

The weakening of the Western Roman Empire's jurisdiction in Spain began in 409 AD, when the Germanic Suevi and

Vandals, together with the Sarmatian Alans crossed the Rhine and ravaged Gaul until the Visigoths drove them into Iberia that same year. The Suevi established a kingdom in what is today modern Galicia and northern Portugal. As the western empire disintegrated, the social and economic base simplified: but even in modified form, the successor regimes maintained many of the institutions and laws of the late empire, including Christianity.

The Alans' allies, the Hasdingi Vandals, established a kingdom in Galicia as well. The Silingi Vandals occupied Andalusia. The Byzantines established an enclave, Spania, in the south, with the intention of reviving the Roman Empire throughout Iberia. Eventually, however, Hispania was reunited under Visigothic rule. The Visigoths adopted the heresy of Arianism and promoted this heresy. Despite their control, the mass of the faithful did not become Arian.

In the 8th century, nearly all of the Iberian Peninsula was conquered (711–718) by largely Moorish Muslim armies from North Africa. These conquests were part of the expansion of the Umayyad Islamic Empire. Only a small area in the mountainous north-west of the peninsula managed to resist the initial invasion.

Under Islamic law, Christians and Jews were given the subordinate status of dhimmi. This status permitted Christians and Jews to practice their religions as people of the book but they were required to pay a special tax and to be subject to certain discriminations.

Conversion to Islam proceeded at a steadily increasing pace. The muladies (Muslims of ethnic Iberian origin) are believed to have comprised the majority of the population of Al-Andalus by the end of the 10th century.

The reconquest of Spain by the Christians started in 722 with the Battle of Covadonga, which led to the creation of the Christian Kingdom of Asturias along the northwestern coastal mountains. Shortly after, in 739, Muslim forces were driven from Galicia, freeing Santiago de Compostela which was incorporated into the new Christian kingdom. Muslim armies had also moved north of the Pyrenees, but they were defeated by Frankish forces at the Battle of Poitiers, Frankia. Later, Frankish forces established Christian counties on the southern side of the Pyrenees. These areas were to grow into the kingdoms of Navarre, Aragon and Catalonia. For several centuries, the fluctuating frontier between the Muslim and Christian controlled areas of Iberia was along the Ebro and Duero valleys.

In 1085 Toledo was captured. Finally, in the 13th century, Cordoba and Seville fell to the Christians. The Crown of Aragon rose to power and Spain became one of the great European nations, leading the expansion into the Americas. (312)

France Becomes Christian

In France, popular tradition holds that conversion started with Mary of Madgelen and others who came with her to France.

The French tradition of Saint Lazare of Bethany is that Mary, her brother Lazarus, and Maximinus, one of the Seventy Disciples and some companions, expelled by persecutions from the Holy Land, traversed the Mediterranean in a frail boat with neither rudder nor mast and landed at the place called Saintes-Maries-de-la-Mer near Arles. Mary Magdalene came to Marseille and converted the whole of Provence. Magdalene is said to have retired to a cave on a hill by Marseille, La Sainte-Baume ("holy cave." baumo in Provençal), where she gave herself up to a life of penance for thirty years. When she was dying she was carried by angels to Aix and into the oratory of Saint Maximinus, where she received the viaticum; her body was then laid in an oratory constructed by St. Maximinus at Villa Lata. (313)

Mary Magdalene's relics were first venerated at the abbey of Vézelay in Burgundy. According to Jacobus de Voragine, these relics were transferred from her sepulchre in the oratory of Saint Maximin at Aix-en-Provence to the newly founded abbey of Vézelay in 771 by the founder of the abbey, identified as Gerard, duke of Burgundy. The chronicler Sigebert of Gembloux , who died in 1112, noted that the relics were removed to Vézelay through fear of the Saracens. There is no record of their further removal to the other St-Maximin; a casket of relics associated with Magdalene remains at Vézelay.

Since September 9, 1279, the body of Mary Magdalene was also venerated at Saint-Maximin-la-Sainte-Baume, Provence. The site attracted such throngs of pilgrims that the earlier shrine was rebuilt as the great Basilica from the mid-13th century, one of the finest Gothic churches in the south of France.

In 1279, when Charles II, King of Naples, erected a Dominican convent at La Sainte-Baume, the shrine was found intact, with an explanatory inscription stating why the relics had been hidden. In 1600, the relics were placed in a sarcophagus commissioned by Pope Clement VIII, the head being placed in a separate reliquary. The relics and free-standing images were scattered and destroyed during the French Revolution. In 1814, the church of La Sainte-Baume, also wrecked during the Revolution, was restored. In 1822, the grotto was consecrated afresh. The head of the saint now lies there and has been the centre of many pilgrimages. (314)

During the third century, France, like much of the Roman Empire, was adversely affected by the Arian heresy. At a Council at Beziers in 356 AD, Arianism as confirmed by most bishops. A few, including St. Hilary of Poitiers and St. Martin of Tours, Bishop of Tours, 372-387, resisted and helped restore the Catholic faith. (315)

In Gaul, Roman rule continued until the invasion of the Franks in the 5th century. In 486, Clovis I, leader of the Salian Franks, and Head of the Merovingian House, defeated Syagrius at Soissons and then united most of northern and central Gaul under his rule. In 496, he converted to Roman Catholicism. This was popular with the people, who wanted to be free of their Arian rulers. With him begins the history not only of the French empire, its government and laws, but also of the French nation, its religion and moral habits. The empire he set up continued for some two hundred years.

By the end of the sixth century the Lombards, Ostrogoths and Visigoths, including the rulers of Spain, were converted from their fourth century Arianism.

As the Merovingian House declined, Charles Martel set up the Carolingian dynasty and began the expansion of the Frankish kingdom. At Tours, he defeated a Muslim army moving into France and effectively stopped their advance through Europe.

Martel's son, Pepin the Short, then became the king of the Franks. He was succeeded by his son, Charlemagne, Charles the Great. Under the rule of Charlemagne, the Carolingian empire reached its peak. His military successes in Spain, Italy and almost all the western area of the old Roman Empire led him to be crowned emperor in 800. His empire enjoyed a high degree of law, order and good government. (316)

Charlemagne was not only an able military leader, but was also a great supporter of education and the arts. During Charlemagne's period, there was a Carolingian renaissance, but shortly after his death the kingdom was divided.

One of the last Carolingian kings of the Franks, Charles III the Simple (893-922), established a peace with the Vikings who had been raiding and plundering his and neighbouring lands. The leader of the Northmen, Rollo paid homage to Charles and was given the Duchy of Normandy. Within a few generations the invaders had integrated into the local population. In 1066, William was the Duke. A good military leader, he had expanded his dominion over neighbouring areas. Soon he decided to conquer Britain. (317)

In other parts of France, the Celts became involved in some of the religious disputes of the times. One was the dispute over the Albigensian heresy. In this, the powerful Counts of Toulouse, the Raymonds, at times supported, then countered the Albigensian heresy. (318)

Celts and the Crusades

One of the great events in which our French ancestors participated was the Crusades. The Redmonds, then known as Raymonds, were among the leaders of the First Crusade.

In 1095, Pope Urban II made an appeal at Claremont, France for soldiers to retake Jerusalem from the Muslims and thereby protect Christian pilgrims against whom atrocities were being committed. His request was supported by the Emperor Alexius 1 Comnenus at Constantinople. A Crusade of the Poor People was quickly organized but it accomplished little. Then a group of professional knights decided to answer the call of the faith. They were led by Raymond IV of Toulouse, Count of St. Gilles, Raymond of Flanders, Robert of Normandy, Godfrey of Bouillon, Bohemund of Taranto and Adhemar of Monteil, bishop of le Puy. They marched into Syria and took the fortress of Antioch in June 1098. Raymond of Toulouse let Bohemund rule Antioch and led the remaining troops to Jerusalem. They conquered the cities of Tripoli, Beirut and Acre.

The battle at Jerusalem lay ahead. By the time they reached the outskirts of Jerusalem, there were some 1,300 knights with 14,000 women and children in tow. Iftikhar, governor of Jerusalem, had poisoned all wells outside the walls. All local food had been brought inside the walls. Only one water source, the pool of siloam, could be used. Food was scarce. Their first attempt to scale the high walls failed. Then supplies arrived at Jaffa. The sailors and craftsmen joined the Crusaders and, with their supplies and some lumber found in a cave, the Crusaders built two siege towers, catapults and a battering ram. On July 13 they moved forward. The Muslims threw sulpher and pitch based fireballs on them. After fighting all day and night, one siege tower burned. The next day, the second siege tower was moved near Herod's Gate. With the Crusaders launching a fire attack against the bales of hay and cotton with which Iftikhar had lined the walls, they breached the walls. With scaling ladders, all then entered the city. Iftikhar fled to the Tower of David. Raymond accepted his surrender and allowed him and a small number to flee Jerusalem. Most of the others were killed, a few were taken as slaves and Jerusalem was pillaged. They ended the conquest with a procession to the Church of the Holy Sepulchre. As Fulcher of Chartes said "They desired that this place, so long contaminated by the superstition of the pagan inhabitants, should be cleansed from their contagion". The holy city of Jerusalem was, once again, in Christian hands. (319)

The British become Christian

The arrival of Christianity into Britain has legends associated with it, as was the case with its arrival in Spain and France. Philip Schaff, in his history of Christianity, notes ten of these:

"1) Bran, a British prince, and his son Caradog, who is said to have become acquainted with St. Paul in Rome, 51 to 58 AD, and to have introduced the Gospel into his native country on his return

2) St Paul (during his captivity between 63 and 67 AD – advocated by Ussher and Stillingfleet; also some say Galatian converts of St Paul visited Britain for trade and spread the religion)
3) St. Peter
4) St Simon Zelotes
5) St Philip
6) St James the Great
7) St John
8) Aristobulus (Romans 14:10)
9) Joseph of Arimathaea, who figures largely in the post-Norman legends of Glastonbury Abbey, and is said to have brought the Holy Grail – the vessel or platter of the Lord's Supper – containing the blood of Christ, to England
10) Missionaries of Pope Eleutherus from Rome to King Lucius of Britain (176-190 AD, this is related by Bede) "(320)

Schaff continues in describing the early development of Christianity. About 208 AD Tertulian declared that "places in Britain not yet visited by Romans were subject to Christ". St Alban died as a British proto-martyr in the Diocletian persecution of 303 AD. Constantine, the first Christian emperor, was born in Britain and his mother, St. Helena, was probably a native of the country. Three British bishops, Eborius of York, Restitutus of London and Adelfius of Lincoln attended the Council of Arles in 314 AD. In the Arian controversy, the British church sided with Athanasius and the Nicene Creed.

Differences developed between the Roman and British practice of the faith. Schaff notes that these were ritualistic and disciplinary. The dating of Easter and running the church through national councils rather than referring to the Pope were two of these. These were resolved over time.

Over the years, the faith was weakened by wars against the Picts of the north, then the Anglo-Saxons, Jutes and Frisians. These invaders gradually drove the Britons to Wales and the borders of Scotland and became masters in Britain.

Among those who struggled against the Anglo-Saxon invaders was the Celtic leader King Arthur, the hero of

Wales and his Round Table, referenced in the Chronicles of Geoffrey of Monmouth. He won many battles against the invaders before being killed in 520 AD.

Britain was restored to Christianity when Pope Gregory 1 sent Augustine to preach and convert there. King Ethelbert, married already to a French Christian, welcomed them. He allowed them to reside in Canterbury, from where they spread the faith.

Augustine demanded the obedience of the Celtic bishops and that they make changes to their current practices, including compliance with the Roman observance of Easter, the Roman form of baptism and that they help to convert the English. They refused and Augustine said they would be punished. A few years later in 613 AD, Ethelfrith the Wild attacked the Britons at Chester and destroyed their army, killed hundreds of priests and monks and destroyed the monastery of Bangor, where more than 2000 monks lived. This destruction caused the loss of the monastery's great library that had been built up over centuries.

The Irish in Ireland become Christian

One of the earliest rulers in Ireland to consider Christianity was Cormac, King of Ireland, who rejected the Druidic religion in favour of Christianity in 266 AD. The *Annals of the Four Prophets* write what happened to him.

"(He) died at Cleiteach, the bone of a salmon sticking in his throat, on account of the siabhradh *genii* which Maelgenn, the Druid, incited at him, after Cormac had turned against the Druids, on account of his adoration of God in preference to them. Wherefore a devil attacked him, at the instigation of the Druids, and gave him a painful death. It was Cormac who composed Teagusc Na Righ, to preserve manners, morals, and government in the kingdom. He was a famous author in laws, synchronisms, and history, for it was he that established law, rule, and direction for each science and for each covenant according to propriety;

165

and it is his laws that governed all that adhered to them to the present time.

It was this Cormac, son of Art, also, that collected the Chroniclers of Ireland to Teamhair, and ordered them to write the chronicles of Ireland in one book, which was named the Psalter of Teamhair. In that book were entered the coeval exploits and synchronisms of the kings of Ireland with the kings and emperors of the world, and of the kings of the provinces with the monarchs of Ireland. In it was also written what the monarchs of Ireland were entitled to receive from the provincial kings, and the rents and dues of the provincial kings from their subjects, from the noble to the subaltern. In it also were described the boundaries and meares of Ireland, from shore to shore, from the province to the cantred, from the cantred to the townland, and from the townland to the traighidh of land. These things are celebrated in Leabhar Na nUidhri. They are evident in the Leabhar Dinnsenchusa. (321)

The next major effort at conversion began in 430 AD. In this year Pope Celestinus the First sent Palladius to Ireland, to propagate the faith among the Irish. Palladius landed in the country of Leinster with a company of twelve men. Nathi, son of Garchu, refused to admit him. However, he baptized a few persons in Ireland, and three wooden churches were erected by him, namely, Cell Fhine, Teach Na Romhan, and Domhnach Arta. At Cell Fhine he left his books and a shrine with the relics of Peter, Paul and other martyrs. On returning to Rome, he contracted a disease in the country of the Cruithnigh, and died thereof. (322)

A year later, Pope Celestine the First sent St. Patrick to convert the Irish. Details of the conversion are provided by the anonymous manuscript *On The Life of St. Patrick*. (323) Patrick had been captured by slave traders and sold to a king in Ireland. After ten years, he bought his freedom and went to Italy. He stayed for thirty years with Bishop German, learning scriptures and developing wisdom and piety. Then he went to Rome. There he was asked to go to Ireland to convert the people. The *Life* provides many details on the struggles between St. Patrick and the Druids who had great influence over the King at Tara, the seat of the Kings of

Ireland. Many opponents of the new religion died in efforts to kill the saint. Yet, he was received well by many who converted to the new faith. After a pilgrimage to Rome, he returned to Armagh, fasted for forty days, then, before celebrating Easter, asked for seven things from an angel:

"seven things are given to me by the Lord, namely, that at Doomsday hell be not shut upon whichsoever of the men of Ireland repenteth before death, were it even for the space of a single hour; that outlanders may not inhabit this island; that the sea may come over it seven years before Doomsday; that seven persons every Thursday and twelve every Saturday I may free from the pains of hell; that whoever shall sing my hymn on the day of his death may be a dweller in heaven, as I promised unto Sechnall; and that on Doomsday I may bring from the pains of hell for every hair of my chasuble, seven of those that shall visit it; and that I myself may be judge over the men of Ireland on Doomsday.' 'All this shall be granted to thee.' said the angel"

St Patrick had great success in Ireland. As Cahill writes:

"Within his lifetime or soon after his death, the Irish slave trade came to a halt, and other forms of violence, such as murder and intertribal warfare, decreased. In reforming Irish sexual mores, he was rather less successful, though he established indigenous monasteries and convents, whose inmates by their way of life reminded the Irish that the virtues of lifelong faithfulness, courage, and generosity were actually attainable by ordinary human beings and that the sword was not the only instrument for structuring a society."(324)

Cahill adds that St Patrick was "the first human being in the history of the world to speak out unequivocally against slavery".

After its conversion, Ireland played a pivotal role in preserving Christianity in Europe as the continent, racked by invasions of pagan groups and weakened internally by the spread of Arianism, entered into severe decline. Cahill described this decline, noting that the Romans had lost northern Africa and much of Spain and Gaul to the Vandals by the 440 AD. Then the Goths and Huns moved westward over the Danube and devastated the eastern provinces. By the early fifth century, the Romans had abandoned Britain. (325)

The Irish remained free and kept their religion. Then they expanded it, building churches and monasteries in many places. In these, they cultivated learning. Cahill quotes John T.McNeill who stated that the breadth and richness of Irish monastic learning derived from the classical authors gave Ireland a "unique role in the history of western culture". They created copies of all the early Irish literature they could find. This created the earliest vernacular literature of Europe to survive. In addition they copied all Greek, Latin and Hebrew works they could find. These included Celtic versions of the Argonautic Expedition, the Seige of Troy, the life of Alexander the Great, the destruction of Jerusalem, the wars of Charlemagne and the Travels of Marco Polo. (326)

Their calligraphy was remarkable. Examples can be seen from the *Book of Kells*, one of the greatest works of the monks, produced around 800 AD. (327)

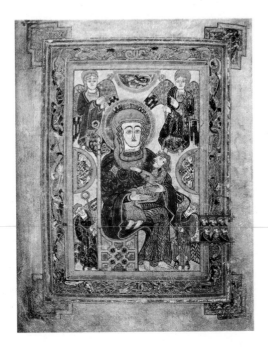

Virgin and Child. This is the oldest extant image of the Virgin Mary in a Western manuscript.

The monasteries of Ireland became refuges to people fleeing the barbarian tribes taking over Europe. They included individuals from the Middle East as well as from all over Europe.

Then in a second stage, the Irish set out to rechristianize Europe. The religious orders they had established were comparable to those established in the East from 356 AD by St Anthony and his successors. The monastic life that he developed spread throughout eastern Asia. (328)

The Irish monks spread their faith throughout Europe, setting up monasteries in the many places they visited. The first great Irish traveler was Columcille, born in 521 AD. In their travels and settlements, these monks reconnected a Europe that had become pagan to the traditions of Christian literacy.

This great legacy has been preserved in numerous sources. As Cahill notes:

"And just as the unyielding warrior Cuchulainn had served as the model of prehistoric Irish manhood, Columcille now became the model for all who would earn the ultimate victory. Monks began to set off in every direction, bent on glorious and heroic exile for the sake of Christ. They were warrior-monks, of course, and certainly not afraid of whatever monsters they might meet. Some went north, like Columcille. Others went northwest, like Brendan the navigator, visiting Iceland, Greenland, and North America, and supping on the back of a whale in mid-ocean. Some set out in boats without oars, putting their destination completely in the hands of God. Many of the exiles found their way into continental Europe, where they were more than a match for the barbarians they met. They whom the Romans had never conquered (and evangelized only, as it were, by accident in the person of Patrick, the imperfect Roman), fearlessly brought he ancient civilization back to its ancient home." (329)

The Irish manuscripts they carried with them ended up in many European libraries. Today they are the great jewels of libraries in England, France, Switzerland, Germany, Sweden, Italy and Russia.

Cahill summarizes the influence of Christian Ireland on Europe in these words:

"Wherever they went they brought their love of learning and their skills in bookmaking. In the bays and valleys of their exile, they reestablished literacy and breathed new life into the exhausted literary culture of Europe. And that is how the Irish saved civilization" (330)

Chapter 9

The Norman Invasions

The Norman Conquest of England

In 1066 the Normans invaded and conquered England.
The Redmonds, then known as Raymonds, were among the invaders. What led to it? (331)
In 1002 King Æthelred II of England married Emma, the sister of Richard II, Duke of Normandy. Their son Edward the Confessor, who spent many years in exile in Normandy, succeeded to the English throne in 1042. This led to the establishment of a powerful Norman interest in English politics, as Edward drew heavily on the Normans for support, bringing in Norman courtiers, soldiers, and clerics and appointing them to positions of power, particularly in the Church.

When King Edward died at the beginning of 1066, the lack of a clear heir led to a disputed succession in which several contenders laid claim to the throne of England. Edward's immediate successor was the Earl of Wessex, Harold Godwinson, known as King Harold II, the richest and most powerful of the English aristocracy. He was elected king by the Witenagemot of England and crowned by Archbishop Eldred of York.

However, he was at once challenged by two powerful neighbouring rulers. Duke William of Normandy claimed that he had been promised the throne by King Edward and that Harold had sworn agreement to this. Harald III of Norway, commonly known as Harald Hardrada, also contested the succession. His claim to the throne was based on a supposed agreement between his predecessor Magnus I of Norway, and the earlier Danish King of England Harthacanute, whereby if either died without heir, the other would inherit both England and Norway. Both William and Harald at once set about assembling troops and ships for an invasion.

Magnus 1 was the first to attack. In fierce fighting with King Harold II, he was defeated.

William attacked next. He assembled a large invasion fleet and an army gathered not only from Normandy but from all over France, including large contingents from Brittany and Flanders. He mustered his forces at Saint-Valery-sur-Somme. The Normans crossed over to England a few days after Harold's victory over the Norwegians, following the dispersal of Harold's naval force. They landed at Pevensey in Sussex on 28 September and erected a wooden castle at Hastings, from which they raided the surrounding area.

Marching south at the news of William's landing, Harold paused briefly at London to gather more troops, and then advanced to meet William. They fought the Battle of Hastings on 14 October. The English army, drawn up in a shieldwall on top of Senlac Hill, withstood a series of Norman attacks for several hours but was depleted by the losses suffered when troops on foot pursuing retreating Norman cavalry were repeatedly caught out in the open by counter-attacks. In the evening the defense finally collapsed and Harold was killed, along with his brothers Earl Gyrth and Earl Leofwine.

English resistance continued in various parts of the country for another five years. By 1071, the Normans were in control.

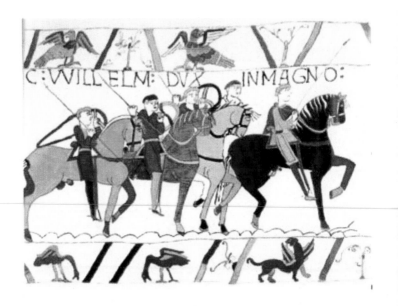

The Bayeux tapestry depicts the battle of Hastings and the events leading to it.

William claimed control of all the land in England and disposed of it as he saw fit. He gave land and titles to a number of his supporters. The Normans soon displaced the native aristocracy in the upper ranks of society.

A survey was done, in 1086, of the wealth of the land, called the Doomsday Book. This survey was the first done since Roman times. By then only 5% of the land remained in English hands.

When Henry II, grandson of William the Conqueror married Eleanor of Aquitane, most of the western part of France came under the British crown.

Within a hundred years, conflict arose between the Norman rulers in England, called the Plantagnets, who ruled England and part of France, and the Capetian kings of France. In 1204 Philip II seized Norman holdings in France. Intermittent fighting over these possessions led to the

175

Hundred Years War. This ended in 1453, when the Plantagnets lost their French possessions in fighting to the French, fighting under Joan of Arc.

Normans Conquer Wales

Initially William the Conqueror was not interested in subduing Wales, but continued attacks by the Welsh and their support for English rebellions, led the Normans to attack in 1071. After lengthy, intermittent fighting, in 1163, Henry II fully subdued the Celts in Wales and accepted homage from the two most powerful leaders of Wales, Rhys ap Gruffydd and Owain Gwynedd. Unlike in England, Welsh prices continued to retain the basic political and geographic structure for some period afterwards. (332)

Normans Conquer Ireland

Almost 100 years after taking England, on May 1, 1169, the Normans attacked Ireland.

In 1166, Dermot MacMurrough, the King of Leinster who had been deprived of his kingdom by Rory O'Connor, the high King of Ireland, for abducting the wife of a lesser king, met Henry II to seek help in recovering his lands in Ireland. Henry II authorized his Lords to assist if they wanted. Richard de Clare, the 2nd Earl of Pembroke, also known as Strongbow, offered to help. Dermot offered his eldest daughter in marriage to Richard and also gave him the succession to Leinster. (333)

The invasion army was led by Raymond (or Redmond) FitzGerald, nicknamed de Gras, meaning Grace. This nickname is sometimes written as Le Gros.

He was a popular military leader, as the following article confirms:

"History scarcely presents a more striking instance of that first and powerful proof of greatness, which lies in an ascendancy over other men's minds, than was exhibited by Raymond le Gros. The soldiers who, without him, were nothing, with him were everything; and Earl Strongbow, says Hollinshed, constrained him to become joint viceroy with himself. Giraldus Cambrensis calls him the "notable and chiefest pillar of Ireland." With heroism so elevated, magnanimity so unsullied, wisdom so profound, and exploits so unrivalled as their unvarnished tale unfolds, Raymond le Gras wanted only a Homer or a Tasso to have been an Achilles or a Rinaldo. In fact, though Strongbow was the head, Raymond was the very soul of the Anglo-Norman enterprise in Ireland. Upon his secession in anger, when Strongbow deferred consenting to his marriage with his sister Basilia de Clare, the war either stood still, or what was worse went back. The repentance of Strongbow was immediate, and his concession complete." (334)

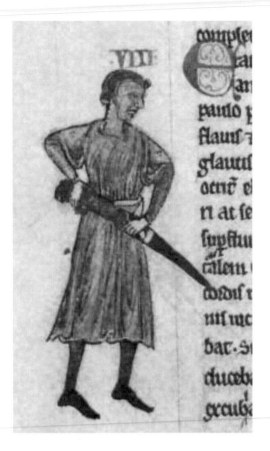

Raymond le Gros in a 13th century manuscript, MS 700 of the National Library of Ireland, illustrating the text of the Expugnatio Hibernica, written by Gerald of Wales, a cousin of Raymond. (335)

Following the conquest, Raymond returned to Wales. After Strongbow allowed him to marry his sister, Basilia, he returned to Ireland to suppress a rebellion that was threatening Waterford. He crushed the rebellion, then extended the conquests to Limerick and other towns. (336) Appointed as the Earl of Pembroke, he became a landowner in Ireland. For, as they had done in England, the Normans took possession of the lands they conquered and divided them up amongst themselves. His property comprised:

"Among these princely grants was that of Grace's country to Raymond le Gros. This consisted of a vast tract of land, comprehending, it is said, the barony of Cranagh, and extending northwards by the liberties of Kilkenny and the river Nore, to the borders of the Queen's County; and thence southwards along the borders of Tipperary and the Munster river to the liberties of Callan : forming a district between eleven and twelve miles in length, and between five and six in breadth. The central situation of Tullaroan, in the district of Grace's country, naturally occasioned the selection of that place for the chief castle of the territorial lords ; some of whom we find styled Baron of Tullaroan, as well as Baron Grace and Baron of Courtstown." (337)

The son of Raymond le Gros, who was called William Fitz Raymond le Gros, or le Gras, or Crassus, lived on those lands. Some descendants have the family name Grace. (338) They built a castle in 1210, which, in the reign of Elizabeth, was designated as "An Grassagh more Ballynacourty," (the great Grace of Courtstown). It is well known in Irish history as the bulwark of early English power. (339)

Chapter 10

Ireland to 1922

Over the next seven hundred years, our ancestors, the Normans, integrated into Irish society and shared with it the challenges posed by the proximity of Britain and its desire to control that land. Jerry Desmond has written a good history of Ireland from the conquest to the twentieth century and this will be the basis of what follows. (340)

Nominally, Strongbow and his Norman troops were acting on behalf of Henry II. Henry wanted Ireland to become part of his Angevin empire, with the Normans serving as feudal underlords. To ensure this, he traveled to Ireland, bringing with him 4,000 well armed troops, and signed the Treaty of Windsor, in 1175, with the Normans and Celtic rulers. Under it Henry took for himself a large portion of Irish land already in Norman hands, including the area around Dublin which later became known as "the Pale". The remaining land already in Norman hands was allocated among the Norman leaders. Finally, Henry agreed to accept Rory O'Connor as Ard Ri (high-king) of the unconquered areas, in western Ireland and western Ulster. O'Connor pledged himself to recognize Henry II as his overlord and to collect annual tribute for him from all parts of Ireland. This treaty was not observed long as O'Connor could not collect the tribute while the Norman barons continued confiscating neighbouring lands.

Henry's son, John I, fought and lost a war against King Philip II of France in 1206. This cost him most of the English possessions in France, including Normandy, Anjou and Brittany. However, he kept Norman-controlled Ireland.

Everywhere they went in Ireland, the Normans built castles and towns, as they had done in England. They also intermarried with Gaelic nobility, establishing the celebrated

Norman-Irish feudal families -- Fitzgerald, Burke, Costello, and Butler -- who ruled much of Ireland under nominal suzerainty from England until late in the 16th Century. Within a few generations, the Normans were as much a part of the Irish landscape as were the Gaels.

The Normans, assisted by a partly Anglo work force, dramatically changed the face of inland Ireland, which previously had been entirely pastoral. Vastly outnumbered by the natives, the Normans congregated in small communities, which gradually evolved in towns, typically centered on a castle and/or church. Indeed, although the coastal towns of Dublin, Wexford, Waterford, Cork, and Limerick were established by the Vikings, the vast majority of inland and other towns and villages in Ireland were founded by the Normans. Munster, under Norman influence, became one of the most French of provinces outside of France itself.

After conquering an area, the Normans typically displaced the Gaelic nobility, or married into it, but the ordinary Irishman was left in peaceful possession of his land to herd cattle and till the soil, just as he had been doing under their native chieftains. The Normans introduced more efficient agricultural practices. They built some of the great cathedrals, including St Patrick's in Dublin, St Mary's in Limerick and St Canice's in Kilkenny.

They installed a strong central government. They struck coinage for Ireland. They introduced English common law, including the jury system. They appointed Sheriffs. And although it served only the Norman-Anglo colony, an Irish parliament modeled on the English one was created in the late 13th century.

Norman-Irish Ireland, comprising about 70% of the island, everything except the Pale and Gaelic Ireland, consisted of the quasi-independent fiefs of the great Norman-Irish lords, who gradually adopted the Gaelic language and culture, and assimilated into Gaelic society. These Norman-Irish lords remained fundamentally loyal to the Crown, but had no interest in becoming part of a feudal monarchy that would strip them of power.

The Norman-Irish lords resisted strong centralized government and benefited when John I was forced to sign the Magna Carta in 1215, incorporating the barons' demands for increased power. The Magna Carta was extended to Norman-Irish lords in 1217. Thereafter, the barons reorganized themselves from a mere advisory body into the Parliament, and over the next 425 years seldom missed an opportunity to grab power away from the Crown, eventually leading to the demise of classic feudalism.

The Norman expansion throughout Ireland slowed in the late 1200s as a result of two major battles, Callann, in 1261 and Ath an Kip in 1270. .

At Callann, the MacCarthys, confined to the south-west corner of Ireland, confronted FitzThomas and the Normans in the mountainous country near Kenmare and defeated them. This stopped the Norman-Irish expansion southward from the upper half of Kerry, and let MacCarthys and O'Sullivans reigned supreme in the south-west corner of Ireland.

At Ath an Kip, to the north, Aedh O'Connor and his Gaelic-Irish fought the Normans under Walter de Burgo, who were expanding their control even further into Ulster, and stopped them. O'Connor had brought in from Scotland, "gallowglasses", professional Norse-Gaelic soldiers, to supplement his own army.

Within a few generations, descendants of the original Normans gradually distanced themselves from the Norman-Anglo way of life and adopted the Gaelic language, dress and culture, becoming so thoroughly assimilated into Gaelic society that they were commonly described as "more Irish than the Irish".

Among these were the Redmonds. As Warre Wells notes:

"Redmonds have for many centuries played an unstained part in the history of the County Wexford and South-Eastern Ireland. They have included landlords and peasants, rebels and officers of the British army, priests and merchants. We may be sure, moreover, that the Redmonds, whatever their origin, did not lack the Gaelic admixture. All the early English settlers in Ireland intermarried with the native population and its descendants. After the Reformation divisions became more acute and intermarriage less frequent; but some of the old English families retained the ancient faith and finally were merged into the Irish nation." (341)

He continues on to note references to the Redmonds in various histories.

"O'Hara in his book on *Irish Families* states that the Redmonds of Ballaghkeene in Wexford had a common ancestor with the noble Geraldines (Dukes of Leinster); this family died out in 1689. Another well-known family of the Redmonds, also extinct, was from Fethard...
Burke's *Landed Gentry* an account of a third family of Redmonds from the same county of Wexford – the Redmonds of the Deeps. Their founder was Edward Redmond, a merchant who flourished in Wexford at the alter end of the eighteenth century." (342)

In the mid-1300s, three extraordinary Norman-Irish earldoms emerged: Desmond and Kildare (each headed by a branch of the Fitzgeralds) and Ormond (headed by the Butlers). These and other Norman-Irish lords were even more secure than English barons in challenging the Crown, because English monarchs never were able to devote to Ireland the resources and attention required to maintain control.

During and after the War of Roses between the English Houses of York and Lancaster, until 1494, governance of Ireland fell largely into the hands of Norman-Irish lords who were considered relatively loyal to the Crown. Initially it was the Fitzgeralds of Desmond, but after 1468, governance fell to the Fitzgeralds of Kildare, whose tenure was called the "Kildare Supremacy". For almost 40 years, the eighth Earl of

Kildare (the "Great Earl") functioned as the uncrowned King of Ireland. He was succeeded by his son, Garrett Og.

Troubles then came with the five monarchs of the 118 year Tudor Dynasty in England, from 1486 to 1603.

Henry VII forced the Irish parliament to adopt Poynings's Law (1494). This law, which was prompted by Ireland's support of the Yorkist side in the Wars of the Roses, gave the English Privy Council a veto over legislation proposed in future Irish parliaments.

Henry VII's son, Henry VIII, was worse. After he split with Rome and set himself up as the head of the church, he summoned Garrett Og, the Earl of Kildare, to England for negotiations intended to expand the Crown's control in Ireland, while curtailing the "Kildare Supremacy". While the Earl was in England, his son, Thomas Fitzgerald, invaded the Dublin Parliament, surrendered the sword of state and announced his independence from Henry. Henry responded by imprisoning Garrett Og in the Tower of London and dispatched an army to Ireland. Henry's army introduced cannons to Ireland and quickly forced Kildare's forces at Maynooth to surrender, after which they were executed. The murders of Thomas and his five brothers terminated the "Kildare Supremacy". Thereafter, no English monarch ever appointed an Irishman as his chief deputy in Ireland. In 1541, Henry declared himself the King of Ireland.

In 1537, the Irish Parliament declared the Anglican religion to be the official religion of the Church of Ireland. Anglicism also became a part of the "English culture" that Henry was forcibly imposing on Ireland. But this complicated the task enormously because there was virtually no indigenous sympathy for "reform" among either the Gaelic-Irish or the Norman-Irish, who remained totally committed to the Pope.

The next ruler, Mary I (r. 1553-58), as a Catholic, officially restored the Catholic religion.

Mary was succeeded by her sister Elizabeth I (r. 1558-1603) who reigned for 43 years, and proved to be one of Ireland's most brutal oppressors.

She crushed all challenges to her authoritarian power. This led to disputes over land and religion in Ireland. Year after year over a great part of Ireland, all means of human subsistence were destroyed, no quarter was given to prisoners who surrendered, and the whole population was skillfully and steadily starved to death.

The Norman-Irish lords generally were intimidated by Elizabeth's "scorched earth" tactics, and reluctantly accepted the "surrender and re-grant" offer first offered by Henry VIII. In Ulster, however, the Gaelic chieftains rejected the feudal land system, the English language, and any other part of Elizabeth's Anglicization program. In 1595, Led by Hugh O'Neill (1550-1615), 2d earl of Tyrone, and his young ally, Red Hugh O'Donnell (1571-1602), they mounted a major rebellion. After some successes, O'Neill was defeated.

O'Neill submitted pursuant to the Treaty of Mellifont on March 1603, six days after the death of Elizabeth, who is credited with completing the re-conquest of Ireland. James I, her successor, pardoned them, but only on condition they accept the "surrender and regrant" program.

The celebrated "Flight of the Earls" occurred four years later. Dissatisfied with their new roles, and still fearing retaliation, O'Neill and virtually the entire remaining Gaelic leadership, 99 leaders in all, secretly boarded a ship at night at Loch Swilley and sailed for the Continent, never to return. The date was September 14, 1607. (343)

The Battle of Kinsale, along with the "Flight of the Earls", marked the end of the old Gaelic order, and established England as conqueror of Ireland. What followed next -- the 17th Century "Plantations" -- were perhaps the most important development in Irish history since arrival of the

185

Celts. They divided Ireland apartheid-like into two hostile camps.

Under these Plantations -- the Ulster Plantation (1609), the Cromwellian Plantation (1652) and the Williamite Plantation (1693) -- 81% of the productive land in Ireland was confiscated from the native Irish (Gaelic-Irish and Norman-Irish alike, but invariably Catholic), and transferred to new immigrants (invariably Protestant) from Scotland and England. The Plantations impacted Ireland in two major ways. First, they introduced into Ireland a new community, eventually 25% of the populace, which differed radically from the natives not only in religion, but also in culture, ethnicity, and national identity. Second, in Ireland's overwhelmingly agrarian economy -- where land equaled wealth and power (and vice versa) -- the Plantations caused a massive transfer of wealth and power to non-native landlords, whose backbreaking rents then thrust 85% of the natives into crushing poverty and degradation. The Plantations are the root cause of the class warfare between rich landlord and poor tenant and religious/cultural clashes that have plagued Ireland since 1610.

The Plantations devastated peasants, who suffered the loss of their property rights under the ancient Gaelic law of gravelkind, which previously had virtually guaranteed them a decent living from the soil. Peasants were allowed to remain as farm laborers or tenant-farmers, but at low wages or backbreaking rents that thrust them into abject poverty.

The first 17th Century plantation, the Ulster Plantation, involved confiscation of three million acres (about 30% of the island), all in six counties in west and central Ulster. The Ulster confiscations were directed almost exclusively at the Gaelic lords and their supporters who had been defeated at Kinsale: O'Neill, O'Donnell, O'Reilly, O'Hanlon, O'Doherty and others. The official plantation indirectly encouraged the much heavier unsponsored migration of working class

Presbyterians from Scotland to Counties Down and Antrim. These migrations permitted eviction of native Catholics in favor of new Presbyterian settlers, whose descendants remain dominant in Northern Ireland even today.

The Norman-Irish lords were largely unaffected by the Ulster Plantation; but soon, on a large scale, they found themselves victims of English confiscation of land based on defects in land titles. Charles I (1625-49) came to an agreement with the lords which confirming title in any person who had possessed land for 60 years or more. This was called The Graces. But after accepting cash from the lords, Charles yielded to pressure from Parliament and reneged on formalizing "the Graces". This led to the rebellion of 1641.

Sir Phelim O'Neill led the Rebellion of 1641, which began with skirmishing in Ulster, during which as many as 12,000 Protestant non-combatants were killed. The rising actually was rooted in disputes over land and to a lesser extent over religion, but O'Neill insisted that his forces were simply supporting the King against a belligerent Parliament. This pressured the Norman-Irish lords, who had Royalist leanings, to join O'Neill's Gaelic forces in an uneasy alliance, the "Kilkenny Confederation". The rebels mounted a seven year insurgency which, if all had gone smoothly, might have led to a permanent accommodation with a divided England. In fact, however, the principal effect of the rebellion was to trigger the English Civil War, in which the king and parliament finally went to war with each other. Parliament's army, led by Oliver Cromwell, a Congregationalist member of Parliament, defeated Charles in a two phase war. Following a trial, Charles I was beheaded in 1649 and the monarchy was abolished.

That same year, Cromwell brought his army to Ireland and quashed the rebellion with a savagery that has become legendary. After the town of Drogheda had surrendered,

Cromwell's troops massacred 3,500 residents, including unarmed women and children. At Wexford, he perpetrated a similar massacre. The rebellion was soon over.

Cromwell and his Puritans spelled disaster for all Catholics, but particularly for the Norman-Irish. Puritans were virulently anti-Catholic and England's traditional tolerance for the Norman Irish quickly became extinct, with both communities now treated as Catholic enemies of England. It was during the Cromwellian era (1649-60) that anti-Catholic animus reached its highest level in Irish history.

The Cromwellian Plantation followed the war. It was the largest and most acrimonious of the confiscations, reducing Catholic ownership of land from 59% to 22% The Cromwellian Plantation took land largely from the Norman-Irish lords, who had joined the rebellion hesitantly and only to show their support for the king, and transferred the land to Cromwell's soldiers and to investors in the war effort.

Among the many that lost their lands at this time were some Redmonds who fought against Cromwell. (344)

By the mid-1660s, the Cromwellian and Ulster Plantations had created a huge landlord class, including the oft-vilified absentee landlords, whose rental income often permitted them to lead lives of leisure, while backbreaking rents had thrust the native Irish into abject poverty, with 85% of the populace living at subsistence level

In 1688-90, the Gaelic-Irish and Norman-Irish Catholics arose in rebellion again when they took sides in a war between two claimants to the English Crown. They supported the hereditary and rightful claimant, James II, against the man who had deposed him, William of Orange. In England, James was seen as representing both Royalists and Catholics, while William represented the Parliamentarian and Protestant factions.

James II converted to Catholicism in 1671, and implemented a series of measures designed to increase the power of the

Crown and to increase the civil rights of Catholics. James recruited a predominantly Catholic army in Ireland, and transferred part of it to England. When a son was born to James in 1688, thereby insuring a Catholic succession, a plot known as the "Glorious Revolution" was hatched to overthrow James II.

James' grand-daughter Mary, and her Dutch Protestant husband, William of Orange, accepted the invitation of several English notables to invade England, to overthrow James and to accede to the throne. When William arrived in England in November 1688, his partisans arose in rebellion in Yorkshire and elsewhere. Meanwhile James' forces deserted, and James himself fled to France. The coup d' etat was bloodless. In 1689, William and Mary were declared joint sovereigns, William III and Mary II. James II had been ousted after only four years.

But James' Catholic army in Ireland remained intact; and in an effort to regain his rightful throne, James promptly began recruiting new Irish and French troops from his exile in France. He promised the Irish that if his war was successful, they would recover their lands and power.

In the first battle, James sent Catholic troops to Derry. Locals resisted and, after a lengthy siege, William's troops arrived to relieve the inhabitants. The Protestants in Derry called themselves the Apprentice Boys. The celebration of a day in their honour is still a major Protestant holiday in Northern Ireland.

In March 1689, James arrived in Ireland to take charge of his army of 25,000. He also presided over a new and largely Catholic Parliament, which voted to overturn the earlier plantations. In June 1690, William of Orange and his army of 36,000 troops attacked.

At the Battle of the Boyne, on July 1, 1690, William's army defeated James' forces. In military terms, it was not a decisive victory, since Irish losses were small and their army lived to fight another day. But James immediately fled back to France.

Under Patrick Sarsfield, the Irish continued the fight for more than a year before suffering a devastating defeat at Aughrim. Finally, Sarsfield negotiated an honorable surrender embodied in the Treaty of Limerick (1691). The treaty allowed Catholics to retain the same religious liberty enjoyed under Charles II, and allowed those who took an Oath of Allegiance, to be pardoned and to keep their property, practice professions and bear civilian arms. The British refused to extend this to the entire Catholic population, thereby facilitating the enactment of anti-Catholic Penal laws, over the objection of King William.

The Treaty also required Sarsfield and more than 10,000 Irish troops to leave Ireland for the Continent. They did so -- the celebrated "flight of the 'Wild Geese'" -- and became legendary soldiers in the armies of France and other continental powers.

There ensued the third and final wave of 17th Century plantations, the Williamite Plantation, which reduced Catholic ownership of land from 22% to 14%.

Almost immediately after the Treaty of Limerick (1691), Anglicans took decisive action to further strengthen their dominant position. Notwithstanding the Treaty, the Irish and English Parliaments, both dominated by Anglicans, enacted a series of "Penal Laws" which, apartheid-like, created a three tier, Anglican controlled society in which (1) Catholics (75% of the population) would be totally excluded from property and power, and (2) Presbyterians (15% of the population) would remain subordinate to Anglicans.

Catholics and Presbyterians alike were required to tithe to the Anglican Church of Ireland, but were officially barred from government employment and military commissions. Catholics alone were barred from elective office, from entering the legal profession, from bearing arms, and from

190

owning a horse worth more than five pounds. Upon the death of a Catholic landlord, his property by law went to his sons in equal shares, unless one of them converted to Anglicanism, in which case the Anglican son received the entire property, along with the right to immediately wrest management from his parents. Catholics were prohibited from purchasing realty, except leases of less than 31 years. Between 1701 and 1778 Catholic ownership of land further declined from 14% to 5%. Catholics were barred from educating their children, except in schools proselytizing for the Anglican religion. Catholic bishops were banned from Ireland, under penalty of death by hanging, disemboweling and quartering. The last of the Penal Laws, enacted in 1727, denied Catholics the right to vote.

In enacting the Penal Laws, the Parliament of England was motivated almost entirely by anti-Catholic animus, but the Parliament of Ireland had additional motivation: preserving the privileged position of the New English "haves" viz-a-viz the native "have nots". Except for the Cromwellian era (1649-60), the period 1692-1740 was the most anti-Catholic in Irish history.

The vast majority of Catholics lived and worked on the land in abject poverty, degradation and despair, with no way out. Their diet consisted almost entirely of the newly introduced potato, plus milk with a herring once or twice a year. Shelter, if any, was a mud hovel with leaky roof and no windows or chimney. Even Catholics who labored full time lived in worse degradation than the poorest beggars elsewhere in Europe. A handful of Catholics achieved middle class prosperity in business -- and their numbers grew as time went by -- but they were exceptions. In terms of compliance with law, Catholics were made criminals under the Penal Laws because they refused to turn in their "illegal" priests, and the draconian injustice of these laws engendered in them a culture of disrespect for the law generally.

Presbyterians congregated in Ulster, where typically they adhered to the culture and religion brought over from Scotland by their ancestors. Close knit and industrious, they responded to discrimination by distancing themselves from Ascendancy culture, becoming a self-reliant community within the larger society. The typical Presbyterian pursued a middle class livelihood in the linen business or in farming.

Anglicans and Presbyterians soon found themselves in serious conflict. The principal problem was that the "established" Church of Ireland, and its Anglican members, treated the Presbyterian Religion as a second class religion, and its members (who generally were less affluent than Anglicans) as second class citizens. Although Presbyterians were treated far better than Catholics -- there were no restrictions on the right to own realty or to bear arms -- they were required to tithe to the Anglican Church of Ireland, and were prohibited from holding government office or military commissions.

The British treated Ireland as a subservient colony, useful primarily for enhancing the prosperity of England. British trade legislation, which typically discriminated against Ireland, was particularly grating. For example, in order to protect English manufacturers, the English Parliament prohibited the export of Irish woolen goods to any country except England, where prohibitive duties made such trade unprofitable. This legislation literally destroyed the Irish woolen industry, to the dismay of merchants of all religions.

In the 1760s, the "Patriot" movement led by Henry Gratton, an affluent and pro-business Anglican, professing loyalty to the King but demanding greater autonomy for Ireland plus concessions to Catholics, emerged as an influential minority in the Irish Parliament. As a result of Gratton's advocacy, a few of the Penal Laws were repealed in the 1770s.

The American Revolution in 1776, led to the formation of the "Irish Volunteers", a militia, consisting almost entirely of

192

well-armed Anglicans, which ostensibly was formed to defend Ireland but which was used adroitly by Gratton to intimidate the British government.

After the American revolution, in which many Irish and Scottish émigrés had fought on the American side, England amended various laws, including Poynings's Law, to give the Irish Parliament full legislative independence, including the right to enact its own trade and tariff policies. This led to an independent Bank of Ireland, a separate Irish postal service, and new government buildings including the Custom House and the Four Courts.

However, independence for Parliament did nothing for the lower and middle classes, Presbyterian or Catholic. Thus Catholics and less affluent Presbyterians, who together made up 90% of the population, found themselves on the same side of the major issues of the day: land reform, Parliamentary reform, elimination of the tithe, and repeal of those penal laws affecting both.

In 1789, the French Revolution ignited existing tensions and pushed Ireland toward similar violent revolution.

Theobald Wolf Tone, an Anglican of modest social standing and the founder of radical republicanism in Ireland, was profoundly influenced by the French Revolution. He demanded parliamentary reform, specifically, a popularly elected one-man-one-vote legislature. To achieve this, he fostered an alliance between Catholics and less affluent Presbyterians. Ultimately, Tone's vision for Ireland was a democratic republic, patterned after the post-revolutionary French Republic. In 1791, with the assistance of Napper Tandy, Tone founded the Society of United Irishmen, peacefully advocating Protestant-Catholic cooperation to achieve parliamentary reform and Catholic emancipation. United Irishmen quickly gained wide support from Ulster Presbyterians, and modest support from some Catholics.

The post-revolution French government declared war on England in 1793. Hoping to secure the loyalty of rebellious Catholics, the British government pressured the reluctant Irish Parliament to repeal some penal laws and to grant Catholics the right to vote.

About 1794, Tone converted from advocate of peaceful Parliamentary reform to violent revolutionary. About the same time, the United Irishmen became a para-military force. In 1796, Tone convinced France to invade Ireland as part of its war effort against England. A French fleet carrying 14,000 troops set sail for Ireland. However, bad weather prevented a landing, and the fleet returned to France.

In 1798, Tone and the United Irishmen again persuaded France to invade Ireland. The plan included coordination of the French invasion with a series of local rebellions. The insurrection in Ulster, led by Henry Joy McCracken, was almost entirely Presbyterian, while the ones in Dublin, Kildare, Carlow, Meath and Queens were nonsectarian.

The rebellion in Wexford was one of the bloodiest confrontations in Irish history. Wexford was an unlikely prospect for insurrection -- no more than 300 United Irishmen and Defenders were operating there -- but violence erupted when Protestant Volunteers, directed to enforce the disarmament order, began flogging Catholics and burning their homes even before the date specified for surrendering arms. Then a Catholic killed a soldier who had burned a barn, and government forces retaliated by burning down another 160 houses. Fully believing that a massacre of Catholics was imminent, Catholics rebelled. Led by Father John Murphy, and armed with little more than pikes against government forces with muskets, the rebels initially took Enniscorthy, then sought to expand into Wicklow. Mass atrocities occurred on both sides. In the end, in 1798, the rebels were routed at Vinegar Hill.

Among those who were accused of participating in the rebellion of 1798 was Father John Redmond. He was a friend of Lord Mount Norris, who had a connection with the United Irishmen. Norrie, in order to divert suspicion from himself, brought charges against the priest, which led to the latter's execution.

John Redmond, who later led the Irish Party, said he had been fascinated by the rebellion of 1798 and added

"I scarcely know a family which cannot tell of a father, or grandfather or some other near relative, who died fighting at Wexford, Oulart, or Ross". (345)

Despite the effective suppression of the local risings, England's Prime Minister, William Pitt, worried about Irish unrest, sponsored an Act of Union, the merger of England and Ireland into a single Parliament. In 1800 the "Act of Union" passed the all-Protestant Irish Parliament, and was quickly ratified by the English Parliament. It refused to emancipate Catholics.

In the early 1800s, Daniel O'Connell (1775-1847), a Catholic advocate of non-violent and lawful political action, emerged as the sole leader of the great masses of peasant and middle class Catholics, who comprised the vast majority of the Irish population.

He pushed for emancipation, which would allow Catholics, to serve in Parliament.

To increase Catholic pressure, he founded the "Catholic Association". The Catholic Association aimed for, and actually attained, grass roots mass membership. It used parish priests to solicit members, and most important of all, it charged a membership fee of one penny per month, which became known as "catholic rent." The amount was so low that even the poorest could afford it, but for their penny, the masses soon came to believe in the association as an empowering institution in which they had a genuine stake.

In the general elections of 1826, as the result of an impressive get-out-the-vote drive funded by Catholic rents and supported by many priests, four sitting anti-emancipation members of Parliament were turned out and replaced by pro-emancipation Protestants. In 1828, O'Connell won a seat, forcing parliament, in 1829, to pass legislation that granted Catholic Emancipation and repealed virtually all of the remaining Penal Laws.

In 1837, O'Connell launched his second great campaign - to repeal the Act of Union of 1800.

Before it succeeded, Ireland suffered the potato famine. A fungus totally ravaged the potato crop in 1845, 1846 and 1848, and partially ravaged it in 1847. Government indifference devastated the Irish people of 1845-49. Throughout this entire four year period of starvation, Ireland was exporting enormous quantities of food. Indeed, up to 75% of the soil was devoted to wheat, oats, barley and other crops which were grown for export, and which were actually exported, all while the populace starved.

The problem was that about half the population -- all wretchedly poor -- worked on farms not for cash wages, but for the right to grow potatoes on tiny plots. They lived on a subsistence diet consisting almost exclusively of potatoes and milk, with a herring once or twice a year. When the potato crop failed, these peasants had neither food for their families, nor cash to buy other food. Initially, only the poor died, victims of starvation. Then as typically happens in conditions of starvation, epidemics of typhus and cholera broke out, felling the affluent along with the poor. In total, about one million died.

Finally, with the 1849 harvest, the potato blight and the famine were over.

After the devastating famine, lower and middle class Irish-Catholics understandably became obsessed with mere survival. They also became bitterly divided over the merits of peaceful politics.

Adherents of Wolf Tone who called themselves "Republicans", advocated an Irish Republic totally separate and independent from England, to be achieved by any means required, including physical force. James Stephens, a Protestant, reorganized Young Ireland into the "Fenian" movement in 1858, with one branch in Ireland, called the Irish Republican Brotherhood, or "IRB" and another in the United States, called the Fenian Brotherhood, later Clan na Gael. The Fenian strategy was to prepare secretly for an armed rebellion to be launched when Britain found itself in a debilitating war or otherwise vulnerable. They sponsored uprisings in 1865 and 1867 in Ireland. In response, England, in 1869, abolished the tithe and repealed the laws that established the Anglican Church as the official church of Ireland.

In the Americas, they initiated attacks against the Canadian colonies in 1866. This pushed Britain to amalgamate the colonies and create the Confederation of Canada.

The Irish continued to press for agricultural land reform. Michael Davitt made it his overriding issue. In 1879, he founded the National Land League, which was not above using intimidation and threats of violence to achieve their ends. They allied with Charles Stewart Parnell (1846-1891), who was elected to the British Parliament in 1875. In 1880, with massive grass roots assistance from Davitt's Land League, a slate of Parnell supporters was elected to Parliament, and Parnell supplanted Isaac Butt as chairman of the Irish party.

The Davitt-Parnell alliance paid dividends almost immediately. Prodded by Parnell, Gladstone and his Liberal government successfully pushed through the Land Act of 1881, which gave fair rents, fixity of tenure and freedom of sale.

Parnell then pushed for Home Rule. However, the House of Lords opposed it and he died before it came to fruition. John Redmond then took over as leader of the Irish party. He remained leader until his death in 1918.

He pushed the English government to spend large amounts of money in Ireland on two new colleges, plus public works projects such as a railroad to western Ireland. Most importantly, the English parliament, in 1903, passed the final piece of comprehensive land reform, the Wyndham Land Act, which permitted tenants to purchase their farms on easy terms over 68 years.

In 1905 Sinn Fein ("we ourselves") was formed by Arthur Griffith (1872-1922). Sinn Fein was primarily an Irish nationalist movement, but it also functioned as a political party. Under Griffith's direction, it advocated a dual monarchy along Austro-Hungarian lines, all to be achieved by passive resistance rather than physical force. Meanwhile, the Irish Republican Brotherhood (IRB) was infiltrating the nationalist and separatist groups, including Sinn Fein, still waiting for the opportunity to foment rebellion if England should find itself in a debilitating war.

In 1910, when neither the Liberal Party nor the Tories won enough seats to form a government without votes from Redmond's Irish party. A deal was struck. Redmond's Irish party cast their votes in favor of the Liberal, Herbert Asquith, for Prime Minister, and he then was able to form a coalition government. In turn, the new government agreed to force through Parliament a bill giving Ireland a separate Home Rule Parliament in Dublin with relatively modest powers over local issues.

Since the electorate was 75% Catholic, the proposed Home Rule Parliament naturally would be dominated by Catholics. Irish Protestants opposed Home Rule, and demanded the separation of Ulster through partition. Then Ulster unionists, to protect against legislative failure, formed an armed paramilitary group, the Ulster Volunteers, to wage war against the proposed new government unless it excluded Ulster. Naturally, supporters of Home Rule -- with the IRB playing a major role -- formed their own paramilitary group, the Irish Volunteers, to counteract the Ulster Volunteers. Ireland seemed to be drifting towards civil war, and Redmond came under increasing pressure to agree to the exclusion of Ulster from Home Rule.

World War I broke out in August 1914, and Home rule was postponed. Home Rule supporters began to demand full or nearly full independence, rather than the limited autonomy provided in the 1914 legislation. The IRB leadership, including Padraic Pearse, Joseph Plunkett and Eamon Ceannt, decided to mount an armed insurrection, even though it might be doomed to failure.

The Rising began on Easter Monday, April 24, 1916, in Dublin. Proclaiming the existence of an Irish Republic, the rebels, 1600 strong, seized and held a number of public buildings, including the General Post Office on Sackville Street, which became command headquarters. The British retaliated. The fighting lasted five days, during which British forces suffered about 500 casualties, including 112 dead. The rebels surrendered on April 29.

The population supported the rebels and in the 1918 election, Sinn Fein won most seats. They met in Dublin and passed a Declaration of Independence and "ratified" the Republic that had originally been proclaimed at the Easter Rising in 1916. They declared themselves to be the Dail Eireann, and passed resolutions declaring that the Dail Eireann had the exclusive power to make laws binding on the Irish people, and that the British Parliament had no jurisdiction over Ireland. They demanded that England evacuate the whole of Ireland. They established Republican courts, which subsequently gained the confidence of the citizenry. The Dail then elected a government, with Eamon de Valera as President and Griffith as Vice President. Collins was appointed Minister of Finance, as well as Commander of the Irish Republican Army (IRA), the name given to the new government's militia, which consisted of former members of the Irish Volunteers.

Following the Dail's 1919 session, guerilla warfare erupted between the IRA, the militia of the new government, about 15,000 troops strong, under Michael Collins and special British forces known as the "Auxiliaries" and the "Black and Tan".

After numerous atrocities, including Bloody Sunday, the British government, responded by enacting the 1920 Government of Ireland Act, establishing separate parliaments for "Northern Ireland" and "Southern Ireland", each with extensive home rule powers. Northern Ireland quickly accepted the legislation, and began a series of brutal pogroms against Catholics.

After months of bitter debate, on January 7, 1922, the treaty passed the Dail on a close vote (64-57), and a provisional "Free State" government was formed to implement the treaty. An election was held. A government that accepted the treaty won the election. The IRA responded by declaring war on the government. The new government's army overwhelmed the IRA and the civil war ended. The Ireland that we now know came into existence, with one free state and with Ulster united within the United Kingdom.

Chapter 11

Emigration around the World

During the centuries of persecution, many Irish left their homeland. This latest Celtic dispersion led to the Irish settling over much of the world during a five hundred year period.
Our ancestors, the Redmonds, were among those who left Ireland in favour of freedom and a better life elsewhere.
So let us now briefly review some of these dispersions.

Europe

The European mainland became a popular destination for Irish fleeing persecution from 1500 to 1900. One of the earliest great waves of emigrants took place with the Flight of the Earls, in 1607, in which many of the Gaelic nobility fled. They went through France and on to Spain. Tadhg O'Cianain, who described their journey in his book *The Flight of the Earls*, in 1609, noted the kindness with which they were met by the French and Spanish, and the animosity of the English diplomats who kept trying to harass them. (346)
Many others followed in their footsteps. One particularly notable group consisted of some 10,000 Irish soldiers who went to the mainland after their defeat by William of Orange in 1690.
Many emigrants went to France, as a common Catholic faith had fostered close ties over the centuries. In this new land, some of the lords and their descendants became well known. One was the French royalist Patrice de Mac-Mahon, who became president of France. Some became military leaders. Among these was a Redmond who became an officer in the regiment of the Chevalier de Dillon in the wars of Louis

XIV. (347) The French Cognac brandy maker, James Hennessy and Co., is named for an Irishman. (348)
After the rebellion of 1797, more Irish went to France. Some joined the army of Napoleon. Among these were some Redmonds and Lyons. After the defeat of Napoleon, some of these men and their families left France for Canada. One, who settled in Frampton, where our ancestors also settled, was Cornelius Lyons. He had fought with Napoleon's army in many battles, including Waterloo. After the defeat of Napoleon, he returned to Ireland, only to find a price on his head. He gathered his family secretly, and then left for Canada. He settled in St. Malachie, near Frampton, in 1823. (349)
Another popular destination for emigrants was Spain, also an ally with a common faith. The Irish were known to have been serving in the Spanish army since at least 1586. Some 40,000 Irish were serving in the regiments of Spain by the year 1650, growing to 120,000 in later years. (350) In Spain and its territories, many Irish descendants can be found with the name Obregón (O'Brien, Irish, Ó Briain), including Madrid-born actress Ana Victoria García Obregón.
From Spain, many moved on to the South American colonies. There some rose to prominent positions in the colonial governments. In the nineteenth century, some helped to liberate the continent.
Bernardo O'Higgins was the first Supreme director of Chile. When Chilean troops occupied Lima during the War of the Pacific in 1881, they put in charge Patricio Lynch, whose grandfather came from Ireland to Argentina and then moved to Chile. (351)
Among those who went to Argentina, perhaps the most famous was William Brown. Creator of the Argentine Navy (Armada de la República Argentina, ARA) and leader of the Argentine Armed Forces in the wars against Brazil and Spain, he was born in Foxford, County Mayo on June 22,

1777 and died in Buenos Aires in 1857. The Almirante Brown-class destroyer is named after him, as well as the Almirante Brown partido, part of the Gran Buenos Aires urban area, with a population of over 500.000 inhabitants.

Cuba was the destination for some. One famous descendant of these immigrants was Che Guevara, whose grandmother's surname was Lynch. Guevara's father, Ernesto Guevara Lynch, said of him: "The first thing to note is that in my son's veins flowed the blood of the Irish rebels".

In Mexico, Irish settlers also became involved in politics and helped to liberate the people from their European overlords. Among these was William Lamport, formerly of Wexford, better known to most Mexicans as Guillen de Lampart, precursor of the Independence movement and author of the first proclamation of independence in the New World. His statue stands today in the Crypt of Heroes beneath the Column of Independence in Mexico City. Some authorities claim he was the inspiration for Johnston McCulley's Zorro.

After Lampart, the most famous Irishmen in Mexican history are probably "Los Patricios". They were Irish who lived in Mexican Texas until the revolution there, when they sided with Catholic Mexico against Protestant pro-U.S. elements. They included the Batallón de San Patricio, a battalion of U.S. troops who deserted and fought alongside the Mexican Army against the United States in the Mexican-American War of 1846 to 1848. Finally, Álvaro Obregón (possibly O'Brian) was president of Mexico during 1920-24 and Obregón city and airport are named in his honour.

Indentured Labour and Slavery in the Americas

Undoubtedly the least pleasant of the stories of emigration are those of the Irish who left their homelands as slaves or indentured labourers. (352)

The Proclamation of 1625 ordered that Irish political prisoners be transported overseas and sold as laborers to English planters, who were settling the islands of the West Indies, officially establishing a policy that was to continue for two centuries. In 1629 a large group of Irish men and women were sent to Guiana, and by 1632, Irish were the main slaves sold to Antigua and Montserrat in the West Indies. By 1637 a census showed that 69% of the total population of Montserrat were Irish slaves. As there were not enough political prisoners to supply the demand, every petty infraction carried a sentence of transporting, and slaver gangs combed the country sides to kidnap enough people to fill out their quotas.

From 1641 to 1653, during Cromwell's wars, some 300,000 Irish were sold as slaves. Most were sent to British plantations in Barbados and other lands. In 1650, for example, 25,000 were sold to planters in St.Kitts. In 1652, 12,000 were sold to planters in Barbados.

Others were transported to Virginia and New England.

One report of 1651 noted that slaves were sold in Barbados for 900 pounds of cotton each

Following the Battle of the Boyne and the defeat of King James in 1691, Irish prisoners were sold as slaves.

Even as late as the 1798 rebellion, Irish prisoners were being sold as slaves in the Colonies and Australia.

The Irish did not accept enslavement readily. Rebellions took place against the British. One in 1649 in Barbados was savagely suppressed. Those who could, fled to the American mainland. For example, many Barbadian born Irish helped establish the Carolina colony. Those shipped initially to Virginia and other mainland colonies, often fled westward to Appalachia and other free areas.

Indeed, it was the difficulty encountered in keeping Irish indentured and slave labour that led planters to prefer slaves from Africa.

Newfoundland

The first recorded Irish presence in present day Canada dates from 1536, when Irish fishermen from Cork travelled to Newfoundland. (352)

Seven English colonies were established by royal charter in Newfoundland between 1610 and 1628, and London-based mercantile companies used Celtic-speaking peasants to settle each one. Many of the early Irish came as servants or indentured labourers. Many came from Waterford and Wexford, which had developed ties with Newfoundland through fishing. Others were from Wales. In 1776, three to five thousand were reported to be leaving annually from these areas on Newfoundland ships, and by 1784 seven-eighths of the population of St John's, Newfoundland, were Irish-born.

The Irish language was commonly spoken in rural areas until the mid-20th century. There is evidence to suggest that as many as 90% of the Irish immigrants to Newfoundland in the 17th and 18th centuries only spoke Irish

Many lived hard lives, receiving little if any pay for the labour they provided to the companies that controlled the fishing industry.

United States

During the 1700s, there was considerable emigration to the American colonies, particularly among the Protestant Scots-Irish, who suffered religious persecution and economic oppression from the Anglicans in Ireland and Scotland. Emigration offered almost a biblical deliverance for them. (354)

Most of the early immigration from Ireland was from Ulster, after the creation of the Ulster Plantation. From 1710 to 1775, over 200,000 people emigrated from Ulster to the 13

Colonies, from Maine to Georgia. The largest numbers went to Pennsylvania. From that base some went south into Virginia, the Carolinas and across the South, with a large concentration in the Appalachian region; others headed west to western Pennsylvania, Ohio, Indiana, and the Midwest.

As a result of the trade between the American colonies and such southern ports as Cork and Kinsale, Catholic Irish immigrated to the new colonies, particularly to Virginia and Maryland, where such names as "New Ireland" and "New Munster" appear.

According to the Dictionary of American History, approximately "50,000 to 100,000 Irishmen, over 75 percent of them Catholic, came to America in the 1600s, while 100,000 more Irish Catholics arrived in the 1700s." Indentured servitude was an especially common way of affording migration, and in the 1740s the Irish made up nine out of ten indentured servants in some colonial regions.

Irish immigrants of this period participated in significant numbers in the American Revolution. The Scotch-Irish were generally ardent supporters of American Independence from Britain in the 1770s. In Pennsylvania, Virginia, and most of the Carolinas, support for the revolution was practically unanimous.

One British major general testified at the House of Commons that "half the rebel Continental Army were from Ireland." One Hessian officer said, "Call this war by whatever name you may, only call it not an American rebellion; it is nothing more or less than a Scotch Irish Presbyterian rebellion."

Mecklenburg County, North Carolina, with its large Scotch-Irish population, was to make the first declaration for independence from Britain in the Mecklenburg Declaration of 1775.

The Scotch-Irish "Overmountain Men" of Virginia and North Carolina formed a militia which won the Battle of Kings Mountain in 1780, resulting in the British abandonment of a southern campaign, and for some historians "marked the turning point of the American Revolution".

Among the many Irish whose deeds are recorded in archives of the revolution was a Mary Redmond of Philadelphia, who spied on the British for Washington's forces, thereby facilitating General Burgoyne's loss in battle and surrender. (355)

So the Scots and Irish, who were being driven from their lands by the British, repaid the British oppressors by becoming the backbone of the armies that liberated the American colonies from British rule.

Indeed, the United States Declaration of Independence contained fifty-six delegate signatures. Of the signers, eight were of Irish descent. Three signers, Matthew Thornton, George Taylor and James Smith were born in Ulster, the remaining five Irish Americans were the sons or grandsons of Irish immigrants: George Read, Thomas McKean, Thomas Lynch, Jr., Edward Rutledge and Charles Carroll, and at least McKean had Ulster heritage. The Carrolls and Fitzsimmons were Catholic, the remainder of Protestant denominations.

After the American revolution, immigration from Ireland grew. Between 1783 and 1812 a total of 100,000 arriving in America. According to the Harvard Encyclopedia of American Ethnic Groups, there were 400,000 U.S. residents of Irish birth or ancestry in 1790 and half of this group was descended from Ulster, and half from the other provinces of Ireland. (356)

By that point few were young servants and more were mature craftsmen. They settled in industrial centers, including Pittsburgh, Philadelphia and New York, where many became skilled workers, foremen and entrepreneurs as the Industrial Revolution took off in the U.S.

In the war of 1812, the Irish joined the Americans in a war to conquer Britain's Canadian colonies. Among those who fought was the grandfather of Charles Stewart Parnell, whom we have discussed above.

With the end of the Napoleonic wars, emigration to the Americas increased. A half million came to American 1815 to 1845; another 900,000 came in 1851-99.

Because British legislation discriminated against United States shipping, and thus kept the cost of passage prohibitively high, most emigrants after 1812, went to British North America, rather than the U.S., travelling in returning Canadian timber ships. The vast majority pushed on from Canada to the United States, where there were family or community links, although increasing numbers now began to stay in the rapidly expanding colony, often encouraged by government grants of land. After the 1820s, as economic depression and natural disasters took their toll, more and more of those leaving were from the labouring classes, the poorest, who somehow managed prices for the passage ranging from £4 to £10 per person.

In 1827, after the government repealed all restrictions on emigration; between 1828 and 1837 almost 400,000 Irish people left for North America. Up to 1832, about half of the emigrants still came from Ulster, but after that date the three southern provinces contributed the majority, and from now on, although a steady stream of Northern Protestants continued to emigrate, encouraged by the established Scots-Irish community, their proportion of total emigration was in continuous   decline.

Up to the 1830s, the favoured route for the emigrants was still to Canada, and from there to the United States. The majority of departures were from Irish ports, with Belfast, Londonderry and Dublin now the most important.

The potato famines accelerated emigration to the Americas. The crops failed in Munster in 1821, and people starved to death in Cork and Clare. There were further crop failures in

1825-30. In 1832 "stark famine" struck Munster and south Leinster. Throughout the early 1830s, cholera repeatedly ravaged the poorest classes, and, in the decade as a whole, the potato crop failed on a local level in eight out of the ten years. Finally, in 1840-1844, the potato crops partly failed three more times. Then, a fungus totally ravaged the potato crop in 1845, 1846 and 1848, and partially ravaged it in 1847.

When the American civil war came, the Irish fought on both sides, often depending on where they lived. For example, those living in Charleston, Savannah and other southern cities, often fought for the confederacy. The majority fought for the Union. At least thirty-eight Union regiments had the word "Irish" in their title.

Many Irish Americans were enthusiastic supporters of Irish independence. The Fenian Brotherhood movement was based in the United States and in the late 1860s launched several unsuccessful attacks on British-controlled Canada. These were known as the "Fenian Raids".

While they failed to free the Canadian colonies from British control, their pressures were among those that led to the Confederation of Canada in 1867.

A total of 36,278,332 Americans, estimated at 11.9% of the total population, reported Irish ancestry in the 2008 American Community Survey conducted by the U.S. Census Bureau. The only ancestral group larger than Irish Americans is German Americans. In addition roughly another 3.5 million, identified more specifically with Scots-Irish ancestry. The Irish are widely dispersed in terms of geography, and occupations. Irish American political leaders have played a major role in local and national politics throughout this period.

Beginning with Andrew Jackson, some twenty-two Irish Americans served as President. They included James Knox Polk, James Buchanan, Andrew Jackson, Ulysses S Grant,

Chester A. Arthur, Grover Cleveland, Benjamin Harrison, William McKinley, Theodore Roosevelt, William Howard Taft, Woodrow Wilson, Warren G Harding, Harry S. Truman, John F. Kennedy, Richard Nixon, Jimmy Carter, Ronald Reagan, George H W Bush, Bill Clinton, George W Bush and Barack Obama. (357)

Settlement in Frampton, Quebec

The Redmonds came over to Canada after the war of 1812. British officers and others involved in the war were given land grants in Quebec, Canada. A region of land, south-east of Quebec City, was ceded to an association whose principal members were Gilbert and William Henderson and Pierre-Edouard Desbarats Other members were demobilized soldiers or pensioners from the army. They developed a number of settlements in this region, including Frampton, St. Malachie and Cranbourne. (358)

After initial, unsuccessful efforts to encourage French Canadian settlers to move into these lands, they fostered Irish, English and Scottish immigration. Irish immigration began in 1806 and reached a peak in the 1830s. Andrew Redmond arrived in the 1820s.

While some of the immigrants remained in this area, many used it as a springboard to move across North America. One of the first groups to leave this area consisted of forty families who moved to the American southwest in the late 1830s. They stopped in St Louis, Missouri for a while, and crossed over the prairies to California. They were among the first Americans to cross the plains and reach and settle in the west coast. They settled in the San Jose valley and other areas. It was on the land of one of these settlers that war was declared on Mexico that resulted in the American takeover of California. (359) Details on the settlement of Frampton and history of the past two hundred years have been published separately by the author. (360)

Religion and the Diaspora

We cannot talk about the Irish emigration around the world without mentioning the spread of the Catholic faith that accompanied it. Just as they had done a thousand years earlier, the Irish carried their faith with them and established Catholic communities everywhere they went. In secular religion, they often dominated local churches, comprising many of the priests and bishops. In the orders of priests, nuns and brothers they spread education and health care wherever they settled as they moved into missionary work in many regions of the world.

Only at the end of time will we fully appreciate how the suffering that led to the emigration produced such a bounty for God in the salvation of millions of souls worldwide for four centuries.

Conclusion

Since Andrew Redmond arrived in Canada, our family has been in Canada seven generations. Andrew, then his son John, then his grandson John lived in Frampton. Henry, great grandson of Andrew, lived in Frampton and Montreal, and his son Patrick, the author, lived in Montreal, then Toronto. My brothers and sisters settled throughout Canada. My family, Siobhan, Michele and Carrie Lee, live in Toronto, as do their five children – Siobhan, Luke, Jamie, Alexander and Zachary.

By the time we arrived in Canada, we were probably 300 to 350 generations removed from Adam and Eve, as discussed earlier in the book.

It has been a great journey through time, filled with travel to new lands, with wars and conquests, with subjugation and liberation.

In the Irish spirit has always been a fierce independence which made our ancestors a formidable and resilient force wherever they lived. As well, there has always been a desire to promote values they perceived as beneficial to themselves and others, reflected during the past two millennia in their promotion of Christianity both during its darkest centuries as well as during its periods of greatest expansion.

Appendix 1

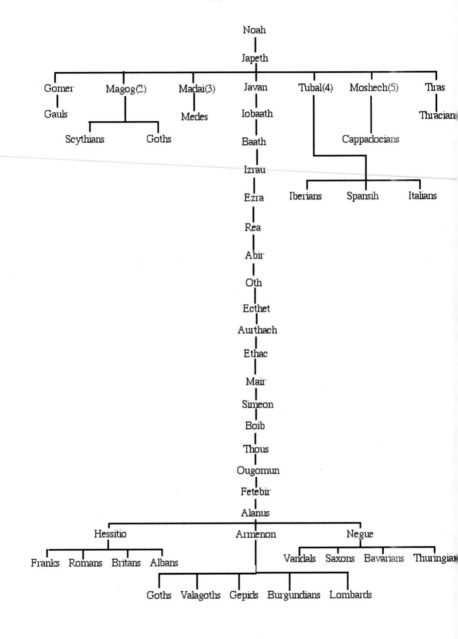

Nennius elaborated on this genealogy in his History of the Britons. (Cooper, op cit, App 3, p.139)

"After the Flood, the three sons of Noah divided the earth into three parts. Shem (settled) in Asia; Ham in Africa, (and) Japheth expanded his borders in Europe. Alanus, of the line of Japheth, (was) the first man who came to Europe with his three sons, whose names were Hessitio, Armenon and Negue. Now, Hessitio had four sons, Francus, Romanus, Britto (and) Albanus. Then Armenon had five sons, Gothus, Walagothus, Gepidus, Burgundus [note: the name Langobardus should have been given here]. (And) Negue had three sons, Wandalus, Saxo (and) Boguarus. Four nations, then, are arisen from Hessitio: the Franks, the Latins, the Albans and the Britons. Then, from Armenon (come) five (nations): the Goths, the Valagoths, the Gepids, the Burgundians (and) the Lombards. (And) from Negue (come) four (nations): the Bavarians, the Vandals, the Saxons and the Thuringians. (And) these nations are subdivided throughout all Europe. Alanus, it is said, was the son of Fetebir, (who was) the son of Ougomun, (who was) the son of Thous, (who was) the son of Boib, the son of Simeon, (who was) the son of Mair, the son of Ethach, (who was) the son of Aurthach, the son of Ecthet, (who was) the son of Oth, the son of Abir, (who was) the son of Rea, the son of Ezra, (who was) the son of Izrau, the son of Baath, (who was) the son of Iobaath, the son of Javan, (who was) the son of Japheth, the son of Noah, (who was) the son of Lamech, the son of Methuselah, (who was) the son of Enoch, the son of Jared, (who was) the son of Mahalaleel, the son of Cainan, (who was) the son of Enos, the son of Seth, (who was) the son of Adam, the child of the living God. I found this teaching in the tradition of the elders."

As can be seen from the chart above, this means that Alanus moved into Europe some eighteen generations, or 450 years after the flood, if we assume 25 years per generation.

214

Cooper notes (p.25) "not one of the names in this list of nations is historically unattested, not even that of the unlikely-sounding Gepids".

Early Irish Genealogy

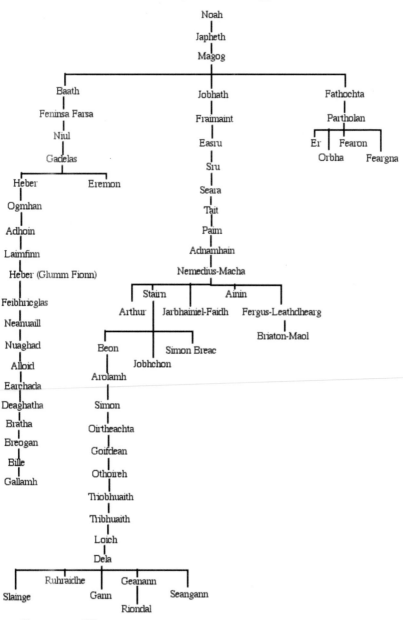

Cooper p.58

Footnotes

Introduction

1. http://www.ibm.com/solutions/genographic/us/en/;
www.nationalgeographic.com/genographic/lan/en/journey.html. IBM
and the National Geographic society are not the only groups going this.
Many companies provide DNA analysis. Do a Google search with the
words *genealogy+y+DNA* to see some of these.
2. https://genographic.nationalgeographic.com/genographic/lan/en/overvie
w; Genetic genealogists are beginning to explore the whole genome – not
being limited to the Y chromosome or mtDNA. Companies such as
23andMe and deCODEme scan hundreds of thousands of markers, which
have come down to us from many ancestral lines, see Ann Turner,
"Satiable Curiosity" in *Journal of Genetic Genealogy*, 5(2); ii-iv, 2009
3. Wells, Spencer, *Deep Ancestry - Inside the Genographic Project*,
(National Geographic: 2006, Washington), pp.36-8
4. Ibid, pp.58-9.
5. This analysis is provided online at
https://genographic.nationalgeographic.com/genographic/index.html. In
order to view it, you need a genographic project ID, which is provided to
everyone who submits a sample. The details noted on each marker is
provided after you enter your project ID
6. Cohen, I.L. "Darwin was Wrong – A Study in Probabilities", *New
Research Publications*, 1984, p.4, quoted in C. StJames, *DNA, The
Ultimate Oopart* available online at http://www.s8int.com/dna1.html
7. Collins, Francis S., *The Language of God*, p. 122; quoted in Joseph
Ratzinger, *Jesus of Nazareth: Holy Week: From the Entrance Into
Jerusalem to the Resurrection* (Ignatius Press San Francisco: 2011).

Chapter 1

8. Wells, op cit, pp.132.
9. https://genographic.nationalgeographic.com/genographic/index.html.,
entry for my Account #.
10. Patricia Balaresque; Georgina R. Bowden; Susan M. Adams; Ho-Yee
Leung; Turi E.King; Zoe H. Rosser; Jane Goodwin; Jean-Paul Moisan;
Christelle Richard; Ann Millward; Andrew G. Demaine; Guido
Barbujani; Carlo Previdere; Ian J. Wilson; Chris Tyler-Smith; Mark A.
Jobling, *"A Predominantly Neolithic Origin for European Paternal
Lineages"* in

http://www.plosbiology.org/article/info%3Adoi%2F10.1371%2Fjournal.pbio.1000285

11. http://www.dailymail.co.uk/sciencetech/article-1244654/Study-finds-Britons-descended-farmers-left-Iraq-Syria-10-000-years-ago.html#ixzz0dBImdMju ; Wells, op cit, p.63 notes that people expanded quickly due to the invention of agriculture in the Karacadag region, a part of Anatolia.

12. Cruciani, Fulvion et al, "A Back Migration from Asia to Sub-Saharan Africa is Supported by High Resolution Analysis of Human Y-Chromosome Haplotypes", *The American Journal of Human Genetics*, vol.70, issue 5, May 2002; also in http://www.sciencedirect.com/science?_ob=ArticleURL&_udi=.

13. Hammer, Michael F.; Tatiana M Karafet; Alan J.Redd; Hamdi Jarjanazi; Silvana Santachiara-Benerecetti; Himla Soodyall and Stephen L. Zegura, "Hierarchical Patterns of Global Human Y-Chromosome Diversity", in http://mbe.oxfordjournals.org/content/18/7/1189.full. They explain this diagram as follows: "Inferences from nested cladistic analysis of Y-chromosome data. Intercontinental signals are indicated by arrows between continent ideograms (note: arrows are not meant to indicate routes of migration), and intracontinental signals are shown by arrows within circles (empty circles for Europe and the Americas denote the absence of intracontinental signals). Solid arrows represent population history events (contiguous range expansions and long-distance colonizations), while population structure processes (recurrent gene flow restricted by isolation by distance and long-distance dispersals) are indicated with dashed arrows (and, in one instance, a dashed line between Asia and Oceania where no polarity could be inferred). The widest solid arrow denotes early range expansion out of Africa at the level of the total cladogram". The cladogram is a tree diagram used to illustrate phylogenetic relationships. For a more detailed explanation, please see http://en.wikipedia.org/wiki/Cladogram

14. Ibid.

15. Wells, op cit, p.132; for a detailed look at the Y chromosome tree phylogeny, see http://ytree.ftdna.com/

16. Ibid, pp.133-140

17. Field, Fred," *The Language Facility – Evolution, Design, or?*" in http://www.ldolphin.org/languagefac.html. Regarding other complex languages, see Taylor, Ian, *In the Minds of Men – Darwin and the New World Order*, 5th ed (TFE Publishing: Zimmerman, MN, 2003), p.169; available online at http://www.creationism.org/books/TaylorInMindsMen/index.htmop cit, p.249.

18. Woolley, Leonard, *The Beginnings of Civilization*, (New York. New York American Library, 1965, p.364, quoted in Curt Sewell, *Biblical Chronology and Dating of the Early Bible*", available at http://ldolphin.org/sewell/sewellchron.html. Sewell was a scientist at Lawrence Livermore Labs.

19. Gould 1977b, 14, quoted in Ian Taylor, op cit, p.169; for a good explanation of Lyell's system of geology, see Turner, op cit., pp.80-1; in support of Gould, Colin Patterson, senior paleontologist at the British Museum of Natural History, wrote, "Gould and the American Museum people are hard to contradict when they say there are no transitional fossils. As a paleontologist myself, I am much occupied with the philosophical problems of identifying ancestral forms in the fossil record. … I will lay it on the line -- there is not one such fossil for which one could make a watertight argument." In James Purloff, *Purloff on Evolution*, in http://mrgreer.tripod.com/purlof.html

20. Ian Taylor, op cit, p.206

21. Hoesch, William A., *"How Coherent is the Human Evolution Story?"* in www.icr.org/article/how-coherent-human-evolution-story/; see also Richard E Green; Adrian W Briggs; Johannes Krause; Kay Prüfer; Hernán A Burbano; Michael Siebauer; Michael Lachmann and Svante Pääbo, "The Neandertal genome and ancient DNA authenticity", in *The EMBO Journal*, v28 (17), Sept 2, 2009 and online at http://www.ncbi.nlm.nih.gov/pmc/articles/PMC2725275/?tool=pubmed

22. Dr. Erick A. Von Fange, *Time Upside Down*, chapters of this book are updated at different times, and one recent update was 2003, p.35. This book can be downloaded from http://www.rae.org/index.html; Dr. T.N. Tahmisian (Atomic Energy Commission USA) in 'The Fresno Bee', August 20, 1959, quoted in N.J.Mitchell, *Evolution and the Emperor's New Clothes*, (Royden Publications, UK, 1983), states "Scientists who go about teaching that evolution is a fact of life are great con-men, and the story they are telling may be the greatest hoax ever. In explaining evolution, we do not have one iota of fact." See http://www.creationism.org/articles/quotes.htm.

23. Richard Leakey (Director of National Museums of Kenya) in *The Weekend Australian*, 7-8 May 1983, Magazine, p. 3 and quoted in *Quotes from Leading Evolutionists*, in http://www.creationism.org/articles/quotes.htm. These quotes are taken from Dr. A. Snelling, *The Revised Quote Book*, Creation Science Foundation, Australia. For details on Ethiopian fossils, see Taylor, op cit, p.241. Lucy is a key fossil in the Ethiopian series.

24. White, T.D., Asfaw, B., DeGusta, D.; Gilbert, H., Richards, G.D.; Suwa, G.; Howell, F.C.; Pleistocene Homo sapiens from Middle Awash,

Ethiopia, summarized in
http://www.ncbi.nlm.nih.gov/pubmed/12802332; see also The Middle
Awash Series, noted in http://www.ucpress.edu/series.php?ser=tmas#.

25. http://www.dailymail.co.uk/sciencetech/article-1341973/Did-humans-
come-Middle-East-Africa- Scientists-forced-write-evolution-modern-
man.html

26. Wells, op cit, pp.173-4; another detailed study claiming East African
origin for Eve is Ian Logan, "A suggested Genome for "Mitochondrial
Eve", in *Journal of Genetic Genealogy*, 3(2): 72-77, 2007.

27. Carter, R.W., Criswell, D, Sanford, J, "The 'Eve" Mitochondrial
Consensus Sequence", in A.A. Snelling ed., *Proceedings of the Sixth
International Conference on Creationism*, (Pittsburgh: 2008), pp.111-116
has the two charts shown.

28. Ibid; see also Robert W Carter, "Mitochondrial diversity within modern
human populations", *Nucleic Acids Research*, 2007 May 35(9): 3039-
3045, available online at
http://www.ncbi.nlm.nih.gov/pmc/articles/PMC1888801/?tool=pubmed.
This has more details on the significance of the macrohaplogroup R; for a
study of mutations, see Lee M. Spetner, *Not by Chance : Shattering the
Modern Theory of Evolution*, Lee M. Spetner: Books.

29. Carter, "The "Eve Mitochondrial Consensus Sequence", p.112-3;
commenting on cladistics, Taylor, op cit, p.153 writes that cladistics
supposes sudden jumps from one ancestral form to another – unprovable
jumps. Nonetheless, they are accepted by the American Museum of
Natural History and the British Museum.

30. Carter, "The 'Eve" Mitochondrial Consensus Sequence", states: "The
human and chimp mtDNA sequences are substantially different, we do
not know the ancestral chimp sequence, and we do not know the degree
of degeneration that has occurred in chimp lineages. Each of these factors
will affect placement of the root." see also Deem, Richard, *Descent of
Mankind Theory: disproved by Molecular Biology*, in
http://www.godandscience.org/evolution/descent.html; Others are
moving that way as well. The International Chimpanzee Chromosome
22 consortium, a team of researchers based in Asia and Europe, has
sequenced a chimpanzee chromosome in unprecedented detail and found
a much larger difference than previously suspected. *Nature*, v.429, p.382,
quoted in http://www.s8int.com/dna4.html.

31. https://genographic.nationalgeographic.com/genographic/lan/en/atlas.htm
l, comments on item 5.

32. Ibid; see also Deem, Richard, op cit; and Caramelli, David; Lucio Milani;
Stefania Vai; Alessandra Modi; Elena Pecchioli; Matteo Girardi; Elena
Pilli; Martina Lari; Barbara Lippi; Annamaria Ronchitelli; Francesco

Mallegni; Antonella Casoli; Giorgio Bertorelle; Guido Barbujani, *"A 28,000 Years Old Cro-Magnon mtDNA Sequence Differs from All Potentially Contaminating Modern Sequences"*, in http://www.plosone.org/article/info:doi/10.1371/journal.pone.0002700.

33. For example, Wells, op cit, p.138.

34. *Fossils, Teeth and Sex: New Perspectives on Human Evolution,* (University of Washington Press, 1987), quoted in David Buchna, *"Lucy's Knee Joint Revisited"*, in http://www.rae.org/lucy.html; Klaus Dona states that an archaeological geneticist confirmed that DNA cannot be recovered from bones older than 10,000 years. See http://www.youtube.com/watch?v=VSmkcn1hJWI; British astronomer Fred Hoyle has stated that the likelihood of life developing spontaneously equals "that of a tornado sweeping through a junkyard and correctly assembling a Boeing 747". Quoted in Lloyd Pye, *"Why Darwinian evolution is flatly impossible"*, in http://www.s8int.com/dna8.html

35. https://genographic.nationalgeographic.com/genographic/lan/en/atlas.html, see 200,000 to 60,000 years chart; see also http://archeology.about.com/od/qterms/qt/qafzeh_cave.htm; Wells, op cit, p.128;

36. Ofer Bar-Yosef, *"Human Migrations: The Cultural Records"*, http://www.wkdialogue.ch/fileadmin/original_presentations/wkd_20060915_ofer_bar-yosef_human_migrations.pdf

37. https://genographic.nationalgeographic.com/genographic/lan/en/atlas.html, see 200,000 to 60,000 years chart.

38. For information on Cro-Magnon and Aurignacian cultures, see http://en.wikipedia.org/wiki/Aurignacian and http://www.elephant.se/cro-magnon.php.

39. Pinhasi, Ron; Joaquim Fort; Albert J. Ammerman, *"Tracing the Origin and Spread of Agriculture in Europe"*, in http://www.plosbiology.org/article/info:doi/10.1371/journal.pbio.0030410 They state:" agriculture is most likely to have originated in the area that today includes north-east Syria, northern Mesopotamia, and part of south-east Turkey near the site of Çayön"; Barbujani; G & L. Chikhi, *"DNAs from the European Neolithic"*, in web.unife.it/progetti/genetica/Guido/pdf/Barbujani-Chikhi.pdf provide a good analysis of the role played by DNA analysis in determining the extent of Neolithic vs. Paleolithic origin of modern European populations. They state that a model of demic diffusion provide "evidence of a major dispersal of people in the Neolithic period". See also Barbujani, Guido & Giorgio Bertorelle, *"Genetics and the population history of Europe"* in

web.unife.it/progetti/genetica/Giorgio/PDFfiles/pnas2001.pdf for further comments on Paleolithic vs. Neolithic; Chikhi, Lounes; Giovanni Destro-Bisol; Giorgio Bertolele; Vincenzo Pascali; Guido Barbujani, *"Clines of nuclear DNA markers suggest a largely Neolithic ancestry of the European gene pool"*, in http://www.ncbi.nlm.nih.gov/pmc/articles/PMC21201/. ; see also Glenn Allen Nolan, Y-DNA HAPLOGROUP I2a (I-P37.2) DYS #385a and 385b at 11 and 17 and the FOMORIANS of IRISH MYTHOLOGY, whose genetic research of his ancestors notes a migratory movement that started some 6000 years ago in http://freepages.genealogy.rootsweb.ancestry.com/~nolenancestry/page1.html

40. Chikhi, Lounes; Richard A Nichols; Guido Barbujani; Mark A Beaumont, " *Y genetic data support the Neolithic demic diffusion model"*, at http://www.pnas.org/content/99/17/11008.full
41. Chikhi, Lounes, et al, *"Clines of nuclear DNA"*.
42. The Basque people entry in http://en.wikipedia.org/wiki/Basque_people, under genetics.
43. Behar. Doran and others, "The Dawn of Human Matrilineal Diversity", in *The American Journal of Human Genetics*, vol.82, issue 5, 24 April 2008, pp.1130-40.
44. Wells. op cit, pp.176-7.
45. US News and World Report, 12/4/1995.
46. Ann Gibbons, "Calibrating the Mitochondrial Clock", *Science*, v.279, pp.28-9, January 2, 1998.
47. Pitman, Sean D., *DNA Mutation Rates and Evolution*, August 2001, updated August 2008, P.6, available online at http://naturalselection.0catch.com/Files/dnamutationrates.html; All the comments from Pitman are from this source.
48. Pitman, op cit.
49. Whitelaw, Robert L., "Time, Life, and History in the Light of 15,000 Radiocarbon Dates", *Creation Research Society Quarterly*, 7:56-71 (1970) quoted in Taylor, op cit, p.305
50. Taylor, op cit, p.307; see also *Isotope Dating Review of Basic principles and Problems*, Greater Houston Creation Association, available online at http://www.ghcaonline.com/Articles/articles.html which notes that Carbon 14 has a half-life of 5730 years; see also http://www.ndt-ed.org/EducationResources/CommunityCollege/Radiography/Physics/carbondating.htm, which discusses Carbon 14 dating and its limitations; see also Larry Vardiman; Andrew A Snelling and Eugene F Chaffin, eds, *Radioisotopes and the Age of the Earth*, 1998, available online at http://www.icr.org/article/radioisotopes-age-earth/; for an interesting

article on Carbon 14 dating, see Mark E. Hall, Towards an absolute chronology for the Iron Age of Inner Asia, in http://www.thefreelibrary.com/Towards+an+absolute+chronology+for+t he+Iron+Age+of+Inner+Asia.-a020586737; Paul Mellars, "A New Radiocarbon revolution and the dispersal of modern humans in Eurasia", *Nature*, vol.439, 23 February 2006; Trevor Major, "Dating in Archaeology: Radiocarbon and Tree-Ring Dating", Apologetics Press, available online at http://www.apologeticspress.org/apcontent.aspx?category=9&article=46 4; see also the excellent articles, audio and video files by Paul Abramson at http://www.creationism.org/mp3/index.htm

51. Taylor, op cit. Taylor writes (pp.241-2) on the Ethiopian fossils that are considered a major potential source of early man that Donald Johanson researched in the Great Rift Valley in southern Ethiopia along the Omo River and uncovered 197 hominid bones, but no skulls. It was announced as Lucy and dated, with potassium-argon dating at 3.1 to 5.3 million years.

52. Robert E. Lee, "radiocarbon: Ages in Error", *Anthropological Journal of Canada*, Vol 19(3), 1981, pp.9-29.

53. Von Fange, Eric, *Time Upside Down*, online version available at http://www.rae.org/indev.html, p.24; (*CRSQ* , 1972, 9:1, p.47).

54. Taylor, op cit, p.324; see also Rev William A Williams, "*The Evolution of man Scientifically Disproved in 50 Arguments*". One of the arguments discusses population. Available online at www.creationism.org

55. Bill Cooper, *After the Flood*, (New Wine Press: Chicester, 1995), pp.51, 67-71. Available online at http://ldolphin.org/cooper/contents.html; Cooper (p.2) took the names listed in Genesis chapters 10 and 11 and after 25 years of work verified that 99% have been recorded in the annals of the ancient Middle East and have survived to the present day. see also Taylor, op cit, p, 273-4; for a good analysis of Ussher and Bible versions of dates; also see Curt Sewell, op cit. For example he notes the three main versions of the Old Testament and gives the dates calculated for the flood for each: Masoretic 1656 AM (anno mundi or year of the world), Septuagint 2262 AM and Samaritan 1307 AM.

56. Taylor, op cit, pp.271-3

57. Cooper, op cit, chapter 9.

58. For further details on location and content of these manuscripts. see Cooper, op cit., 32,46, and 139. The History by Nennius deserves comment. In 597 AD Augustine visited the king of Kent with instructions to bring the English under the dominion of the Papacy. In 604 AD Augustine, the Roman Bishop, ordered the massacre of the scholars and spiritual leaders of the Welsh at Bangor. This led to the neglect and loss

of many of the books and chronicles maintained by these monks. Fortunately, Nennius gathered all that remained and included them in his History of the Britons. They included some of the most important documents of the ancient world that we have today, such as the genealogy noted in Appendix 1.

59. Cooper, op cit, p.56
60. *Chronicum Scotorum*, Anonymous, A Chronicle of Irish Affairs, from the earliest times to AD 1135, with a supplement containing the events from 1141 to 1150, translated by William M Hennessy, (London, 1866) Gearoid MacNiocaill, electronic edition compiled by Beatrix Farber & Ruth Murphy; CELT, University College, Cork, 2003; online copy at http://www.ucc.ie/celt/online/T100016.html; manuscript at Dublin Trinity College Library, 1292. Before AM 1599.
61. Moore, Laoise T.; Brian McEvoy; Eleanor Cape; Katherine Simma and Daniel G. Bradley, "*A Y-Chromosome Signature of Hegemony in Gaelic Ireland*", in http://www.ncbi.nlm.nih.gov/pmc/articles/PMC1380239/

Chapter 2

62. Genesis 1:26-31; 2:7, 2:21-23
63. Emmerich, St. Anne Catherine, *The Life of Jesus Christ*, (TAN books and Publications Inc.: Rockford, Ill, 2004) Vol.1, pp.6-18, 26, 29.
64. Cooper, op cit, Appendix 12
65. *The Collected writings of St Louis Marie de Montfort, God Alone*, (Montfort Publications: Bay Shore, NY, 2008) p.59; see also Beriault, Francine, *Gatherings of Love with God's Action, Through His Instrument, The Girl of My Will in Jesus*, Collection of Teachings, (Sherbrooke: Editions Saint-Raphael, 2010) vol.4, p.77
66. http://www.divinewillinfo.org/qa.html
67. Stokes, Whitley, editor, *The Fifteen Tokens of Doomsday*, London, British Library Additional MS 30512, folio 95a1-98a2. Description from the website of the British Library, available online at http://www.ucc.ie/celt/published/T207002/index.html
68. *Saltair na Raan*, manuscript RAWL B 502, fn19-40 in the Bodleian J and other Oxford Libraries, Oxford, ed by Whitley Stokes writing attributed to Oengus the Culdee in the ninth century; available on Google library archives at http://www.archive.org/stream/saltairnarannac00rawlgoog/saltairnaranna c00rawlgoog_djvu.txt , XL The penance of Adam and Eve, , lines 1483-1628; IV Preface 1629-1932.
69. Genesis 6:2,4-6

70. Beriault, op cit, v.3, pp.80-2; Klaus Dona states that a book, written by a son of a Spanish conqueror who married an Inca queen, states they had found large skeletons along the coast that they concluded were from devils, so they destroyed them. See http://www.youtube.com/watch?v=VSmkcn1hJWI

71. Genesis, 6:5-8

72. The Holy Bible, Douay-Rheims version, An Historical and Chronological Index to the Old Testament, p.298.

73. Cusack, Margaret Anne, *An Illustrated History of Ireland*, 1868, 2nd edition, pp. 25-6, book available online at http://www.libraryireland.com/HistoryIreland/Title.php; published in facsimile by Bracken Books, London, 1987; see also a summary in http://www.archive.org/details/anillustratedhi00cusagoog

74. *Saltair na Raan*, op cit, Preface, line1969

75. Emmerich, op cit.

76. *Saltair na Raan*, op cit, preface IV lines 2217-2228; Preface V 2229-2240

77. https://genographic.nationalgeographic.com/genographic/lan/en/atlas.htm l, comments on item 5. Ibid; see also Deem, Richard, op cit; and Caramelli, David; Lucio Milani; Stefania Vai; Alessandra Modi; Elena Pecchioli; Matteo Girardi; Elena Pilli; Martina Lari; Barbara Lippi; Annamaria Ronchitelli; Francesco Mallegni; Antonella Casoli; Giorgio Bertorelle; Guido Barbujani, "A 28,000 Years Old Cro-Magnon mtDNA Sequence Differs from All Potentially Contaminating Modern Sequences", in http://www.plosone.org/article/info:doi/10.1371/journal.pone.0002700.; Green, Richard E. Johannes Krause, Susan E. Ptak, Adrian W. Briggs, Michael T. Ronan, Jan F. Simons, Lei Du, Michael Egholm, Jonathan M. Rothberg, Maja Paunovic & Svante Pääbo, Analysis of one million base pairs of Neanderthal DNA", in *Nature*, 444,pp.330-336 (16 November 2006)

78. https://genographic.nationalgeographic.com/genographic/index.htm

79. Taylor, op cit, pp.216-7, quoting Thom, 1971 and Prideaux, 1973;

80. The drawing and other information come from http://en.wikipedia.org/wiki/Prehistory of France, Upper Palaeolithic.

81. *Annala Rioghachta Eireann*: Annals *of the kingdom of Ireland by the Four Masters, from the earliest period to the year 1616. Edited from MSS in the Library of the Royal Irish Academy and of Trinity College Dublin published as the Annals of the Four Masters,* offered online by University College, Cork and Seoirse Ó Luasa, An Caifé Liteartha, An Daingean, who donated a copy of the Annals of the Four Masters to the

225

CELT Project. Available online at http://www.ucc.ie/celt/published/T100005A/index.html; see folio 2242.1

82. MacFirbis, Duald, *Chronicum Scotorum*, compiled at the College of St. Nicholas, Galway, 1650, Kal.v.f.1 10 Anno mundi 1599; see also Cusack, chs.2-3

83. *Cin oj Drom Snechta*, quoted in O'Curry, Tradition, p.13 and Cusack, op cit, ch 3, p, 29.

84. Times Online, The Times, January 9, 2009, *Archaeology Ireland* 22 No.3:18-21 at http://www.timesonline.co.uk/tol/life_and_style/court_and_social/article 5477636.ece; this is quoted in Nolan Y-DNA Haplogroup 12a (I-P37.2) DYS #385a and 385b at 11 and 17 and the *Formorians of Irish Mythology*, available online at http://freepages.genealogy.rootsweb.ancestry.com/~nolenancestry/page1f.html

85. Nolan, op cit.; see also Ireland's History in Maps, http://www.rootsweb.ancestry.com/~irlkik/ihm/ancient.htm

86. Dona, Klaus, *Dinos and Humans Together*, at: http://www.rense.com/general92/dino.htm; see also http://www.youtube.com/watch?v=XmMwo1Xzgus&feature=related; he has an interview at http://www.youtube.com/watch?v=VSmkcn1hJWI; and http://www.youtube.com/watch?v=syWq6_oVhD0&feature=related has the pre-Sanskrit script. It is entitled Klaus Dona, *The Hidden History of the Human Race*.

87. Paul Abramson, audio and video files on http://www.creationism.org/mp3/index.htm

88. Job 40:10-28; 415-25.

89. Cooper, op cit, chapters 10-11

90. Ibid, ch 11, pp.85-91

91. Ibid, ch 10, p.78; The Times, 21st July 1977.

92. Plato, *Critias,* translated by Benjamin Jowett, available online at http://www.activemind.com/Mysterious/Topics/Atlantis/timaeus_and_critias.html

93. Plato, *Timeaus*, translated by Benjamin Jowett, available online at http://www.activemind.com/Mysterious/Topics/Atlantis/; see also comments by Paul Drockton on Atlantis. He notes they worshipped satan and believed in supremacy of science and the human mind, http://www.moneyteachers.org/Atlantis.html

94. Quoted in http://www.s8int.com/water6.html; they refer to MaltaDiscovery.com for further information; see also Jonathan Gray, *Archaeological Newsflash* #112 for discussion of a city off the coast of Peru. http://www.beforeus.com/first.php

226

95. Bennett, Jim & Scott Mandelbrote, *The Garden, The Ark, The Tower, The Temple: biblical metaphors of knowledge in early modern Europe*, Catalogue published to accompany the exhibition of the same name held in the Bodleian Library Exhibitions Room, 2nd February to 2nd May, 1998; Website by Jessica Ratcliff; quoting Walter Raleigh, *The Historie of the World in Five Bookes,* London, 1614, quoted in http://www.mhs.ox.ac.uk/gatt/catalog.php , cat 80, p.80 and based on *The Holy Bible ...Illustrated with Chorographical Sculps. by J. Ogilby,* 2 vols, Cambridge, 1660

96. Cory, *Ancient Fragments*, London, 1832, p. 26 *ff.* quoted in Budge, E.A. Wallis *The Babylonian Story of the Deluge and the Epic of Gilgamish*, 1929; Original title *The Babylonian Story of the Deluge as told by Assyrian Tablets from Nineveh*, revision by C.J. Gadd; available online at http://www.sacred-texts.com/ane/gilgdelu.htm; George Smith published, in 1872, the eleventh tablet of the Epic of Gilgamish, which described the deluge; this version is a variation of the text cited above

Chapter 3

97. Genesis, chapter 5.

98. Genesis 6:8

99. Genesis 6:10; 7:7

100. Brown, Walter, In the Beginning: Compeling Evidence for Creation and the Flood, Centre for Scientific Creation, 2008; available online at http://www.creationscience.com/onlinebook/; for he video, see http://www.youtube.com/watch?v=X16SE-N-8ys

101. Parker, Chris, *"After the Flood; A Graveyard Planet"*, in http://s8int.com/WordPress/?p=1726; see also the interesting video by Joe Taylor, called *Mt Blanco and Fossils* at http://www.creationism.org/mp3/index.htm

102. Smith, George, *The Chaldean Account of the Deluge*, Transactions of the Society of Biblical Archaeology 2 (1873), pp.213-34, available online at http://www.sacred-texts.com/ane/chad/chad.htm; for a very interesting video on the Epic of Gilgamesh, see http://www.youtube.com/watch?v=C8iR7p5eSbQ&NR=1; see also Mark Edward Lewis, The flood Myths of Early China, (SUNY: 2006)

103. Shown in http://www.youtube.com/watch?v=C8iR7p5eSbQ&NR=1

104. James Perloff is quoted in http://www.youtube.com/watch?v=C8iR7p5eSbQ&NR=1 ; see also www.rapitflybeats.net; creation science website http://creationwiki.org/James_Perloff; Perloff wrote *Tornado in a*

junkyard-The Relentless Myth of Darwinism, available at WorldNetDaily.com

105. Siculus, Diodorus, *The Library of History*; Loeb Classical Library Edition, 1935, 12 volumes, Greek texts and facing English translation: Harvard University Press, 1933 thru 1967. Translation by C. H. Oldfather thru Volume 6; Vol. 7 by C. L. Sherman, Vol. 8 by C. Bradford Welles, Vols. 9 and 10 by Russell M. Geer, Vol. 11 by F. R. Walton. ; edited and available online by Bill Thayer at http://penepole.uchicago.edu/Thayer/E/Roman/Textx/Diodorus Siculus/home.html, Book 1, 10. see also http://www.pantheon.org/articles/d/deucalion.html

106. Genesis 9:19 Noah is spelt Noe; Cham is often spelled Ham; Sem is often spelled Shem

107. Cooper, op cit, ch.2, p.18.

108. Genesis 10:2.

109. Cooper, op cit, Appendix 3, pp.127-32.

110. Genesis, 11:1-8.

111. http://bible.cc/genesis/11-2.htm, Clark's Commentary

112. http://bible.cc/genesis/11-2.htm

113. Historical and Chronological Index to the Old Testament in the *Douay-Rheims Bible*, p.298-9; this bible was the Latin Vulgate bible translated into Latin from the original languages by St. Jerome (342-420 AD)

114. http://bible.cc/genesis/10-8.htm, Clark's Commentary on the Bible

115. Smith. George, *The Chaldean Account of Genesis* (1876), p.313 Princeton Theological Seminary Library; available online at http://www.archive.org/details/chaldeanaccount00smit; Cooper, op cit, Appendix 2, p.122

116. Cooper, Appendix 2, p.122; an interesting article on the Tower of Babel is A.R. George, *The Tower of Babel: archaeology, history and cuneiform Texts*", available online at http://eprints.soas.ac.uk/3858/2/TowerOfBabel.AfO.pdf and quoted in http://en.wikipedia.org/wiki/Etemenanki fn.1

117. Tower of Babel in http://en.wikipedia.org/wiki/Tower_of_Babel, and check Josephus, "Ant." i. 4, § 2

118. http://en.wikipedia.org/wiki/Tower_of_Babel; for a listing of the libraries which have fragments of Orosius, *Historiae,* see http://www.hf.uib.no/i/klassisk/orosius.html

119. Smith. op cit; Siculus, Diodorus, op cit, the editor of the book series writes in fn 24: According to Herodotus (1.181) it had eight stories, but E. Unger (Babylon (1931), pp191 ff. finds evidence for only seven (cp. the Reconstruction, p383). The height of this great structure was nearly 300 feet, and in the course of time there gathered about it the

Hebrew myth of the Tower of Babel (cp. The Cambridge Ancient History, I, pp503 ff.).; Semiramis was a consort of Nimrod, believes Alexander Hislop, The Two Babylons, 1853, quoted in http://en.wikipedia.org/wiki/Semiramis".; http://www.archive.org/details/chaldeanaccounto00smit; and http://www.archive.org/stream/chaldeanaccounto00smit/chaldeanaccount o00smit_djvu.txtChaldean account of genesis, p.48

120. Cooper, op cit, pp.25-6; An interesting study of the Y chromosome in Anglo-Saxon Britain shows closeness between Anglo-Saxons and Danes and distance between these two and the Welsh, reflecting the differences in lines of descent from Japheth; see Weale, Michael E; Deborah A Weiss; Rolf F Jager; Neil Bradman; Mark G, Thomas, " Y chromosome evidence for Anglo-Saxon Mass Migration", in http://mbe.oxfordjournals.org/content/19/7/1008.full

121. Douay Rheims Bible, Historical Commentary, p.298-9

122. Chronicum Scotorum, p.2; it uses AM, meaning Anno Mundi, Year of the World.

Chapter 4

123. Cusack, op cit, p.137

124. Cooper, op cit, map in Appendix 3, text pp.129-30

125. Rice, Tamara Talbot, The Scythians, (Praeger: New York, 1957) online copy available at http://www.questia.com/PM.qst?a=o&d=5855314, p.33 quoted in The United States and Britain in Bible prophecy, (United Church of God, 2001) available online at http://www.beyondtoday.tv/booklets/US/scythians.asp 1961, p.33.

126. Justinus, Marcus Junianus, Epitome of the Philippic History of Pompeius Trogus translated, with notes, by the Rev. John Selby Watson. (London: Henry G. Bohn, York Street, Convent Garden, 1853). Book 2.1. 2.3. available online at http://www.forumromanum.org/literature/justin/english/introduction.html); see also http://www.attalus.org/translate/justin7.html

127. Justinus, op cit, Book 2.1

128. Herodotus, The Histories of Herodotus of Halcarnassus, translated by George Rawlinson, (Omphaloskepsis: Ames, Iowa, 2000) Book 4 discusses the Scythians, pp.1-8 online copy available at www.omphaloskepsis.com/ebooks/pdf/hrdts.pdf ; he lived in the 5th century BC (c.484 BC – c.425 BC). He has been called the "Father of History" since he was the first historian known to collect his materials systematically, test their accuracy to a certain extent and arrange them in

a well-constructed and vivid narrative; see
http://en.wikipedia.org/wiki/Herodotus
129. Cooper, op cit, Appendix 3, commentary on Gomer, p.129; Appendix 3, commentary on Madai, p.130; see also http://www.livius.org/cg-cm/cimmerians/cimmerians.html
130. Justinus, Marcus Junianus, *Epitome*. Book 2.3.
131. Justinus, book 2.3
132. Diodorus, 2.43
133. Herodotus, op cit, Book 4. 1.105: Jeremias 4:29, 5:16-7.
134. Justinus, Book 2.3
135. http://en.wikipedia.org/wiki/Scythia
136. Herodotus, op cit, book 4
137. Herodotus, op cit, book 4
138. http://en.wikipedia.org/wiki/Scythia
139. Ibid.
140. http://en.wikipedia.org/wiki/Scythia
141. Herodotus, Book 4, pp.18-22; 40-1; 49
142. http://en.wikipedia.org/wiki/Scythia
143. Photographic print of Scythian War Chariots from Mary Evans, available from http://www.amazon.co.uk/Photographic-SCYTHIAN-CHARIOTS-Mary-Evans/dp/B001NRSH8Q
144. Justinus, Book 2.1 , 2.3 in http://www.forumromanum.org/literature/justin/english/trans2.html)
145. Diodorus, book 2.46
146. http://www.timelessmyths.com/classical/trojanwar.html
147. Cusack, op cit, pp.37-8; Herodotus, book 1. vii. c. 89.
148. www.bibleorigins.net/ ExodusRedSeaCrossingMapElKraieh.html; Douay Rheims Bible, Historical Index, p.298 ; http://answers.yahoo.com/question/index?qid=20080406104456AAhmI3 w
149. Cusack, op cit, quoting Nennius, pp.52-3; Cooper, op cit, pp.64-5
150. Herodotus, book 5, pp.54-5 discusses the Greeks importing the Phoenician script
151. Cusack, op cit, pp.55 quoting *Procopius.—Hist. Gen. d'Espagne*,vol. i. c. 1. p. 4; http://en.wikipedia.org/wiki/Canaan
152. Rankin, op cit, p.7.
153. Cusack, op cit, p.39; Herodotus, op cit, book 4, pp.34-5 mentioned the Phoenicians sailing around Africa and having the sun upon their right hand. The circumnavigation of Africa by a Phoenician ship, in the reign of Neco, about 610 B.C., is credited by Humboldt, Rennell, Heeren, Grote. and Rawlinson. Of their voyages to Cornwall for tin there is no question, and it is more than probable they sailed to the Baltic for amber.

It has been even supposed that they anticipated Columbus in the discovery of America. Niebuhr connects the primitive astronomy of Europe with that of America, and, therefore, must suppose the latter country to have been discovered.—*History. of Rome*, vol. i. p. 281. This, however, is very vague ground of conjecture; the tide of knowledge, as well as emigration, was more probably eastward.

154. Rankin, David, *Celts and the Classic World*, (Croom Helm Ltd. 1987) online copy available at http://books.google.com/books?id=fdqk4vXqntgC&printsec=frontcover &dq=%22celts%22&q=&hl=en#v=onepage&q&f=false, pp.2-5.

155. Picture from http://www.michaelbradley.info/articles/megalithic_movers.html

156. http://en.wikipedia.org/wiki/Hecataeus_of_Miletus; he lived from 550 BC to 490 BC.

157. Cahill, Thomas, *How the Irish Saved Civilization*, (Doubleday: Toronto1995), op cit, p.79

158. Justinus, book 41.1

159. Ibid, book 41.1-3

160. http://creationwiki.org/Magog; the reader may find *The Forgotten Tribes of China* by Kevin Sinclair of interest in this area of study.

161. Rankin op cit, p.32

162. Ibid, p 30-1.

163. Ibid, p.31 quoting Myles Dillon 1947 and 1975

164. Ibid, pp.32-3.

165. Hall, op cit.

166. Keyser, Christine, Caroline Bouakaze, Valery G. Nikolaev; Daniel Montagnon, Tatiana Reis and Bertrand Ludes, "Ancient DNA provides new Insights into the history of south Siberian Kurgan people", in *Human Genetics*, Volume 126, Number 3, 395-410, abstract. Quoted in http://www.springerlink.com/content/4462755368m322k8/?p=087abdf3e df548a4a719290f7fc84a62&pi=0

167. http://en.wikipedia.org/wiki/Scythians, quoting Keyser, Christine "Ancient DNA".

168. Ibid, quoting Bouakaze, 2009:"Pigment phenotype and biogeographical ancestry from ancient skeletal remains: inferences from multiplexed autosomal SNP analysis", *International Journal of Legal Medicine*, vol. 123, no. 4; Ricaut, F. et al. 2004. "Genetic Analysis and Ethnic Affinities From Two Scytho-Siberian Skeletons". *American Journal of Physical Anthropology*. 123:351–360; Clisson, I. et al. 2002. "Genetic analysis of human remains from a double inhumation in a frozen kurgan in Kazakhstan" (Berel site, Early 3rd Century BC). *International Journal of Legal Medicine*. 116:304–308; Rice, op cit, p.178

169. http://en.wikipedia.org/wiki/Scythians, quoting *Spiegel Online* Jan 12, 2011, available online at http://www.spiegel.de/international/0,1518,433600,00.html
170. http://en.wikipedia.org/wiki/Scythians
171. Rankin, op cit, p.26; (181) Ibid, p.30; he quotes Wagner 1971: 247ff
172. http://www.unc.edu/celtic/catalogue/stbrigid/Tricephalic_Head.html - it has three faces
173. Rankin, op cit, pp.30-1.
174. http://www.civilization.ca/cmc/exhibitions/civil/egypt/egtut01e.shtml
175. http://en.wikipedia.org/wiki/Tutankhamun
176. http://www.eutimes.net/2010/06/king-tuts-dna-is-western-european/
177. dsc.discovery.com/videos/king-tut-unwrapped; http://www.youtube.com/watch?v=Q7RSMGMU2jc&NR=1 discusses the DNA results; http://heritage-key.com/blogs/ann/king-tut-unwrapped-tutankhamun-mummy-forensics-air-discovery-channel; http://www.youtube.com/watch?v=S-Jjb94G5ls and http://www.youtube.com/watch?v=jr-HR-ckKX8&feature=related, this second one shows the DNA.; this is the key video explaining the DNA http://www.youtube.com/watch?v=2wccgN467E8 see also Michael Tsarion interview with Jeff Rense at http://www.youtube.com/watch?v=Q7RSMGMU2jc&NR=1
178. http://www.eutimes.net/2010/06/king-tuts-dna-is-western-european/ ; this video explains it in detail http://www.youtube.com/watch?v=2wccgN467E8 ; website of Whit Athey at http://www.hprg.com/hapest5/ and the *Journal of Genetic Genealogy*, which Athey edited at http://www.jogg.info/
179. http://www.youtube.com/watch?v=Q7RSMGMU2jc&NR=1
180. http://www.youtube.com/watch?v=2wccgN467E8
181. http://en.wikipedia.org/wiki/Nefertiti
182. Tyler-Smith et al 2007
183. http://en.wikipedia.org/wiki/Tutankhamun
184. http://www.eutimes.net/2010/06/king-tuts-dna-is-western-european/
185. http://en.wikipedia.org/wiki/Tutankhamun
186. http://en.wikipedia.org/wiki/New_Kingdom
187. The following description of Tutankhamun is taken from http://en.wikipedia.org/wiki/Tutankhamun

Chapter 5

188. https://genographic.nationalgeographic.com/genographic/index.html., entry for my Account #.
189. Rankin, op cit, pp.7-8; http://en.wikipedia.org/wiki/Prehistory_of_France

190. Rankin, op cit, pp. 7-8.
191. http://en.wikipedia.org/wiki/Prehistory_of_France
192. Rankin, op cit, pp.15-6
193. http://en.wikipedia.org/wiki/Prehistory_of_France
194. Rankin, pp.15-6; see also Neustupny and Neustupny 1961:152
195. Rankin, op cit, pp.15-6
196. Rankin, op cit, pp.15-6
197. Rankin, op cit, p.8 quoting Herodotus 2.33
198. Rankin, op cit ,pp.9-10; he quotes Momigliano 1975:51)
199. http://freepages.genealogy.rootsweb.ancestry.com/~nolenancestry/page1.html
200. http://en.wikipedia.org/wiki/Celts
201. http://www.cornwallinfocus.co.uk/culture/celts.php
202. This section is based on Rankin, op cit, pp.9-12
203. http://en.wikipedia.org/wiki/Celts, who quotes Sarunas Milisauskas, *European Prehistory: a Survey*, page 363. Springer, 2002 http://books.google.com/?id=31LFIITb3LUC&pg=PA363&dq=Hecateau s+of+Miletus+celt&q=Hecataeus%20of%20Miletus%20celt. Retrieved 2010-06-07.; Waddell, op cit, p.105 quoting Strabo I,2,27.
204. Rankin, op cit.
205. Quoted in Rankin, op cit, p.36
206. Rankin, p.39-40 quoting Justin 43.5ff
207. Diodorus, op cit, book 5.32
208. http://freepages.genealogy.rootsweb.ancestry.com/~nolenancestry/page1.html; Nolan, *1000 Years of O'Nolan History in Ireland and the New World*, in http://freepages.genealogy.rootsweb.ancestry.com/~nolenancestry/page1.html
209. Diodorus, Book 5.25-31;
210. Ibid, Book 31
211. Cusack, op cit, p. 88; she quotes Strabo, 1. iv. p. 197; Suetonius, *V. Cla.* ; Pliny, *Hist. Nat.* 1. xxv. c. 9. Pliny mentions having seen the serpent's egg, and describes it.
212. Hennig, R, "Die Anfänge des kulturellen und Handelsverkehr in der Mittelmeerwelt," *Historische Zeitschrift*, 139 (1928), 1-33; he quoites Diodorus, 2.47.
213. http://en.wikipedia.org/wiki/Prehistory_of_France
214. Schaff, Philip, *History of the Christian Church*, Vol IV, Medieval Christianity, AD 590-1073, pp.15-6; available online at http://www.ccel.org/ccel/schaff/hcc4.i.ii.xvi.html
215. Cooper, op cit, pp.30-1
216. http://en.wikipedia.org/wiki/List_of_Celtic_tribes

217. Diodorus, op cit, Book 5.33
218. Rankin, op cit, p.19
219. Livy (Titus Livius) *The History of Rome*, Book 5, para 34 online version available at http://www.maryjones.us/ctexts/classical_livy.html); this remarkable history comprises 142 books; Livius lived from 59 BC to 17 AD; also available as a published version Titus Livius. *History of Rome*. Editor Ernest Rhys Translator Rev. Canon Roberts. Everyman's Library. E.P. Dutton and Co. New York: 1912; http://en.wikipedia.org/wiki/Lucius_Tarquinius_Priscus
220. Cooper, op cit, ch 4, p.31
221. Cremin, Aedeen. *The Celts in Europe*, (Lansdowne Publishing, 1997)
222. Livy, op cit, para 34
223. Justinus, op cit, book 24.4.
224. Livy, op cit, para 34-5.
225. Justinus, op cit, book 20.5
226. Livy, op cit, para 37
227. Ibid, para 48; see also Justinus, op cit, 38.4; it was also commented on by Diodorus Siculus in Book XIV.113-117
228. Rankin, op cit, p.12
229. Justinus, op cit, Book 24.4
230. http://en.wikipedia.org/wiki/Gallic_invasion_of_the_Balkans
231. http://en.wikipedia.org/wiki/Gallic_invasion_of_the_Balkans; http://en.wikipedia.org/wiki/List_of_Celtic_tribes
232. http://en.wikipedia.org/wiki/Gallic_invasion_of_the_Balkans
233. Justinus, op cit, Book 24.4-25-9.
234. http://en.wikipedia.org/wiki/List_of_Celtic_tribes quoting sources such as J. J. Wilkes, *The Illyrians*, 1992.
235. *In Cath Catharda, The Civil War of the Romans*, anonymous, translated by Whitley Stokes Electronic edition compiled by Janet Crawford, Benjamin Hazard, Beatrix Färber, Funded by University College, Cork and The HEA via the LDT Project, available online at http://www.ucc.ie/celt/published/T305001/index.html; Chapter 20 is entitled *The Adventure of Sextus Pompeius, and the Predictions of Thessalian Erictho, and the Prophecy of the infernal Spectre* , pp.296-7.
236. http://en.wikipedia.org/wiki/Gallic_invasion_of_the_Balkans
237. Ramsay, William Mitchell, *A Historical Commentary on St Paul's Epistle to the Galatians*, (London, 1900) new version edited by Mark Wilson, (Kregel Publications, 1997) ebook available at http://www.koboBooks.com/eBook/-historical-commentary-St-Pauls-Epistle/Book-ir3Msl-AL0CW15aKJGCIDA/page1.html, see pp,40-52.; see also Rankin, op cit, p.15; http://en.wikipedia.org/wiki/List_of_Celtic_tribes has the map

238. Justinus, op cit, Book 25.9-10 and Book 38.4
239. Josephus, Flavius, *The Wars of the Jews*, Book 1.xxxiii, available online at http://www.maryjones.us/ctexts/classical_josephus.html#origin
240. http://en.wikipedia.org/wiki/Galatia
241. The map comes from http://en.wikipedia.org/wiki/Galatia
242. http://en.wikipedia.org/wiki/Galatia; http://www.newadvent.org/cathen/06336a.htm; http://en.wikipedia.org/wiki/Dying_Gaul
243. Josephus, op cit, Book 2.xvi
244. http://en.wikipedia.org/wiki/Galatia

Chapter 6

245. Cooper, op cit, p.36, then pp.63-4 for Formorians.
246. Rankin, op cit, p.12
247. Nolan, Godfrey, (http://www.ibiblio.org/gaelic/celts.html, site maintained by Seàn O Miadhachàin (Godfrey Nolan)
248. http://en.wikipedia.org/wiki/List_of_Celtic_tribes
249. http://www.cornwallinfocus.co.uk/culture/celts2.php and http://www.cornwallinfocus.co.uk/culture/celts3.php
250. The description of the La Tene culture comes from http://www.3dhistory.co.uk/00PreHistory.htm
251. All references to the Celts are found in Caesar, op cit, Book 5, chapter 12, 14; Book 6, chapter 13, 14, 15, 16, 17, 18, 19; Book 7, chapter 22
252. http://www.britainexpress.com/History/Celtic_Britain.htm
253. Ibid.
254. Caesar, op cit, Books 5, 6, 7; http://www.cornwallinfocus.co.uk/culture/celts6.php
255. Caesar, op cit, Books 5, 6, 7; http://www.britainexpress.com/History/Celtic_Britain.htm
256. Cahill, op cit, p.79.
257. Nolan, Glenn Allen, op cit.
258. Chronicum Scotorum, p.3
259. Annals of the Four Masters, AM 2859.
260. Cooper, op cit, pp.62-3
261. Waddell, L. Austine, *The Phoenician Origin of Britons, Scots and Anglo Saxons Discovered by Phoenician and Sumerian Inscriptions in Britain by Pre Roman Briton Coins*, 1924, p.102.
262. Cooper, p.61; Annals of the Four Masters, M2520.0; *Chronicum Scotorum*, p.5
263. Cusack, op cit, pp.40-1; Waddell, op cit, p.79 chapter 10 also states it was later, around 390 BC

264. Walsh, Dennis, *Ireland's History in Maps, Neolithic, Bronze and Iron Ages*, in http://www.rootsweb.ancestry.com/~irlkik/ihm/neolithic.htm
265. *Annals of the Four Masters*, M2820.1, Ibid, 2850.1, 2859; Cooper, op cit, pp.62-3
266. Ibid.
267. Ibid.
268. Ibid., AM2859, AM3066, Am3370.2; Cusack, op cit, p.31; Conell MacGeoghegan's translation of the Annals of Clonmacnois, quoted by O'Donovasn, p.11 and quoted in Cusack, op cit, p.32.
269. Ibid., AM3303.1
270. Ibid.
271. Cusack, op cit, p.44
272. Ibid.
273. Nolan, Glenn Allen, op cit. he quotes Researchers Trace Roots of Irish and Wind Up in Spain, an article of March 23, 2000, by Nicholas Wade of the New York Times; Basques are Brothers of the Celts, an article of April 3, 2001, by Robert Highfield of The Daily Telegraph; and "We are not Celts at all but Galacians", an article of September 10, 2004, by Brian Donnelly of The Herald (London).
http://www.magoo.com/hugh/irishkings.html; The Milesian Genealogies describes all the families and their origins in Spain, see http://www.rootsweb.ancestry.com/~fianna/history/milesian.html, compiled and edited by Pat Traynor from the original 1892 edition of John O'Hart's Irish Pedigrees. See also http://www.magoo.com/hugh/irishkings.html
274. Cooper, op cit, pp.64-5
275. *Chronicum Scotorum*, op cit, AM 2544.
276. *Annals of the Four Masters*, op cit, M3500.1
277. Cusack, op cit, p.51
278. Cusack, op cit, pp.49
279. Walsh, op cit.
280. *Annals of the Four Masters*, M3656.2
281. Cahill, op cit, p.142; photo taken from http://en.wikipedia.org/wiki/Gundestrup_cauldron
282. Walsh, op cit.
283. Cooper, op cit, pp.30-1
284. Map taken from http://en.wikipedia.org/wiki/List_of_Celtic_tribes
285. Cahill, op cit, p.136

Chapter 7

286. http://en.wikipedia.org/wiki/Strabo

287. For a full list of the Celtic peoples of Cisalpine Gaul, see http://en.wikipedia.org/wiki/List_of_Celtic_tribes
288. For a listing of the groups, see http://en.wikipedia.org/wiki/List_of_Celtic_tribes; http://en.wikipedia.org/wiki/File:Map_Gallia_Tribes_Towns.png
289. Diodorus, op cit, Book 1.4
290. Caesar, Julius, *The Gallic Wars*, Translated by W. A. McDevitte and W. S. Bohn, offered online at http://classics.mit.edu/Caesar/gallic.mb.txt, Book 1, chapter 1,p.1
291. The following description of the wars is taken from Ibid, Book 1; Book 2 chapter 4, 6, 35; Book 3, chapter 9
292. Caesar, op cit, Book 3, chapter 13;
293. Ibid, Book 7, chapter 76; Book 8, chapter 46, 49 and http://www.cornwallinfocus.co.uk/culture/celts1.php
294. Ibid, Book 4, chapter 20, 24, 33; Book 5, chapter 8, 11
295. Ibid.
296. http:www.cornwallinfocus.co.uk/culture/celts4.php
297. http://www.cornwallinfocus.co.uk/culture/celts4.php
298. Cusack, op cit, pp.59-60
299. Rankin, op cit, pp.17-18
300. Ibid, p.15
301. http://en.wikipedia.org/wiki/Galatia; Livy, XXXVIII, xvi; the wars are referred to in I Mach., viii; http://www.newadvent.org/cathen/06336a.htm
302. http://en.wikipedia.org/wiki/Galatia This article incorporates text from Chisholm, Hugh, ed (1911). *Encyclopedia Britannica* (Eleventh ed.). Cambridge University Press.)

Chapter 8

303. http://www.newadvent.org/cathen/11567b.htm
304. Galatians 4:14; Ramsay; http://www.newadvent.org/cathen/06336a.htm quoting Lightfoot, *Galatians* (4th ed., London, 1874); the new Advent series was edited by Kevin Knight; Beth Ste Marie transcribed this article on Galatians; based on Aherne, C. (1909). "Epistle to the Galatians" in *The Catholic Encyclopedia*. (New York: Robert Appleton Company); Ramsay, op cit, p.478; Epistle of St Paul to the Colossians 3:10-11
305. http://www.newadvent.org/cathen/06336a.htm
306. Ramsay, op cit, pp.322-3
307. Ibid, p.170
308. Comentarii in Epistolam ad Galatos, 2.3, composed c. 387

309. Strobel, Karl, "The Galatians in the Roman Empire: historical tradition and the ethnic identity in Hellenistic and Roman Asia Minor", *Ethnic Constructs in Antiquity*, Number 13, Amsterdam university press, 2009; Nixon, L.F., *The Archaeological Record of the Galatians in Anatolia*, M.Sc. thesis, The University of british Columbia, 1977.

310. http://www.wadsworth.com/history_d/templates/student_resources/0534 600069_spielvogel/InteractiveMaps/timeline_maps/map7_3.html

311. http://en.wikipedia.org/wiki/Way_of_St._James; http://www.red2000.com/spain/santiago/history.html

312. Http://en.wikipedia.org/wiki/Spain; http://www.andalucia.com/history/romans.htm

313. http://en.wikipedia.org/wiki/Mary_Magdalene; see also http://www.newadvent.org/cathen/09761a.htm

314. http://en.wikipedia.org/wiki/Mary_Magdalene; see also http://www.newadvent.org/cathen/09761a.htm

315. http://www.newadvent.org/cathen/07349b.htm has a good map showing this.

316. Schaff, op cit; http://xenophongroup.com/montjoie/norman.htm; http://www.justfrance.org/france/france-history.asp; Wallbank, p.215

317. Wallbank, pp.300-315

318. Wells. Warre B., *A Biography of John Redmond*, (Nisbet & Co: London, 1919). pp.2-6

319. McFall, J. Arthur, "Taking Jerusalem: Climax of the First Crusade" in http://www.thehistorynet.com/MilitaryHistory/articles/1999/0699_text.ht m; see also Runciman, Steve, *The First Crusade*

320. Schaff, op cit, pp.15-6; 15-20; 24-5

321. *Annals of the Four Prophets*, M266.1

322. Ibid., M430.2

323. Ibid, M431.2; anonymous work *On the Life of St Patrick* gives a good account of this. (tr Whitley Stokes, 1876, electronic edition compiled by Ruth Murphy, CELT: Corpus of Electronic Texts: a project of University College, Cork College Road, Cork, Ireland (2000) (2010) available online at http://www.ucc.ie/celt/published/T201009/index.html, p.39

324. Cahill. Thomas, *How the Irish Saved Civilization*, (Doubleday: Toronto1995, p.110, 114

325. Ibid, pp.36-7, 160

326. Ibid, p.165; http://www.newadvent.org/cathen/08614b.htm

327. http://en.wikipedia.org/wiki/Book_of_Kells has these three pictures

328. Cusack, op cit, p.17; Cahill, op cit; details on the work of St Anthony can be found in Rev. Herman Bernard Kramer, *The Book of Destiny*, (Rockford: Tan, 1955) pp.191-2.

329. Cahill. op cit, p.171

330. Ibid, pp.187-8

Chapter 9

331. The following account is taken from
    http://en.wikipedia.org/wiki/Norman_conquest_of_England
332. http://en.wikipedia.org/wiki/Norman_invasion_of_Wales
333. http://en.wikipedia.org/wiki/Richard_de_Clare,_2nd_Earl_of_Pembroke
334. http://www.libraryireland.com/articles/CourtstownCastleDPJ1-
    22/index.php
335. http://en.wikipedia.org/wiki/Raymond_FitzGerald;
336. http://en.wikipedia.org/wiki/Raymond_FitzGerald; see also
    http://www.libraryireland.com/JoyceHistory/Raymond.php see also
    Brooks, Eric St. John, "An Unpublished Charter of Raymond le Gros",
    The Journal of the Royal Society of Antiquaries of Ireland, Seventh
    Series, Vol. 9, No. 3 (Sep. 30, 1939), pp. 167-169 , (article consists of 3
    pages) , Published by: *Royal Society of Antiquaries of Ireland* , Stable
    URL: http://www.jstor.org/stable/25510204
337. Wells, Warre B., op cit, pp.27-8
338. http://www.libraryireland.com/articles/CourtstownCastleDPJ1-
    22/index.php
339. http://www.libraryireland.com/articles/CourtstownCastleDPJ1-
    22/index.php

Chapter 10

340. Desmond, Jerry, *Concise History of Ireland,* 2000, available online at
    http://jerrydesmond.tripod.com/index-2.html
341. Wells, Warre, op cit, p.29.
342. Ibid, p., 29
343. O'Ciannain, Tadhg, *The Flight of the Earls,* (1607-1609) CELT project,
    translated with notes by Paul Walsh, 1st ed, (St. Patrick's College:
    Maynooth, 1916), available online at
    http://www.ucc.ie/celt/published/T100070/index.html
344. Wells, Warre, p.29-30; http://en.wikipedia.org/wiki/John_Redmond
345. Wells, Warre, p.30

Chapter 11

346. O'Ciannain, op cit.

347. Wells. Warre, pp.27-9.
348. Desmond, op cit; http://en.wikipedia.org/wiki/Irish_diaspora; much of the following section is based on this source.
349. Redmond, Patrick, *Irish life in Rural Quebec: A history of Frampton*, (Adams Press: Chicago, 1977), p.13. available at the Quebec Family History Society Library, HG/154.01/R42/1970, at http://www.qfhs.ca/lib.html.
350. http://freepages.genealogy.rootsweb.ancestry.com/~nolenancestry/page1.html
351. http://www.kavanaghfamily.com/articles/2003/20030618jfc.htm; Irish Times. April 6, 2011, on Spain and South America, see also http://www.irishtimes.com/ancestor/magazine/emigration/emig2.htm; http://en.wikipedia.org/wiki/Irish_diaspora
352. http://www.kavanaghfamily.com/articles/2003/20030618jfc.htm and http://www.irishtimes.com/ancestor/magazine/emigration/pre-fam.htm; are the sources for the section on slavery
353. http://en.wikipedia.org/wiki/Newfoundland_Irish; A good review of Irish emigration to Newfoundland is John Mannion, *Tracing the Irish: A Geographical Guide*, in http://www.inp.ie/?q=node/40
354. http://www.irishtimes.com/ancestor/magazine/emigration/pre-fam.htm; the following section on the Americas is based on this source.
355. http://colonialancestors.com/revolutionary/women.htm
356. http://en.wikipedia.org/wiki/Scotch-Irish_American; http://en.wikipedia.org/wiki/Irish_Americans
357. http://en.wikipedia.org/wiki/Irish_Americans
358. Kirouac, Rev. J., *Histoire de la Paroisse de Saint-Malachie* (Quebec: Proulx, 1909)
359. Redmond, op cit, p.69
360. Ibid.

Bibliography

Abramson, Paul "*What about the dinosaurs*", and others in
http://www.creationism.org/mp3/index.htm

Aherne, C "Epistle to the Galatians" *The Catholic Encyclopedia*
(New York: Robert Appleton Company, 1909)

Anonymous *Annals of Clonmacnoise*, from the earliest period to
1408. An English translation was made by Connell
MacGeoghegan in 1627; see
http://www.libraryireland.com/JoyceHistory/Annals.ph
p

Anonymous *Chronicum Scotorum, A Chronicle of Irish Affairs,
from the Earliest Times to AD 1135, with a supplement
containing the Events from 1141 to 1150*, edited and
published by William M. Hennessey (London, 1866) ;
reprinted Wiesbaden, 1964; Edited and translated by
Gearoid MacNiocaill, available from CELT ,
University College, Cork, 2003; online copy at
http://www.ucc.ie/celt/online/T100016.html;
manuscript at Dublin Trinity College Library, 1292;
this manuscript was compiled about 1650 by Duald
MacFirbis, see
http://www.libraryireland.com/JoyceHistory/Annals.ph
p

Anonymous "Historical and Chronological Index to the Old
Testament", *The Holy Bible, Douay-Rheims Version*,
(Tan Books: Rockford, 2000)

Anonymous *In Cath Catharda*, The Civil War of the Romans,
translated by Whitley Stokes, electronic edition
compiled by Janet Crawford, Benjamin Hazard,
Beatrix Farber, University College, Cork and the HEA
via the LDT project, available online at
http://www.ucc.ie/celt/published/T305001/index.html;
Chapter 20 is entitled *The Adventure of Sextus
Pompeius, and the Predictions of Thessalian Erictho,
and the Prophecy of the infernal Spectre.*

Anonymous "Isotope Dating Review of Basic principles and
Problems", Greater Houston Creation Association,
online at http://www.ghcaonline/Articles/articles.html
and

241

| | www.ghcaonline.com/Articles/Isotope_dating/Isotope_ |
| Anonymous | *On the Life of St. Patrick*, translated by Whitley Stokes, electronic edition compiled by Ruth Murphy; available online at http://www.ucc.ie/celt/published/T201009/index.html; edition used in digital version *Three Middle-Irish Homilies on the Lives of Saints Patrick, Brigit and Columba*, edited by Whitley Stokes; 1st ed privately published in Calcutta, 1877. |

www.ghcaonline.com/Articles/Isotope_dating/Isotope_
Dating_080830.pdf

Anonymous   *On the Life of St. Patrick*, translated by Whitley Stokes, electronic edition compiled by Ruth Murphy; available online at http://www.ucc.ie/celt/published/T201009/index.html; edition used in digital version *Three Middle-Irish Homilies on the Lives of Saints Patrick, Brigit and Columba*, edited by Whitley Stokes; 1st ed privately published in Calcutta, 1877.

Anonymous   *Saltair na Raan*, manuscript RAWL B 502, fn19-40 in the Bodleian J and other Oxford Libraries; writing attributed to Oengus the Culdee in the 9th century; edited by Whitley Stokes; available online at CELT, http://www.ucc.ie/celt/published/G202001/index.html

Anonymous   *The Babylonian Story of the Deluge and the Epic of Gilgamish*; Original title *The Babylonian Story of the Deluge as told by Assyrian Tablets from Nineveh*, also *titled The Babylonian Legend of the Deluge as told to the Hero Gilgamish by his ancestor Uta-Napishtim, who had been made immortal by the gods*, translated by E.A. Wallis Budge 1929; revision by C.J. Gadd; available online at http://www.sacred-texts.com/ane/gilgdelu.htm; George Smith published, in 1872, the eleventh tablet of the Epic of Gilgamesh, which described the deluge; available online at http://www.sacred-texts.com/ane/chad.htm and http://www.archive.org/details/chaldeanaccount00smit

Anonymous   *The Fifteen Tokens of Doomsday*, London, British Library Additional MS 30512, fo 95a1-98a2; edited by Whitley Stokes, available online at CELT, http://www.ucc.ie/celt/published/T207002/index.html

Balaresque, Patricia; Georgina R. Bowden; Susan M. Adams; Ho-Yee Leung; Turi E.King; Zoe H. Rosser; Jane Goodwin; Jean-Paul Moisan; Christelle Richard; Ann Millward; Andrew G. Demaine; Guido Barbujani; Carlo Previdere; Ian J. Wilson; Chris Tyler-Smith; Mark A. Jobling, "*A Predominantly Neolithic Origin for European Paternal Lineages*" in http://www.plosbiology.org/article/info%3Adoi%2F10.1371%2Fjournal.pbio.1000285

242

Barbujani; G & L. Chikhi, *"DNAs from the European Neolithic"*, in web.unife.it/progetti/genetica/Guido/pdf/Barbujani-Chikhi.pdf

Barbujani, Guido & Giorgio Bertorelle, *"Genetics and the population history of Europe"* in web.unife.it/progetti/genetica/Giorgio/PDFfiles/pnas2001.pdf

Bar-Yosef, Ofer *"Human Migrations: The Cultural Records"*, http://www.wkdialogue.ch/fileadmin/original_presentations/ wkd_20060915_ofer_bar-yosef_human_migrations.pdf

Behar, Doran; Quintana-Murci, Lluis; Scozzari, Rosaria; Makkan, Heeran; Tzur, Shay; Comas, David; Bertranpetit, Jaume; Tyler-Smith, Chris; Wells, Spencer R: Rosset, Saharon; Mitchell, Robert John; Villems, Richard; Soodyall, Himla; Blue-Smith, Jason; Pereira, Luisa; Metspalu, Ene, "The Dawn of Human Matrilineal Diversity", in *The American Journal of Human Genetics*, vol.82, issue 5, 24 April 2008

Beriault, Francine, *Gatherings of Love with God's Action, Through His Instrument, The Girl of My Will in Jesus*, Collection of Teachings, (Sherbrooke: Editions Saint-Raphael, 2010) vol.4

Bouakaze, C., et al. (2009), "Pigment phenotype and biogeographical ancestry from ancient skeletal remains: inferences from multiplexed autosomal SNP analysis", *International Journal of Legal Medicine*, vol. 123, no. 4

Brooks, Eric St. John, "An Unpublished Charter of Raymond le Gros", *The Journal of the Royal Society of Antiquaries of Ireland,* Seventh Series, Vol. 9, No. 3 (Sep. 30, 1939)

Brown, Walter   In the beginning: Compelling Evidence for Creation and the Flood, Center for Scientific Creation, 2008; online copy available at http://www.creationscience.com/onlinebook/ Brown, Walter, *The Flood*, at http://www.youtube.com/watch?v=X16SE-N-8ys

Buchna, David,   *"Lucy's Knee Joint Revisited"*, in http://www.rae.org/lucy.html

Caesar, Julius   *The Gallic Wars*, translated by W. A. McDevitte and W.S. Bohn; offered online at http://classics.mit.edu/Caesar/gallic.mb.txt; the Internet classics archive by Daniel C. Stevenson, Web Atomics

World Wide presentation is copyright 1994-2000, Daniel C. Stevenson, Web Atomics

Cahill, Thomas, *How the Irish Saved Civilization*, (Doubleday: Toronto, 1995)

Caramelli, David; Lucio Milani; Stefania Vai; Alessandra Modi; Elena Pecchioli; Matteo Girardi; Elena Pilli; Martina Lari; Barbara Lippi; Annamaria Ronchitelli; Francesco Mallegni; Antonella Casoli; Giorgio Bertorelle; Guido Barbujani, "*A 28,000 Years Old Cro-Magnon mtDNA Sequence Differs from All Potentially Contaminating Modern Sequences*", in http://www.plosone.org/article/info:doi/10.1371/journal.pone.0002700

Carter, Robert W.; Criswell, D.; Sanford, J.; "The 'Eve" Mitochondrial Consensus Sequence", in A.A. Snelling ed., *Proceedings* of the Sixth International Conference on Creationism, (Pittsburgh, 2008).

Carter, Robert W. "Mitochondrial diversity within modern human populations", *Nucleic Acids Research,* 2007 May 35(9): 3039-3045, available online at http://www.ncbi.nlm.nih.gov/pmc/articles/PMC1888801/?tool=pubmed.

Chikhi, Lounes; Giovanni Destro-Bisol; Giorgio Bertolele; Vincenzo Pascali; Guido Barbujani, "Clines of nuclear DNA markers suggest a largely Neolithic ancestry of the European gene pool", *Proceedings of the National Academy of Sciences*, 1998 July 21; 95(15) 9053-9058, available online at http://www.ncbi.nlm.nih.gov/pmc/articles/PMC21201/

Chikhi, Lounes; Richard A Nichols; Guido Barbujani; Mark A Beaumont, " Y genetic data support the Neolithic demic diffusion model", *Proceedings of the National Academy of Sciences*, August 20, 2002, vol.99, no.17, 11008-11013. Available online at http://www.pnas.org/content/99/17/11008.full

Clisson, I; Keyser, C.; Francfort, H.-P.; Crubezy, E; Samashev Z.; Ludes, B., "Genetic analysis of human remains from a double inhumation in a frozen kurgan in Kazakhstan", (Berel site, early 3rd century BC), *International Journal of Legal Medicine*. 2002 116:304–308

244

Cohen, I.L.   "Darwin was Wrong – A Study in Probabilities", *New Research Publications*, 1984

Cooper, Bill   *After the Flood*, (New Wine Press: Chicester, 1995), pp.51, 67-71. Available online at http://ldolphin.org/cooper/contents.html;

Cremin, Aedeen. *The Celts in Europe*, (Lansdowne Publishing, 1997)

Cruciani, Fulvion, Santolamazza, P.; Shen, P.; Macauley, V.; Moral, P.; Olckers, A.; Modiano, D.; Holmes, S.; Destro-Bisol, G.; Coia, V.; Wallace, D.C.; Oefner, P.J.; Torroni, A.; Cavalli-Sforza, L.L.; Scozzari, R.; Underhill, P.A.; "A Back Migration from Asia to Sub-Saharan Africa is Supported by High Resolution Analysis of Human Y-Chromosome Haplotypes", *The American Journal of Human Genetics*, vol.70, issue 5, May 2002; also in http://www.sciencedirect.com/science?_ob=ArticleUR L&_udi=.

Cusack, Margaret Anne, *An Illustrated History of Ireland*, 1868, 2nd edition, p.17 available online at http://www.libraryireland.com/HistoryIreland/Title.php ; published in facsimile by Bracken Books, London, 1987; see also a summary in http://www.archive.org/details/anillustratedhi00cusago og

Deem, Richard,   *Descent of Mankind Theory: disproved by Molecular Biology*, in http://www.godandscience.org/evolution/descent.html

Desmond, Jerry, Desmond's *Concise History of Ireland*, 2000, available online at http://jerrydesmond.tripod.com/index-2.html Dona, Klaus http://www.youtube.com/watch?v=VSmkcn1hJWI;

Dona, Klaus   *Dinos and Humans Together* at http://www.rense.com/general92/dino.htm;

Emmerich, St. Anne Catherine, *The Life of Jesus Christ*, (TAN Books and Publications Inc.: Rockford, Ill, 2004) Vol 1

Field, Fred   " *The Language Facility – Evolution, Design, or?*" in http://www.ldolphin.org/languagefac.html

George, AR   The Tower of Babel: archaeology, history and cuneiform Texts", available online at http://eprints.soas.ac.uk/3858/2/TowerOfBabel.AfO.pd f and quoted in http://en.wikipedia.org/wiki/Etemenanki fn.1

245

Gibbons, Ann, "Calibrating the Mitochondrial Clock", *Science*, v.279, pp.28-9, January 2, 1998.

Gray, Jonathan *Archaeological Newsflash #112*

Greater Houston Creation Society *Isotope Dating Review of Basic principles and Problems*, available online at www.ghcaonline.com/Articles/Isotope_dating/Isotope_Dating_080830.pdf

Green. Richard E; Adrian W Briggs; Johannes Krause; Kay Prüfer; Hernán A Burbano; Michael Siebauer; Michael Lachmann and Svante Pääbo, "The Neandertal genome and ancient DNA authenticity", in *The EMBO Journal*, v28 (17), Sept 2, 2009 and online at http://www.ncbi.nlm.nih.gov/pmc/articles/PMC2725275/?tool=pubmed

Hall, Mark E. "Towards an absolute chronology for the Iron Age of Inner Asia", in http://www.thefreelibrary.com/Towards+an+absolute+chronology+for+the+Iron+Age+of+Inner+Asia.-a020586737

Hammer, Michael F.; Tatiana M Karafet; Alan J.Redd; Hamdi Jarjanazi; Silvana Santachiara-Benerecetti; Himla Soodyall and Stephen L. Zegura, "Hierarchical Patterns of Global Human Y-Chromosome Diversity", in http://mbe.oxfordjournals.org/content/18/7/1189.full.

Hennig, R. "Die Anfage des kulturellen und Handelsverkehr in der Mittelmeerwelt", *Historische Zeitschrift*, 139 (1928).

Herodotus, *The Histories of Herodotus of Halcarnassus*, translated by George Rawlinson, (Omphaloskepsis: Ames, Iowa, 2000) ; Book 4 discusses the Scythians; available online at www.omphaloskepsis.com/ebooks/pdf/hrdts.pdf; Herodotus lived in the 5th century BC (c.484 BC-c.425 BC). He has been called the Father of History since he was the first historiam known to collect his materials systematically, test their accuracy to a certain extent and arrange them in a well-constructed and vivid narrative; see http://en.wikipedia.org/wiki/Herodotus

Hoesch, William A. "*How Coherent is the Human Evolution Story?*" in www.icr.org/article/how-coherent-human-evolution-story/

Kramer, Rev. Herman Bernard *The Book of Destiny*, (Rockford:Tan, 1955)

Josephus, Flavius *The Wars of the Jews*, available online at http://www.maryjones.us/ctexts/classical_josephus.htm l#origin

Journal of Genetic Genealogy*, edited by Whit Atley, available online at http://www.jogg.info/

Justinus, Marcus Junianus *Epitome of the Philippic History of Pompeius Trogus*. translated with notes, by the Rev. John Selby Watson. (London: Henry G. Bohn, 1853) available online at http://www.forumromanum.org/literature/justin/english /introduction.html see also http://www.attalus.org/translate/justin7.html

Keyser, Christine, Caroline Bouakaze, Valery G. Nikolaev; Daniel Montagnon, Tatiana Reis and Bertrand Ludes. "Ancient DNA provides new Insights into the history of south Siberian Kurgan people", in *Human Genetics*, Volume 126, Number 3, 395-410, abstract. Quoted in http://www.springerlink.com/content/4462755368m32 2k8/?p=087abdf3edf548a4a719290f7fc84a62&pi=0

Kirouac, Rev. J. *Histoire de la Paroisse de Saint-Malachie* (Quebec: Proulx, 1909)

Leakey, Richard *The Weekend Australian*, 7-8 May 1983, Magazine

Lee, Robert E., "radiocarbon: Ages in Error", *Anthropological Journal of Canada*, Vol 19(3), 1981, pp.9-29.

Lewis, Mark Edward *The Flood Myths of Early China*, (SUNY. 2006)

Livy (Titus Livius) (59BC – 17 AD) *The History of Rome*, 142 books; Book 5, Section 17, available online at http://www.maryjones.us/ctexts/classical livy.html; published version Titus Livius, History of Rome, ed Ernest Rhys, translated by Rev. Canon Roberts, (New York: Everyman's Library, E.P. Dutton and Co. 1912)

Logan, Ian, "A suggested Genome for 'Mitochondrial Eve", in *Journal of Genetic Genealogy*, 3(2): 72-77, 2007.

Mannion, John *Tracing the Irish: A Geographical Guide*, in http://www.inp.ie/?q=node/40

McFall, J. Arthur "Taking Jerusalem: Climax of the First Crusade", in http://www.thehistorynet.com/MilitaryHistory/articles/ 1999/0699_text.htm

Montfort, St. Louis Marie de, *The Collected Writings of St. Louis Marie de Montfort, God Alone*, (Bay Shore: Montfort Publications, 2008)

Moore, Laoise T.; McEvoy, Brian; Cape Eleanor; Simma, Katherine; Bradley, Daniel G. "A Y-Chromosome Signature of Hegemony in Gaelic Ireland" , The American Journal of Human Genetics, 2006 February; v.78 (2): 334-338; available online at http://www.ncbi.nlm.nih.gov/pmc/articles/PMC138023 9/

Nixon. L.F.,   *"The Archaeological Record of the Galatians in Anatolia"*, M.Sc. thesis, The University of British Columbia, 1977.

Nolan. Glenn Allen, *1000 Years of O'Nolan History in Ireland and the New World*, in http://freepages.genealogy.rootsweb.ancestry.com/~nol enancestry/page1.html

Nolan. Glenn Allen,   *Nolan Y-DNA Haplogroup I2a(I-P37.2) DYS #385a and 385b* at 11 and 17 and the *Formorians of Irish Mythology*, available online at http://freepages.genealogy.rootsweb.ancestry.com/~nol enancestry/page1.html

Nolan. Godfrey   http://www.ibiblio.org/gaelic/celts.html, site maintained by Sean O'Miadhachain

O'Ciannain, Tadhg, *The Flight of the Earls*, (1607-1609), CELT Project, translated with noted by Paul Walsh, 1st ed (Maynooth: St. Patrick's College, 1916), available online at http://www.ucc.ie/celt/published/T100070/index.html

O'Clery, Michael, Conary and Cucogry and O'Mulconry, Ferfesa , *The Annals of the Four Masters*, 1632-1636; translated by John O'Donovan, see http://www.libraryireland.com/JoyceHistory/Annals.ph p; O'Donovan, John, tr.; electronic edition compiled by Emma Ryan, published by CELT, Corpus of Electronic Texts, a project of University College, Cork, Ireland; online copy available at http://www.ucc.ie/celt/published/T100005A/index.html

Ogilby, J.   *The Holy Bible ...Illustrated with Chorographical Sculps.,* 2 vols, Cambridge, 1660

Parker, Chris   *"After the Flood; A Graveyard Planet"*, in http://s8int.com/WordPress/?p=1726

248

Perloff, James   *Tornado in a Junkyard-The Relentless Myth of Darwinism*, available at WorldNetDaily.com

Perloff, James   *Tornado in a Junkyard*, video interview online at http://www.youtube.com/watch?v=hIWthzqE_h0

Pinhasi, Ron; Joaquim Fort; Albert J. Ammerman, *"Tracing the Origin and Spread of Agriculture in Europe"*, in http://www.plosbiology.org/article/info:doi/10.1371/journal.pbio.0030410

Pitman, Sean D., *DNA Mutation Rates and Evolution*, August 2001, updated August 2008, P.6, available online at http://naturalselection.0catch.com/Files/dnamutationrates.html

Plato   *Timaeus and Critias*, 360 BC, translated by Benjamin Jowett, available online at http://www.activemind.com/Mysterious/Topics/Atlantis/ timaeus_and_critias.html

Purloff, James   *Purloff on Evolution*, in http://mrgreer.tripod.com/purlof.html

Pye, Lloyd,   *"Why Darwinian evolution is flatly impossible"*, in http://www.s8int.com/dna8.html

Raleigh, Walter, *The Historie of the World in Five Bookes,* London, 1614, quoted in http://www.mhs.ox.ac.uk/gatt/catalog.php

Ramsay, William Mitchell, *A Historical Commentary on St Paul's Epistle to the Galatians*, (London, 1900) new version edited by Mark Wilson, Kregel Publications, 1997) ebook available at http://www.kobobooks.com/ebook/-historical-commentary-St-Pauls-Epistle/book-ir3Msl-AL0CW15aKJGCIDA/page1.html

Rankin, David *Celts and the Classic World*, (New York: Routledge, 1998)

Ratzinger, Joseph *Jesus of Nazareth: Holy Week: From the Entrance into Jerusalem to the Resurrection*, (San Francisco: Ignatius Press, 2011)

Redmond, Patrick *Irish life in Rural Quebec: A History of Frampton*, (Adams Press: Chicago, 1977)

Ricaut, Francois-X; Keyser-Tracqui, C; Cammaert, Laurence; Crubezy, Eric; Ludes, B,. "Genetic Analysis and Ethnic Affinities From Two Scytho-Siberian Skeletons", *American Journal of Physical Anthropology*. April 2004, 123:351–360

Ricaut, Francois-X; Keyser-Tracqui, C; Bourgeos, J.; Crubezy, E.;
Ludes, B, "Genetic Analysis of a Scytho-Siberian
Skeleton and Its Implications for Ancient Central Asian
Migration, *Human Biology* – Vol 76, no 1, February
2004, pp.109-125

Rice, Tamara Talbot, *The Scythians*, (Praeger: New York, 1957) online
copy available at
http://www.questia.com/PM.qst?a=o&d=5855314

Schaff, Philip   *History of the Christian Church*, Vol IV, Medieval
Christianity, AD 590-1073, available online at
http://www.ccel.org/ccel/schaff/hcc4.i.ii.xvi.html

Siculus, Diodorus, *The Library of History*; Loeb Classical Library
Edition, 1935, 12 volumes, Greek texts and facing
English translation: Harvard University Press,
1933 thru 1967. Translation by C. H. Oldfather thru
Volume 6; Vol. 7 by C. L. Sherman, Vol. 8 by
C. Bradford Welles, Vols. 9 and 10 by Russell M.
Geer, Vol. 11 by F. R. Walton. ; edited and available
online by Bill Thayer at
http://penepole.uchicago.edu/Thayer/E/Roman/Textx/
Diodorus Siculus/home.html, Book 1, 10. see also
http://www.pantheon.org/articles/d/deucalion.html

Spetner, Lee M., *Not by Chance : Shattering the Modern Theory of
Evolution* , (Lee M. Spetner: Books, 1997)

Smith. George "The Chaldean Account of the Deluge", *Transactions of
the Society of Biblical Archaeology 2* (1873) 213-34,
available online at http://www.sacred-
texts.com/ane/chad/chad.htm also at Theological
Seminary Library; available online at
http://www.archive.org/details/chaldeanaccounto00smi
t

Snelling, Dr. A., *The Revised Quote Book*, Creation Science Foundation,
Australia.

StJames, C   *DNA, The Ultimate Oopart*, available online at
http://www.s8int.com/dna1.html

Strobel, Karl   "The Galatians in the Roman Empire: historical
tradition and the ethnic identity in Hellenistic and
Roman Asia Minor," *Ethnic Constructs in Antiquity*,
no.13, Amsterdam University Press, 2009.

Tahmisian, Dr. T.N., in '*The Fresno Bee*', August 20, 1959

Taylor, Ian   In *the Minds of Men - Darwin and the New World
Order*, 5th ed, (TFE Publishing: Zimmerman, MN,

2003), p.351 available online at
http://www.creationism.org/books/TaylorInMindsMen/
index.htm

Taylor, Joe   Mt Blanco and Fossils, in
                     http://www.creationism.org/mp3/index.htm

Traynor, Pat   compiled and edited by *The Milesian Genealogies*, see
                     http://www.rootsweb.ancestry.com/~fianna/history/mil
                     esian.html, edited from the original 1892 edition of
                     John O'Hart's *Irish Pedigrees*. See also
                     http://www.magoo.com/hugh/irishkings.html

Turner, Ann,   "Satiable Curiosity" in *Journal of Genetic Genealogy*,
                     5(2); ii-iv, 2009

Vardiman, Larry, Andrew A Snelling and Eugene F Chafifin, eds,
                     Radioisotopes and the Age of the Earth, 1998.
                     available online at
                     http://www.icr.org/article/radioisotopes-age-earth/

Von Fange, Dr. Erick A., *Time Upside Down*, 2003, p.35. available
                     online at http://www.rae.org/index.html

Waddell, Lawrence Austine *The Phoenician Origin of Britons Scots &
                     Anglo-Saxons Discovered by Phoenician and Sumerian
                     Inscriptions in Britain by Pre Roman Briton Coins*,
                     (Williams & Norgate 1924)

Wallbank, T. Walter, Alastair M Taylor, Nels M. Bailkey, *Civilization
                     Past and Present*, Vol 1, 5th ed, (Scott, Foresman &
                     Co: Chicago, 1965)

Walsh, Dennis   *Ireland's History in Maps, 1996-2009*, online at
                     http://www.rootsweb.ancestry.com/~irlkik/ihm/neolithi
                     c.htm

Weale, Michael E; Deborah A Weiss; Rolf F Jager; Neil Bradman; Mark
                     G, Thomas, " Y chromosome evidence for Anglo-
                     Saxon Mass Migration", *Molecular Biology and
                     Evolution*, Vol 19, Issue 7: pp.1008-1021 available
                     online at
                     http://mbe.oxfordjournals.org/content/19/7/1008.full

Wells, Spencer, *Deep Ancestry: Inside the Genographic Project*,
                     (Washington: National Geographic: 2006,), pp.36-8

Wells, Warre B.*A Biography of John Redmond*, (London: Nisbet & Co,
                     1919)

White, T.D., Asfaw, B., DeGusta, D.; Gilbert, H., Richards, G.D.; Suwa,
                     G.; Howell, F.C.; "Pleistocene Homo sapiens from
                     Middle Awash, Ethiopia", *Nature*, 2003 Jun 12;

423(6941): 742-7 summarized in
http://www.ncbi.nlm.nih.gov/pubmed/12802332
Williams, Rev William A., *"The Evolution of man Scientifically
Disproved in 50 Arguments"*. Available online at
www.creationism.org
Woolley, Leonard, *The Beginnings of Civilization*, (New York: American
Library, 1965), p.364, quoted in Curt Sewell, *Biblical
Chronology and Dating of the Early Bible"*, available
at http://ldolphin.org/sewell/sewellchron.html